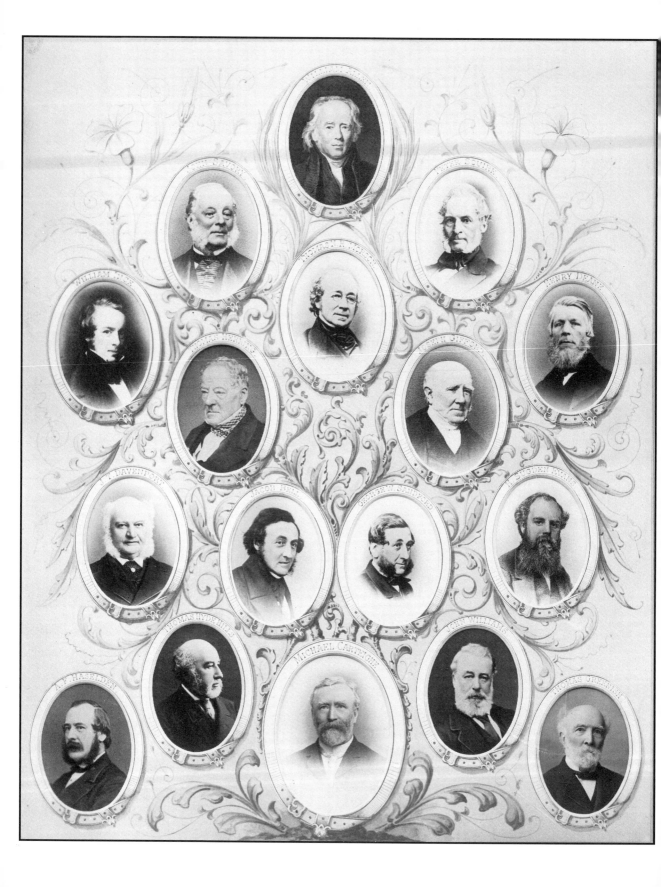

ROYAL PHARMACEUTICAL SOCIETY
OF GREAT BRITAIN
1841 – 1991
A Political and Social History

ROYAL PHARMACEUTICAL SOCIETY OF GREAT BRITAIN
1841 – 1991

A Political and Social History

S.W.F. Holloway

With illustrations chosen by
Kate Arnold-Forster *and* Nigel Tallis

London
THE PHARMACEUTICAL PRESS
1991

British Library Cataloguing in Publication Data
Holloway, S.W.F.
  Royal Pharmaceutical Society of Great Britain
  1841-1991.
  1. Great Britain. Pharmacology, history. Royal
  Pharmaceutical Society of Great Britain
  I. Title
  615.06041

  ISBN 0-85369-244-0

Copies of this book may be obtained through any good bookseller or, in any case of difficulty, direct from the publisher or the publisher's agents:

The Pharmaceutical Press
(Publications division of the Royal Pharmaceutical Society of Great Britain)
1 Lambeth High Street, London SE1 7JN, England

Australia

The Australian Pharmaceutical Publishing Co. Ltd.
40 Burwood Road, Hawthorn, Victoria 3122, *and*
Pharmaceutical Society of Australia
Pharmacy House, P.O. Box 21, Curtin, ACT 2605

Germany, Australia, Switzerland

Deutscher Apotheker Verlag
Birkenwaldstrasse 44, D-7000 Stuttgart

India

Arnold Publishers (India) Pte. Ltd.
AB/9 Safdarjung Enclave, New Delhi 110029

Japan

Maruzen Co. Ltd
3–10 Nihonbashi 2-chome, Chuo-ku, Tokyo 103

New Zealand

The Pharmaceutical Society of New Zealand
124 Dixon Street, P.O. Box 11 – 640, Wellington 1

U.S.A.

Rittenhouse Book Distributors, Inc.
511 Feheley Drive, King of Prussia, Pennsylvania 19406

To Future Generations
of Pharmacists

Contents

Foreword

The Royal Pharmaceutical Society of Great Britain has reached its 150th anniversary year in 1991. In this 150 years, the Society has grown from a small association of proprietor chemists and druggists into a worldwide body representing nearly 38,000 pharmacists working in the community, the hospital service, industry and academia.

The Society was established with a clear purpose: to guide the development of the pharmaceutical profession into a body of qualified practitioners with legal responsibilities to uphold professional status and standards.

Today there is widespread recognition of the important role played by pharmacists throughout healthcare. Earlier this year the Secretary of State for Health, William Waldegrave, wrote to me saying:

"I congratulate the Society on reaching its 150th anniversary. The achievements of those 150 years have been remarkable. The public and the Government rightly hold the pharmacist, and the Royal Pharmaceutical Society, in high esteem."

The Society's membership can be proud to have achieved so much in accordance with their founders' objectives. This significant anniversary is also a time to look ahead to the challenges and change that pharmacy is well-placed to tackle.

The Council is delighted that this first full history of the Royal Pharmaceutical Society has been written by Sydney Holloway, whose interest in the history of the profession stretches back over many years.

Generous support for this publication has come from Boots Pharmaceuticals, Glaxo Pharmaceuticals Ltd., Merrell Dow Pharmaceuticals Ltd. and the Wellcome Foundation Ltd.

Linda J. Stone
President

Preface

On 11 May 1988 the President was pleased to announce to the members that the Queen had granted the title Royal to the Pharmaceutical Society of Great Britain. This book recounts the story of the Pharmaceutical Society from its foundation in 1841 to the present day. More attention is given to the first hundred years than to the last fifty. The difficulty of digesting the mass of material relating to the recent history of the Society and the fear of treading on too many toes has determined the chronological balance of the book. Other imbalances stem from my ignorance. No attempt has been made to deal comprehensively with the Society's contribution to the development of pharmaceutical science, education and practice. The book might best be described as a political chronicle. It describes the purposes for which the Society was founded, the efforts made to fulfil them and the ways in which it was helped or hindered by other institutions. As mine is the first attempt to write a history of the Society, a primary aim has been to provide a straightforward narrative account of the Society's development based on an investigation and interpretation of the most reliable sources. At the same time I have tried to locate the work of the Society within a broad historical and social context.

Although the Council of the Royal Pharmaceutical Society has met all the expenses not only of publication but of authorship as well, this is not an official history. I have been given complete freedom to tell the story as I found it. The Officers of the Society have done everything possible to facilitate my task and have kept nothing secret from me, but they neither exercised any censorship nor even saw what I had written.

This book is based on the printed and manuscript archives of the Royal Pharmaceutical Society and in particular upon the volumes of the *Pharmaceutical Journal* and the Council Minutes. From necessity it draws more on the public record than on the private papers of pharmacists. The almost total absence of correspondence and personal papers relating to the Society's affairs is a lacuna which can never be filled. Since I had only two years to collect the material for and write this volume, it has not been possible for me to explore every possible source. There comes a time when the ruthless but arbitrary decision has to be made to search no more. My consolation is to think of the satisfaction later writers will derive from discovering the errors in my story.

This book could not have been written without my drawing on the work of other authors, most of them unknown to me except through their writings. Although I have limited the notes strictly to a bare recital of sources, I hope my debt to their work will be obvious from these references. Each reference is intended to be an acknowledgment of much needed help.

S.W.F HOLLOWAY
London House
26 September 1990

Acknowledgments

This book could not have been written without the encouragement and support of Bernard Silverman, President of the Pharmaceutical Society from 1987 to 1989, and John Ferguson, the Secretary and Registrar. Bernard Silverman suggested I write it and he and John Ferguson made it possible for me to do so. At an early stage in my research I received help and encouragement from Desmond and Susan Lewis. Desmond Lewis, who was Secretary and Registrar from 1967 to 1985, could and should have written this history himself. Had he done so, it would have been more readable and better informed. Pamela North, Head of the Library and Technical Information Service, and Kate Arnold-Forster, Curator of the Museum, not only made it easy for me to use the library and archives of the Society but never failed to revive my flagging spirits. The illustrations used in this book, chosen by Kate Arnold-Forster and Nigel Tallis, were selected from the Museum collection of the Royal Pharmaceutical Society, and I am grateful to the Society for permission to use them. I value greatly the help and friendship I received from all the staff of the Library, Museum, and Technical Information Service. John Fowler, editor of the *Journal of Pharmacy and Pharmacology* was kind enough to read drafts of some early chapters and made helpful comments. Elizabeth Foley, secretary of the Statutory Committee and Robert Dewdney, head of the Society's Education Division, gave up their valuable time to answer my questions, as did Mr E.J.R. Hill of Walker Martineau, solicitors. Before I started work on this book and before he became a member of Council, Michael Burden introduced me to a group of Leicester pharmacists who were good enough to share their thoughts with me. Also in Leicester, Ilya Neustadt and Tom and Susie Whiteside came to my rescue when I really needed help. The Vice Chancellor (Dr K.J.R. Edwards) and the Executive Pro-Vice Chancellor (Professor G. Bernbaum) of Leicester University kindly arranged for me to have unpaid leave of absence.

The preparation of this book took two years and for most of that time I lived in Room 174, London House, Bloomsbury. I will always be grateful to the Director (David Emms) and the Warden (John Pepper) for granting me the privilege of joining that stimulating fellowship of international scholars in Mecklenburgh Square. Four of my fellow residents were particularly supportive of my work: Professor Tom Jones from Connecticut, U.S.A., Dr William Pomeranz from Cleveland, Ohio, David Davis from St. John's, Newfoundland and Dr Guglielmo Caporale from Naples, Italy.

Finally I wish to thank the men who constructed the Grand Union Canal who, without any intention of doing so, contributed so much to my mental and physical health.

S.W.F Holloway

List of Illustrations

CHAPTER ONE

Jacob Bell

Prima luce—At first light

John Bell and 338 Oxford Street—Friends, family and pharmacy—Early education and apprenticeship—Artistic circles and London Society—The practising chemist and the world of science—Anaesthesia

"Towards the end of 1798, John Bell opened his shop". It was an ordinary act of historic importance. Every pharmacist appreciates the significance of opening the doors of one's first shop. The culmination of a lengthy period of preparation and training is but the beginning of an enterprise undertaken with anxiety and expectation. When John Bell opened the doors of his unpretentious shop in a sparsely populated area of London's West End, he knew full-well its importance for his own career; but he could never become aware of its wider historical significance. Today that opening is justly celebrated as the *fons et origo* of the Pharmaceutical Society of Great Britain. John Bell's assiduous application transformed the little shop in Oxford Street into one of the most splendid retail establishments in London. Jacob Bell, his eldest surviving son, inherited the business that, throughout his life, yielded the substantial sums he used to found and advance the interests of the Pharmaceutical Society.

Jacob Bell was born into a world of pharmacy and Quakerism. Both his parents came from long-established Quaker families. His mother, Eliza (d.1839) was the eldest daughter of Frederick Smith (1757–1823), chemist and druggist, of 29 Haymarket, London, to whom his father, John Bell (1774–1849) had been apprenticed. The obituary Jacob Bell wrote of his father in 1849 remains the primary source of our knowledge about his family: but, as a source, it needs to be read with care.[1] The memoir is a portrait in words: the details are not intended to be historically accurate, they are used to convey the impress of the father.

Before embarking in business as a chemist and druggist, Frederick Smith held for many years a position in the Post Office with an annual salary of nearly £1000: but he was sacked in 1783 when, as Jacob Bell explains, his religious objection to both capital punishment and oath-taking prevented his giving evidence in a case of robbery. Although entirely without training as a chemist and druggist, he took over his father-in-law's shop in the Haymarket and made a success of it. The custom of adulterating medicines was so prevalent at the time that Smith did not allow his religious scruples to interfere with it. Red precipitate was mixed with red lead, glauber salts were sold as nitre for horses, and both genuine and adulterated horse powders were prepared. There was a small room almost exclusively used for

1

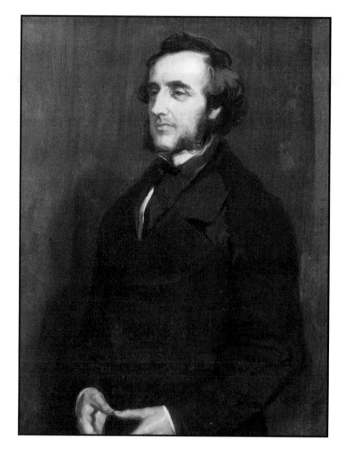

1 *Oil portrait of Jacob Bell by his friend Sir Edwin Landseer RA, 1859. This was painted in two hours, at one sitting, three days before Bell's death. It was presented by the artist to Thomas Hyde Hills, who bequeathed it to the Society in 1891.*

"russifying" rhubarb, i.e., cutting and filing East Indian, to imitate the more expensive Turkey, rhubarb. Once the business was firmly established, Frederick Smith paid his son Edward to run it, while he retired to Croydon, devoting the rest of his life to public and benevolent objects and the affairs of the Society of Friends. Edward, doubtless as a token of gratitude and respect, commissioned his friend, the then famous artist Benjamin Robert Haydon (1786–1846), to portray his parents. The picture, *The Quiet Hour*, which depicts a Quaker and his wife devoutly reading the Bible by lamplight, is now in the library of the London Society of Friends.[2]

Religious principles were also responsible, according to Jacob Bell's account, for a change of occupation and fortune in the Bell family. John Bell's father (also called Jacob) had been a prosperous mastmaker at Wapping Wall prior to the American War of Independence (1776–83). His unease at supplying materials for a purpose so much at variance with the principles of the Society of Friends led him to withdraw from the enterprise and become a hosier, at which, we are told, he was much less successful. His brother-in-law and former partner, James Sheppard, found it possible to salve his own conscience and carry on the profitable business of making masts. This version of events must be treated with scepticism. When our first Jacob Bell married Sarah Sheppard, the daughter of James, a shipwright of Wapping Wall, Shadwell in September 1771, he was termed "Hozier and citizen and Longbow Stringmaker".[3] At that time he was living at Fish Street Hill, in the parish of St. Leonard's, Eastcheap, where his first six children were born. By July 1780, however, when his fourth daughter, Martha Collinson, was born, he was living at Nut Tree House, Plaistow, West Ham. It was here that his fourth and fifth sons, Peter Collinson and Jacob were born. His fifth daughter, Katherine, was born at Wapping Wall, Shadwell in 1785 and at this time he was described as "a mastmaker". His sixth daughter, Rebecca, was born at Great Ilford in Essex.[4] We can be certain, then, that the eighteenth-century Jacob Bell changed his occupation. He started out as a hosier like his father, uncle, and elder brother, but became a mastmaker some eight years after his marriage to a shipwright's daughter. The move had more to do with the strength of Quaker family ties than the pangs of Quaker conscience. The timing was commercially adept: the demands of war made shipbuilding a prosperous industry.

John Bell was born on 4 December 1774 and received a good classical education at the famous Quaker academy in Tottenham kept by Thomas Coar. His father intended him to enter the medical profession and as a preliminary step he was apprenticed to Frederick Smith in the Haymarket. During his apprenticeship he attended the lectures of Dr. Pearson on chemistry, materia medica, and the practice of physic and subsequently Dr. Hooper's lectures delivered in the private school of medicine in Blenheim Street at the premises of Joshua Brookes, the noted surgeon. His nervous temperament, the reduced circumstances of his father, and his fear of too great an exposure to the temptations of the world are adduced to explain why he abandoned the idea of becoming a medical practitioner. Perhaps he realised, as many did, that just as much money could be made without bothering to obtain qualifications. Within a year of completing his apprenticeship and while still under 24 years of age, John Bell commenced business as a chemist and druggist at 338 Oxford Street. His father, whose financial decline seems to have been shortlived, took up the lease of the shop for him, lent him £400 to prepare and stock it, and added, in the autumn of 1799, a further £250 in the form of an apprenticeship premium for the younger brother (yet another Jacob). Young Jacob's contribution to the success of his brother's business was not inconsiderable. The assistance and encouragement of a youthful, hard-working member of the family, made zealous by the expectation of an eventual partnership, must have been invaluable at the start. Indeed, it was he who defined the distinctive quality of the Bell enterprise. At a time when, and in an area where, most retail establishments indulged in the fabrication of cheap medicines, the young Jacob "maintained without flinching that it was not only possible but expedient as a matter of policy to defy competition in price and make the quality of the medicines the primary consideration". Although this sound amalgam of ethics and commerce became the avowed policy of the business, Jacob was not rewarded with a partnership. Instead, his brother suggested he start up in some other part of London: before he could do so, however, he died of consumption in October 1805, aged 22.

The Oxford Street shop was an immediate success. In his father's obituary, Jacob Bell relates anecdotal evidence to the contrary, but he did not intend it to be taken seriously. In less than twelve months John Bell had taken on an apprentice and a shopboy and managed to persuade his uncle, James Sheppard, to lend him £100 for structural improvements. He astutely let off surplus accommodation to lodgers and kept a tight rein on recurrent expenditure. Soon after the second year he was able to pay off the £500 capital he had borrowed from his father and uncle. In the winter of 1800 he took Thomas Zachary as an apprentice for a premium of £125, followed in the next few years by Robert Ellwood (premium £100) and Henry Cockfield (premium £250). All three came from good Quaker families. His son tells us that "in taking apprentices, he was never tempted by a high premium, and, in fact, rather preferred those who had nothing to pay, under the idea that . . . they would be more likely to prove docile and tractable". But John Bell had other ways of ensuring the co-operation and loyalty of his workforce. "In the domestic regulations of the establishment he was remarkably strict, prohibited the assistants from going out in the evening under any pretence without express permission, and would not allow any deviation from the rules and regulations which were drawn up in writing". A copy of these regulations, written down in 1810, but obviously already in force for several years, has been preserved.[5] The detailed specification of duties carefully graded in an hierarchy of seniority and responsibility and the precision of the daily and weekly timetables, weighted by the degree of difficulty of the tasks, foreshadows modern job descriptions and time-and-motion studies. Scientific management preceded scientific pharmacy. Bureaucratic rules and regulations are not necessarily the product of the size of an organization: a family firm can spawn them just as readily as I.C.I.

What was the basis of this early success? Clearly John Bell worked hard himself and made certain those who worked under him did likewise. Nothing very ambitious was attempted. "He did not profess to be an operative or analytical Chemist, but confined his attention to the retail and dispensing business, and adopted certain fixed principles to which he rigidly adhered, as being at the same time in accordance with his conscientious feelings, and calculated to gain the confidence of the public". Being a very strict Friend, "he used to stand behind his counter with his cocked hat on", wondering "whether it would be possible to carry out to the full extent what he considered to be the principles of strict honesty". His earlier basic medical training was put to good account. "Without any attempt on his part to encourage counter practice, he was frequently applied to by the poor for advice . . . and, much against his inclination, he acquired some little repute as a doctor among that class of customers". Had he so desired, he could have asserted his right to be registered as an apothecary practising before the 1815 Act. Instead he aligned himself against the apothecaries, and became, in 1813, a member of the committee of prominent metropolitan chemists and druggists responsible for securing exemption for the trade from the operation of the penal clauses of the Apothecaries Act.[6]

By 1802 John Bell was doing so well he felt confident enough to marry. His marriage was blessed with eight children, Sarah (born 1804), John (1806), Eliza (1808), Jacob (1810), Anna (1811), Frederick John (1814), Maria (1816) and James (1818). "He continued for some years", wrote Jacob Bell, "to devote unremitted personal attention to his business, which increased beyond his expectations". In 1806 the shop was enlarged and, by that time, three apprentices and two general utility men were kept fully employed, in either the front shop or the "elaboratory" at the rear. By 1819, however, many of the details of running the business had become irksome, so he took from his staff two of his former apprentices, Thomas Zachary and John H. Walduck, both Quakers, and admitted them as partners. The name of the firm became John Bell and Co. Thomas Zachary took charge of the shop and John Bell went to live on his fine country estate, the Clock House at West Hill, Wandsworth, whence he drove daily in a pony-trap to Oxford Street. Increasingly he devoted his time to "benevolent and charitable objects especially in connexion with the Society of Friends". The business continued to advance steadily under its extended management. The development of Regent Street by John Nash between 1813 and 1820, and the growing popularity of the Harley Street area among physicians, transformed the prospect. Although prescribing continued to be important, dispensing and retail sales formed a large and expanding sector. The shop acquired a wide reputation. Every preparation was made on the premises: the laboratory, although attached to a retail shop, was as completely equipped as that of a wholesale house. It was this laboratory that was immortalised in the 1850s by William Henry Hunt's watercolour. By the 1820s John Bell and Co. had become well known throughout the Quaker community. Former apprentices and assistants settled down in various parts of the country and sent their own apprentices to gain experience in the old shop. 338 Oxford Street became, in effect, a private school of pharmacy providing a thorough grounding in all aspects of the trade. The students comprised not only indentured apprentices (paying premiums of £250 – £300) but also short-term pupils of various kinds.[7] Among the latter were medical students fulfilling the requirement to attend a course of practical pharmacy. Several men who later made their mark in the annals of pharmacy received their early education at 338 Oxford Street, including Theophilus Redwood, John Mackay, Robert Alsop, Henry Deane, Thomas Southall, H.C. Baildon, George Nelson, George Francis, and John Garle.

"Towards the end of 1798, John Bell opened his shop". These words are taken from Jacob Bell's obituary of his father. The memoir tell us perhaps as much about the son as the father. Not only is it a portrait of the man who had such a profound influence on his son's formative years but in the manner of its composition the author reveals the nature of those influences. The memoir displays in its writing an impressive combination of objectivity, psychological insight and deep affection. The events that are recorded, the features that are highlighted, as well as the style and tone of the overall picture reflect the depth of the father's legacy and the intensity of the son's struggle to free himself from it. Many illustrations of that Quaker discourse by which sound business decisions are precipitated by the elaboration of religious principles are provided: the tenets of Quakerism and the practice of pharmacy are shown to possess an elective affinity. Yet, throughout, there is an awareness of the gap between principles and behaviour, an appreciation of the way in which intentions are mocked by outcomes, a sense of the gentle ironies of life.

Jacob Bell begins by justifying the very act of an editor publishing, in his own journal, a memoir of his father. It was only undertaken, he claims, at the suggestion of several members of the Pharmaceutical Society "who considered that an account of the early life of a Chemist who had been above half a century in the business might be instructing as well as useful". This obituary is no mere act of piety: its purpose is as didactic as any Quaker tract. His father's life is offered as "a practical illustration of the result of a strict adherence to conscientious principle, even under apparently unfavourable circumstances" and as "an

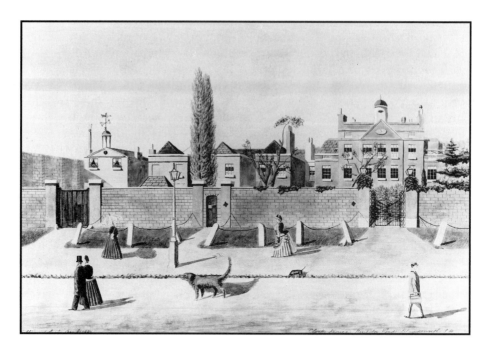

2 *Primitive watercolour view of 1887 showing Clock House, Kingston Road, Wandsworth, the former residence of John Bell. This building was later demolished to make way for the Putney branch of the London and South-Western Railway.*

encouragement to young men under similar circumstances''. The lessons that the young are expected to draw from this life are not, however, unequivocal. The meek, the industrious, and the pure in heart and drugs are shown to be blessed; but am I really my brother's keeper? What moral were the young intended to draw from the following episode?

> About this period, [my father's] attention was directed to the subject of intemperance, and its lamentable effects on the lower classes. Being in the habit of distributing tracts to the poor in favour of total abstinence, he considered it his duty to try the experiment himself, by way of example ... During this time his health was not uniformly good ... and he was advised to try the effect of a more stimulating regimen. For some time he was unwilling to deviate from his abstinent resolve, but Dr. Wilson ... suggested a plan which overcame the scruple. The wine was put up in two-ounce bottles, and sent from the shop as a medicine. Finding the effect beneficial, he afterwards submitted, under medical orders, to take a glass of wine in the usual way.

Was the lesson, perhaps, to learn to handle with tact and skill the sensibilities of one's father?

Jacob Bell makes use of a private journal his father kept in 1797 at the age of 22 to illuminate "the peculiar constitution of his mind". "His chief desire appeared to be to escape 'the snares and temptations of the world', and to adhere strictly to the path of duty.

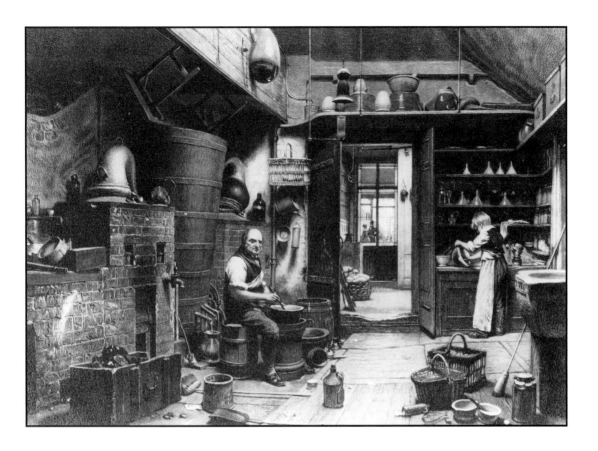

3 *Mezzotint by J.G. Murray after the watercolour by W.H. Hunt (1790–1864), of the old "elaboratory" of 338 Oxford Street, the premises of John Bell & Co., in the 1840s. The seated figure is a portrait of John Simmonds, who had been the laboratory man at the business from its opening in 1798.*

He was conscious of a natural irritability of temper, which it was his constant endeavour to subdue". His bouts of "despondency and contrition", his sense of "his incapacity to 'cope with the world'" were joined by "diffidence and nervous temperament". His deep sense of sin and guilt, his lack of resolution and confidence, and the profound distrust of his own motivation are all recurring themes of Quaker biography and seem to be traits characteristic of a certain Quaker mentality. The self-interrogation and inquisition of the conscience are part of the terrifying sense of the isolation of the individual, naked before God. They are, at the same time, preliminary to the search for rational control of both the self and the world: the fountain head of that self-mastery which is fostered by a strict education and expresses itself in the diligence, discipline, and endeavour that are encapsulated in the concept of "vocation".

The craft of the chemist and druggist was a particularly attractive occupation for the devout member of the Society of Friends. Ownership of a small, independent, family-based business provided a peculiarly satisfying milieu for the expression of the Quaker personality. To understand why this was so, it is necessary to consider the implications for ordinary, everyday activity of commitment to the Quaker creed. As Christians and Protestants, Friends placed each man's salvation ultimately in his own personal relation to God. Protestantism gave priority to the individual conscience and set it up as a judge above all traditional authority. The exercise of private judgment was not only a right but a duty. The distinctive character of Quakerism arises from its emphasis on the fact of God making himself directly known in the heart of every human being. This experience is the Light of Christ, since in Christ the character of the Light is shown uniquely and supremely. The Light made known in the heart is the primary religious authority; the Light will, of course, be recognized and checked with reference to the knowledge of God, and particularly of Christ, found in the Bible; but the Bible is secondary in authority to the Spirit. The acknowledgment that God's Spirit is given to all results in an organization of the church based on the priesthood of all believers and a social outlook based on the sacredness of every personality. Traditional authorities and traditional hierarchies of rank and deference are dissolved by such beliefs. Moreover, there can be no division of life into the sacred and the secular. Quakers emphasize the potentially sacramental nature of every part of life. Man has been created to fulfil God's purposes in the ordinary routines of daily life. Mundane activity is a sacred duty. A man's behaviour in this world is indicative of his inner spiritual life.

An understanding of the personality structure and behavioural patterns engendered by this set of beliefs may help to explain why so many successful chemists and druggists in the late eighteenth and early nineteenth centuries were Quakers. Few situations offered so clearly the prospect of congruence between personality and career, between belief and activity. Proprietorship of one's own family-based business provided a sense of independence and personal responsibility, of being one's own master. The success of the enterprise could be seen to be closely related to the efforts and character of the owner. Profits acted as a barometer of personal achievement. Diligence, discipline and commitment were likely to be rewarded; and success was recorded with precision by the balance-sheet. Rational planning and resource management brought dividends denied to those who followed the traditional rituals of economic life. The individual made the crucial decisions. Such satisfactions were characteristic of any small scale family business. The role of chemist and druggist was especially fulfilling for it was a position with ethical and social responsibilities, providing opportunities for the exercise of individual judgment based on acquired knowledge and special skills.

In the late eighteenth century members of the Society of Friends were a people apart, peculiar in their way of dress, their forms of worship and their sober, austere, earnest way of life. The leather breeches, drab coat, buckled shoes and broad brimmed hat came to be regarded and adopted as a badge of their calling. Legal disabilities and religious discrimination prevented them holding public office, attending the English universities, and entering certain professions. These restrictions forced them to establish their own schools and academies and to direct their energies to entrepreneurial activity. Endogamy made virtuous what was almost a necessity. Thus Quakers came to form an extensive but closely-knit community within the wider society. The close association of religious beliefs, business activities and family life gave them a reputation for honesty, integrity, and fair-dealing, as well as for thrift and hard work. Although as businessmen Quakers traded with the outside world, most of their business associates and partners were chosen from among the members of their own Society, often indeed from their own kin: and they took in as associates, apprentices and employees, Friends and the children of Friends. Bonds of Friendship lubricated sentiments of trust, personal probity and family reputation. The Quaker network stretched throughout Britain and overseas to North America. It operated as an elaborate system of social control and mutual aid. Finance, knowledge and personnel flowed along its arteries. The Quaker community provided more extensive facilities and more intense supervision than the wider society. For some, however, the greater range of opportunities offered may have been more than offset by the weight of obligations demanded.

John Bell as an individual and as the bearer of the Quaker faith had a profound influence on his eldest surviving son. From this source can be traced Jacob Bell's self-discipline, the watchful control of his emotions, his deep inner strength and sense of purpose, his perseverance and drive. Yet in many ways Jacob and his father were poles apart. In contrast to his father's timidity and lack of confidence, Jacob had an exuberance and sense of adventure. While John Bell was withdrawn and inward-looking, his son was a master of the arts of friendship. From an early age Jacob revealed abilities and tendencies which led him to question and ultimately to reject many aspects of his father's way of life. He abandoned the Quaker mode of speech and dress before cutting himself free from the obligations of membership. Paradoxically, it was the financial success of the business John Bell created that provided the means for his son to develop the interests and abilities which lured him out of the confines of the meeting-house and dispensary into the temptations offered by politics and the arts. Yet one of Jacob Bell's greatest achievements was to carry over into the practice of modern, secular, scientific pharmacy the Quaker sense of inner commitment and ethical conduct.

When he was twelve years old, Jacob Bell was sent to the school of his uncle, Henry Frederick Smith, at Blackwell, near Darlington, where he stayed for about four years.[8] The school deserved its high reputation with wealthy Quakers: it was once described as "a collegiate school where the sons of Friends could have the advantage of a good education without the exposure of University life".[9] At school Jacob began to display his literary and artistic talents as well as signs of independence and detachment. When he was sixteen he wrote lengthy essays on the two social issues which most quickened Quaker consciences at the start of the nineteenth century, war and slavery.[10] His condemnation of the waste of human and other resources in war was retained throughout his life and was to be vehemently reiterated in 1851 at the conclusion of his Society of Arts lecture on the Great Exhibition.[11] In less serious mood, he composed facetious dialogues in the then fashionable burlesque-heroic style and illustrated them with clever pen-and-ink sketches. The overbearing solemnity of a volume of Quaker tracts was once punctured by the young man's playful caricatures of its authors and by an unflattering portrait of Jacob Bell himself "trying to understand this queer book".[12] Another early literary production, undertaken with school friend Lawson Ford, was a manuscript periodical devoted to a humorous, at times grotesque, presentation of school news and gossip, under the whimsical title, "Bellford Gazette".

On leaving school, Jacob was apprenticed in his father's business. His father, at that time (1827), had two partners, one of whom, Thomas Zachary, lived on the premises in Oxford Street. Jacob was put under his immediate control and was made to submit to all the regulations to which apprentices and young assistants were then subjected. In those days the young men started work at eight in the morning and were kept busy until eleven at night. None was allowed to leave the premises in the evening without special permission; but those off duty were free to go out in the morning before breakfast. Evenings were spent either in the counting-house at the back of the shop or in the bedrooms where each apprentice had a desk and a few shelves to keep personal reading material. At breakfast and teatime no conversation was permitted since all were expected to read. The bookcase in the dining room contained a few religious tomes together with A.T. Thomson's *London Dispensatory*, Thomas's *Practice of Physic*, and a few other works of this kind. Most of the apprentices, however, did their reading in general literature; Jacob, encouraged by Theophilus Redwood and Robert Alsop, read mainly chemistry books.[13]

Even during these arduous days, Jacob Bell's joyful appreciation of the comic side of life broke through. He kept a copiously illustrated journal in which, as Redwood observed, "various members of the household, including even some of those in authority, if their exercise of discipline clashed with the laxer ideas of the young master, figured in some caricature representations". His cleverly titled manuscript, *List of Fractures made during the Apprenticeship of Jacob Bell*, has lively pen-and-ink illustrations and delightfully recalls the day-by-day life in an early nineteenth century pharmacy. Many straightforward accidents occur; one bottle is smashed against a mortar, another by the cork being driven in too far, the bottom of a mortar is knocked out by the pestle, a drawer is pulled out too far and its contents scattered on the floor, breakages of window panes and oil lamps seem almost routine. Some incidents hint at malice aforethought: a galley-pot crushed in a cork-press; "an old fool of a pill pot" tossed into the rubbish bin; a bottle deliberately dropped on the counter while Jacob asserts, "There, see, it won't break", and a companion observes, "Ah, but it has!" What a contrast there is between all this and his father's morose journal of 1797! During his pupilage, the heir of the house went out of his way to develop warm and intimate relations with his fellow apprentices and the assistants. He worked alongside them in a relaxed and happy way, encouraging their ambitions and promoting their education and welfare. After his death he was recalled in terms of great affection by such diverse ex-residents as Henry Deane, John Mackay and Theophilus Redwood.

After an initial period of the full rigours of apprenticeship, Jacob was gradually given more freedom. He attended lectures on chemistry at the Royal Institution and on the practice of physic at the recently-opened King's College. On becoming the occupant of a larger bedroom, he immediately converted it into a laboratory by installing a furnace and other chemical apparatus. At about this time he also developed an interest in the study of comparative anatomy and demonstrated his skills as a manipulator by the successful preparation of animal skeletons. These tissue-removing exercises were usually carried out at his father's house in Wandsworth "where bitter denunciations sometimes arose when the odious effluvium of some dead monkey, rat or porcupine, undergoing its term of maceration, penetrated unbidden the quarters of the family". Jacob must have aroused the disapproval of the family on other occasions. The story, which he often told, of a youthful prank is recounted by W.P. Frith in his autobiography.[14] In those

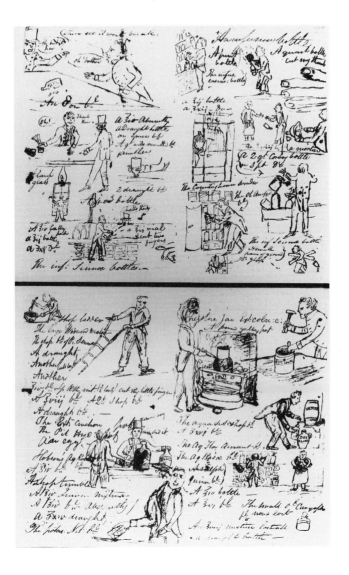

4   *Humorous illustrations from* A List of Fractures made during the apprenticeship of Jacob Bell. (Motto) 'Save the Pieces!', *a diary kept by the young Jacob Bell to record the early years at his father's pharmacy.*

days, at Quaker "meeting", the men sat on one side of the chapel, and the women on the other.

> Bell disliked this arrangement, and finding remonstrance of no avail, he disguised himself in female attire, and took his place in the forbidden seats. For a time all went well, but a guilty conscience came into play on seeing two of the congregation speaking together and eyeing him suspiciously the while; he took

fright, and catching up his petticoats, he went out from "meeting" with a stride that proclaimed his sex.

Frith adds that for this he was "expelled from the community". His membership may, indeed, have been temporarily suspended, but it was not until he was forty-five that Jacob Bell was "discarded by the Quakers". On 23 August 1855, the Kingston Monthly Meeting disowned him, "having for a considerable time past habitually absented himself from our religious meetings".[15] Jacob Bell's keen sense of theatre and his delight in the ridiculous often coloured his version of the more prosaic events in his life.

In his youth his studies were not confined to subjects appertaining to pharmacy. From an early age he had manifested an aptitude for drawing and now he was given leave to attend classes at the famous school of art run by Henry Sass and to receive lessons in oil painting from Henry Perronet Briggs. Briggs, who was a Quaker and a cousin of Jacob, became a close friend. Bell purchased the most successful of his Shakespearean paintings, *Othello relating his adventures to Desdemona*, and was responsible for commissioning other work by him. Briggs produced, in 1833, a portrait of John Bell (an engraving of which appeared as the frontispiece of the *Pharmaceutical Journal* for 1848/49) and later, having designed the membership certificate of the Pharmaceutical Society, painted the well known portrait of its first holder, the eminent Quaker scientist and philanthropist, William Allen, F.R.S. When Briggs died in 1844, at the age of 52, he left his two children under Jacob Bell's guardianship, and Bell's sister, Eliza, looked after them in the house at Langham Place: the son died young and the daughter became the wife of a vicar in Kent.[16] Bell was Briggs' executor and several letters survive showing how conscientiously he carried out his duties. He wrote around to those whose portraits Briggs had painted, or to their relatives and friends, inquiring whether they wished to purchase the paintings. Lord Wharncliffe replied from Curzon Street, in March 1844, that, although he did not want his own portrait, he was enclosing eighty guineas for that of the Duke of Wellington. The unsold paintings went to auction at Christie's.

The eminent Victorian artist, W.P. Frith, also became a close friend. In his autobiography, he gives an account of Jacob's short but eventful career at art school.

> When Bell first appeared at Sass's, he wore the Quaker coat; but finding that the students showed their disapproval in a marked and unpleasant manner—such, for instance, as writing "Quaker" in white chalk across his back—he discarded that vestment . . .
>
> . . . on one fatal Monday morning, after witnessing an early execution at Newgate, he drew the scaffold and the criminal hanging on it . . . We were grouped round the artist listening to an animated account of the murderer's last moments when Sass appeared.
>
> The crowd of listeners ran to their seats and waited for the storm. Mr. Sass looked at the drawing, and went out of the studio—a pin might have been heard to drop. Bell looked round and winked at me. Sass returned, and walked slowly up to Mr. Jacob Bell, and addressed him as follows: "Sir, Mr. Bell; sir, your father placed you under my care for the purpose of making an artist of you. I can't do it; I can make nothing of you. I should be robbing your father *if I did it*. You had better go, sir; such a career as this," pointing to the man hanging, "is a bad example to your fellow-pupils. You must leave, sir!"

"All right," said Bell, and away he went, returning to the druggist's shop established by his father in Oxford Street ...

Although Jacob Bell gave up the idea of becoming an artist himself, he remained devotedly attached to and a liberal patron of art, as well as the friend of artists during his life. It was Bell who commissioned Frith to paint his masterpiece, *Derby Day*.

> Mr. Jacob Bell had desired me to paint an important picture for him so soon as I found a subject agreeable to his taste and my own. On seeing the sketch of the *Derby Day*, no time was lost in deliberation, for I was commissioned to paint a picture five or six feet long from it, at the price of fifteen hundred pounds; the copyright being reserved to me, and a reasonable time conceded for the loan of the picture for engraving ... Before the picture was begun, the copyright for the engraving was purchased by Mr. Gambort, who agreed to pay fifteen hundred pounds for it.
>
> The owner, Mr. Bell, was also very useful to me in procuring models. Few people have a more extensive acquaintance, especially amongst the female sex, than that possessed by Jacob Bell; and what seemed singular, was the remarkable prettiness that distinguished nearly all these pleasant friends. I had but to name the points required, and an example was produced.
>
> "What is it to be this time?" he would say. "Fair or dark, long nose or short nose, Roman or aquiline, tall figure or small? Give your orders."
>
> The order was given, and obeyed in a manner that perfectly astonished me. I owe every female figure in the *Derby Day*, except two or three, to the foraging of my employer.

The viewing of *Derby Day* at the Royal Academy attracted so many visitors that Bell had to persuade the President and Council to protect it with a rail, thus according it a privileged status that aroused the envy of Frith's fellow artists.

By the age of twenty-five, Jacob Bell had acquired an impressive collection of modern art. Frith relates an anecdote, which must have originated with Bell, which shows how religious sanction could be obtained from his father by defining his pleasures as business. Frith wrote of Bell:

> It is reported of his father, a rigid Quaker, who watched with disapproval his son's purchases of pictures, that he said to him one day:
>
> "What business hast thou to buy those things, wasting thy substance?"
>
> "I can sell any of *those things* for more than I gave for them, some for twice as much."
>
> "Is that verily so?" said the old man. "Then I see no sin in thy buying more."

Jacob Bell's artistic talent and sensibilities brought him into contact with men in whose society he found pleasures excelling even those of artistic production. His own perceptive powers were quickened and enhanced, but, above all, he discovered that he was able to stimulate and harness the zeal of his artistic friends. He became their ministering angel. Bell made himself indispensable as patron, adviser, and friend. He unashamedly admired their talents and openly celebrated their achievements. He modestly and discreetly made available to them his commercial acumen and business skills. He revelled in their company:

13

he felt invigorated by their presence. Although he maintained a lively and extensive correspondence with a wide range of people in the world of art, only a few of the letters now survive. These, nonetheless, provide a glimpse of that world. In April 1847 we find the famous caricaturist George Cruikshank trying to persuade Bell to drop in on the private showing of the watercolours of Valentine Bartholomew, whose flower paintings gave Queen Victoria such pleasure and who is now remembered for his views of Windsor. John Frederick Tayler, an etcher, illustrator and painter of Scottish landscapes, asks Bell to take a look at his new painting, "a picture of some importance". Tayler, like Bell, had taken lessons at Sass's. Another artist, David Gibson, seeks Jacob's opinion of his latest creation, intended for next year's Academy exhibition, and thanks him for sending him a "capital" canvas. Clarkson Stanfield, the marine and landscape painter, urges Bell to mount his horse and gallop up Hampstead Heath to visit him at his new home, aptly called "The Green Hill". Jacob, a fine horseman, gave up hunting only at his father's insistence. E.M. Ward and C.R. Leslie, two eminent Victorian artists who benefited from Bell's patronage, write to make arrangements for their paintings to be engraved. Charles Landseer seeks his advice on a commission he has received for an Aesop picture: should he accept and at what price? Count D'Orsay, portrait painter, friend of Napoleon III and glittering socialite, enquires in 1844 about the possibility of buying Edwin Landseer's Comus fresco (which Bell, however, kept for himself) and four years later sends a bust of Lord George Bentinck, glowing after the application of one of Bell's special polishes.

The artist with whom Bell was most closely associated and on whose work he had most influence was undoubtedly Sir Edwin Landseer (1802–1873). Landseer was already an established painter when Bell first made his acquaintance. Early in his life Landseer made his way into the highest ranks of society. A fellow of the Royal Academy by the age of thirty, he rapidly became the close and privileged companion of the Royal family and of several aristocratic families. Yet his most intimate friend and valued adviser was the son of a Quaker shopkeeper. When Landseer's poor health in 1840 led his medical advisers to suggest a holiday on the Continent, Jacob Bell accompanied him on his journey through Belgium and along the Rhine to Geneva where they stayed together for more than four months. On the return journey they stayed at the Hotel Meurice in Paris for a few days. The impact "this metropolis of dissipation" had on them was vividly recorded in a letter written in December 1840:

> I almost died of the Louvre yesterday and have not dared go out at all today . . . for fear of seeing anything. When I have recovered from the excitement of the Louvre I shall go out and put myself in jeopardy by looking at something else. Having with me a man of the right sort of metal who has never seen Paris before increased what I have to go thro'—In fact we are obliged to support each other under it all—for whether we turn to the pictorial, the tasteful, the intellectual, the sensual or the tout ensemble department there's always a something to drive one mad. What a place this is for spending money. What a lucky thing to be run aground with only just enough to pay our way home! . . . We are delighted to hear that the Queen has favored the nation with a ditto of her little self.

Landseer was never happier than in the company of Jacob Bell and spent as much time as he could spare at Bell's house in Langham Place. Landseer had a town house in St. John's Wood but purchased a country house adjacent to the The Clock House in

Wandsworth. His most productive period was from 1840 to 1860 when Bell's influence was at its height: after Bell's death Landseer suffered increasingly from bouts of depression and mental illness. From 1840 Bell took control of Landseer's business affairs which he managed with zeal and discretion, rescuing him from the clutches of the picture dealers. His services were invaluable in conducting the negotiations for the sale of Landseer's pictures and of the right to take engravings from them. Bell's correspondence with the engravers H. Graves and Co., of Pall Mall, between the years 1841 and 1859 reveals how astutely Landseer's affairs were managed. In March 1841 we find Graves agreeing to pay 600 guineas "for copyright for engraving purposes" of two pictures, the Duke of Beaufort's dog and *Horses Drinking*. In 1857 the copyright of *Uncle Tom and His Wife For Sale* and *Scene at Brae Mar* was secured for £1,300 and, in the same year, £1,200 was paid for the right to engrave *Saved*. The agreements ensured that Sir Edwin retained a significant measure of control over the final product. The engraver was either chosen or approved by the artist who received proofs from time to time for touching. No impressions were to be published until Sir Edwin had approved, in writing, the final proofs.[17]

Jacob Bell performed a useful service to Landseer and other artists by his advice and help on the question of how copyright affected them. Bell sought the opinions of his good friend, Thomas Talfourd, the leading authority on copyright law and the man mainly responsible for the 1842 Copyright Act. Buttressed with Talfourd's counsel, Bell was successful in helping artists realise their rights in the reproduction of their works. Regarding the subject of copyright from a strictly commercial point of view, he appreciated the full value of the privilege and was able to secure for artists the monetary rewards which belonged to them but which they had not previously exploited.

Bell had considerable influence on the evolution of Landseer's art. It has been suggested that it was a common love of animals, especially of dogs and horses, which originally drew the two men together. Bell undoubtedly encouraged Landseer to become the outstanding animal painter of the nineteenth century, a success that owed much to the way he endowed the animals in his pictures with human emotions and character. Bell's acute commercial sensibility led him to direct Landseer towards the subjects and mode of presentation that found favour with the new bourgeoisie whose growing wealth made them keen to decorate their walls with paintings and engravings. Bell himself purchased some of Landseer's best works, including *The Maid and the Magpie, Alexander and Diogenes*, *The Defeat of Comus, Highland Dogs, Dignity and Impudence, Shoeing*, and *The Sleeping Bloodhound*. *Shoeing*, which was exhibited at the Royal Academy in 1844, contains portraits of Bell's bay mare "Old Betty", his bloodhound "Laura", and his personal farrier. In his *Memoirs of Sir Edwin Landseer*, F.G. Stephens relates a typical Jacob Bell anecdote. The dog in the painting, *The Sleeping Bloodhound*, died by falling some thirty feet from a parapet at the Clock House. Hoping to secure a sketch of his favourite hound, Bell carried the lifeless dog from Wandsworth to Landseer's home in St. John's Wood. Reporting Landseer's reaction, Bell said:

> The sight of the unfortunate hound suddenly changed an expression of something approaching vexation (at the interruption during his daily occupation) into one of sorrow and sympathy, and after the first expression of regret at the misfortune, the verdict was laconic and characteristic—"This is an opportunity not to be lost; go away; come on Thursday, at two o'clock." It was then about midday, Monday. On Thursday, at two o'clock, there was "Countess" as large as life, asleep, as she is now.[18]

15

Thus art follows life. Any artist capable of meeting such deadlines deserves fame and fortune!

Jacob Bell was one of the leading patrons of British art in the first half of the nineteenth century. At his home in Langham Place he formed a collection of paintings most of which had been executed by artists who were his personal friends. "The drawing room . . . was a gallery of art", recalled Joseph Ince in 1891. "The walls were hung, or rather hidden, by a collection of modern paintings".[19] In April 1859 he exhibited the majority of this impressive collection in the rooms and for the benefit of the Marylebone Literary and Scientific Institution, of which he was President. Bell prepared the catalogue himself: at the time it was recommended as "a model . . . to all future compilers of catalogues". So popular was the exhibition that £200 was raised and the Institution was relieved of about two-thirds of its liabilities. In his Will Bell left the finest examples from the Collection to the National Gallery. In addition to the works of Sir Edwin Landseer, the bequest included paintings by Charles Landseer, Rosa Bonheur, C.R. Leslie, William Etty, E.M. Ward, G.B. O'Neill, William Fettes Douglas, Frederick Lee and Thomas Cooper, and W.P. Frith's *Derby Day*. At the time of his death the value of his bequest to the nation was put at between £18,000 and £20,000.

At the beginning of the nineteenth century, London had recently gained its reputation as an important centre for the buying and selling of paintings and the English were relative newcomers to the ranks of enthusiastic European art collectors. Jacob Bell was in many ways a pioneer in his extensive patronage of British artists: he set an important precedent in channelling wealth from newly tapped urban sources into the increasingly buoyant art market. During the industrial revolution works of art became symbols central to the process of the cultural integration of the upper ranks of British society. Patronage of the arts celebrated a new cultural identity that bound together the core of the propertied classes, royalty, aristocracy and the metropolitan bourgeoisie. As they became involved in new forms of economic activity and embraced the imperatives of commercialization, so they elaborated new forms of cultural unification. Within this new consensus, subtle gradations of status were linked to manifestations of civilised behaviour: virtue came to be measured by the delicate balance of taste. Connoisseurship of painting gained new significance as taste became a matter of pressing concern; for central to the discourse on virtue was informed appreciation of art.

At his private residence, 15 Langham Place, Jacob Bell gave many brilliant parties for his artistic, literary, musical and theatrical friends. During the years 1837–1843, three of Bell's associates worked together in the production of a new magazine, Bentley's Miscellany. Charles Dickens wrote both *Oliver Twist* and *Nicholas Nickleby* for the magazine, George Cruikshank (1792–1878) designed the cover and supplied many of the illustrations, and Samuel Lover (1797–1868) was a founder and early contributor. Bell found Lover a particularly attractive person for he mirrored his own sense of humour and diverse talents. Lover was a painter of miniatures, a composer of songs and ballads, a popular novelist, a musician, dramatist, and theatrical entertainer. Born near Dublin, he moved to London in 1835 and soon became an established part of the artistic, literary and theatrical scene. He painted Lord Brougham in his Chancellor's robes; wrote a novel, *Rory O'More, A National Romance*, and successfully adapted it for the stage; composed a burlesque opera *Il Paddy Whack in Italia*; and triumphantly toured America and Canada with his "Irish

Evening", an entertainment of songs, recitations, and stories, written and performed by himself. Lover, it was said, "possessed those typical qualities usually called Irish".[20]

The MacIans, like Samuel Lover, were friends of Bell with feet in both theatrical and artistic camps. It is not known how Bell first became acquainted with Robert Ronald MacIan (1803–1856). He may well have viewed the young Scot's exhibition at the Suffolk Street Gallery in 1835 and he would certainly have seen his landscape at the Royal Academy exhibition of 1836. Bell may well have got to know MacIan first as an actor, for he would have seen him on the stage at Covent Garden in 1838 and at Drury Lane the following year, and invited him and his wife to one of his parties during the season. MacIan's wife, Fanny, was at least as talented as her husband. She taught in the female school of design at Somerset House and was an accomplished artist, exhibiting at the Royal Scottish Academy, British Institution and the Royal Academy. Like her husband, she specialised in depicting scenes from Scottish history: her best known work is *Highlander defending his family at the Massacre of Glencoe*, his is, probably, *The Battle of Culloden*. Jacob Bell was a close friend and had encouraged Robert to abandon the stage and devote himself entirely to painting. The Library of the Pharmaceutical Society possesses three amusing letters from Bell to the MacIans in 1844, requesting the return of a pair of Highland pistols. Typically each letter is illustrated in Bell's own facetious way with imaginative pen-and-ink sketches.

Over the years Bell entertained many famous guests at Langham Place. His gatherings were small scale and intimate compared to the lavish annual parties given by his friend, Benjamin Lumley (1811–1875). Lumley was for twenty years director of Her Majesty's theatre, where Bell had a box throughout the season. Lumley's fetes, in the grounds of his Fulham villa, were

> one of the salient events of the "London Season" ... coronet, pen, brush, throat
> of priceless value, and lithesome limbs, all joined amidst rich illuminations and *feux
> de Bengale*, in one *grande ronde* of unrestricted hilarity and enjoyment.[21]

Bell's gatherings were less grandiose but more frequent. Between 1838 and 1856 Jacob Bell and his guests were privileged to see, at Her Majesty's, the first performances in England of many of the greatest Italian operas: Donizetti's *Lucia di Lammermoor* (1838), *Lucrezia Borgia* (1839), *Don Pasquale* and *Linda di Chamounix* (1843) and *La Figlia del Reggimento* (1847) with Verdi's *Ernani* (1845), *Nabucco* (1846), *Attila* (1848) and *La Traviata* (1856). Thanks to Lumley, Bell would also have heard the London performances of Jenny Lind, the great Swedish soprano. Lumley was a man of many parts and opera was not the only interest he had in common with Bell. Trained as a solicitor, Lumley had practised as a Parliamentary agent before taking up theatre management. He published in 1838 the standard work on *Parliamentary Practice on Passing Private Bills*. His knowledge of the procedures of the House of Commons would prove of value to Bell later in his career.

Just as other Quakers found that religious discipleship brought unanticipated commercial rewards so Jacob Bell discovered that his love of art had consequences which were unintended but welcome. He bought pictures out of admiration and friendship: they became a sound investment. By the cultivation of his artistic connexions, he was enabled to throw off the impediment of his philistine, petit-bourgeois origins and lay claim to the possession of cultural attainments that secured his acceptance in the higher ranks of society. There was no calculation in this transformation. Bell inherited from his father a belief in the basic equality and dignity of all men and a healthy disrespect for inherited rank and titles. His assessment of merit was based on personal achievement and he expected to be judged by the same criterion. It was almost entirely the force of his own character that enabled Bell to achieve for himself the distinguished position he held among his contemporaries. He was not of high birth nor had he powerful connexions: he had neither rank nor family influence to recommend him. He made his mark in the higher ranks of Victorian society in spite of his background and the unpretending occupation of a chemist and druggist. Yet he was, to an important degree, favoured by circumstances. His father, by assiduous application and disciplined management, had established, during his long life, a business in Oxford Street capable of sustaining its own growth. It not only enabled its founder to amass wealth enough to leave his children affluent but it continued to realise very handsome profits throughout the life of his son. Jacob Bell had the good sense to retain the principal share of the enterprise until the day of his death. Had he achieved nothing else, he would have been remembered as the head of a famous firm of dispensing chemists, the excellence of whose drugs gave them a European reputation.

When Jacob started work as an apprentice with the firm, there were, in association with his father, two partners, Thomas Zachary and John H. Walduck. Both junior partners retired in 1836 and Jacob Bell and one of his younger brothers, Frederick John, took their places. Little is known about Frederick John. He joined the Microscopical Society on its foundation in 1840 and was instructed in the use of the microscope by Dr. J.S. Bowerbank, a noted exponent, who lived in Islington. Frederick was a founder member of the Pharmaceutical Society and one of its first auditors. His connexion with the firm ended in 1847. The other surviving brother, James, had been trained as an architect, so when the founder of the business died in 1849, Jacob became the sole proprietor. Despite all the other calls on his time and attention, he seems to have personally superintended the business. By that date there were at least ten assistants and apprentices living and working at 338 Oxford Street under the direct supervision of George Baggett Francis, who had served his apprenticeship there and was now chief of the laboratory. Mrs. Francis was the housekeeper: hence it was that George Bult Francis (1850–1929), a founder of British Drug Houses, came to be born at 338 Oxford Street. The man in daily charge of the business was Thomas Hyde Hills (1815–1891). Hills had been apprenticed to Mr. Thorby of Brighton, himself an old Bell's man. In 1837 he came to London and was engaged as a junior assistant at Bell's.

> Jacob Bell took a great fancy to him. They were about of an age, Bell being then
> in his 27th year and Hills in his 22nd. Mr. Bell had a house in Langham Place,
> and had begun to draw round him the artistic and literary circle with which he was
> identified until the end, and which Thomas Hyde Hills kept up until death thinned
> the ranks of Jacob Bell's friends. Not very long after Mr. Hills had entered 338
> Oxford Street Jacob Bell invited him to his house in Langham Place for a few days'
> visit, and there Mr. Hills remained until his friend's death in 1859.[22]

After serving in the front shop for eight years, Hills was appointed superintendent of the laboratory in 1845. As an associate of the Pharmaceutical Society, he attended classes at the School of Pharmacy and became a Ph.C. in 1848. Hills became so indispensable in the management of the business that in 1852 he was taken into partnership. In his Will, Bell left his partner his own (2/3rds) share of the business, including the goodwill and the stock, manufacturing implements, stores, and the additional premises in Queen Street.

All who worked at 338 Oxford Street testified that Jacob Bell was an exceptionally kind and considerate employer. Although the shop was open seven days a week from eight in the morning till eleven at night, careful arrangements were made to allow assistants and apprentices time for recreation, religious observance and study. Even though the laboratory and dispensary themselves constituted a school of practical pharmacy, every encouragement was afforded the staff to attend lectures and courses, both before and after the establishment of the Pharmaceutical Society's School of Pharmacy. The subsequent careers of those who worked under Bell bear witness to the fact that the Oxford Street shop provided a thorough preparation for survival in a highly competitive world. Bell had a deep sense of justice and fair play: this in turn inspired loyalty and affection in those who worked for him. He demonstrated his confidence in the ability of his assistants by delegating much responsibility to them. They responded by devoting themselves to the success of the firm. Thomas Hyde Hills became a partner, George Francis was in charge of the laboratory, Francis Middleton supervised the dispensing, and John Barnard became, in effect, Bell's personal secretary. On Bell's death, they were generously rewarded: Francis, Middleton and Barnard each received £500.

Jacob Bell's shop in Oxford Street, in the very heart of the West End, was probably the most prestigious pharmaceutical business in Britain. In common with many chemists and druggists throughout the country, there was a thriving retail business: this involved a certain amount of counter prescribing, the preparation of family recipes and the restocking of family medicine chests, and the sale of a great range of remedies, special, standard, and proprietary. A letter written by Robert Browning, the poet, in 1856 relates how, shortly after arriving at 39 Devonshire Place, Elizabeth sent him out to get some of her indispensable morphine, which he obtained from his old friend, Jacob Bell. The practice that distinguished the high-class establishments like Bell's from the run-of-the-mill chemist's shop was the dispensing of physician's prescriptions. Bell and Co. developed a special relationship with the leading London physicians. They recognized that prescriptions taken to 338 Oxford Street would be accurately dispensed with unadulterated materials; that the dispenser would be trained to adhere strictly either to the London Pharmacopoeia or to the specific indications of the prescriber; and that patients would be handled with deference and sensitivity. Jacob Bell took his responsibilities as a dispensing chemist very seriously. "On principle", he affirmed, "a prescription should either be prepared correctly or it should not be prepared at all, and in all cases of doubt application should be made to the prescriber".[23] Many of the procedures followed at 338 Oxford Street anticipated modern good practice. Someone who had worked for the firm for many years bore testimony to "the extreme caution always exhibited by him in matters of doubt". No dubious prescription would be dispensed "without a previous interview with the prescriber and an explanation of the unintelligible preparations". The writer continued:

> And here I would, from experience, recommend most earnestly the plan pursued at Mr. Bell's establishment in this respect to all our fraternity; many an accident would thus be avoided, many a patient benefited, whilst no one is injured. In cases where the prescriber is not to be met with, some "ruse" should be adopted by which to screen the patient from danger, without, of course, compromising the character

of the medical man. If there be no means of communicating with the writer, some other practitioner might, under the circumstances, consider and advise in the matter.[24]

Chemists and druggists, in Bell's view, had important social responsibilities. He would readily have supported the comments of Dr. John Scoffern expressed in 1847:

> Society is not content to regard them as mere dispensing machines: they are expected to be competent to pass a judgment on the general qualities of a medicine and to be equal to the task of detecting any glaring mistakes. This is what society requires of them.[25]

Jacob Bell spent much of his life trying to ensure that they would be able to meet those requirements.

The fact that Jacob Bell was himself a practising pharmacist governed his sympathies. When the new edition of the London Pharmacopoeia appeared in 1836, he welcomed most of the revisions: the introduction of the alkaloids (morphia, aconitina, strychnia and veratria), several preparations of iodine, hydrocyanic and phosphoric acids; the inclusion of explicit instructions for testing the strength of preparations and for detecting impurities; and many other new features.[26] However, he urged that the Pharmacopoeia must be regarded, not "as a criterion of the progress of chemical discovery", but "as a simplified medium of communication between the prescriber and the compounder of medicine".[27]

> The main objects in revising a Pharmacopoeia should be its simplification, the rejection of useless formulae, the avoidance of ambiguous terms, and to facilitate the prescribing and compounding of medicine.
>   In reforming a Pharmacopoeia the object of the work should be kept constantly in mind, namely, the accurate administration of medicine ... the names employed should be such as will be easily understood, applicable to the substances to which they refer, and not liable to be confounded with one another when written in prescriptions, with the ordinary contractions.

Unfortunately, there were, in the new edition, needless alterations in "the terms or strength of the preparations", and changes in nomenclature which were "capricious, unnecessary, and practically inconvenient". He concluded that "in looking over the present and former editions, it appears as if pains had been taken to mystify the subject, to overburthen the memory, and to puzzle those for whose use it is published".[28] Already, at the age of 27, Jacob Bell was articulating the needs of the dispensing chemist.

The scientific papers Bell contributed to the Pharmaceutical Society's proceedings are unmistakably the work of a practising chemist and druggist. A list of the titles alone indicates their bent. "Practical remarks on decoctions and infusions" (1841), "On the distilled water of bitter almonds" (1841) "Mr. Liston's isinglass plaster" (1841), "Apparatus for preparing extracts in vacuo" (1841), illustrated by James Bell, architect, "Adulteration of senna" (1842), "Some preparations of balsam of copaiva" (1843), "On hemidesmus indicus" (1843), "Remarks on some peculiarities in extemporaneous prescriptions" (1844), "Oil of lavender" (1848), "Calamine" (1848), "The relative produce of taraxacum root at different periods of the year" (1851), "Notes on several preparations of the Pharmacopoeia" (1859) and "Concentrated infusions and decoctions, liquors and fluid extracts" (1859). Not even by the standards of the time of their publication would these papers be regarded as contributions to science. Several of them were heavily criticized at the meetings. Bell had no illusions about his credentials as a scientist. His papers were intended to encourage other practising chemists and druggists to make contributions to the Pharmaceutical Society's scientific meetings. "He makes no pretensions to the character of a man of science", declared *The Chemist* in 1850, and went on to assert that his lack of scientific skill and experience constituted a major deficiency in the editor of a scientific journal.[29] The judgment of a rival can scarcely be disinterested. It is, nonetheless, true that *The Chemist* deserved its reputation as a scientific periodical superior to the *Pharmaceutical Journal* during Bell's editorship. *The Chemist*, however, depended primarily on translations of German and French work: the policy of the *Pharmaceutical Journal* was to encourage British contributions. In any event, Bell was not conceited enough to rely entirely on his own judgment as editor. He worked in close but informal association with Dr. Jonathan Pereira, the leading authority on materia medica, and Theophilus Redwood, a close friend and expert in pharmaceutical chemistry. The letters that Pereira wrote to Bell during the years 1844 to 1853 reveal the extent to which the editor was assisted, guided, admonished and encouraged by his physician friend.

Recognition of his own limitations did not dampen Bell's enthusiasm for science. He was elected an honorary member of several foreign scientific societies and to fellowships of the Chemical, Linnaean and Zoological societies of London. He was an ardent supporter of the Royal Institution: summaries of its monthly meetings were carried by the *Pharmaceutical Journal* throughout his period as editor. Bell held regular scientific soirées at his home in Langham Place: he seemed to enjoy the company of eminent scientists as much as that of his artistic friends. An informed knowledge of science had become, by the beginning of Queen Victoria's reign, as much an emblem of civilisation as connoisseurship of the arts. Participation in formal gatherings of experts in natural philosophy, botany, zoology, geology and chemistry provided confirmation of both bourgeois and intellectual status. Within the culture of science, the separate discourses of scientific disciplines were being constructed. None felt the exhilaration of living in this era more readily than Jacob Bell: none found its atmosphere more stimulating.

"In the year 1846 great interest was excited among medical men and pharmacists, as well as generally among the public", relates Theophilus Redwood, "by the introduction of a method of producing insensibility to pain while important surgical operations were being performed. This was effected in the first instance by the inhalation of the vapour of ether".[30] "This is now the all-engrossing subject", declared Peter Squire, the Queen's pharmacist, in January 1847, "and the public attention is daily called to the several operations which have been performed without the accompaniment of the severe pain heretofore experienced".[31] Most of the leading metropolitan chemists and druggists immediately became involved in the introduction of anaesthesia. The design of inhalers for the administration of sulphuric ether and the search for volatile fluids, with the analgesic qualities of ether but without its disadvantages, were the focus of their concern. William Hooper, a chemist and druggist of Pall Mall East, constructed the apparatus for the first anaesthetic use of ether in this country, the extraction of "a firmly fixed molar tooth" on 19 December 1846. Two days later, when Robert Liston at University College Hospital amputated a thigh, "the ether vapour was administered by means of an ingenious apparatus extemporaneously contrived by Mr. Squire of Oxford Street".[32] A detailed description of

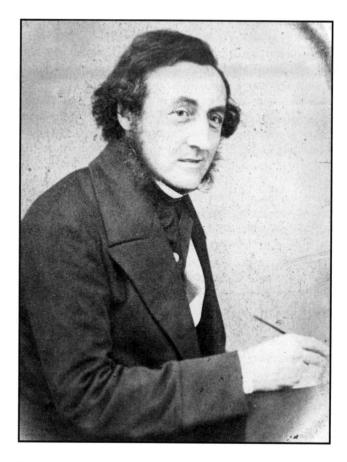

5 *Jacob Bell as editor of the* Pharmaceutical Journal. *An albumen paper copy print of 1891, from a daguerreotype portrait of the mid 1840s.*

this apparatus with a simple diagram was published in the December 1846 issue of the *Pharmaceutical Journal*. In the course of the following months much time and thought were devoted by pharmacists to improving methods of administering ether. During the spring of 1847 the pages of the medical journals were full of descriptions and illustrations of these early types of inhaler. Members of the Pharmaceutical Society exhibited and discussed their own designs at their January meeting in 1847. Jacob Bell's own apparatus consisted of a common green quart bottle into which a little water was introduced with the ether. A flexible tube joined the flask to a mouthpiece and a valve box. The mouthpiece was made of glass to allow it to be easily cleaned. "Some persons might object to apply to their mouths a pad or wooden tube saturated with moisture from the patient who used it last".[33] Set behind the mouthpiece was the valve box, comprising alternately acting inspiratory and expiratory non-return valves, formed from glass discs, each resting on a short piece of tubing. "By watching the movements of these valves, which are contained in a transparent glass tube, the operator can at once detect any defect in the adjustment of the mouth-piece. If this does not fit properly, or becomes displaced so as to allow the air to be drawn in at the sides, the valves do not act".[34] At the meeting of the Pharmaceutical Society Bell observed "that most of the instruments hitherto recommended had been constructed with the view of making the most perfect apparatus without reference to expense. He thought it was also desirable to contrive a means of attaining the result as economically as possible". Cost effectiveness was combined with adaptability. "This apparatus could easily be put together by a surgeon in the country who could not command the facilities of a London hospital". *The Medical Times* described Bell's inhaler as "having the merit of efficiency, compactness and elegance".[35]

Between 25 January and 26 March 1847 twenty-two operations were performed at the Middlesex Hospital under the influence of ether supplied by Jacob Bell and using his apparatus for its inhalation. "In every case in which the ether was fairly inhaled, perfect insensibility was produced", reported J. Henry Rogers, the acting house surgeon.[36] The first "operation without pain" reported from the Middlesex Hospital was a long and difficult lithotomy performed by J. Moncrieff Arnott on 25 January 1847. Arnott had been a good friend of Bell for more than six years. In May 1841 he had expressed his approval of Bell's plans for the constitution of the Pharmaceutical Society at one of the famous tea-parties at Bell's house. The operation at the Middlesex was justifiably described at the time as one "where the efficacy of the ether was put to as severe a test as it had yet been subjected".[37] The patient, an Irishman aged 68, "was made to inhale the vapour of ether, from an apparatus contrived for the purpose by Mr. Jacob Bell, who assisted Mr. Tomes in administering it".[38] John Tomes, surgeon-dentist at the hospital, and Jacob Bell acted together as the first anaesthetists at the Middlesex. Bell had earlier worked with Tomes, later Sir John, doyen of British dentists, in administering anaesthetic to dental patients at the hospital.[39] During these experiments, chloroform, albeit in a dilute form, was used as an anaesthetic for the first time, nine months before James Young Simpson proclaimed its virtues.

After the establishment of ether, many persons up and down the country were trying out all likely volatile fluids. It is not surprising that Jacob Bell should try out the effect of chloric ether: its composition and medicinal use had been the subject of papers in the early numbers of his *Pharmaceutical Journal*. In 1843 Alexander Ure had contributed a misleading paper on terchloride of carbon and in the same year Redwood's lecture on the preparation of ethers added confusion rather than light.[40] But, in March 1846, Dr. Jonathan Pereira authoritatively distinguished between chloride of olefiant gas (then often called chloric ether) and terchloride of carbon or chloric ether.[41] Simpson, in his famous pamphlet recommending the use of chloroform, made use of Redwood's revised account of the composition and manufacture of chloroform which was derived from Pereira's paper.[42] There can be no doubt that the chloric ether used as an anaesthetic by Bell in January 1847 was a mixture of chloroform with about six or eight parts of rectified spirit. He himself described it as consisting of chloroform with about 80 per cent of alcohol.[43]

"The introduction of the so-called chloric ether, in the year 1847, by the late Mr. Jacob Bell", said Alfred Coleman, dental surgeon to the Metropolitan Free Hospital, in a paper read before the Odontological Society in 1862, "has, I think, failed to receive the merit it deserves".

Mr. Bell employed it at the Middlesex Hospital where several Dental operations were performed under its agency. Had the nature of this compound been fully known at the time, the cause of uncertainty in its action would have been discovered, and chloroform brought under the notice of the profession. This discovery, however, was left for Dr. Simpson, of Edinburgh ...[44]

Although Bell was fully aware of the fact that chloric ether was "less powerful in its effects than sulphuric ether", it never seems to have occurred to him to try it in a more concentrated form.[45]

In November 1847 when Simpson announced his discovery, Dr. Roderick Macleod, the editor of the *London Medical Gazette*, noted that "Mr. Bell successfully employed the vapour of chloric ether as a substitute for that of sulphuric ether as early as February". He continued:

... the liquid employed by Mr. Bell was the identical compound recommended by Dr. Simpson, i.e., chloroform, or perchloride of formyle, which has been extensively sold in London as chloric ether or terchloride of carbon ... Soon after ether-inhalation was introduced, Mr. Bell tried chloric ether, and found it to answer. It was employed at the Middlesex Hospital, but as it is more expensive than sulphuric ether, it has not lately been so much in request. Dr. Simpson's preparation appears to be of a more concentrated kind than that usually sold ... There is not, therefore, that novelty in the use of this agent, which the reports in the medical journals would have the profession to suppose. At the same time, it is evident, from Dr. Simpson's paper, that this gentleman was not acquainted with the prior experiments of Mr. Bell.[46]

Jacob Bell was closely associated with the Middlesex Hospital. He was a subscribing governor for many years, and between February 1846 and the end of 1848 he was a member of the medical committee. That he was responsible for the use of chloric ether in the Middlesex is not surprising: but it is also probable that he was instrumental in introducing it to St. Bartholomew's. In 1871 and again in 1877, Dr. Michael Cudmore Furnell claimed in the *Lancet* that he had brought chloric ether to St. Bartholomew's during the summer of 1847 where it was used for operations performed by both William Lawrence and Holmes Coote.[47] This part of the story is not disputed: but Furnell's claim that he, while a pupil of Bell, discovered the analgesic effects of chloric ether and drew Bell's attention to them is scarcely credible. As editor of the *Pharmaceutical Journal*, Jacob Bell would have acquired as much knowledge of chloric ether as anyone in Britain, and as proprietor of one of the leading pharmaceutical establishments he would have been involved in its routine manufacture and sale. Furnell's story that in 1847 he stumbled across "a covered and neglected bottle" labelled chloric ether, "away in a dark storeroom", must have been the product of an inventive memory. It is far more probable that Jacob Bell's success at the Middlesex led him to suggest that his young student Furnell should try it out at St. Bartholomew's.

When Jacob Bell drew the attention of readers of the *Pharmaceutical Journal* to Simpson's discovery, he pointed out that chloric ether had already been tried with success at some of the London hospitals. "It was found to be more agreeable to the taste than sulphuric ether, and less apt to produce coughing, and irritation of the organs of respiration. In other respects the operation of the two agents corresponded". He added that he had himself repeatedly administered both of them together.[48] Dr. John Snow, in 1855, recalled that "when chloroform was first administered in London in 1847, it was inhaled from its solution, in about seven parts of spirit, under the name of chloric ether".[49] In 1897, Dudley W. Buxton, the anaesthetist at University College Hospital, referring to "the use by Jacob Bell and Mr. Lawrence in London . . . of chloric ether or chloroform dissolved in spirits of wine", concluded that "had Bell only gone one step further chloroform would have been an accepted anaesthetic".[50] And, of course, Jacob Bell, rather than James Young Simpson, would today be remembered as the person responsible for the introduction of chloroform as an anaesthetic. However, the essential advance, for which Simpson deserves the credit, was not the idea of trying chloroform, but the provision of proof that not only did it produce anaesthesia, but, in crucial respects, it was superior to ether.

Jacob Bell was not the only chemist and druggist acting as an anaesthetist in 1847. Benjamin Ward Richardson, in his biographical introduction to John Snow's book, *On Chloroform and Other Anaesthetics*, recounts the following story. One day, on coming out of one of the London hospitals, Snow met a druggist whom he knew, "bustling along with a large ether apparatus under his arm". After exchanging greetings, the druggist (probably Peter Squire) urged Snow not to detain him. "I am giving ether here and there and everywhere and am getting quite into an ether practice".[51] The discovery of anaesthetics was one of the major pharmaceutical advances of the nineteenth century: it was the first occasion on which the synthetic products of the organic chemist were used to produce a therapeutic effect of major importance. Theophilus Redwood accounted for the original involvement of pharmacists in the administration of anaesthetics in these words:

> It was the duty of the qualified pharmacist to seek out and prepare the best chemical compounds for the production of these anaesthetic effects, and it was not inconsistent with this position that he should assist in producing and applying the vapour, as these involved the exercise of some amount of chemical knowledge and manipulative skill.[52]

The prospect, however, of chemists and druggists working alongside consultant surgeons in hospital operating theatres was too much for the self-appointed guardians of the privileges of the medical professions. Such activities were taken to indicate an intention to usurp the legitimate duties of medical practitioners. As the Pharmaceutical Society was anxious to avoid exciting any such suspicions, pharmacists made no attempt to defend their colonization of this newly opened territory. They withdrew gracefully, leaving the field to house surgeons and hospital porters!

At the start of 1841, Jacob Bell had just returned from a four month holiday on the Continent with Edwin Landseer. While they were in Geneva, Jacob had been taken ill with a severe attack of quinsy (peritonsillar abscess) which detained them for six weeks. For health reasons, he would have been well advised "to take things easy", to ensure that the coming year was not a strenuous one. There was no need for him to work. He received a handsome income, more than enough to allow him to relax and enjoy the pleasures of life without let or hindrance. He was surrounded by almost everything than can make life pleasant: an ample number of intimate and caring friends and a wide circle of brilliant and famous acquaintances, in whose company he revelled. He had a great variety of tastes and pursuits and means enough to gratify and follow them. Art, literature, music, theatre, scientific activities, hunting and riding, the merry-go-round of "high society": his interests and talents encompassed all of these. He moved with ease in the highest ranks of society.

Within the higher echelons of early Victorian society, certain attributes were greatly valued: kinship of a long-established, aristocratic family; education at the ancient English universities; and adherence to the faith of the Established Church. Such values were firmly entrenched within, and constantly threatened from without. Having gained a precarious entrée to the Establishment, Jacob Bell must have been sorely tempted to cover his tracks, to conceal his social origins and the source of his wealth. "It is a truth universally acknowledged, that a single man in possession of a good fortune, must be in want of a wife". An eligible bachelor, he might have married the daughter of a high-status family. He had, by now, lost his religious conviction and identification with the Society of Friends: his detached, secular frame of kind would have presented no obstacle to conversion to Anglicanism. He owned a small country estate in Surrey and a resplendent town house in Langham Place. He cherished an art collection that many country gentlemen would have envied. By shrewd investment, he could have severed all connexion with the world of the shopkeeper and turned his back on the degrading retail trade. He could have made himself "a gentleman".

He did none of this. In the spring of 1841 he took up the cause to which the best years of his life and his most vigorous exertions were devoted: the foundation and development of the Pharmaceutical Society of Great Britain. This was a venture which would make onerous calls upon his time, wealth and energy, which would reward him with accusations and insults, and which would eventually drag him to an early death. Far from being ashamed of and humiliated by his background, Jacob Bell proclaimed his origins and sought to make every chemist and druggist in the land proud of earning a living from such an honourable calling. Although intellectually and socially estranged from the Society of Friends, he was deeply influenced by his Quaker upbringing. The idea that life remains unfulfilled unless dedicated to the pursuit of a worthy cause was deeply imbedded in his psyche. His father and both his grandfathers had retired from business to devote themselves to benevolent and charitable objectives. William Allen, on reaching a state of financial security, spent the rest of his days working for the emancipation of slaves, the education of the poor, and the reformation of prisons. His partner, John Thomas Barry, abandoned his post to promote the abolition of capital punishment. Robert Alsop sold his business to consecrate his life to religion and social amelioration. The dictates of Quaker conscience forced these men to abandon pharmacy to seek inner peace and fulfillment in the pursuit of religious and philanthropic ends. Jacob Bell was too much of a Quaker not to feel the same need to make sense of his life by dedicating himself to work for the welfare of his fellow men. He responded to the same inner imperatives, but in a different way. He was too worldly-wise, too detached, too civilised to become a missionary for religion. His scepticism, his rationalism, his intellectualism, his abhorrence of bigotry and fanaticism, all militated against the adoption of religious enthusiasm. Instead of abandoning pharmacy, he made pharmacy his cause. The progress of pharmacy as a science and as a profession became his secular mission and gave his life its meaning.

Jacob Bell

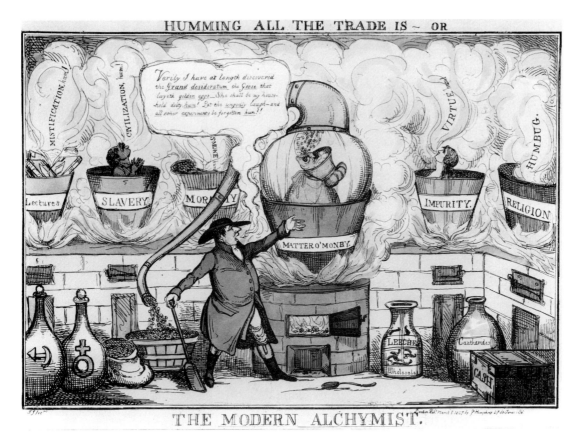

6 Humming all the trade is — or the modern alchemist. *Drawn and etched by T.H. Jones, published by G. Humphrey, 27 St. James's Street, London, 8 March 1827.*

This hand coloured etching is one of several fierce satires produced at the time of William Allen's third marriage accusing him of hypocrisy and humbug. Allen appears as an alchemist in Quaker dress, depicted standing in his laboratory surrounded by crucibles containing personifications of his many interests. The central alembic contains a head of Mrs Birkbeck, from whose mouth spouts a fountain of gold coins.

NOTES AND REFERENCES TO CHAPTER ONE

The following abbreviations are used throughout the reference lists: Bell and Redwood = J. Bell and T. Redwood, *Historical Sketch of the Progress of Pharmacy in Great Britain* (1880); *C.&D.* = *Chemist and Druggist*; *P.J.* = *Pharmaceutical Journal*

1. *P.J.* 8 (1848–9) 589–95
2. G.E. Bryant and G. P. Baker (eds.) *A Quaker Journal* (1934) vol.1, 43, 46, 49–50

3. Juanita Burnby, "The family history of Jacob Bell", *P.J.* 230 (1983) 582–4
4. Bell Family Bible
5. *C. & D.* 53 (1898) 160–5
6. Bell and Redwood 49
7. E.g. indenture for Francis Robert Gunter, for a term of 5 years and 8 months from 21 April 1837, premium paid to Jacob Bell being £299-19s.
8. *Journal of the Friends Historical Society* 22 (1925) 21–2, 87–8
9. *Ibid.* 19 (1922) 105–7.
10. *P.J.* 1 [2] (1859–60) 153–60. The author of the obituary was Daniel Hanbury.
11. *The Chemical Record and Drug Price Current*, 20 December 1851, 361–2
12. Tracts 444, The Library, Friends House, London.
13. Bell and Redwood 282–5.
14. W.R. Frith, *My Autobiography and Reminiscences* (1890) 28–9, 183, 188, 192–5.
15. Kingston Monthly Meeting minutes (1853–65) 135. The Library, Friends House, London.
16. Volume MM 176. The Library, Friends House, London.
17. British Museum Additional Ms. 46140, and the letters of Sir Edwin Landseer and Charles E. Lewis to Jacob Bell, now in the Royal Institution, London.
18. F.G. Stephens, *Memoirs of Sir Edwin Landseer* (1874) 97.
19. *C. & D.* 38 (1891) 546
20. A.J. Symington, *Samuel Lover* (1880)
21. Benjamin Lumley, *Reminiscences of the Opera* (1864) 323.
22. *C. & D.* 53 (1898) 164
23. *P.J.* 6 (1846–7) 500
24. *Pharmaceutical Times* 2 (1847) 163
25. *Pharmaceutical Times* 2 (1847) 119
26. Bell and Redwood 75
27. *Lancet* 1838–9 (2) 748–9
28. *Lancet* 1836–7 (1) 708–10
29. *The Chemist* new series 1 (1849–50) 469–71
30. Bell and Redwood 182
31. *P.J.* 6 (1846–7) 350
32. Barbara M. Duncum, *The Development of Inhalation Anaesthesia* (1947) 131–2
33. *P.J.* 6 (1846–7) 355
34. *Lancet* 1847 (1) 185
35. *Medical Times* 16 (1847) 306
36. *Lancet* 1847 (1) 367
37. *London Medical Gazette* new series 4 (1847) 218
38. *Lancet* 1847 (1) 133
39. O.P. Dinnick, "My Victorian Predecessors at the Middlesex Hospital", *Proceedings of the History of Anaesthesia Society* 5 (February 1989) 13–21
40. *P.J.* 3 (1843–4) 170–2, 369–71, 490–5.
41. *P.J.* 5 (1845–6) 412–4.
42. *P.J.* 7 (1847–8) 278
43. *P.J.* 7 (1847–8) 279
44. Alfred Coleman, *Anaesthesia: considered especially in reference to operations in Dental Surgery* (1862) 4
45. *P.J.* 6 (1846–7) 357 footnote.
46. *London Medical Gazette* new series 5 (1847) 939 footnote.
47. W. Stanley Sykes, *Essays on the First Hundred Years of Anaesthesia* (1960, 1961) I, 162–4; II 168–77.

48. *P.J.* 7 (1847–8) 277
49. *Lancet* 1855 (1) 108
50. *Lancet* 1897 (2) 1370
51. Barbara M. Duncum, *The Development of Inhalation Anaesthesia* (1947) 18
52. Bell and Redwood 183.

CHAPTER TWO

The Chemist and Druggist,
1750–1870

Dolore urgente—If the pain is severe

The origin of the chemist and druggist—The commercialisation of society—The rise of the chemist and druggist in London and the provinces—The high-class establishment—The middle-order chemist—Self-medication and the professionalisation of medicine—Medical botany—Chemists and druggists and the labouring classes—The absence of fraternity

Chemists and druggists emerged as a distinct branch of the medical profession during the eighteenth century. Their emergence is part of the commercialisation of Georgian society.[1] During the third quarter of the eighteenth century many sectors of British society experienced a period of rising prosperity. There was an increase in the number and wealth of the middling classes, i.e. of merchants, tradesmen, shopkeepers, clerks, farmers and skilled craftsmen. For the first time such groups found themselves with money to spare after meeting the necessities of life. Following the example of their social superiors, they spent more on consumer goods and services. A consumer revolution occurred: a greater proportion of the population than in any previous society was able to enjoy the pleasures of acquiring material possessions. Men, and particularly women, bought as never before. Objects, which for centuries had been the exclusive possessions of the few, came to be within the reach of the many and within the reasonable expectation of the majority. What had once been regarded as "luxuries" came to be seen as "decencies" and "decencies" were now considered "necessities". Goods which had once been available only on holidays and festivals through the agency of markets, fairs and itinerant pedlars were increasingly to be had any day of the week through the additional agency of an ever-growing network of shops. The eighteenth century saw an increasing proportion of the population living in towns with a concomitant spread of fixed-premise retailing and rise of urban shopping precincts.

The birth of a consumer society elicited notice from British and foreign observers. Arthur Young in 1771 spoke of universal luxury and thirty years later Dibden wrote of the prevailing opulence of all classes. The Gottigen professor, G.C. Lichtenberg, thought that the luxury and extravagance of the lower and middling classes in England during the 1770s had "risen to such a pitch as never before seen in the world". "England surpasses all the other nations of Europe in luxury", wrote the historian J.W. von Archenholz in 1791, "and the luxury is increasing daily!" "All classes", he added, "enjoy the accumulation of riches, luxury and pleasure". Most visitors from abroad were astonished by "the inveterate national habit of luxury of the English". These eloquent comments are not to be taken as the considered findings of social investigation: there remained a mass of poverty in eighteenth-century England. Nonetheless, something out of the ordinary was clearly thought to be happening. One of the characteristics of a consumer society is that its riches are spread out for all to see. The superficial impression was of universal affluence, the reality was a revolution in consumer behaviour. The propensity to consume was unprecedented: it penetrated to the lower reaches of society and had a dramatic impact on the economy. Before the eighteenth century it had not been thought possible that consumers at all levels of society might acquire new wants and find new means of generating purchasing power. The idea of man as a consumer with unlimited appetite driving the economy to new levels of prosperity and destroying all traditional barriers to the wealth of nations was a construction of eighteenth-century economists. "Consumption is the sole end and purpose of all production", wrote Adam Smith in 1776, "and the interest of the producer ought to be attended to only so far as it may be necessary for promoting that of the consumer. The maxim is ... perfectly self-evident". A century before it had been inconceivable.

The producers and sellers of goods should not be viewed as merely responding to these changes: they played a substantial part in bringing them about. They helped to release the public's latent consuming capacity. Changes in commercial techniques and the development of promotional skills both fed and fed upon the appetites of the consumer. Chemists and druggists were a product of the consumer revolution. Medicine, both orthodox and fringe, expanded as part of the general growth of the service sector. A perusal of the few surviving eighteenth-century account books provides evidence of increasing outlays by middle-class families not only on items such as library subscriptions, music lessons and hairdressing, but also payments for health care. The husband, who had been helped into the world by the village midwife, now booked the surgeon-apothecary to deliver his wife's babies; women, whose grandmothers had collected herbs to brew family receipts, now bought proprietary medicines for their ailments.[2]

Chemists and druggists were both medical practitioners and shopkeepers. Whereas apothecaries might practise without a shop—and many increasingly did so—the shop was the defining characteristic of the chemist and druggist. Much of what we know about the early chemists and druggists is dependent upon that fact. In contrast to many other practitioners of medicine, chemists and druggists are easily identifiable: they have a fixed location, their shops. The rise of the chemist and druggist is inseparable from the introduction of new forms of retailing. In order to make inroads into the domain of the apothecary and to stave off the competition of the pedlars, chapmen, and hawkers, the chemist and druggist had to adopt new techniques for the sale of drugs. Primarily this involved the launch of a new type of retail establishment. The old apothecary's premises in the seventeenth and early eighteenth century did not correspond to our idea of a shop: a better description would be a combination of work-shop, storeroom, surgery and living room. In contrast, the chemist and druggist gave prominence to the retail side of his activities. He went out of his way to make his premises attractive to the customer. He took advantage of the new plate glass for his windows instead of the old ring or bottle glass. By adopting the new shop fronts with the larger twelve by sixteen inch window panes, he made his presence in the high street felt. The old small diamond lattice windows precluded an arresting display: the new window panes were decorated with jars of water-white glass holding coloured liquids.[3] These rapidly became the symbol of the trade; the chemist and druggist's equivalent of the barber's pole and the pawnbroker's balls. By the 1840s the fact was widely acknowledged. "From the middle of the panes glare huge, coloured glasses, yellow, red and blue, having inscribed upon them certain talismanic characters", wrote the Hungarian physician, J.E. Feldman, in 1842.[4] Readers of Dickens will recall that when Tom Pinch, assistant to Seth Pecksniff went to Salisbury to meet a new apprentice, he filled in time "window-shopping" including the "chemists' shops, with their great glowing bottles". By 1843, the year in which *The Life and Adventures of Martin Chuzzlewit* appeared, enterprising London chemists were beginning to adopt new window arrangements. Charles Knight, surveying the London scene that year, was sure that "most London walkers will remember the time when the large red, and green, and yellow bottles, shedding a ghastly light on the passer-by, were the chief indications of the presence of a druggist's shop".[5] Since the shops were open from seven in the morning till eleven at night, the lights behind the coloured bottles guided customers to the door during the winter months. To draw further attention to their shops the more ambitious chemists and druggists began, in the closing decades of the eighteenth century, to encroach upon the public footpaths with bow-windows. Matthew Hinton ran foul of the Chester city authorities in 1767 for projecting his shop-window in Lower Bridge Street.[6] Elsewhere, however, the new style establishments sprang up without restriction.

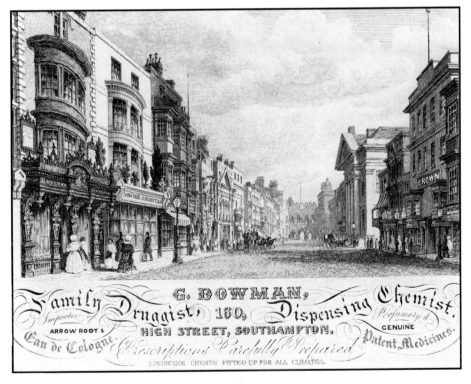

7 *Illustrated tradecard of George Downman, Dispensing Chemist and Pharmaceutist, 160 High Street, Southampton.*

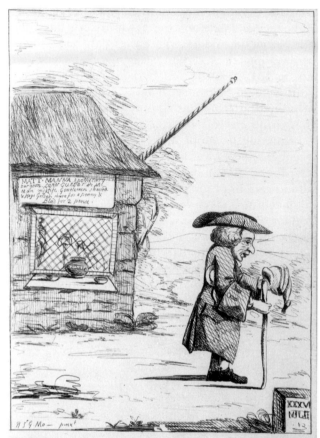

MATTHEW MANNA. A COUNTRY APOTHECARY.

8   Matthew Manna. A Country Apothecary. *Drawn by R.St.G. Mansergh and etched by M. Darly, published by M. Darly, Strand, 11 October 1773.*

The time-honoured practice of pharmacy by the apothecary obtained its characteristic features from origins in the pre-industrial urban economy. The guild system, with its strict control over who might practice a given craft, who might be trained, how one was to be trained, and how the craft was to be practised, provided the framework within which the apothecary operated. By the mid-eighteenth century the guild system, as the predominant mode of urban economic and social organisation, was in ruins. Adam Smith believed that the guild system had driven out arts and manufactures from the greater part of towns-corporate: bad work and high prices had been the effects of its monopoly. The chemist and druggist was one of the beneficiaries of its collapse. Breaking away from guild restrictions and discarding the mentality based on co-operation and regulation, the chemist and druggist celebrated the values of free trade and open competition. The fundamental tenets of his philosophy began with the belief in the unrestricted right of every man to follow

34

whatever occupation or profession is most congenial to his temperament or best calculated to put money in his pocket. Ordinances and statutes which created reserved occupations were repressive because they interfered with and are contrary to the prerogatives of the individual. The regulation of a trade must be left to the judgment of those who pursue it and to the sovereignty of the consumer. The need to attract custom, rather than adherence to communal standards, was the driving force behind the activities of the chemist and druggist. He inaugurated a two-fold freedom: his own liberty to dispense whatever pharmaceutical preparation he may wish, to whomever he may wish, without interference from physicians or fellow-traders; and the liberty of the public to purchase and use whatever medication it may choose.[7]

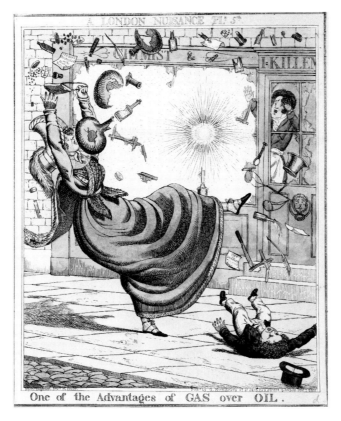

9   One of the Advantages of Gas over Oil. *Drawn and etched by Richard Dighton, published by G. Humphrey, 27 St James's Street, London, 7 February 1822.*
This hand coloured etching, plate number five in the series A London Nuisance, *satirised the new hazards of illumination by burning coal gas. The depiction of the premises of "I. Killem, Chymist & [Druggist]", evidently purports to represent one of the chemists and druggists of Bond Street.*

The chemist and druggist was one of the group of small traders who succeeded in exciting new wants and making available new goods to the eighteenth-century public. By boosting demand, they helped to create a new consumer market of unprecedented size and buying power. Chemists and druggists were busy, inventive, profit-seeking businessmen, whose eager advertising, active marketing and inspired salesmanship did much to usher in a new type of society in eighteenth-century England. During the last fifteen years of the century, the consumption of excised commodities in mass demand, such as tobacco, soap, candles, printed fabrics, spirits and beer was increasing more than twice as fast as the population. While population increased fourteen per cent in this period, tea consumption increased by ninety eight per cent and that of printed fabrics by one hundred and forty two per cent.[8] By 1780 the value of sales of patent medicines was estimated at £187,500 a year. The government, confident that this trade would continue to expand, imposed a stamp tax on "quack medicines" in 1783. It was not removed until 1941![9]

TABLE 1 *Numbers of Chemists and Druggists at Various Dates in Selected Towns*

BOLTON		BRISTOL		HUDDERSFIELD	
1822	7	1775	3	1790	2
1834	14	1793–4	12	1822	5
1851	29	1819	29	1828	6
		1826	44	1837	9
		1835	56	1847	14
		1845	61	1853	16
		1851	114		

LEEDS		LEICESTER		LIVERPOOL	
1822	20	1822	11	1822	52
1834	40	1835	22	1834	113
1841	49	1841	27	1846	161
1848	72	1850	34	1851	188

MANCHESTER		MERTHYR TYDFIL		NOTTINGHAM	
1822	52	1822	2	1806	13
1834	94	1835	7	1822	17
1841	145	1850	16	1825	22
1851	195			1835	51
				1841	56
				1850	63

NORWICH		SHEFFIELD		WAKEFIELD		YORK	
1822	17	1750	1	1790	2	1822	2
1839	32	1774	3	1822	6	1834	28
1851	30	1797	10	1828	10	1841	24
		1817	17	1837	13	1848	30
		1833	38	1847	20		
		1838	50	1853	19		
		1841	56				

Sources: David Alexander, *Retailing in England during the Industrial Revolution* (1970) 239
John Austen, *Historical Notes on Old Sheffield Druggists* (Sheffield, 1961) 10, 11, 15, 26, 35, 68.
P.S. Brown, *Med. Hist.* 24 (1980) 297–314
Irvine Loudon, *Medical Care and the General Practitioner 1750–1850* (1986) 135
Hilary Marland, *Med. Hist.* 31 (1987) 415–439

TABLE 2 *Number of Registered Medical Apprentices*

	1711–17	1793–99
Apothecaries	594	110
Surgeon-Apothecaries	28	335
Surgeons	184	330
Chemists and Druggists	11	273

Source: J.G.L. Burnby, *A Study of the English Apothecary* (1983)

The number of chemists and druggists in England increased markedly in the years after 1780: all sources, literary and statistical, agree on this. Trade directories, themselves a product of the commercialisation of society, can be used to indicate the trend. As sources for statistics they need to be used with caution. Other evidence reveals that chemists and druggists were under-reported in eighteenth-century trade directories. In their infant days, directories concentrated upon the more established enterprises. More reliable data have been derived from the Inland Revenue apprenticeship records, seventy-two large volumes, now in the Public Records Office, covering (with gaps) the period May 1710 to January 1811. From these the names and some details of both masters and apprentices can be extracted. These records obviously do not provide a complete record of masters and apprentices, still less of chemists and druggists. Tax evasion was easier in the eighteenth century than today. Although the decline of guild regulation undermined the necessity for apprenticeship, the exemptions provided under the Medicine Stamp Acts for regularly apprenticed vendors may have restored its attractiveness and encouraged its official registration. The statistical evidence is summarised in the tables. Both sets of data indicate a marked increase in the number of chemists and druggists during the eighteenth century, and literary evidence—primarily the anguished response of the rival apothecaries—suggests that the general rise occurred from about 1780. From that date, not only was there an increase in the absolute number of chemists and druggists throughout the urban areas of Britain, but there was a growth in numbers *relative* to the rising population and *relative* to the still growing number of other medical practitioners. Chemists and druggists rapidly became established as a new species of homo medicus: they made a major contribution to the health needs of both the urban and rural population.

The rise of the chemist and druggist began in London. The size and character of London was a prime factor in the creation of a consumer society. The growth of the city, from 200,000 inhabitants at the beginning of the seventeenth century to 900,000 by the end of the eighteenth, made it unique in Europe. By 1700 London had already become the largest European city and had no serious rival in Britain. Seven per cent of England's population lived there in 1650: eleven per cent in 1750. No other city in Europe housed such a large proportion of a country's population. The influence of London was felt by an even greater number of people: estimates suggest that during the eighteenth century one in six of the English population had some experience of living in the capital.[10] James I's prophecy, that "soon London will be all England", began to have the ring of truth. In London prosperity and competition led to refinement and specialisation. The capital was the breeding ground of new arts and crafts, the centre of novel forms of conspicuous consumption, the shopwindow and workshop for the whole nation. The emergence of the chemist and druggist can be traced to London in the early years of the eighteenth century. The London Directory of 1715 records that in the area from Holborn to Aldgate there were nine apothecaries, two chemists and thirty-nine druggists. In 1721 the Society of Apothecaries failed to enlist the support of the College of Physicians in its attempt to curb the activities of the druggists: in 1748 the Society, now acting on its own, was still unable to bring the chemist and druggist to heel. A critic of the Society observed that there were already over a hundred chemists and druggists in town.[11] By 1763 J. Mortimer wrote that the number of chemists and druggists in London "almost exceeds belief".[12] As they grew in number, so the range of their activities spread. "Within the last thirty-five years", wrote one authority in 1818, "a new order, the dispensing Druggist or Chemist, has arisen, which is very similar to what the Apothecary was a century and a half ago. We believe that prior to 1788 there were not, in all London, more than half a dozen Druggists who dispensed medicines from Physicians' prescriptions. There are now of this description, above 600! Many of them keep assistants to prescribe, to bleed, and to take the management of minor surgical cases; and few or none refuse to take charge of any casualty to which they may accidentally be summoned as medical or surgical practitioners".[13] Samuel Gray, in his *Supplement to the Pharmacopoeia* (1818), observed that the shops of chemists and druggists "are in general confounded with those of the Apothecaries". The only distinction that Gray could discover was that, whereas medical practice was the principal object of the "modern" apothecary, "with the Chemist and Druggist, or old Apothecary, retail and dispensing are principal, and medical practice mostly confined to the counter". Dr. G.M. Burrows despairingly declared that "it had indeed become difficult to define who was, or who was not, an Apothecary".[14] To assist the public, proprietors wishing to stay behind the counter simply styled themselves, in directories and advertisements, as "chemists and druggists". Thus the famous Plough Court pharmacy was run, from 1715, by Silvanus Bevan, who called himself "an apothecary", but from 1765, when it came under the management of Timothy Bevan, the premises were styled "Druggists and Chemists".[15] The continuous existence of a pharmacy business in Derby has been traced from the mid-seventeenth century. Up to 1764 the premises were run by a succession of "apothecaries"; from then on, the proprietor was styled "druggist"; by the early nineteenth century he was referred to as a "dispensing chemist". Similarly, in Chester, a pharmacy had existed since the Restoration. Until 1722 it was run by apothecaries, but then Peter Ellames, "apothecary and druggist" took over, and in turn his sons carried on the business, simply calling themselves "druggists".[16] An ill-defined process of differentiation was occurring. The apothecary who became the general practitioner was one side of the coin. During the seventeenth century he began to move out of his shop and turned himself into a dispensing physician and later into the eighteenth-century "surgeon-apothecary and man midwife". By the nineteenth century he had collected credentials from the College of Surgeons and the Society of Apothecaries and called himself a general medical practitioner; he began to insist on being paid for giving advice; the back room of his house became his "surgery". The other side of the coin was the chemist and druggist. For him the practice of medicine meant the sale of commodities (drugs and chemicals) and, to further his trade, he made the shop the focus of his innovating activities. His growing expertise in producing the materia medica led him along the path to advising and prescribing. Differentiation led to de-differentiation: which side of the coin was which?

The prosperity of London encouraged the sub-division of pharmaceutical labour. In London, wrote Jacob Bell in 1843,

> we have Operative Chemists, Dispensing Chemists, Manufacturing Chemists, Wholesale Druggists, Saline Chemists, Chemists and Druggists who give their attention to particular classes of preparations; others who cultivate the sale of horse and cattle medicines; others who are between wholesale and retail, and supply Apothecaries with drugs. The nature of the retail trade also varies according to neighbourhood and the rank of the customers.[17]

Even by the middle of the eighteenth century, some degree of specialisation had emerged. John Toovey, druggist and chemist, whose shop was at the sign of the Black Lion in the Strand, ran a typical retail establishment. His advertisements announced that he prepared

> all sorts of Chemical and Galenical Medicines, ... the very best French and English Hungary Waters, Lavender and Mineral Waters, Daffy's and Stoughton's Elixir, etc. Wholesale and Retail ... Physicians Prescriptions made ... Chests of Medicines for Gentlemen and Exportation.[18]

By the end of the century all major towns had shops like Toovey's. By that time, too, provincial wholesale druggists had emerged: but the London wholesalers maintained their grip on the business throughout the nineteenth century. The papers of the eighteenth-century wholesale druggist, William Jones, have fortunately survived and provide a good picture of his varied activities.[19] He began in 1746 with a modest shop near Drury Lane, but, in 1757, took over the business of Elim Walter, chemist, at 24, Great Russell Street, near Covent Garden. An inventory of 1761 allows us to form a good impression of the premises he acquired. They comprised a shop, a counting house, a laboratory, warehouses, vaults, cellars, a cockloft and living quarters for the family, apprentices, servants and lodgers. The shop incorporated the best modern features. The front, with its two glazed sash windows, splendid door, obelisks, lamps and signboard with a red cross, was designed to attract custom. The interior had two buck's heads for decoration and was illuminated by a brass chandelier with two sconces and furnished with three desks, two stools, a bookcase and a safe. Dispensing was done at two counters, beneath each of which a nest of drawers held the standard equipment of weights, labels, containers and leather for plaster and blister spreading. Each counter had its own beam scale with copper pans and there were eight hand balances. The shop was full of drugs. In the centre were the hundredweight sacks and casks of senna, gum arabic, peruvian bark, myrrh, and Glauber's salts. Other dry goods were stored in 53 shop boxes in the ten casks behind the counters, in 150 species glasses (some with brass caps), and in the nests of drawers under both windows. The liquids were kept on six front shelves and in 150 glass stoppered bottles in a large glass case. Behind the shop, the laboratory was equipped with a still, retort, digester, presses, oil jars, sand baths, a wind furnace and syrup and plaster pans. The drugs and chemicals were kept separately: the chemicals in the large vault and the drugs in various warehouses, one of which was equipped with a pulley and tackle for handling the heavy packages. Throughout his highly successful career, Jones maintained his retail shop, dispensing the prescriptions of eminent physicians like Sir Francis Milman and Sir Gilbert Blane, vending tenpennyworths of manna, sassafras, laudanum and chamomile flowers, and selling his specialty, Tincture of Peruvian Bark, at 3/6d a bottle. He even dealt in fire insurance and lottery tickets. But wholesale was his forte.

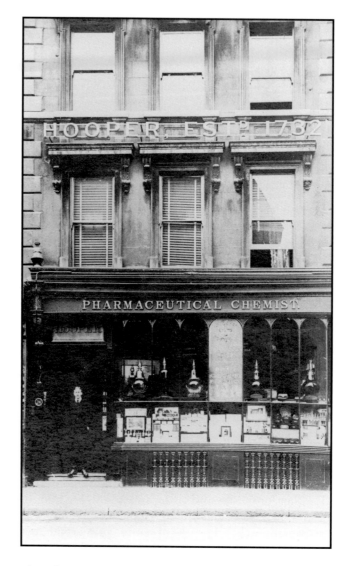

10   *The premises of W. Hooper & Co., at 24 Russell Street, Covent Garden, c. 1900. Established in 1732, the business was taken over in 1757 by William Jones, an early chemist and druggist. This was one of the oldest continuously occupied pharmacies in England until its demolition in 1908. The exterior shown here, though remodelled in the 1870s, preserves the shop's original sign of the red cross.*

William Jones supplied Dr. Robert James with the antimony and cream of tartar used in the production of the famous patent medicine, Dr. James' Fever Powders (nearly two million doses of which were sold within a twenty-year period): the order book for 1772 itemizes "the usual 500 lb of antimony" for Dr. James. When John Hunter urged Edward

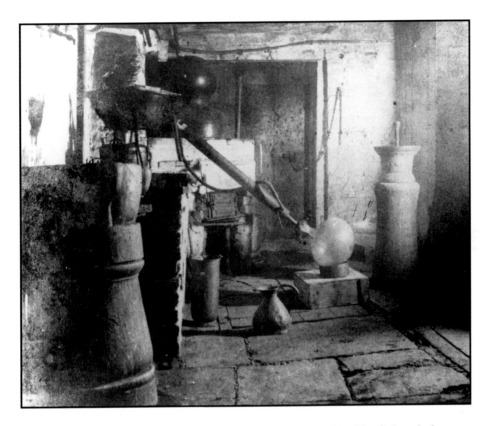

11 *Interior of the laboratory of W. Hooper & Co., c. 1900. The fittings had changed remarkably little since the eighteenth century. A large sixty gallon still appears in the centre of the photograph, and a Whitechapel bell-metal mortar can be seen on the right.*

Jenner to set up "Jenner's Tartar Emetic" as a proprietary remedy, it was William Jones who came to mind as the best person to market it. By then, Jones had developed a large export trade with France, Gibraltar, the West Indies, Canada and the East India Company. Within England, he took advantage of the business opportunities created by the newly-founded voluntary hospitals and secured contracts to supply drugs, chemicals and appliances to the infirmaries at Chester, Stafford, Hereford and Salisbury as well as several London hospitals. He regularly sold drugs valued at nearly £200 per year to Westminster Hospital. An indication of the renown of his firm is the fact that he was able to secure apprenticeship premiums of £200 when the going-rate for London apothecaries was between £50 and £100. Twice a year, William Jones would leave his son and partner, John, in charge of affairs in London and ride around the Midlands and the West Country, drumming up custom. In Bristol he would stay with the surgeon, William Barrett, F.S.A., and in Bath with the apothecary, surgeon and botanist, William Sole, F.L.S., of Trim Street. He traded wholesale with surgeons, apothecaries and druggists throughout the region. Jones purchased his drugs direct from the warehouses in Leadenhall Street and Tower Hill: he obtained chemicals from W. Henry Durbin of Bristol and Matthew Saunderson of Sheffield. In the eighteenth century, success as a wholesaler was dependent upon the simultaneous assumption of the role of financier. Before the growth of the banking system, and in a society chronically short of specie, the granting and receiving of trade credit was an essential lubricant of the economy. Jones' banking activities became a very considerable part of his business. We find him managing executor and trustee accounts; investing clients' surplus funds in government securities; handling India Bonds for widows, spinsters and country clergymen; arranging the payment of stamp duty, land tax and poor rate for his customers; granting a mortgage to John Hunter on the lease of his property at Earls Court; acting as banker to Lord Portsmouth, the Dukes of Bedford, Kingston and Newcastle, and the Earls of Harcourt and Effingham; and dealing, inevitably, in inland bills of exchange. The latter were the customary means by which tradesmen, shopkeepers, middlemen and manufacturers paid for commodities and raw materials, especially when they came from outside the locality. A provincial purchaser of London goods would draw the bill on a Londoner with whom he had credit. Discounting bills of exchange was a risky but highly profitable business.

The time-lag between the rise of the chemist and druggist in London and in the provinces was nearly half a century. Richard Smith, junior, of Bristol (1772–1843), surgeon to the Bristol Infirmary, gives a vivid account of their emergence in Bristol during the 1790s in his *Bristol Infirmary Biographical Memoirs*. The sudden appearance of their shops all over the city was remarkable. A Mr. Jackson was the first to open "a *splendid* shop—he had immensely large and elegantly painted jars in the windows". Jackson did a thriving trade and his apprentices soon set up on their own account. "'Dispensing Establishments' soon began to multiply everywhere". The Bristol physicians, who had little reason to protect the apothecaries, recognised the advantages in having their prescriptions dispensed by specialists in pharmacy. They "began to inform their patients that there was no need of their paying eighteen pence to an apothecary when the draught might be had for sixpence elsewhere—and that if a physician were alone employed he would have no inducement to order such a load of 'apothecary's stuff'". The apothecaries soon found that "families where they had been in for a good thing for many years ... slipped from their fingers altogether". Some physicians colluded with the chemists, attending at stated hours in their shops to give free advice and splitting the income for the medicines dispensed. What happened in Bristol happened all over England. Chemists and druggists sprang up providing a new and cheaper form of medical care in competition with the apothecaries. In 1818 a correspondent to *Monthly Magazine* wrote from Ipswich:

> I have a family of four children and until I grew wiser by experience I annually paid 20 or 30 pounds for their little ailings, for which I now get medicine for about as many shillings at a neighbouring druggist.[20]

The profits to be made from the sale of drugs and medicines had brought prosperity to the apothecaries. "There is no branch of business, in which a man requires less money to set him up, than this very profitable trade", wrote Robert Campbell in 1747.

> Ten or twenty pounds, judiciously applied, will buy gallipots and counters, and as many drugs to fill them with as might poison the whole Island. His profits are

unconceivable; five hundred per cent is the least he receives; the greatest part of his out-laying is in viols, small boxes, and cut paper; and these are often worth ten times what they contain.[21]

In this passage Campbell refers to the old-style retail apothecary: what he says applies equally to the new-style chemist and druggist. The collapse of the guild system and the increased purchasing power of the middle classes opened the floodgates to this new breed of tradesman. By the 1780s it was becoming relatively easy for an individual seeking to set up as a retail druggist to borrow capital. Provided he could demonstrate his probity, sobriety and reliability, and as long as he had some assets to begin with, no matter how small, he would generally be deemed a sound risk. By far the most important credit mechanism in the eighteenth century was the simple financial accommodation or trade debt. Members of the extended family lent money to their kin to establish them in business: suppliers of raw material gave credit to merchants who extended it to tradesmen. The granting and receiving of trade credit was a far more important source of funds than banks. The merchant, therefore, occupied the central position in the credit structure and his decisions regarding credit were crucial. The enormous expansion of British overseas trade in the eighteenth century had the by-product of increasing the volume and types of drugs imported. The wholesale druggists in London, Bristol and Liverpool had the opportunity of greatly augmenting their stocks: thus importers, drug brokers, and wholesalers were keen to find new retail outlets.

In the second half of the eighteenth century wholesalers eager to extend credit met up with a host of young men eager to launch into business. These men had served apprenticeships and were now employed as assistants. "A journeyman of this trade", wrote Robert Campbell, "has but small encouragement: fifteen or twenty pounds a year is as much as they can get, and are rarely wanted". The decline of the guilds and the growth of the retail trade offered these men an end to their frustration. The consumer revolution was for them a truly liberating experience: it provided the opportunity to set up in business on their own account. The rise in the number of lads being apprenticed to chemists and druggists after 1760 is an indication of the excellent prospects for setting up as one's own master. Credit and debt were almost universal in the eighteenth century.[22] Trade credit was available in the normal course of business and was vital to the chemist and druggist whose trade was rapidly expanding. The young men who sought independence by becoming proprietors of chemist shops found themselves caught up in an elaborate and extremely fragile web of credit. The acute shortage of specie in the eighteenth century made such a situation inevitable. The cash shortage—especially the supply of small denominations—was so acute that commerce could not have continued, still less expanded, without working credit. The extraordinary difficulties created by the lack of specie probably account for the flexibility and ingenuity of the credit arrangements in Georgian England. The shortage of small change led chemists and druggists to issue their own form of coinage known as "tokens". These were generally the size of the old penny or shilling and their values were of that order, the higher values being of silver. A Brighton chemist and druggist, I.B. Phillipson, was issuing silver tokens, value one shilling, as late as 1811 or 1812.[23] Since they could be ultimately exchanged only at the place of issue, they bound the customer to the shopkeeper just as strongly as the tradesman was bound in debt to the wholesaler.

The ready market for the chemist and druggist was shown by the rapid increase in their numbers: but not all who entered the trade were successful. John Acton (1799–1872) noted in his diary that, between 1824 and 1838, seventeen druggists in Sheffield went bankrupt and nineteen left the business.[24] The level of commercial skill needed to excel was very much higher than is often realised. John Howard (1726–1790) estimated that in 1776 there were nearly two and a half thousand Englishmen in prison for debt and most of them were tradesmen, shopkeepers, and small masters. The high level of bankruptcies (623 in 1773, 634 in 1779) provides a grim reminder of those who, in responding to economic opportunity, found only financial disaster. Even in the commercially buoyant years some businessmen failed through incompetence or ill-luck: in the dark days of depression it required ingenuity and abundance of entrepreneurial skills to survive.[25]

The success of the chemist and druggist depended upon his ability to meet his customer's needs: the sovereignty of the consumer determined his life and work. British society during the late eighteenth and early nineteenth century was a multi-layered structure in which "the several ranks of men slide into each other almost imperceptibly". The rapid urbanisation which occurred after 1780 was accompanied, however, by a gradual process of residential segregation. Aikin noted that the flight to the suburbs by the middle classes had begun in Manchester as early as 1795 and by the 1840s demarcated residential zones were found in all sizeable towns.[26] The diversity of neighbourhoods accounts for the heterogeneity of chemists and druggists. They were highly differentiated, economically and socially. Although, as a whole, they were thriving, there were many levels of prosperity and many divisions within the ranks. It has been customary to assume that chemists and druggists occupied within the class structure a residual position between the middle and the working class, i.e., that they constituted a cohesive social stratum located within the lower middle classes. Such an assumption precludes a clear understanding of their activities. Chemists and druggists were, of necessity, integrated into the communities they served and their class identity was a reflection of those constituencies. A great gulf stretched between the well-established, substantial wholesaler-cum-manufacturer-cum-retailer and the small corner-shopkeeper, scraping a living little better than that of his working-class customers. A series of gradations between these extremes reflected the character of the neighbourhood and the social and economic status of the clientele. The diversity of communities determined the variety of methods and styles of practice. Opportunities for business varied from area to area, from metropolitan to provincial, from urban to rural, from central shopping precinct to working-class parish, from middle-class suburb to industrial slum. The occupation of chemist and druggist was regulated by the mechanisms of the market economy. Entry at any level was restricted by the requirement of capital: survival needed good fortune and special skills. Breaking into the better-class market was far from easy. Extensive premises were required for storage and safekeeping of materials, for workshops and laboratories, and for living quarters for assistants, apprentices and domestic servants and even, perhaps, for porters and errand boys. The purchase or renting of such places in fashionable town centres, the cost of equipping them, purchasing stock and materials, paying rates, all necessitated a hefty initial capital outlay. In April 1710 Anthony Kingsley, a druggist of Newgate Street, London, took into partnership his apprentice, Edward Pincke, and Anselm Beaumont, a journeyman druggist. Between them, they put up capital totalling £8,000.[27] In 1747, when Thomas Corbyn went into partnership with Morris Clutton, they each put up nearly £2,000 in capital.[28]

Chemists and druggists were an amorphous group. The poor corner-shopkeeper stood out at one end of the spectrum: at the other were the high class establishments of which Jacob Bell's shop in Oxford Street provides a metropolitan example and the firm of Ferris, Brown & Score, a provincial one. By 1841 Ferris, Brown & Score was the leading firm of chemists and druggists in Bristol.[29] The business originated in 1770 when Mr. Tillendam, a member of the Society of Friends, opened a shop in Union Street. After his death his widow carried on the business until her retirement early in the nineteenth century. She was succeeded by John Fry, another Quaker and a member of the famous family of cocoa and chocolate manufacturers. He had been apprenticed in 1782 for a premium of £63 to Thomas Sparkes, a druggist of Exeter in Devon. Under Fry's direction the shop flourished and additional premises in Castle Street had been acquired by 1796. Later he took into partnership Richard Ferris and James Gibb, who had served an apprenticeship with his brother William Fry, a Bristol distiller and druggist.[30] The firm then became styled Fry, Gibbs and Ferris. The partnership continued until 1825 when Gibbs decided that pharmacy did not provide sufficient scope for his business ability and forsook it to devote his attention to railways and the large-scale manufacture of alkali. Gibbs' place in the firm was taken by George Brown: by then it had set up one of the earliest plants in the country for the production of aerated waters. Fry retired in 1833 and the name became Ferris, Brown & Capper. When the original building was destroyed by fire in 1834, not only were new premises acquired in Union Street, but a branch was opened at The West Mall, Clifton, under the supervision of George Brown. A few years later further expansion took place with the opening of a branch in Clevedon. The firm was now the leading chemists in the Bristol area and its status was established when it secured the appointment as suppliers of medicines to King William IV. The warrant was renewed in 1840 when Ferris, Brown & Score were appointed chemists to Queen Victoria. Richard Ferris became the first president of the Bristol branch of the Pharmaceutical Society. By 1851 Ferris & Score, as the firm was then known, employed 13 men and had 7 resident assistants or apprentices. The firm advertised extensively in the local press: its name was associated in 1851 with newspaper advertisements for at least thirty-seven different proprietary medicines.

Ten years earlier, in September 1841, the firm published a 52 page booklet entitled, *Directions for the Family Medicine Chest, and a Catalogue of Drugs and Chemicals, Select and Miscellaneous Articles, Patent Medicines, etc., etc.* The book, printed in London, was aimed at middle-class customers: the blue semi-stiff covers, gilt edging and gilded royal coat-of-arms were meant to impress. The text provides a good idea of the services an elite pharmaceutical establishment offered its clientele. First and foremost, this is a guide to self-medication. It enables the reader to prescribe for herself and her household. The booklet describes the fitting up of a medicine chest and points out that "any of the medicines indexed as for the medicine chest may be had separately". The equipment for the chest is given as a graduated wine glass, glass pestle and mortar, glass funnel, lancet, lint, spatula, scales and weights. Forty medicines and articles are listed for inclusion in the chest. They include adhesive plaster, blue pill, cream of tartar, Dover's powder, grey powder and Dr. James' powder. Each item is given a monograph in the catalogue describing the properties and giving the dosage. Dr. James' powder, for example, is described as having the properties of a febrifuge and sudorific; the dose is given as gr. 3–6 twice a day in the form of a pill. The information is provided that:

in recent colds, if a dose be taken and after it a basin of gruel, it will generally afford much relief by producing perspiration; it is a valuable medicine in eruptive diseases as measles, small-pox, fever, etc., but in all cases for which it is required, the bowels should first be attended to.

The catalogue is designed to introduce customers to new remedies. Among "select preparations" is found "Kreosote", described as having been recently discovered by M. Reichenbach, and to have the power speedily to arrest caries of the teeth. It was, however,

> highly important that the substance should be employed in a state of the utmost purity, and entirely free from certain deleterious principles naturally mixed with it in the compounds from which it is obtained; and for this purpose that their friends and the public may be protected, Ferris, Brown & Score have attached their seal to every bottle sold by them as a guarantee for its purity.

The customer is reminded of the advantages of dealing with a substantial firm.

> As manufacturers and importers, we are enabled to pledge ourselves to use and sell only such drugs and preparations as are of the purest character, whilst the extent of our consumption is a guarantee not only of their being good but fresh.

The small, purely retail, chemist may offer his wares more cheaply but they are likely to be both adulterated and stale.

> To secure accuracy and dispatch, our establishments are divided into separate departments, each superintended by a responsible confidential assistant, and the whole under our constant unremitting personal care.

Promptness and accuracy in dispensing customers' own receipts, or physicians' prescriptions are assured.

> The Dispensing Department will, as usual, claim their special care; and for this purpose, Mr. Ferris has fixed his residence on the Premises, where he will be at all times accessible. The most vigilant attention is given to the dispensing of prescriptions, with which no other department is permitted to interfere.

The comparison implied is not primarily with the dispensing of lesser chemists but more significantly with that of the general practitioner. The apothecary, in spite of his training in pharmacy, was often absent on his rounds and would leave his young apprentice or unqualified assistant in charge of his dispensary. The Bristol firm of chemists and druggists could boast:

> In fine, our object in the management of our business is under a deep conviction of the responsibility involved, and with a view to require the confidence of our friends and the public, to devote to it our undivided attention, and for this purpose we have fixed our residences on the premises, where we are accessible at all hours.

Another good example of a high-class chemist's business is the one owned during the 1830s by Thomas Henry Dunn in Highgate village near London.[31] Dunn had been in business before moving in 1830 to impressive new premises on a site previously occupied by the White Lion tavern: the old wine cellars were adapted as a storeroom and the arresting new shop front incorporated the inn's six fluted Ionic columns. Highgate, then as now, was a very fashionable and exclusive residential area and Dunn owned the only chemist's shop there. His customers included the Earl and Countess of Mansfield, who lived at Caen Wood (Kenwood), the Earl of Burford, the Duke and Duchess of St. Albans, Sir Thomas Coutts, the banker, Sir Robert Chester, George Basevi, the architect of the FitzWilliam Museum, Cambridge, Charles Knight, the publisher and founder of the *Penny Magazine*, Michael Faraday, Rev. T.H. Causton, the Vicar of St. Michael's, and Rev. Dr. Dyne, the Headmaster of Highgate School. Patients from far and near came with their prescriptions: from Colney Hatch, Crouch End, Finchley, Friern Barnet, Holloway, Hornsey, Kentish Town, Muswell Hill and Whetstone, even from Blackheath and St. Albans. There were some half-a-dozen doctors practising in Highgate during the 1830s, but Dunn made up prescriptions from eminent medical men in Piccadilly, Oxford Street and the City of London. Among the prescribers were four presidents of the Royal College of Surgeons, Mr. J. Andrews, Sir Benjamin Brodie, Sir Anthony Carlile and Sir Astley Cooper, and leading members of the medical establishment like Sir Charles Clarke, Sir Benjamin Travers, Sir William Adams and Sir William Prout.

The high status of the neighbourhood and clientele explain the prominence in the business of prescription-dispensing. Few other establishments would have been so heavily involved in dispensing the prescriptions of physicians and surgeons. The surviving prescription books reveal that during the last six months of 1840 over 1,800 prescriptions were dispensed of which 800 were new and the rest repeat prescriptions. Unfortunately, entries representing repeated prescriptions only appear in the books from July 1840 onwards: up to that date only new prescriptions were noted. In 1830 there were 275 new prescriptions, in 1831 433, in 1840 905, and in 1841 889. It is probable (assuming a constant rate of repeat to new prescriptions) that during the 1830s Thomas Dunn was dispensing an average of between 800 and 1,000 prescriptions a year. At this time the prescription belonged to the patient who would take it to the chemist to be dispensed as often as needed. Dunn's pharmaceutical skills were widely recognised. In one prescription, John Elliotson, F.R.C.P., professor of the practice of medicine at University College London, testified to the dispensing skills of "my friend Mr. Dunn" who, he adds, "will be particular about the Colchicum". Elliotson knew a thing or two about pharmacy: his father was a chemist and druggist. Even in Highgate, the dispensing of prescriptions would not have been enough to keep the business afloat. Dunn, like other chemists, prescribed over the counter, dispensed family receipts, sold drugs, chemicals and proprietary medicines, made up veterinary preparations, and retailed a wide range of non-pharmaceutical goods. He also acted as a surgeon, cupping and bleeding patients on request.

The high-class pharmaceutical establishments were located in the central urban shopping precincts of major cities or in upper class residential areas. The building itself was impressive, often incorporating distinctive features within its architecture and with modern interior fittings. The establishment was large: it included storerooms, a laboratory and workshop, a counting house, and residential accommodation for assistants, apprentices, and domestic servants. In addition, porters, shopmen and errand or delivery boys would be employed. The business might be owned and controlled by one person or, more likely, as a partnership. Throughout the country, the principal retail firms were also manufacturers and wholesalers. Preparations for their own shops and for wholesale were manufactured in their laboratories: drugs and chemicals were supplied to hospitals, dispensaries, general

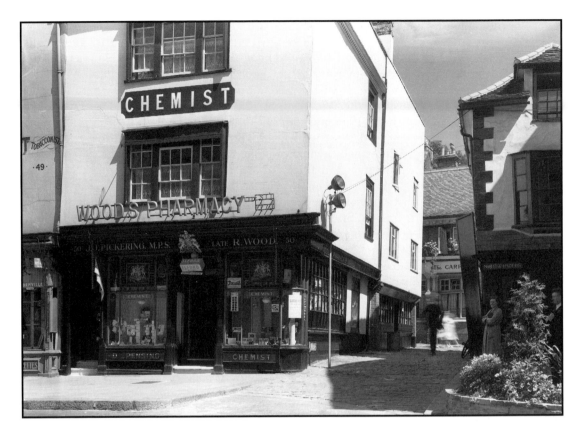

12 *Woods Pharmacy Ltd., 50 High Street, Windsor, Berkshire, 1953. Established in 1770, at the time this photograph was taken in 1953 the business was run by J.J. Pickering MPS.*

practitioners and lesser chemists. The business was primarily pharmaceutical but surgical instruments, soda and mineral waters, perfumery and toilet preparations were also sold. The high-class shops had a virtual monopoly of the dispensing of physicians' prescriptions: but they also dispensed family receipts, prescribed over the counter, supplied medicine chests to families, ships and institutions, sold spectacles, and performed surgery and dentistry. In the eighteenth century the complexity of their business relationships led some of them to undertake financial services: in the nineteenth century their probity, respectability and economic solidity made them valued as agents for fire and life insurance.

The leading chemists and druggists were substantial businessmen making large profits and leaving considerable fortunes. An analysis of wills shows that chemists and druggists were capable of amassing just as much if not more than manufacturers, farmers and professional men like attorneys and physicians. George Hall, for example, owned a high class shop in Kirkgate, Huddersfield. By the time he was forty, in 1851, he had an assistant

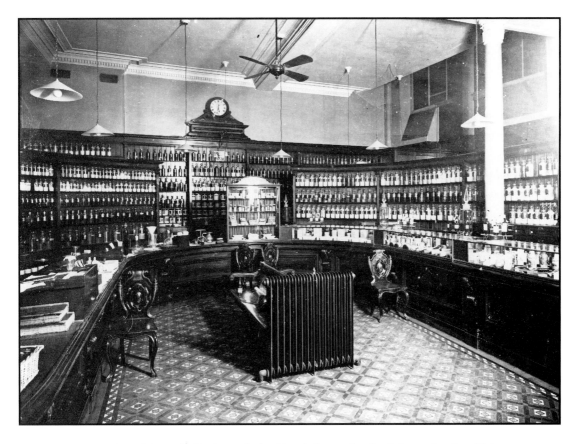

13 *Interior of Allen & Hanburys Ltd., Plough Court, Lombard Street, London. Taken in 1927, it shows the immaculate appearance of this "establishment" up-market business.*

and three apprentices and employed two general servants in his shop. He lived out of town at Longwood House in the prosperous suburb of Fartown, where he farmed twenty-eight acres. Investing in land and farming it increased his wealth and status. By 1891 he owned ninety-two acres and was employing five agricultural labourers and two domestic servants.[32] The level of apprenticeship premiums is indicative of the rewards to be gained in a trade. By the last quarter of the eighteenth century parents needed to find £250 to bind their sons to a leading London druggist and even in the provinces £200 might be necessary. In London, hospital surgeons could command as much as £500 but attorneys and leading apothecaries rarely received more than 150 guineas. General practitioners, in both London and the provinces, took on apprentices for premiums of £50.

Far from being insignificant or marginal members of the local community, the well-established chemists and druggists had high status within it. "In most towns", observed Jacob Bell in 1852, "some of the most intelligent and respected inhabitants are chemists. We continually find them filling responsible offices, such as mayor, magistrate, guardian of the poor, etc., and also connected with sanitary committees and local institutions of a scientific and useful description. They are not usually addicted to politics, but it will be generally found in any town where a chemist enters into such matters, he holds a prominent position in the committee of his party".[33] George Hall was a member of the Huddersfield Town Council and a committee member of the Infirmary. George Earle, a chemist and druggist who built a splendid brick house with sinuous bow fronted shop windows at 58, High Street, Winchester in 1774, held a number of public offices including those of pavement commissioner, bailiff, alderman, justice of the peace and constable. He was mayor of Winchester four times between 1790 and 1805. His son John became mayor in 1828–9 and again in 1831–2. Thomas Goadsby, a chemist and druggist with a shop near the Albert Bridge in Manchester, became a commissioner of police in 1839, served as a councillor from 1844 to 1857, first for the Exchange ward and then for St. James ward, was made an alderman in 1857 and was elected mayor of Manchester in 1861. Chemists and druggists played a significant part in the civic and political life of Leicester, a medium-sized East Midlands industrial city with a population of 51,000 in 1841.[34] The mayor in 1804, and an alderman for many years, was Edmund Swinfen. From their premises in the Market Place, Edmund and his father trained at least fourteen apprentices. Thomas Woodward, the son of one of the Swinfen apprentices, and himself a chemist and druggist, became a councillor. William Evans Hutchinson, a Quaker and in business as a chemist in Gallowtree Gate until 1839, was an alderman for three years from 1835 and councillor from 1841 to 1850: he left pharmacy in 1839 and later became chairman of the Midlands Railway Company. Joseph Goddard, who took over Hutchinson's business in Gallowtree Gate, transferred from nearby Market Harborough. He had been an assistant for several years in a leading London pharmacy. He soon established himself in Leicester and was a councillor in the early 1850s. He was the originator of the well-known metal polish that bears his name. Thomas Cooper and Henry Pickering were other Leicester chemists and druggists to serve on the town council. All those who became councillors were active in civic affairs in other ways, serving as members of Parish Select Vestries, an organ of local government, or on the Board of Guardians administering the Poor Law.

In the work of modern medical historians, the chemist and druggist is consistently referred to as an "unorthodox" or "irregular" or "para-medical" or "fringe" practitioner, part of the "medical periphery", and even as a "quack", lumped together with folk-healers, medical botanists, wise-women, midwives, bone-setters, and mountebanks.[35] A moment's reflection reveals how wide of the mark such assessments are. There was nothing unorthodox about the pharmacy practised by the majority of chemists and druggists: it was the same pharmacy as that practised by apothecaries and used by physicians and surgeons. It was the pharmacy of the three Pharmacopoeias of London, Edinburgh and Dublin. Indeed, the research and activities of the leading chemists and druggists were responsible for introducing new drugs, new chemicals, and new processes into medical practice: they also developed methods for detecting impurities. Physicians were quick to recognise that the dispensing of the chemist and druggist was based on greater knowledge and performed with greater expertise than that of the apothecary. An apprenticeship served with a leading chemist and druggist was unquestionably a superior education in up-to-date pharmacy than that received by a general practitioner's apprentice. In 1837 the staff of the London Hospital insisted that a chemist and druggist be engaged as "being more likely to be skilled in the making of medicines than an apothecary". This decision was taken after complaints that the apothecary had made three serious mistakes in dispensing in one day.[36] A letter in *The Chemist* in 1840 claimed that

> a striking proof of the *superior* accuracy of druggists' dispensing, is shown in the fact of young men, educated in the business, being in almost all cases preferred in the public hospitals—*at Apothecaries' Hall itself*—and in hundreds of private surgeries.[37]

When, in 1843, Henry Wentworth Acland, later Regius Professor of Medicine at Oxford, wanted to study practical pharmacy, he made arrangements to do so in the chemist and druggist shop in Mayfair owned by John Lloyd Bullock.[38]

There was, as we have seen, nothing marginal about the status of the leading chemists and druggists within their local communities: their ranking in the local prestige-scale was far higher than that of the general practitioner. The chemist and druggist relied upon the careful cultivation of a local reputation for his success: his livelihood depended upon the long term judgment of the general public. Sixty-five per cent of the chemists and druggists in Bristol in 1851 were locally born and trained: their shops were further guarantees of permanence and reliability.[39] To describe chemists and druggists as "irregular" or "fringe" practitioners is to make a nonsense of the English language. Instead of artificially buttressing his practice by acquiring irrelevant paper qualifications, the chemist and druggist grounded his reputation on local public opinion. "That in every profession the fortune of the individual should depend as much as possible upon his merit and as little as possible upon his privilege", wrote Adam Smith in 1774, "is certainly for the interest of the public".[40] But not, of course, in the interest of the less successful competitors, as the whining of the apothecaries from 1794 onwards shows.

Before 1858 chemists and druggists were as much part of the medical profession as apothecaries. In 1747 Robert Campbell described "the profession of physic in all its branches", i.e., "the physician, surgeon, chymist, druggist, and apothecary". The Apothecaries Act of 1815 specifically authorised chemists and druggists "in the buying, preparing, compounding, dispensing, and vending drugs, medicines, and medicinal compounds, wholesale or retail". In the words of Justice Park in May 1828, "The object of the act was to keep the business of apothecary distinct from the other branches of the profession". He saw "four degrees in the medical profession, physicians, surgeons, apothecaries, and chymists and druggists". "Each is protected in his own branch, and neither must interfere with the province of the other", he concluded.[41] Four of the nine Bills introduced for the regulation of the medical profession in the years between 1840 and 1850 included chemists and druggists as part of the profession. In 1842 Jacob Bell wrote an historical reflection on "the position which pharmacy occupies or ought to occupy as a branch of the medical profession". Chemists and druggists were not finally excluded from the medical profession until the 1858 Act: to describe them before that date as "para-medical" or part of the medical periphery is anachronistic and misleading. Apothecaries or general practitioners frequently referred to chemists and druggists as "quacks". The insecure often find in others their own faults. The ranks of general practitioners teemed with "quacks": among the leading candidates for the accolade must be those who were afraid to appear in their true colours, those who falsely claimed to be "surgeons" with only a licence from Apothecaries' Hall, and those who purchased degrees *in absentia* from Scottish and German universities to convert themselves into "physicians".[42] There was not a single allegation made against chemists and druggists in the nineteenth century that could not be made with equal or greater force against the general practitioner.

The chemists and druggists whose shops occupied the middle ground between the high-class establishments and the poor corner-shops were typified by their ability to improvise. Whereas the high-class practitioners were linked by the dispensing of prescriptions to the practice of physicians and surgeons, the majority of chemists never saw a physician's prescription and had little occasion to dispense them. Before the introduction of the 1911 National Insurance scheme, ninety per cent of all dispensing took place in general practitioner's surgeries.[43] Chemists and druggists served the public directly. The staple parts of their pharmaceutical trade were vending drugs without prescription, supplying the ingredients of family receipts, restocking medicine chests, selling veterinary and patent medicines, and producing their own medicinal preparations. The importance of the sale of horse medicines in Victorian cities is easily forgotten. The horse did not disappear from the city streets until the 1930s: the coming of the railway, far from diminishing the importance of the horse, substantially increased the amount of horse traffic in towns. It has been estimated that late Victorian society required one horse for every ten persons (men, women and children). By 1902 there were about three and a half million horses in Britain, most of them working in urban areas.[44] By producing and selling horse remedies, chemists and druggists performed the same functions as present-day garages: they kept the urban transport system running. For human beings, chemists and druggists made up mixtures, draughts, pills, powders, liniments, lotions, ointments, drops, electuaries, gargles and plasters. They took natural barks, herbs, leaves, flowers, roots and seeds and crushed, boiled, infused and strained them. They dealt with all manner of aches, pains, bruises and strains. They let blood and applied leeches. They bandaged wounds, lanced boils, reduced abcesses and inflammations and treated ulcerated limbs. They sold and fitted surgical appliances. They drew teeth and sold spectacles. Some even practised midwifery. They were general medical practitioners, advising and prescribing over the counter and even visiting patients.

In order to survive and prosper each chemist and druggist had to respond to the business opportunities in his own area. He had to adopt a market strategy flexible enough to provide services and goods neglected by other practitioners and tradesmen. He had to be prepared to practise a wide range of medical skills and to sell a diversity of products. There is no such creature as the typical chemist and druggist and no such thing as the typical shop. The combination of skills and goods not only varied from shop to shop but also over time. Chemists and druggists were always on the look-out for new lines and new types of custom. Such strategies might lead an individual to greater diversification or to greater specialisation. The range of goods sold by nineteenth-century chemists is well illustrated by the following "poem", distributed as an advertising hand bill in 1844 by an early member of the Pharmaceutical Society who displayed his diploma "handsomely framed, glazed, and elevated on a stand".

> If drugs you would have of the very best sort,
> Go to Judson's, the Chemist, where they may be bought,

And fine patent medicines for woman or man,
Horse, cattle and pig drinks the best that you can;
Genuine sheep ointment the strongest that's made,
In preparing of which Judson can challenge the trade.
If tea you would have of the finest in kind,
The price and the palate he'll suit to your mind:
He's fine Turkey coffee the best in the mart,
To warm both the stomach and gladdened the heart:
If wines are your object, both strong, good, and old,
His is the shop where the purest are sold;
They'll cheer up the spirits and be a reliever
From cholera morbus or typhus fever.
His segars and snuffs are the rarest indeed,
And as for tobacco the pure foreign weed.
If spices, vinegar, or pickles you'd buy,
Just step into Judson's, have a little, and try
Figs, oranges, lemons, or sugar-candy.
Barley-sugar, and most sweets that are handy,
Lozenges, nuts, muscatels, almonds, and prunes,
Fifes, flutes, and violins for playing your tunes.
If such you may want the best you can get,
As none ere sold better in Hertfordshire yet.
The young and the old may be suited to taste,
With fish-sauces, capers, or anchovy paste;
Also tooth, clothes, nail, plate, hair brushes, and oil,
Perfumery, hair pins, and combs free from soil.
Jewellery cheaper by twenty per cent
Than many could buy if to London they went.
Stationery in all its various branches,
Engraving performed as fashion advances.
A large stock of snuff-boxes, rich, good, and rare,
And Rowland's maccassar for oiling the hair.
Fancy soaps of all sorts for beauty and smell,
Cold creams for the hands and face—lip-salve as well.
His paints, oils, and colours the richest in shade,
And as to quality the best that are made.
Ready money, remember, kills flying, they cry,
The which you must pay for whatever you buy.[45]

The distinction between medicines and drugs on the one hand and food and drink on the other was not as clear cut then as it is now. Nor was their production as specialised or on such a large scale. When a chemist sold tobacco, snuff, tea, coffee, mineral and soda waters, ale, spirits and wines, his customers might be buying them, like their purchases of drugs and medicines, for health reasons. Moreover, the preparation of medicines from herbs, drugs and chemicals led easily to the production of mustards, vinegars, sauces, pickles, confectionery, cosmetics, perfumery, furniture cream and polishes. The needful equipment, manufacturing techniques and even the ingredients overlapped. Alfred Bird (1811–1878), a chemist and druggist in Bell Street, Birmingham, made a baking powder before he invented Bird's eggless custard powder, which soon took the public fancy and has retained it ever since. Two chemists and druggists in partnership in Broad Street, Worcester, John H. Lea and William Perrins, spent two years experimenting with different kinds of sauces before they sold their first bottle of "Worcestershire" sauce in 1830.[46]

Chemists and druggists made extensive use of advertising not only in the local newspapers but also via the medium of handbills, trade cards, prescription envelopes and medicine wrappers and labels. The prescription envelope, used to return the patient's prescription after it had been copied into the prescription book, was widely used to advertise the shop from the early nineteenth century. The arrival of a new chemist in a town would be advertised in the local press and by a distribution of handbills. On setting up in Sheffield in 1807 Joshua Gillat sought "the favour of the public which he will endeavour always to merit by serving his friends in the best manner and on the lowest terms. Prescriptions made up with the greatest care, accuracy and neatness". In 1818 John Earle drew the attention of "the Nobility, Gentry and the Public in general", by means of an advertisement in the *Hampshire Chronicle*, to the services he supplied:

> Physicians' and family prescriptions dispensed with neatness and accuracy; Painters and families supplied with oils and colours on reasonable terms; Fish sauces of all kinds, genuine teas, wax candles and spices of the best qualities, genuine patent medicines.

In January 1827 the *Wakefield and Halifax Journal* carried the news that W. Clater, chemist and druggist, had commenced business at the Market Place, Wakefield and that he "respectfully informs the nobility, gentry, and inhabitants of Wakefield, and its vicinity, that he has ... laid in an entire, fresh, and extensive assortment of all kinds of drugs, chemicals and galenicals".[47]

During the nineteenth century chemists and druggists usually had their own range of proprietary medicines, their own special lines and preparations. Many famous brand names were first manufactured by provincial chemists. "Eno's Fruit Salt" was the creation of James Crossley Eno (1820–1915), who had a pharmacy in Newcastle-upon-Tyne; Arthur Oglesby of Barnsley used his skill to manufacture "Nurse Harvey's Gripe Mixture"; and "Kompo" was originally formulated by a Leeds chemist and druggist.[48] Since successful specialties could bring fame and fortune, the formulae were closely guarded. Upon retirement or death the chemist's collection of recipes and prescriptions were handed over to his heirs or successors in business. Edmund Swinfen of Leicester stated in his will:

> The recipes and prescriptions from whence my nostrums or proprietary medicines are prepared are to be given to my son Richard and I have instructed and informed him respecting the true and genuine composition and preparation thereof. And I have not made known or revealed the mode of preparing the same to any other person whatsoever.[49]

In 1832 when G.B. Reinhardt took over his father's shop he announced that the business would continue in the premises near the old church, Wakefield,

> whereat may be had, as usual, faithfully prepared from the recipes of the late G.B. Reinhardt, his invaluable medicine, *Balsam of Horehound*, for curing coughs, colds, asthmas, hooping cough, declines, and consumptions. Also his truly valuable and never failing medicine for the cholera morbus, or vomiting and purging; and also his excellent medicines for worms; all of which medicines, from trial and

LOZENGES

SOLD BY

JOHN BELL,

Chymist,

No. 338, OXFORD STREET,

OPPOSITE

GREAT PORTLAND STREET.

———

Acidulated Rose Lozenges, for Coughs, &c.
Aniseed ditto.
Anodyne Pectoral, ditto.
Anti Acid, or
Absorbent ditto for Heartburn, &c.
Aromatic Steel ditto.
Bath ditto.
Black-Currant ditto, for Sore Throats, &c.
Burnt Sponge, ditto.
Candied Horehound, for Hoarseness, &c.
Cachou de Rose Lozenges.
Ching's Worm, ditto.
Dawson's Pectoral ditto.
Ginger ditto.
——— Candy.
——— Pearls.
Horehound Lozenges.
Ipecacuanha ditto, for obstructed Expectoration, &c.
Lavender ditto.
Lemon ditto.
Magnesia ditto.
Nitre ditto, for Sore Throats, &c.
Paregoric ditto.
Patirosa or Rose ditto.
Pectoral ditto from the Balsom of Tolu.
Peppermint ditto.
——— Candy.
——— Pearls.
Pontefract Cakes.
Poppy Lozenges.
Refined Liquorice.
Sulphur Lozenges.
Tamarind ditto.

. * Prescriptions and Family Recipes carefully prepared.*

14 *Hand bill advertising lozenges available from "John Bell Chymist", c. 1798–1819.*

experience, have obtained very high reputations, and can only be prepared by G.B. Reinhardt, as he is the sole possessor of his late father's recipes.[50]

The fact that secret and exclusive formulae and techniques of preparation were passed on from generation to generation suggests how competitive yet how traditional the trade was.

Some chemists, beginning with sales of their secret remedies in their own shops, found a wider outlet in their neighbourhood, and then launched out on a regional or even nation-wide scale with extensive advertising and large-scale manufacture.

The sale of proprietary medicines expanded rapidly in the eighteenth century. For the person who could raise the funds for the necessary advertisements secret remedies promised a large financial harvest. Advertisements for pills, ointments, plasters, mixtures, elixirs and appliances flooded the press: the distribution of broadsheets reinforced the impact. By the mid-nineteenth century chemists and druggists were the largest retail outlets but they faced much competition in the sale of patent medicines from booksellers, stationers, printers, newspaper proprietors, drapers, tailors, grocers, publicans and hairdressers. Among the long-lived medicines were Goddard's Drops (seventeenth century), Hooper's Female Pills (patent 1743), Dr. James' Fever Powder (patent 1747), Joshua Ward's Paste and Godfrey's Cordial, both introduced in the eighteenth century. In the early nineteenth century they were joined by such favourites as Morison's Pills, Holloway's Pills and Ointment, and Page Woodcock's Pills. Most chemists stocked vast ranges. W.P. England of Huddersfield and F. Cardwell of Wakefield, for example, advertised the sale of Brande's Bronchial Sedative, Woolley's Pectoral Candy, Dr. Locock's Pulmonic Wafers, Holloway's Ointment and Dr. Bright's Pills of Health.

The chemist and druggist's shop was the context in which patent medicines and orthodox medication were brought together. The boundary between the two was never clear-cut. In the eighteenth century an established physician had patented a fever powder and later patentees included five persons described as physicians, surgeons, or apothecaries.[51] Studies of the patent medicines most often advertised in eighteenth-century newspapers have indicated that their composition closely paralleled that of the official preparations used by regular practitioners.[52] They shared the same active ingredients such as opium, as a pain-killer, and antimony, which induced sweating to reduce fever. A study of medicines advertised in the eighteenth and nineteenth centuries for treating the diseases of women suggests the similarity of proprietary and orthodox medicines.[53] Contemporary writers had earlier made the same point. In 1856, Dr. Henry Letherby of the London Hospital reported that analysis showed a large class of advertised medicines were "almost identical in their composition with the common Aperient Pills, which are dispensed at the public hospitals". By selling patent medicines, the chemist and druggist helped to further the advertisers' aim of identifying their products with regular medicine. A recent systematic sample of advertisements for 100 medicines in seven Bristol newspapers published in 1851 and 1861 shows that (1) the title of "doctor" was included in the names of 28 medicines (2) the proprietor described himself by this title or as a surgeon in 17 instances, (3) use in orthodox medicine was claimed for 16 medicines, (4) medical authorities were quoted in the text of 11 advertisements, (5) 4 advertisements included testimonials allegedly from medical men. In short, the advertisements for fifty preparations sought to associate them with regular medicine.[54] By marketing the products, the chemist and druggist reinforced that effort. The government stamp duty may also have worked to the same end: the stamps seemed to imply official approval of the product.

Proprietary medicines were purchased by all social classes in the nineteenth century. Friedrich Engels, in his classic description of Manchester in 1844, noted that

large numbers of patent medicines are sold as cures for all sorts of actual and imaginary complaints. Morrison's Pills, Parr's Life Pills, Dr. Mainwaring's Pills and thousands of other pills, medicines, and ointments which are all capable of curing all the illness under the sun ... So the English workers now gulp down their patent medicines, injuring themselves while filling the pockets of the proprietors.[55]

George King, a medical practitioner from Bath, however, asserted in 1844 that "it is not the lower classes of the community that buy and patronize the advertised nostrums, but the higher and educated". The proprietors of patent medicines used elementary consumer psychology. The real secret of their remedies was the promise to meet needs which orthodox medicine failed to supply: to cure fatal diseases like cholera and consumption, to restore lost youth and vigour, or to treat embarrassing conditions like venereal disease and unwanted pregnancies. Samuel Solomon's Balm of Gilead was sold as a cure for the manifold ill-effects of masturbation: Hooper's Female Pills were a thinly disguised abortifacient.

The financial loss to the medical practitioner was only one of the grounds for his objection to the sale of proprietary medicines. Like all forms of self-medication, their large-scale use meant that a substantial area of health care escaped control by the medical profession. The popular reputation of patent medicines implied a reservoir of therapeutic knowledge that could be tapped directly by the layman. The success of patent remedies was derived from two sources: the self-diagnosing, self-help health care tradition, and the newly constructed consumer desire for novelties and miracle-cures.[56]

The tradition of family self-medication was deeply rooted among the populace. In pre-industrial Britain, the sufferer habitually played an active and sometimes a decisive role in interpreting and managing his own state of health. Self-diagnosis and dosing were standard practice at all levels of society and the laity regularly dispensed medicine to friends, family and servants. Nowadays many people automatically go to the doctor as soon as they feel ill: in pre-industrial society no one routinely called in the doctor, even when they were seriously ill. No one believed that medical men had a monopoly of knowledge of diagnosis and therapy. Ordinary people thought, with good reason, that they could understand illness and treat it just as effectively as the doctor. So when someone felt ill, they reflected on their symptoms and formed their own diagnosis; they then usually administered medical self-help.

Until at least the mid-nineteenth century, folk medicine, a strange amalgam of medicine, religion and magic, was an integral part of lower-class culture. It is misleading to think of it as something employed by the poor for want of better means or as merely residuary to the activities of the medical practitioner. It was used more frequently and regarded more highly by the mass of the population than the advice of doctors. Magical practices survived in rural areas until late in the nineteenth century. "We have white-witches, and black-witches, charmers of burns and scalds, casters of nativities, and foretellers of the fate of parturient women", reported one observer of country practice in 1846. In 1850 a child died of burns in the Forest of Dean after being treated in turn by three "wise women", the last one pronouncing a "mysterious charm", in which the parents had implicit faith. In 1853 a sawyer, dying of erysipelas, persuaded two friends to carry him over a bridge near Bristol, so that, by crossing water, he would be freed from the power of the witches he believed had brought about his illness. In 1858 a woman from rural Somerset travelled to Bristol to consult a "cunning man" because she believed her pigs were bewitched.[57] Pre-industrial beliefs and traditions survived the rapid urbanisation of the nineteenth century. Migrants from the countryside brought their folk practices and herbal remedies with them. Even for town dwellers the countryside was close at hand and many retained traditional knowledge of hedge and field plants; some would leave the town when no work was available to gather wild herbs for medicines and cordials. A general practitioner from the Pennines believed that medical herbalism was "the study of every rustic". He recorded in 1841 that he had often seen in workingmen's cottages collections of more than thirty specimens, the "medical virtues" of which were known to the cottagers who distilled them for tinctures, infusions and fomentations.[58]

By the end of the seventeenth century, however, medical magic seems to have disappeared among the literate middle class and gentry: its demise is a facet of the long-term withdrawal of patrician from plebian culture which has been traced by modern historians. Two types of evidence support this conclusion. The *Gentleman's Magazine* was a widely-read miscellany which carried, during the course of the eighteenth century, hundreds—if not thousands—of pieces on medical matters. A popular feature was the inclusion of local and family cures sent in by readers (e.g. goose grass as a fortifier, salt water bathing to make wens disappear). But a careful search of its pages, from its foundation in 1731 to beyond the end of the eighteenth century, provides not the slightest indication of the continued use of magical healing, even for such desperate conditions as cancers. A parallel exercise involved working through more than twenty manuscript family recipe books from the eighteenth century. It was common for literate families to keep such books, often for generations, recording cooking recipes and household hints as well as medical remedies. Although such remedies were gleaned from a gamut of local sources, not a trace of medical magic is to be found.[59]

Archdale Palmer, Lord of the manor of Wanlip in Leicestershire, kept up his recipe book for fourteen years, from 1658 to 1672. Archdale enlisted the aid of his wife, daughters, daughters-in-law, cousins, friends, neighbours, servants, physicians, apothecaries, farriers, clergymen, soldiers and even "Grace Savell, a Madwoman" to supply the receipts he needed. A minister from Ireland told him how to cure tooth-ache, Lady Hartopp of Dalby Hall instructed him in the making of biscuits. Remedies for "mother-fits", chilblains, measles, rickets, and sore eyes are interleaved with ways of preparing treacle-water, sugar roses, and cordial lozenges and brewing wines from raisins, elder, plums and poppies. One of the first recipes in England for making coffee is included: the new beverage, tea, is recommended for treating "a fit of the vapours".[60] The recipe book of James Woodhead of Netherthong, near Huddersfield, written about 1818, reveals how great the impact of the chemist and druggist was on family self-medication. Woodhead's book contains some forty remedies. Oil of cloves is recommended for tooth-ache, spirits of turpentine and castor oil for obstructions of the "testines" and turmeric for liver complaints: a recipe for "female pills" contains iron, aloes and antimony. All these ingredients would be obtainable from the local chemist and druggist.[61]

The rise of the chemist and druggist can be seen as an aspect of the adaptation of folk medicine to urban, industrial society. In the seventeenth century well-bred families had bottles of home-brewed purges, vomits, pain-killers, cordials, febrifuges and tonics ready in the kitchen. By the late-eighteenth century middle-class families were starting to stock up with drugs or proprietary medicines bought from the chemist and druggist. By then both

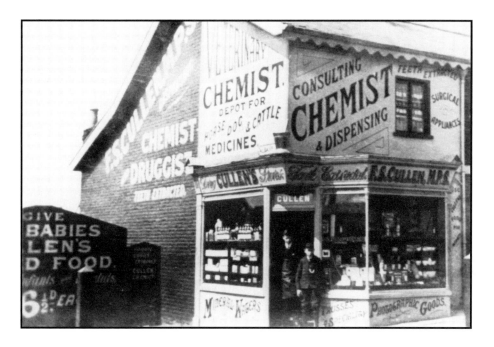

15 *Cullens Drug Store, Norfolk, 1890s. A pharmacy heavily decorated with advertising and illustrating the wide range of products and services offered: "Trusses a speciality— photographic goods—teeth extraction — veterinary chemist".*

rich and poor were making use of his services for the compounding of family receipts. Those who could afford them would purchase a family medicine chest, with its book of instruction providing "a description of the names and qualities of the medicinal compositions contained" therein, "with an account of their several uses and the quantities proper to give at each dose".[62] At the time that domestic medicine chests became popular, new self-help manuals began to be published. John Wesley's *Primitive Physick, or an Easy and Natural Method of Curing Most Diseases* was first published in 1747. It contains remedies for virtually every disease known to man. By "primitive" Wesley meant "easy to administer" and therein lay its success. Laid out alphabetically, like a dictionary, it listed in simple English seven or eight—sometimes more—cures (one thousand and twelve in all) for each ailment. For over a hundred years it was a best seller: it sold more copies than any other medical handbook of its time.[63] The religious and populist tone of its preface and the evangelical career of its author must have contributed to its tremendous success. William Buchan's *Domestic Medicine; or the Family Physician*, first produced in 1769 was also an immediate and great success. By the time of his death in 1805, nineteen large editions amounting to at least 80,000 copies had been sold.[64] The extent of self-medication in early Victorian England is suggested by the continued popularity of this type of literature. In 1847 Buchan's *Domestic Medicine* was still being republished, at least six new or reprinted editions of Wesley's

Primitive Physick appeared in the 1840s, while the edition of Cox's *Companion to the Family Medicine Chest and Compendium of Domestic Medicine* published in 1846 was described as the thirty-fourth. Just how widespread the use of domestic recipes was is demonstrated by the regularity with which chemists and druggists advertised their skills in making them up. The art of dispensing was used on family receipts, not on doctors' prescriptions. All drugs could be obtained over the counter; there was no control, no concept of prescription-only medicines.

The power of the consumer in the eighteenth century was felt not only by the chemist and druggist but by all branches of the medical profession. The fee-paying patient or consumer of medicine, not the medical practitioner, had the upper hand and determined the conditions on which service was rendered. Today the doctor commands professional authority: he has the backing of his professional organization, the prestige of science, and the power of the modern state. He commands the apparatus of modern scientific medicine with its diagnostic technology, laboratory tests, and complex systems of therapy: he is supported by consultants, specialists, supplementary professions, and the labyrinthine bureaucracy of the hospital. The patient expects a great deal of him. This was far from the case in the eighteenth century. Scepticism about medicine was high: the occupation's prestige low. Physicians were caricatured in prints and pilloried in novels and plays.[65] The aristocratic and wealthy sick played an assertive and even dominant role in clinical consultations. By virtue of the wider social basis of their power, such "patients" were in a position to define their own needs and the manner in which those needs were to be met. Faced by rich, powerful, critical, demanding and arrogant patrons, the physician was forced into the role of lackey and sycophant. Samuel Johnson sometimes gave orders to his doctors: on one occasion, against his physician's advice, he insisted that his surgeon bleed him. Dr. Thomas Percival, in his *Medical Ethics* (1803), cautioned physicians to fall in with the wishes of their wealthy patients to have particular medicines prescribed. "The trouble about people of consequence", Diafoirus remarks in Moliere's *Le Malade Imaginaire*, "is that when they're ill, they absolutely insist on being cured". Diaries of eighteenth-century patients reveal that they frequently ignored their doctor's advice and had no compunction about dismissing him if he tried to be bossy. They would shop around for whatever practitioner or treatment suited their purse and inclinations. Among the rich, the eighteenth-century physician was expected to be, above all else, a gentleman, socially accepted in the circles among which his patrons moved. Elegance and wit were of greater importance than technical competence: a good bedside manner was the sine qua non of success.

In the eighteenth century self-diagnosis and self-medication were the norm. But by the end of the century some medical men were seeking ways of curtailing that freedom. Thomas Beddoes (1760–1808), an Edinburgh-trained physician practising in Bristol, was an early exponent of views which became typical of professional middle-class radicals in the early nineteenth century. Politically they were hostile to both rich and poor. They abhorred the corruption and inefficiency of aristocratic government: they had contempt for the ignorant, ungovernable masses. Society needed re-organizing along rational, scientific lines. Beddoes, for example, supported the phase of the French Revolution which swept away feudalism and enhanced the power of the bureaucratic middle class. In Britain the franchise, the legal system, the prisons, the police force, the poor law, educational institutions, all required reformation, all needed to be made more systematic, more rational. Professional men of science should have greater influence in the running of society. More planning, more regulation, more discipline were needed to bring society under control. Beddoes was appalled by the democratic tendencies of the commercial revolution. The medical profession had to free itself from the control of the consumer. Before there could be an increase in the collective prestige of the profession and the establishment of ethical codes and standards, the free market in medicine had to be swept away. The essence of quackery is patient self-help, the conspiracy between buyer and seller that produces obsequious doctors anxious to give their patients what they ask for, and commercially-minded drug sellers. The patient should be firmly under the doctor's control. There should be more medical students taking five-year courses, more experimental hospitals, more preventive medical institutions, more centralised, statistically-based information on public health. The experts should be in control. Beddoes was utterly hostile to any form of popular medicine and, indeed, to any medical activity not engaged in by formally qualified practitioners.[66]

Between 1794 and 1858 the medical reform movement changed the meaning of self-medication. In the seventeenth and eighteenth centuries there was little antagonism between medical self-help and orthodox medicine. It was the growing professionalisation of medicine that made self-medication "unorthodox" and "unprofessional". The medicine of the laity became "quack" medicine, i.e. medicine beyond the control of the qualified. The medical reformers during the exclusionist era of early Victorian professionalisation succeeded in converting the people's medicine into "fringe" medicine. The continuity of lay medicine became, therefore, something more than the precarious survival of old habits: it was converted into a form of determined opposition to expertise and professionalism. It became an expression of popular resistance to the cultural aggression of the professionalisation of medicine. Early opposition surfaced in John Wesley's preface to his *Primitive Physick*, but in the 1840s complete philosophies of resistance to orthodox medicine appeared. The movements which engendered them were essentially defensive: attempts to maintain rights and privileges under threat. They were closely linked to other divisions within British society, to increasing class consciousness and conflict, and to the deepening religious antagonisms. Working men who saw their crafts destroyed by the capitalist organisation of industry, who saw their children's education being taken over by "alien" Church schools, who saw their traditional recreations being restricted by the new police force, who felt that their former freedom and autonomy were being undermined by the growing surveillance of the state, such men found it difficult to see the growing professionalisation of medicine as progress. Greater power and more privileges for the medical profession seemed to imply less and fewer for the ordinary working man.

The preface to *Primitive Physick* is decidedly anti-professional: Wesley defends the right of "every man of common sense" to "prescribe either to himself or his neighbour". In earlier times, he argues, physic, like religion, was traditional; every father handed down to his sons

> what he had himself in like manner received, concerning the manner of healing both outward hurts, and the diseases incident to each climate, and the medicines which were of the great efficacy for the cure of each disorder.

But now medicine has become an abstruse science. Doctors take advantage of their situation by charging exorbitant fees, by writing books no layman can understand and by needlessly complicating prescriptions. "As theories increased", wrote Wesley, "simple medicines were more and more disregarded and disused: till in a course of years the greater part of them were forgotten". Medicine should be restored to its ancient simplicity:

> ... neither the knowledge of Astrology, Astronomy, Natural Philosophy, nor even Anatomy itself, its absolutely necessary to the quick and effectual cure of most diseases incident to human bodies: nor yet any chimical, or exotic, or compound medicine, but a single plant or root duly applied.

The populism and anti-professionalism of *Primitive Physick* must have been an important and continuing influence among working men. Wesley was quoted with approval by those who attacked established medicine during the 1840s. Medical botany or Coffinism was the most significant social movement of the 1840s to express its opposition to professional medicine by defending the traditional right of every man to be his own physician.

Alfred Isaiah Coffin came to England from Troy, New York State, in 1838, initially to London, then to Hull. By 1848 he was established in Manchester where he stayed about two years before moving back to London. Coffin was a purveyor of a system of herbal remedies, called medical botany, devised by Samuel Thomson in North America, where it attained considerable popularity during the 1830s and 1840s. Coffin went on lecture tours in the north of England with the aim of setting up local societies, members of which had to possess his book, *The Botanic Guide to Health*, which cost six shillings. Coffin tried to secure the active involvement of ordinary people in the organisation. The local societies were democratically run with elected committees whose responsibility it was to see that one or more members visited and prescribed for all the sick who sought the help of the Society: another member kept stock of the Society's collection of roots and herbs. At each weekly meeting, members reported on their successes and discussed any difficult cases, in order "that the people may mutually assist each other in the study of Medical Botany". Meetings began with a lecture from one of the members. At Whitsun each year a general convention of all the local societies of the British Friendly Medico-Botanic Association was held. Constituent societies were established in several towns in Lancashire and Yorkshire in the late 1840s. Coffin also operated through agents, chemists and druggists who prescribed and sold his remedies, and whom he supplied from premises in Manchester. He published a fortnightly penny review, *Coffin's Botanical Journal and Medical Reformer* (1849–59), containing news of and comments on the progress of the movement.[67] Coffin was not the only one to popularise the Thomsonian system. The brothers George and John Stevens were active in Bristol and the Midlands. John Skelton, a London shoemaker and a leading Chartist throughout the 1840s, studied under Coffin in Manchester during the spring of 1848. That summer he went with Coffin on a missionary tour of Rotherham, Sheffield, Blackburn, Bacup, Ramsbottom, Oldham, Wakefield, Barnsley, Stockport, Birmingham, Manchester, Derby, Nottingham and Leicester. In the 1850s he practised in Leeds and later Manchester: between 1852 and 1855 he published a monthly periodical, *Dr. Skelton's Botanic Record and Family Herbal*.[68]

Medical botany had a considerable following among factory operatives, craftsmen, artisans, tradesmen and shopkeepers in the North and Midlands. The organization and ideology appealed to intelligent working men, deeply interested in radical politics, religious dissent and self-improvement. "Despite irregularities, social disadvantage, educational drawbacks, the working men in many places have made a noble stand in defence of their rights, duties, and privileges", reported D.W. Heath, a lecturer from the Nottingham Medico-Botanic Society in 1853. There was a close association between the Coffinites and religious non-conformity. A writer in the *Carlisle Patriot* claimed that the chief feature of Coffinism "is the almost total monopoly of it by religious dissenters of the most zealous castes". Coffin's meetings were held in Wesleyan or Primitive Methodist chapels. He recommended total abstinence from alcohol and was presented with addresses of thanks and more useful gifts by temperance groups. Coffin wrote that he felt under great obligation to many members of the Society of Friends and was presented with a pair of spectacles by the Leeds quakers.[69]

Coffinism was aggressively anti-establishment. The therapeutic procedures and medicines of the medical profession were positively harmful: "thousands perish under their hands who would otherwise have survived", claimed Coffin. "Mercury, opium, alcohol, and the use of the lancet", he continued, "are of themselves sufficient to account for the speedy depopulation of a world". The professional attitudes and social pretensions of doctors were attacked with equal vigour:

> the licensed to kill enters the house of sickness, and, at the bedside, takes in charge, with the authority of law, his exclusive right over the prostrate victim, whose blood he draws, whose frame he tortures, whose bowels he secretly poisons, and whose disease he cures, or, at his will, prolongs; but kill or cure, his charge is made, in amount wholly at his own discretion; and should his depletion be the cause of death, nothing can be said against it, it was done according to rule ...

For centuries the medical profession had been accumulating power and now had "the prescriptive right of killing or curing at pleasure". Doctors "vainly imagined themselves to be the only rightful oracles of the science". But now was the time to "throw off the yoke of medical despotism". The "so-called science of medicine", wrote John Skelton, is "imposed upon society, and supported by law" and its practitioners "being so respectable and respectably connected ... cannot possibly be wrong". Yet it is, in fact, "one huge deception alike injurious to all". The poor and the needy must be released from "medical bondage".

Coffin believed that medical knowledge must be demystified and medical practice deprofessionalised.

> That which has been falsely termed science in medicine, is no more than a tissue of incongruities, interwoven with the obsolete and unmeaning language of the schools of antiquity, invented for no end, save the final prostration of the human intellect at the shrine of monopoly, in order to dignify and confer wealth on a few individuals, and to support institutions which have thus grown upon us. The learned have combined together for the purpose of throwing dust into the eyes of the people, in support of which fallacy they have invented a language peculiar to themselves.

When stripped of "the false airs of pedantic learning" there is nothing in medicine beyond the reach of the ordinary mind. It was not "a difficult, abstruse, mysterious science": it only seemed so because "of its being a sealed profession". Medicine should be simplified and popularised. It was outrageous that new academies were being set up to clothe in mystery the secrets of nature. But the system of medical botany had been freed "from all technicalities" and was "so easy to be understood that every member of society may learn it if disposed". "There is now actually in existence a complete system of medical treatment which each individual can take into his own hands with little trouble, and almost without expense—a system at once embracing all that is safe and good in all others known". Botanic medicine was the people's medicine: "the common sense of the people, when in possession of a true theory of medicine, will be found quite capable of curing all diseases to which they are subject". With the aid of Coffin's *Botanic Guide*, "every father can now discharge the duties of physician to his own household".[70].

The essence of medical botany was democratic self-care, i.e. the idea that all human beings are obliged to care for each other. The founding of local societies was seen as a way in which "the people may mutually assist each other": and evening schools were set up for mutual instruction, to help "the poorest of his fellow countrymen to help themselves". Medicine was a subject which all should be equally taught and in which the advantages and duties are mutual. Professionalism in medicine is anti-democratic; it involves the privatisation of public knowledge; it is a crime against humanity. "To mystify, shut up in the schools, and make private property of that knowledge, which of all others ought to be universally taught, is a wrong the deepest and most injurious to society". The professionalisation of medicine, like the enclosing of the common land, deprived the ordinary man of his birth-right.[71]

The medical profession was uncompromising in its hostility towards the Coffinites: both class and professional interests drove it to react vigorously. The Thomsonian system was recognized as a comprehensive challenge to the established position and the swelling pretensions of the orthodox practitioner. The idea that working class people might practise and prescribe with little more instruction than that to be garnered from mutual discussion groups, a few lectures and Coffin's manual, denied the medical reformers' case for prolonging training and tightening qualifying requirements. The general practitioners' leaders, already engaged in power struggles with the medical corporations, were determined to resist this new attack on their proprietary rights and privileges. The battlefield was chosen with care: when medical botanists were charged with manslaughter, the cards were stacked heavily against the defendants. Only regular practitioners could be called on to establish the cause of death at inquests and the medical press provocatively refused to recognise medical botanists except by their previous occupations. The notion that former cotton-spinners, bricklayers or stonemasons might practice medicine was regarded as self-evidently absurd. But the medical profession was over-zealous. The *Pharmaceutical Journal* commented that, at some inquests, "the medical witnesses have apparently endeavoured to prove too much", and the judge in one trial commented that "if people were to be tried on the judgement of old practitioners for acting contrary to received notions, there would never be any improvement in medicine".[72]

The responses of chemists and druggists to the Thomsonian movement provide a striking illustration of the amorphous character of their profession in early Victorian England. The leading establishments in London and the provinces went along with the medical profession's labelling of Coffinites as dangerous quacks and imposters, but refrained from joining in the hue and cry for their legal suppression. At the other extreme, several chemists and druggists became medical botanists themselves, selling and prescribing the authorised remedies. Thomas North Swift, a "druggist and botanist" of Huddersfield acted as an agent for Dr. Skelton during the 1860s and 1870s. Jesse Boot's great pharmaceutical empire began

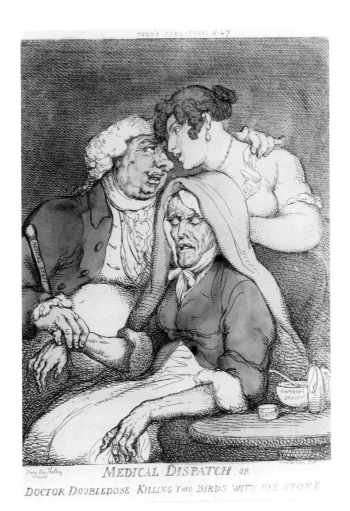

16 Medical Dispatch or Doctor Doubledose killing two birds with one stone, *drawn and etched by Thomas Rowlandson (1756–1827).*

as a medical botany business in Nottingham. His father John, a local Wesleyan preacher, was a follower of Coffinism and called his shop the "British and American Botanic Establishment". He advertised vegetable remedies, both retail and wholesale, and made himself available for consultation at his shop on Mondays, Wednesdays and Saturdays.[73] The majority of chemists and druggists were distinctly unsectarian: they happily embraced each and every system of health care. While the high-class firms trod the straight and narrow, the lesser brethren followed the bypaths to fields such as medical galvanism, phrenology, hydropathy, homeopathy as well as medical botany. Most tried to maintain an eclectic approach to medical theories and systems. A chemist and druggist might well sell Morison's pills, for example, without necessarily subscribing to his medical theories. James

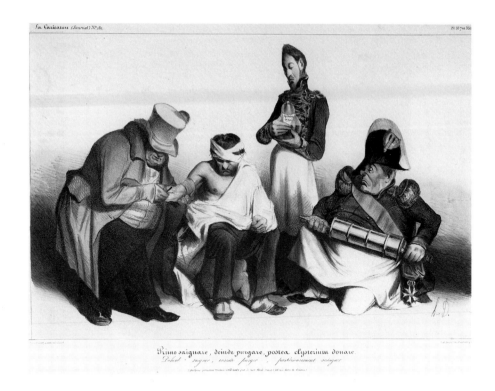

La Caricature (Journal) Nº 161.

Primo saignare, deinde purgare, postea clysterium donare.

17 Primo Saignare, deinde purgare, postea clysterium donare [*First to bleed, then to purge, finally to give clyster*] *drawn by H. Daumier (1808–1879), lithographed by Bequet, published 5 December 1833.*

The scene shows Louis Philippe giving first aid to Wernet, the postman, run down by the King's carriage and satirises the misfortunes of France, symbolised in Wernet's accident.

Morison, "The Hygeist", surfaced in 1821 with his own system of medicine, which postulated a common cause of all diseases and a universal vegetable pill (minerals and chemistry were explicitly rejected) to cure them. Morison's hygiene movement retained its support well into the 1860s under the slogan: "Blood of Man is the Life—Diseases arise from impurities in the blood—Cleanse the Blood, and you banish disease".[74] Most proprietors of patent medicines were anxious to gain by implied association with orthodox medicine, but Morison was openly and aggressively hostile to professionalism. "The old medical science is completely wrong" the title-page of one of his publications declared. Like the medical botanists, he challenged the medical profession in theory and practice.[75] But those who sold his pills rarely swallowed his doctrines. Chemists and druggists managed to hunt with the hounds and run with the fox at the same time.

The working-class culture, which became the breeding ground of Coffinism, was the source of life for the small corner-shop chemist and druggist. Although he met the health needs of the labouring classes during the nineteenth century, he was subjected to

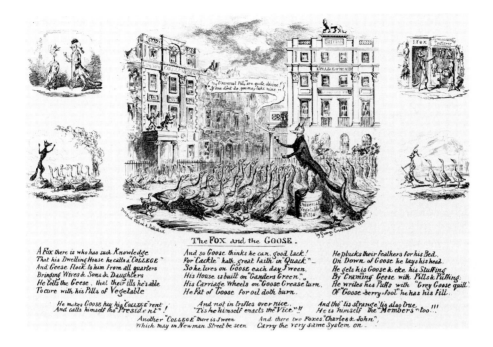

The FOX and the GOOSE.

A Fox there is who has such Knowledge
That his Dwelling House he calls a "COLLEGE"
And Geese Flock to him from all quarters
Bringing Wives & Sons & Daughters
He tells the Geese, that their ills he's able
To cure with his Pills of Vegetable

He makes Goose hay his "COLLEGE" rent,
And calls himself the "President".!

Another "COLLEGE" there is 'tween
Which may in Newman Street be seen

And so Goose thinks he can, good lack!
For "Cackle" hath great faith in "Quack" –
So he lives on Goose each day 'tween.
His House is built on "Ganders Green",
His Carriage Wheels on "Goose Grease turn.
He Fat of Goose for oil doth burn.

And not in trifles over nice.
'Tis he himself enacts the "Vice".!!

And there two Foxes "Charles & John",
Carry the very same System on.

He plucks their feathers for his Bed,
On Down of Goose he lays his head.
He gets his Goose & eke his Stuffing
By Cramming Geese with Pills & Puffing.
He writes his Puffs with "Grey Goose quill",
Of "Goose-berry-fool" he has his Fill.

And tho' 'tis strange 'tis also true,
He is himself the "Members" too.!!!

18   The Fox and the Goose *designed and etched by George Cruikshank (1792–1878) in 1833.*

  The British College of Health was established in 1828 by James Morison and used to defend his system of medicine and promote his proprietary products. It is one of the buildings depicted here along with the rival establishment, the London College of Health, managed by physicians.

remorseless criticism then and is still scorned by modern historians. He was perceived, and is now portrayed, as an uneducated, ignorant opportunist, guilty of foisting himself off as a medical practitioner on the gullible poor, and causing untold injury to the health of his customers, particularly defenceless women and children. His practice is represented as a combination of primitive physic and pharmacy, minor surgical operations crudely carried out, and occasional unskilled man-midwifery. That working-class patients preferred to spend their hard-earned and meagre wages buying medicine from the local druggist rather than attending charitable dispensaries or receiving treatment under the poor law is taken as evidence of their own irrationality and ignorance. The evidence, however, on which such accusations rest, derives from the observations of individuals who had neither the ability nor the desire to make sense of what they saw, except in their own blinkered way and for their own hostile purposes. The illiterate, bungling, positively dangerous chemist and druggist is a stereotype invented by interested parties in the nineteenth century and perpetuated by uncritical historians.[76]

  There are considerable difficulties in studying corner-shop chemists. Unlike their more prosperous and enduring contemporaries, they have not bequeathed records of their daily activities to the archivist. They are, therefore, difficult to get at: neither the sources nor the appropriate methodological tools have been available. In the absence of any detailed analysis, our understanding has been inherited directly from the blanket condemnation by nineteenth-century medical practitioners who had a particular interest in denigrating the ordinary chemist and druggist. It will not be possible to gain a realistic view of the contribution of the chemist and druggist to the nation's health in the nineteenth century without first sweeping away the distortions produced by modern historians' uncritical acceptance of certain types of evidence. This evidence, derived primarily from the parliamentary select committees on medical poor relief of 1844 and 1854, and supplemented by snippets from novels and the medical press, must first be reviewed.

Nineteenth-century criticisms of chemists and druggists tended to elaborate the theme that their ill-informed prescribing and indiscriminate sale of medicines and drugs, usually adulterated, constituted a major public health hazard. Much concern was expressed in parliamentary reports about the danger to the sick of resorting to druggists. The term "druggist" was the word used to describe the villain of the piece; but it is clear from the context that the person in mind was the chemist and druggist in working-class neighbourhoods. Polemicists often make use of the "unacceptable" behaviour of one segment to denigrate a whole group. In 1854, Thomas Gilbert, superintendent registrar for Bristol, stated in his evidence to the Select Committee on medical relief, that many children died because the difficulty their parents had "of getting medical aid, leads them either to doctor them according to an old Woman's directions, or to take them simply to druggists, who know nothing about the disease, and get them a little quackery".[77] Gilbert was conscientiously repeating the authorised version which had first been told to the 1844 Select Committee, in great detail, by Henry Wyldbore Rumsey (1809–1876). Rumsey was a highly intelligent man; fellow of the Royal College of Surgeons by examination, elected F.R.S. in 1874. In 1835 he had been appointed honorary secretary of the poor law committee of the Provincial Medical and Surgical Association (now the B.M.A.). He performed the duties of that office with exemplary energy and devotion and soon became the undisputed authority on the medical services of the poor law and the indomitable champion of the poor law medical officer. "To him State Medicine was not a word; it was the central idea of his life", as his obituary oddly put it.[78]

Rumsey believed that the poor law medical officer was overworked and underpaid: that the ratepayers' contribution to the poor law medical services had to be substantially increased. He set out to demonstrate that the present underfunded service left gaps that were filled by incompetent and dangerous practitioners. To do this, he circularised poor law medical officers to provide evidence of unqualified practice. Having obtained returns from 42 places, he presented the evidence to the 1844 Select Committee, which he used as a platform to publicize the P.M.S.A.'s views on the poor law medical service. Not unexpectedly, the downtrodden poor law medical officers discovered that their direct competitors for private practice, the chemists and druggists, were the cause of all the trouble. In Hull, approximately one-quarter of the population was said to use the services of the prescribing druggist; in Shrewsbury it was common for the poor to visit druggists in the early stages of disease; in Southampton "quite as many of the poor are prescribed for by druggists as by regular practitioners"; in Brighton, as many people received treatment from druggists as from the hospitals, dispensary and medical clubs together. From Wolverhampton it was reported that:

A very large proportion of fatal cases among children were not seen by medical
men, and often not even by druggists, the mothers merely applying for remedies
at the druggist's shop.

This was also the case, "to a lamentable extent", in Reading, where a third of the
druggists even visited the sick. In Wakefield "probably from 4,000 to 5,000 poor resort
annually to the druggists", and in Lincoln "the retail druggists have considerable practice
among the poor, both in chronic cases and in the early stage of acute complaints; minor
operations are also performed by them".

In his evidence before the Select Committee, Rumsey quoted at length from the report
of Mr. Dorrington, a Manchester surgeon:

It is perfectly frightful to contemplate the loss of life amongst young children and
infants arising from the practice of numerous druggists in the poorest parts of the
town. Any one who is much amongst the poor, and who sees as much of the disease
of infants as I do, cannot fail to be horror-struck at the immense loss of life
constantly taking place from this shameful practice. It is one of those crying abuses
that deserves the most earnest attention of the legislator and philanthropist. Those
who have been accustomed to life as it is in agricultural districts and small market
towns, have no notion of the fearful extent to which human existence is played with
in large towns, and in no way so barefacedly as in this. Adults may have a right
to hazard their own lives by going to ignorant druggists or professed quacks, but
they most assuredly have none to risk that of the helpless children . . . and as moral
restraints are not sufficient to prevent this, legal ones of great stringency are
imperatively needed. I speak decidedly and warmly on this point, because I am
daily brought into contact with the miserable consequences of the present state of
things.

Rumsey claimed that the difficulties of obtaining proper medical advice induced "the
multitude" to flock to the druggist's shop:

I do not say it is the only cause; the ignorant and uninformed have a natural
tendency to seek benefits of all kinds from inferior sources. Then the easy access
to the druggist's shop, vying with the gin palace in its tempting decorations, attracts
those who prefer spending a few pence, to encountering the formalities and delay
attendant on an application to a qualified practitioner. Then the speedy
apprehension of the case by the druggist's shopman, a glance being sufficient to
satisfy him both as to its nature and treatment, and his ready selection of some drug
as a certain cure for the malady of the customer, all this tells wonderfully on the
ignorant of all classes. The inevitable results to the community are fearful loss of
life and destruction of health.[79]

Historians have sought to confirm the validity of Rumsey's appraisal of chemists and
druggists and their working-class customers by referring to an odd assortment of similar
comments. G. Wilson, a Leeds general practitioner, in a letter to the *Lancet* in 1854,
describing the extent of unqualified practice in his area, complained that the "lower
extreme" of a general practitioner's potential practice was effectively closed to him by the
prescribing druggists.

These people sell to the working class for a few pence whatever to themselves seems fit and proper for all manner of diseases, never leaving their crowded shops, and of course living at no expense for horse, carriage, etc., *while all their receipts are in ready money*. But when the patient has spent all his ready cash, what then? Why, he goes to the regular practitioner, where he gets credit for months, years, or very frequently *for ever*.[80]

In 1857 a *Lancet* editorial drew attention to the growing numbers of druggists:

Hanging about the suburbs of town, infesting its central parts, ... these people absorb much money and destroy many lives and much health.

Their popularity is explained by the fact that:

Large towns consist almost entirely of operatives who look upon physic as a trade,—and a poor one too,—who have not the ability to form any opinion as to the proficiency of their betters in point of general education—who rather like some one of their own class—who have a strong belief in a natural gift for doctoring, and above all, believe most fervently in cheap physic, cheap advice, and cheap visits.[81]

Historians have even relied on fiction to colour their image of the chemist and druggist. A scene in Elizabeth Gaskell's novel, *Mary Barton*, which purports to describe working-class life in mid-nineteenth century Manchester, is claimed as authentic. In the story, John Barton goes to a druggist for medical assistance on behalf of a workmate stricken with typhus fever, prior to attempting to obtain an infirmary order. Barton described the case to the druggist, who

proceded to make up a bottle of medicine, sweet spirits of nitre, or some such innocent potion, very good for slight colds, but utterly powerless to stop, for an instance the raging fever of the poor man it was intended to relieve.

Nonetheless,

Barton left the shop with comfortable faith in the physic given him; for men of his class, if they believe in physic at all, believe that every prescription is equally efficacious.

This material has been quoted at length because of its value as evidence, not of the activities of chemists and druggists, nor of the attitudes of their working-class customers, but of the preconceptions and prejudices of nineteenth-century medical men and their middle-class allies, and, a fortiori, of present-day medical historians.

Without any critical analysis, historians have been content to regurgitate this material and to endorse the value judgments contained within it. The *Lancet*, under the editorship of Thomas Wakley (1795–1862), was an unrelenting advocate of the rights of the "surgeon in general practice". Its violent and intemperate attacks on the medical corporations and on dispensing druggists made it notorious in its day. *The Chemist* rightly observed that "the only class at which its venom is not levelled is that in which most abuses exist". It is now an invaluable guide to the nineteenth-century general practitioner's view of the medical world: its observations on chemists and druggists have to be interpreted in that light. Elizabeth Gaskell's account of working-class life was truly fictitious: it was based on neither experience nor empathy. Maria Edgeworth, in a letter to the author of *Mary Barton* in 1848, described the novel as a contribution to the growing science of political economy.[82] She was right: it paints the working class exactly as the bourgeois political economists imagined them to be. The cultural barriers separating Victorian middle-class novelists from the labouring classes were too dense for Mrs. Gaskell to penetrate. Her sympathies lay, in any case, with the medical profession: her uncle was Dr. Peter Holland, a physician who lived at Knutsford in Cheshire. The views and evidence of H.W. Rumsey were unashamedly selective. He was, in effect, counsel for the prosecution. As a member of the jury, one notices the inconsistencies and internal contradictions which, in spite of the prevailing hostile bias, trickle through his evidence.

Rumsey's case was that the poor placed themselves in danger by consulting druggists rather than regular practitioners. He asserted, but did not attempt to demonstrate, that the consequence was suffering and loss of life. It may have been that Rumsey was shrewd enough to realise what we indeed now know—that in terms of the quality of treatment supplied, its scientific status, and its success rate, there was nothing to separate the practice of chemists and druggists from that of regular medical practitioners. Rumsey was certainly aware of the thesis that linked the high death rate of children and adults with insanitary living conditions rather than access to medical care. With the benefit of hindsight and more than a century of research, it is clear that the practice of medicine, whether regular or irregular, made little impact, positive or negative, on the high rates of mortality. The main dangers to the health of the population were poverty, malnutrition, over-crowded slums, contaminated water, inadequate sanitation, excessive hours of work, and unhealthy and dangerous work environments. The main stumbling block for Rumsey was the alleged difference in quality of the medical treatment provided by druggists and the poor law medical service. The case for increasing public expenditure on the poor law service was that the poor had to be rescued from the malpractice of druggists: the case for improving the terms and conditions of service of the poor law medical officers was the inadequacy of the treatment they were able to offer. Rumsey presented evidence in support of both arguments. The evidence for the second proposition is the more convincing for being first hand: evidence by poor law medical officers about their own activities.

The salary of the poor law medical officer included the cost of drugs for patients. Rumsey argued that the sick poor could not be properly treated until medicines were provided at a separate cost to the ratepayer: at existing low salaries doctors were of necessity induced to withhold necessary expensive medicines such as "quinine, sarsaparilla, castor oil, tinctures and aromatics". Cheap substitutes had to be resorted to; "a worse description of drugs than could be safely applied to private patients". Joseph Rogers, founder and president of the Poor Law Medical Officers' Association, admitted that his members commonly used cheap substitutes, that they averted their eyes from the sufferings of the poor rather than prescribe opium costing thirty-two shillings a pound. The story was repeated by witness after witness before the Select Committees.[83] The poor, in their ignorance, asserted Rumsey, bought drugs, which he believed were likely to be adulterated, from the chemist. The underpaid poor law medical officer was forced to supply the poor with adulterated drugs. The druggist was not qualified to diagnose and prescribe: the overworked poor law medical officer sent his raw apprentice or unqualified assistant to look after the poor. Was it ignorance that led the poor to prefer the chemist and druggist? Or did they know at least as much as Dr. Henry Wyldbore Rumsey?

Rumsey's case had an inescapable but damning logic: general practitioners, who took on the job of poor law medical officer, had one set of standards for private patients and another, inferior, set for the poor. Rumsey argued that this was the fault of the contract system: the inference was that doctors were cruel and dishonest. The ethical superiority of the educated general practitioner over the profit-seeking chemist and druggist was neither apparent nor real. The inconsistencies which break the surface in Rumsey's evidence are manifestations of a fundamental contradiction in the principles of the reformed poor law system; a contradiction which the poor law medical officers incorporated into their own thinking. Rumsey and his fellow doctors had condemned the old indulgent poor law system as "bad in principle, worse in practice ... spreading idleness, vice and destitution". They welcomed the move from the benevolent, paternalistic attitudes towards the poor to the punitive principle of "less eligibility" enshrined in the Poor Law Amendment Act of 1834. To destroy the culture of dependency, the living standards of those in receipt of poor relief were to be made lower than those of the worst paid labourer in employment. Rumsey believed the principle of "less eligibility" was right and proper, while simultaneously admitting that medical treatment "is always expensive ... a luxury beyond the poor man's reach".[84] If the independent labourer could not afford medical relief, it could only be provided to the pauper in a form so debased that both doctor and patient would be degraded. Rumsey and his friends in the Provincial Medical and Surgical Association wanted the best of incompatible worlds. As members of the middle class, they believed in maintaining a dual system of work incentives: low taxation for themselves and the scourge of poverty for the working class. As members of the medical profession, they believed in providing treatment under conditions and to standards defined by themselves. An acceptable standard of medical relief for the poor would undermine the principle of "less eligibility" and lead to an increase in public expenditure: its necessary corollary was the provision of publicly-funded medical care for all who could not afford it.

Chemists and druggists existed whenever there was a sufficient local demand for them. The precise nature of this demand was one which nineteenth century middle-class observers failed to appreciate. Their implicit notion was that if "qualified" general practitioners made their services available to all sections of the population, their evident superiority would be universally recognized, and working-class demand would simply be converted away from the chemist and druggist. The issue, however, was not so straightforward. In the first place the practice of resorting to the druggist's shop was not confined to the poor. G. Wilson, the prescient surgeon from Leeds already cited, remarked,

> Nor is the druggist system confined to the poor, for very many indeed of the middle classes go to the druggist first, and only send for the surgeon when a certificate of the cause of death seems likely to be wanted for the registrar.[85]

Jacob Bell, with greater wisdom and knowledge, wrote,

> Many persons who are quite aware of the difference between an Apothecary and a Chemist, object to calling in a medical man on every trivial occasion. They resort to their own nostrums and family receipts, and in the application of these remedies the Chemist is sometimes consulted, not as a medical man, but as a person who, from his constant manipulation of medicines, is supposed to know something about their effects.[86]

72

Working-class attachment to the chemist and druggist was even more tenacious. Even when free medical treatment and drugs were made available through voluntary hospitals, charitable dispensaries and the poor law, the working class obstinately chose to endanger their chances of recovery by visiting the chemist's shop. Medical men, as we have seen, were not slow to offer their personal explanations for this phenomenon. The ignorance of the working class allowed them to be lured by incessant advertising, tempting decorations, easy access and instant diagnosis. Whenever a Victorian middle-class writer found the behaviour of his inferiors incomprehensible, he ascribed the ignorance to them rather than to himself. We must try to do better than that.

The poor patronised the local chemist and druggist rather than be patronised by the regular medical profession. Among working people there was a strong current which rejected the elitism of those in authority and distrusted the services of professionals. Professionalisation of middle-class occupations was experienced by the labouring classes as a form of authoritarian regulation and social control: an attempt to impose alien values and to undermine traditional practices and freedoms. This was manifested in various spheres and, everywhere, met working-class resistance. Anti-professionalism is seen clearly in the continued support for working-class private venture (common-day) schools long after the provision of elementary education by the voluntary societies and the state; in the numbers of adults who attended humble mutual improvement societies rather than the civically approved Mechanics' Institutes; in the working-class preference for local preachers and an unpaid ministry rather than the "hireling priests" of the Established Church. When on trial, radicals like Thomas Cooper elected to conduct their own defence rather than be defended by a barrister. The Coffinites, with their slogan, "The People their own Physician", and the patronage of the corner-shop chemist harmonised well with such anti-authority, anti-professional attitudes. The thick underfelt of working-class hostility towards the medical profession has never been fully exposed. Working people's experience of charitable dispensaries, voluntary hospitals and the poor law medical services was humiliating and stigmatizing. In 1804 Thomas Beddoes, whose advocacy of professional medicine we have already noted, was forced to concede that the experience of

> medical charities shows that the sick are constantly flying off before they have a chance of due benefit. I take this to be a want of proper understanding. All has hitherto been conducted in a style of authority. It has been too much mere dumb show between doctor and patient.[87]

Forty years later, *The Chemist* observed

> It must be admitted, that the humiliation, neglect, and frequent insult, which the poor experience at the hands of both officials and pupils at the dispensaries ... causes them to evince the greatest reluctance to avail themselves of the assistance there offered.[88]

Acceptance as a patient by dispensaries and hospitals required a letter of recommendation from a governor or a subscriber, who gave priority to their own servants and employees. Recommendation was always dependent on an appropriate display of deference and servility. Once admitted to an infirmary patients were

> always required to conduct themselves in an orderly and respectful manner; they are aware on entering a hospital that they must comply, unhesitatingly, with their

advice, and abide by the directions of the medical officers; if the slightest difficulty occurs they are immediately discharged.

In the first half of the nineteenth century, hospital surgery was, in every sense, a traumatic experience for the tortured victim. Authoritarian surgeons were able to exploit for their own ends the highly vulnerable situation of the poor patient.[89]

Insensitive treatment of the sick poor was followed by callous dissection of the pauper dead. Popular hostility towards the medical profession was significantly increased by the 1832 Anatomy Act which provided for anatomists to be supplied by the bodies of the poor who died without money to pay for funerals. Until 1832 the only legal source of cadavers for anatomical dissection had been a restricted number of hanged felons. The inadequacy of this source became more acute as schools of anatomy expanded during the eighteenth century. The use of dissection as a dire punishment derived its meaning from a shared belief in the importance of post-mortem reverence for the corpse. In popular funeral rituals the significance attached to the corpse was grounded in beliefs which linked the care of the mortal remains with the fate of the soul. For the working classes the Anatomy Act added to the horrors associated with the workhouse: death on the parish meant desecration of the body. The state used the needs of the medical profession to make poverty a social and moral crime.[90]

The Anatomy Act was an early legislative indication of the shift from the benevolent attitudes of the old poor law to the harsh principles of 1834. The stigmatizing of poverty and the resultant reluctance of the poor to apply for relief was a deliberate device of the government to create the impression that the amount of "real" poverty was minimal and declining and that the provision of services for the poor was adequate. Yet in Bradford, for example, with a population of 132,000, the annual number of cases of illness treated under the poor law system in the 1840s amounted to less than one per cent of the population, and those treated by the charities to less than three per cent. Only one in six of the sick poor in Bradford received any form (charitable or publicly-funded) of medical poor relief when the total number of sick poor was probably about 40,000 cases a year. Throughout the period after 1834, the stigma of pauperism was a powerful disincentive for those in need of medical relief. Those who were prepared and able to find such relief were harshly treated. In 1909 a witness before the *Royal Commission on the Poor Laws* stated:

> The tradition of the service is that every pauper is to be looked on as being such through his or her own fault, and the tendency is to treat the case accordingly . . .
> I believe that the tradition, as to the pauper, is that he is a shade only from the criminal . . . Now, to this tradition the Medical Officers tend, like other officers, to become a victim, and the tendency is that the case of sickness is treated as a 'pauper' and not as a 'patient'.[91]

Spokesmen for the medical profession liked to give the impression that doctors were in the habit of treating the poor without payment. H.W. Rumsey, who became expert at compiling statistics illustrative of the medical profession's humanity and sense of duty, argued that the poor law service was merely an inadequate supplement to the doctors' charitable efforts. In Liverpool in 1834 a quarter of the population received some form of medical poor relief, 23 per cent from medical charities and only 2 per cent from the poor law surgeons. Similarly, in the Newark area, in 1843, 40 per cent of the population received "gratuitous treatment". "Legal medical relief reached little more than one-sixth of the destitute sick", reported Rumsey, "nearly five-sixths being left to the charitable feelings of a profession which certainly does not luxuriate in the marrow of English opulence".[92] Financial insecurity made some doctors less than charitable. An inquest at Finsbury, London in 1862 on a two year old child named Richard Clarke provides striking evidence of this. When the child became ill, his father rushed to the local general practitioner, Henry Buss, M.R.C.S., who refused, however, to come until the father signed a note binding him to pay five shillings for the doctor's visit. The doctor's response on being implored to hurry was: "Are you prepared to pay? Have you got five shillings?" Although the child was dead by the time the reluctant doctor arrived, Clarke paid him his fee. Buss defended himself by saying that he was obliged to act thus to guard against imposition. He had to live by his profession. Those who could not pay ought to apply to the parish doctor. The Coroner remarked that the course pursued by Dr. Buss was not peculiar to that gentleman. The jury expressed "their regret that medical men should refuse to attend the poor without guaranteed payment. The jury consider that as such refusals are frequent, the fees for first visits should be paid by the Poor Law". General practitioners frequently took poor men to court for failing to pay fees. In 1841 a chimney-sweeper was put in prison for failing to pay a doctor's bill of £2-2s-6d, although the apothecary owed him as much for sweeping his chimneys.[93] In 1853 a Sheffield surgeon brought an action to recover his bill of £4-11s-6d, which the defendant, a working man, pleaded was excessive, he having been charged for 21 days' attendance in an unsuccessful treatment of diarrhoea.[94] *The Chemist* sympathised with working men who sought the aid of general practitioners. "Hapless are the poor creatures who apply to these men: they are drenched and charged and . . . if they cannot pay them—and what poor mechanic or labourer can?—are summoned in scores to the petty courts and made to rue their fate: such practices we have too often seen among the low fraternity about Shoreditch and Ratcliffe Highway".[95]

The Chemist mounted a vigorous campaign against counter prescribing chemists and druggists but realised that the doctors' harsh treatment of the defaulting poor went a long way to account for their ubiquity:

> The difficulty and the justice of the question of Chemists practising behind their counters appear to involve the following considerations: The excessive charges of medical men, which totally preclude the poor from applying to them for advice, and the almost certainty that if they do and cannot pay, their doom be a prison, through the instrumentality of the Court of Requests. Hence it will be evident that they are the sole or chief cause of that evil of which they so loudly and so continually complain, and the poor are therefore driven to seek the best advice they can get from Chemists . . .[96]

On another occasion, the editors of *The Chemist*, Charles and John Watt, concluded:

> Much better for the poor is it that chemists should do their best for them for a few pence paid at once, than that they should become liable to extravagant charges, and be compelled to discharge the debt by death in a prison![97]

The clumsy attempts by the medical profession to suppress medical botany did nothing to lessen working class hostility towards doctors. Several of the cases against working-class Coffinites had evidently been concocted by local medical men in order to put a stop to what they considered improper interference with the profits of their profession. When the medical botanist, John Wood, was found not guilty of manslaughter, loud clapping broke out "which continued for some time before it could be suppressed by the officers of the court". The release of Ellis Flitcroft, a Coffinite imprisoned for one month for acting as an apothecary, was described as the occasion for a triumphant procession, "drawn by four horses, and accompanied by Dr. Coffin and others, the temperance band playing through the streets". They were preceded by several banners and a flag inscribed "Release of the persecuted Flitcroft".

The corner-shop chemist and druggist drew support from working-class disenchantment with the medical establishment. Counter prescribing, like the advice of the medical botanists, stood in marked contrast to the authoritarian treatment meted out by many doctors. Reports of the trial of John Wood note that he carefully explained the proposed course of treatment to obtain approval before proceeding; and another Thomsonian practitioner, John Stevens, advised full discussion with the patient and his friends before starting treatment. Working men appreciated being treated as fellow human beings rather than as pauper criminals or hospital teaching fodder. Chemists and druggists offered their customers a degree of power and control over their treatment which was entirely absent in publicly-provided medical care. The corner-shop chemist was the product, not of working class ignorance, but of a culture, which although physically and financially constrained, valued independence and self-determination. The chemist's shop was attuned, in atmosphere and organisation, to the demands of that culture. "Thousands of persons apply daily to chemists for worm powders and other simple medicines", wrote a pharmaceutical chemist in 1864, "many of these customers are in a wretched state of poverty, and their children more than half-dead for want of proper food and attention; and in a great majority of cases they would rather pay the chemist a few pence than be sent to any public institution, or be contemptuously treated by a charity doctor".[98]

The chemists and druggists who met the health needs of the working class during the first half of the nineteenth-century had a hard life. The line between success and failure was a tenuous one: their own standard of living was scarcely higher than that of their customers. Running these small corner-shops was never easy: every member of the family was expected to help. The shop was said to be open from seven in the morning till eleven at night; in reality it never closed. The chemist was expected to deal with every emergency: he was general medical practitioner, surgeon, dentist and even man-midwife. The minimum amount of capital was invested in the business: the maximum amount of labour was required of all members of the family. The service was unpretentious, the shop itself simple, but it played a key role in community life. The corner-shop chemist was dynamically involved in the culture of the working class community. He was, in a real sense, a community pharmacist. The few general practitioners who tried to develop private practice among the labouring population did not generally live among them. For personal and professional reasons, general practitioners had their homes among the middle classes. In 1851, in Bristol as a whole, the number of chemists and druggists equalled that of medical practitioners; but in the poorer districts of Bedminster and the parish of St. Phillip and Jacob there were sixteen chemists and druggists and only five general practitioners.[99] The chemist and druggist lived and worked among the poor and identified himself with them: he shared their language and customs, their understandings and prejudices, their thinking and lifestyle. Knowing one's customers was a crucial part of the business.

The idea that chemists and druggists were ignorant and dangerous was a myth deliberately created by general practitioners who could not compete in open competition with them. In the eighteenth century, apprenticeship was the normal method of training for both the lesser professions and crafts and trades: attorneys, surgeons, and apothecaries as well as druggists, drapers, grocers, coachmakers, saddlers, and boot-and-shoe makers all qualified through apprenticeship. It was not until the nineteenth century that the lower branches of law and medicine turned to paper credentials as a means of differentiating themselves from the skilled trades. The higher branches, the ancient liberal professions of divinity, law, and physic, found no use for written examinations and little use for examination of any sort until well into the nineteenth century. A classical education and the right social connexions were the qualifications needed to become a clergyman, barrister or physician. Eighteenth and early nineteenth century physicians were not trained to perform a professional function but to live a suitably leisured and cultured life-style. They were "remarkable for their literary tastes and their association with the world of wealth rather than for professional skill or scientific eminence".[100] What medical education they did receive was more a form of trained incapacity than a method of acquiring effective ways of treating illness. The medical systems and theories they imbibed constituted barriers to scientific understanding. Apprenticeship, with all its faults, involved the tyro in the empirical acquisition of practical skills directly relevant to the treatment of disease.

Most chemists and druggists had, like general practitioners, served apprenticeships or shorter periods of training with established practitioners. Many worked as assistants before setting up on their own account. No one could hope to survive in such a highly competitive trade without a combination of manual skills, business sense and a considerable practical knowledge of medicine and pharmacy. Like other skilled or craft retailers, chemists and druggists were involved in processing and even producing the goods they sold. Such men required specialist knowledge to set up in business: their survival depended on their developing and extending their knowledge and skills through daily practice. It is, of course, part of the strategy of professionalisation to place greater value on book-learning and credentials than on manual skills and practical intelligence: but a man might satisfy the examiners at the College of Surgeons and Apothecaries Hall—and they were easily satisfied—but fail to convince the public of his worth. As Jacob Bell observed, "the diploma of the Apothecary is looked upon by the poorer classes more as a symptom of a longer bill than as a test of higher qualification".[101] There is no reason to believe that the early nineteenth-century chemist and druggist knew less about disease or was less capable of treating it effectively than any university-educated physician or doubly-qualified surgeon-apothecary. Untrammelled observation, personal experience, manual dexterity, and identification with and knowledge of the patient and her environment were more important assets than formal education and paper qualifications. Chemists and druggists were the most popular members of the medical profession. Few who fell ill failed to visit their shops. They dealt with far more patients than any other branch of the profession. They were the providers of primary health care for the whole population. Moreover, until 1913, the chemist and druggist carried out his work without any form of financial assistance from either the state or charities: on the contrary, he contributed increasingly to public funds through rates, taxes and the sale of duty-bearing goods.

* * *

"The Pharmaceutical Society at the outset had one very serious difficulty to contend with", observed Jacob Bell near the end of his life, "namely, the entire absence of fraternity and disposition to pull together, which was the proverbial characteristic of the chemists and druggists".[102] This lack of solidarity was the product of the system of social relationships in which they were implicated. Chemists and druggists were cut off from one another by marked differences in income, wealth, status and power. Instead of forming a coherent social stratum, their social positions mirrored the class and status divisions of the wider society. The substantial manufacturer-cum-retailer inhabited a different social world from that of the poor corner shopkeeper. They were enmeshed in distinct social networks, which determined the type and range of their activities, at work and in the community. More fundamentally, their involvement in these networks gave rise to their different conceptions of what constituted the core components of their occupational role.

In the daily routines of their working life, chemists and druggists, instead of being drawn into close contact with one another, were thrown apart and isolated. Their shops were, in general, scattered and dispersed: where they were huddled together in central shopping areas, proximity engendered rivalry rather than co-operation. The chemist and druggist spent his days serving his customers and working alongside the members of his family and (usually) his assistants and apprentices. They, rather than his fellow chemists, influenced his attitudes and expectations. The long hours worked and the involvement of the family tended to give the enterprise a socially withdrawn and even introverted character. Family relationships were moulded by the constraints of the business: wife and children were an integral part of the labour force. Few chemists could afford the luxury of separating home and work.

Jacob Bell believed that "the cold, shy reserve, almost amounting to suspicion", which was characteristic of chemists and druggists, stemmed from the isolation from one another in which they lived and worked. Their business does, at times, seem to have been conducted in an atmosphere of distrust and insecurity. The carefully guarded recipes passed on from father to son or favoured apprentice; the danger that sharp practices like adulteration might be exposed; the fear of loss of public confidence, a sure deathblow to any business; these were grist to the mill of secrecy. Their whole way of life encouraged chemists and druggists to look on one another as competitors rather than as brothers. The social order was perceived in terms of individualistic notions of personal achievement and initiative. The explanation of a man's success was sought for in the qualities which distinguished him from his fellows: his greater knowledge, special skill, his business acumen, his greater discipline or determination. The values embedded in the occupation celebrated individual difference rather than collective social action. Moreover, there was little or no occasion for chemists and druggists to meet one another: indeed, there were precious few opportunities for any form of social intercourse outside of work. Jacob Bell observed that most chemists and druggists never attended meetings and seldom read pamphlets. Until the publication of *The Chemist* in January 1840 there was no regular medium of communication between opinion-formers and the rank and file. The absence of a pharmaceutical press both reflected and reinforced the lack of occupational consciousness. Similarly, apprenticeship as a system of training reinforced isolation and individualism. Institutional education in schools and colleges brings pupils together to share common experiences and allows the development of an "esprit de corps" which can serve as the embryo of professional consciousness. Apprenticeship brings together master and pupil and individualises the learning process.

78

The pupil identifies, not with his fellow students, but with his master.

Jacob Bell noted that the "absence of sympathy or tendency towards any kind of union or social communication" was a widely-observed feature of the trade. Although collectively, chemists and druggists faced the same difficulties and would have benefited from each other's advice and help, each one experienced his problems as unique to himself and sought individual solutions. The isolated nature of the work environment inhibited the perception that he shared common interests with others. The daily routine served merely to increase the potential for hostility towards one another. Hence there developed a cautious isolationism in which the solitary practitioner guarded the secrets of his trade by keeping his own counsel and declining the company of possible rivals and competitors. The occupation was, indeed, prized for its ethos of independence and autonomy. A major attraction was the chance it offered to be one's own master.

Chemists and druggists emerge from the evidence as less a mutually supportive brotherhood than a crowd of individualists in which the class divisions and discriminations of society at large were repeated in a microcosmic form. The key feature is the absence of any network of co-operative relationships. Given the absence of cohesion within the pharmaceutical body and the lack of any sense of occupational solidarity, it is perhaps surprising that an association such as the Pharmaceutical Society was ever established. Jacob Bell recalled that:

> When the undertaking was at first proposed, it was considered by many persons to be chimerical and fruitless. It was said that there was in the trade no public spirit—no disposition to unite in any measures for the general benefit—that the jealousy prevailing between individuals would be an obstacle to any union among them; and it was a common remark that ... "the chemists would not pull together for six months.[103]

Establishing the Pharmaceutical Society was a very personal project. No one who had taken the trouble to investigate its feasibility would have considered undertaking it. The most cursory market research would have signalled failure. That the Pharmaceutical Society was actually founded was due to the vision and perseverance of one man. It became Jacob Bell's mission and vocation.

NOTES AND REFERENCES TO CHAPTER TWO

1. N. McKendrick, J. Brewer and J.H. Plumb, *The Birth of a Consumer Society* (1982)
2. Roy Porter, *Disease Medicine and Society in England 1550–1860* (1987) chapter 4
3. J.K. Crellin and J.R. Scott, *Glass and British Pharmacy 1600–1900* (1972)
4. J.E. Feldman, *Quacks and Quackery Unmasked* (1842) 12–15
5. Charles Knight (ed.) *London* (1843) vol.5 391
6. J.G.L. Burnby, *A Study of the English Apothecary from 1660 to 1760* (1983) 59
7. David L. Cowen, "Pharmacy and Freedom" *American Journal of Hospital Pharmacy* 41 (1984) 459–67
8. Peter Mathias, *The Transformation of England* (1979) 162
9. George Griffenhagen, *Medicine Tax Stamps Worldwide* (Milwaukee, 1971) 6–13
10. E.A. Wrigley, "A simple model of London's importance in changing English society and economy, 1650–1750", *Past and Present* 37 (1967) 44–60

11. Bell and Redwood 28.
12. J. Mortimer, *The Universal Director* (1763) 18
13. *Authentic Memoirs, . . . of the most eminent Physicians and Surgeons of Great Britain* (1818) xiii
14. Bell and Redwood 45, 68–9
15. E.C. Cripps, *Plough Court. the story of a notable pharmacy* (1927) and D. Chapman-Huston and E.C. Cripps, *Through a City Archway: the story of Allen and Hanburys, 1715–1954* (1954)
16. J.G.L. Burnby, *A study of the English Apothecary* 57–9
17. Bell and Redwood 119
18. J.G.L. Burnby, *A Study of the English Apothecary* 53
19. G.M. Watson, *The Business of an Eighteenth Century Chemist and Druggist*, typescript, RPSGB Library, 1958. A shorter version was published as "Some eighteenth-century trading accounts" in F.N.L. Poynter (ed.) *The Evolution of Pharmacy in Britain* (1965)
20. Irvine Loudon, *Medical Care and the General Practitioner 1750–1850* (Oxford 1986) 133–4
21. R. Campbell, *The London Tradesman* (1747) 64, 63
22. B.L. Anderson, "Money and the structure of credit in the eighteenth century", *Business History* 12 (1970) 85–101
23. Leslie G. Matthews, *History of Pharmacy in Britain* (1962) 317
24. J. Austen, *Historical Notes on Old Sheffield Druggists* (Sheffield 1961) 68
25. N. McKendrick, J. Brewer and J.H. Plumb, *The Birth of a Consumer Society* (1982)
26. J. Aikin, *Description of the Country from Thirty to Forty Miles Round Manchester* (1795) quoted in Asa Briggs, *The Age of Improvement* (1959) 64
27. Leslie G. Matthews, *History of Pharmacy* 215
28. Roy Porter and Dorothy Porter, "The rise of the English drugs industry: the role of Thomas Corbyn" *Med.Hist.* 33 (1989) 286
29. "A Bristol pharmacy passes", *C. & D.* 163 (1955) 146–7
30. P.J. and R.V. Wallis, *Eighteenth Century Medics* (2nd edition, Newcastle Upon Tyne, 1988)
31. A.E. Bailey, *Early Victorian Pharmacy*, typescript, R.P.S.G.B. Library, 1958. A shorter version was published as "Early nineteenth-century pharmacy" *P.J.* 185 (1960) 208–12
32. Hilary Marland, "The medical activities of mid-nineteenth-century chemists and druggists with special reference to Wakefield and Huddersfield", *Med.Hist.* 31 (1987) 415–439
33. *P.J.* 12 (1852–3) 98
34. J.K. Crellin, "Leicester and 19th century provincial pharmacy", *P.J.* 195 (1965) 417–20; *C. & D.* 2 (1861) 358–60
35. H. Marland, *Med.Hist.* 31 (1987) 415–439; Irvine Loudon, "The vile race of quacks with which this country is infested", in W.F. Bynum and Roy Porter (eds.) *Medical Fringe and Medical Orthodoxy, 1750–1850* (1987) 106–28
36. Edward Morris, *A History of the London Hospital* (1910) 175
37. *The Chemist* 1 (1840) 282
38. J.B. Atlay, *Sir Henry Wentworth Acland, A Memoir* (1903) 96, 325
39. P.S. Brown, "The providers of medical treatment in mid-nineteenth-century Bristol", *Med. Hist.* 24 (1980) 297–314
40. Adam Smith, *The Wealth of Nations*, edited by J.R. McCulloch (Edinburgh 1863) 585
41. S.W.F. Holloway, "The Apothecaries' Act, 1815: a reinterpretation", *Med. Hist.* 10 (1966) 124–9
42. S.W.F. Holloway, "Medical Education in England, 1830–1858", *History* 49 (1964) 299–324
43. *P.J.* 6 [2] (1864–5) 375, 11 [2] (1869–70) 404–8, 189 (1962) 33–5
44. F.M.L. Thompson, *Victorian England: The Horse-Drawn Society* (1970)
45. *The Chemist* 5 (1844) 322
46. Leslie G. Matthews, *History of Pharmacy* 238–9

47. H. Marland, *Med. Hist.* 31 (1987) 432

48. A. Wright, "Some Yorkshire Proprietaries", *Pharm. Hist* 10 (1980) 6–8

49. J.K. Crellin, *P.J.* 195 (1965) 419

50. H. Marland, *Med.Hist.* 31 (1987) 433

51. P.S. Brown "Medicines advertised in eighteenth-century Bath newspapers", *Med. Hist* 20 (1976) 152–68

52. P.S. Brown, "Some treatments of skin disease in eighteenth-century Bath", *International Journal of Dermatology* 21 (1982) 555–9.

53. P.S. Brown, "Female pills and the reputation of iron as an abortifacient", *Med. Hist.* 21 (1977) 291–304

54. P.S. Brown, "Social context and medical theory in the demarcation of nineteenth-century boundaries" in W.F. Bynum and Roy Porter, *Medical Fringe and Medical Orthodoxy, 1750–1850* (1987) 216–233

55. F. Engels, *The Condition of the Working Class in England*, translated and edited by W.O. Henderson and W.H. Chaloner (Oxford 1958) 117–8

56. Roy Porter, *Disease, Medicine and Society*

57. P.S. Brown, "Herbalists and medical botanists in mid-nineteenth-century Britain with special reference to Bristol", *Med. Hist.* 26 (1982) 405–20.

58. *Lancet* 1840–1 (2) 424

59. Roy Porter, "Medicine and the decline of magic", *Strawberry Fare* Autumn 1986, 88–94

60. Grant Uden (ed.) *The Recipe Book 1659–1672 of Archdale Palmer, Gent.* (Wymondham, 1985)

61. H. Marland, *Med. Hist.* 31 (1987) 429

62. British Library (BM 1507/1722). Booklet dated 1780.

63. G.S. Rousseau, "John Wesley's 'Primitive Physic' (1747)", *Harvard Libraray Bulletin* XVI (1968) 242–256

64. C.J. Lawrence, "William Buchan: medicine laid open", *Med. Hist.* 19 (1975) 20–35

65. Kate Arnold-Forster and Nigel Tallis, *The Bruising Apothecary, Images of Pharmacy and Medicine in Caricature* (1989)

66. Michael Neve, "Orthodoxy and Fringe: medicine in late Georgian Bristol" in W.F. Bynum and Roy Porter, *Medical Fringe and Medical Orthodoxy, 1750–1850* 40–55

67. John V. Pickstone, "Medical botany (self-help medicine in Victorian England)", *Manchester Literary and Philosophical Society, Memoirs and Proceedings* 119 (1976–7) 85–95

68. J.F.C. Harrison, "Early Victorian radicals and the medical fringe" in W.F. Bynum and Roy Porter, *Medical Fringe and Medical Orthodoxy, 1750–1850*, 198–215

69. P.S. Brown, *Med. Hist.* 26 (1982) 405–20.

70. P.S. Brown, in W.F. Bynum and Roy Porter, *Medical Fringe and Medical Orthodoxy, 1750–1850*, 216–233

71. Logie Barrow, "Democratic epistemology: mid-19th century plebian medicine", *Society for the Social History of Medicine Bulletin* 29 (1981) 25–9

72. *P.J.* 9 (1849–50) 101 and 10 (1850–1) 383: *The Times* 25 March 1850

73. Stanley Chapman, *Jesse Boot of Boots the Chemists: a study in business history* (1974) 32–7

74. Virginia Smith, "Physical puritanism and sanitary science: material and immaterial beliefs in popular physiology, 1650–1840", in W.F. Bynum and Roy Porter, *Medical Fringe and Medical Orthodoxy, 1750–1850*, 174–197

75. William H. Helfand, "James Morison and his pills", *Transactions of the British Society for the History of Pharmacy* 1 (1974) 101–35.

76. Ruth G. Hodgkinson, *The Origins of the National Health Service: The Medical Services of the New Poor Law, 1834–1871* (1967) 120–2, 136–7, 257–60, 364–7
H. Marland, *Med. Hist.* 31 (1987) 415–439

77. *Select Committee on Medical Relief* 1854 (348) XII Q.723
78. Irvine Loudon, *Medical Care and the General Practitioner* 235–48, 318–9
79. *Select Committee on Medical Poor Relief*, 3rd Report, 1844 (531) IX Q.9121
80. *Lancet*, 1854 (1) 458
81. *Lancet*, 1857 (2) 326
82. R.D. Waller, "Letters addressed to Mrs. Gaskell by celebrated contemporaries", *Bulletin of the John Rylands Library* XIX (1935)
83. Ruth G. Hodgkinson, *The Origins of the National Health Service* 120–2 364–5, 367
84. Irvine Loudon, *Medical Care and the General Practitioner* 237
85. *Lancet* 1854 (1) 458
86. *P.J.* 4 (1844–5) 249
87. T. Beddoes, *Rules of the Medical Institution for the Relief of the Sick and Dropping Poor* (Bristol, 1804) 93
88. *The Chemist* 3 (1842) 123
89. Ivan Waddington, "The role of the hospital in the development of modern medicine: a sociological analysis", *Sociology* 7 (1973) 211–224
90. Ruth Richardson, *Death, Dissection and the Destitute* (1987)
91. M.A. Crowther, "Paupers or patients? Obstacles to professionalisation in the Poor Law medical services before 1914", *Journal of the History of Medicine and Allied Sciences* 60 (1984) 33–54
92. Irvine Loudon, *Medical Care and the General Practitioner* 242
93. *The Times* 22 June 1841; *C. & D.* 3 (1862) 336–7
94. *Dr. Skelton's Botanic Record and Family Herbal* (1853) 314
95. *The Chemist* 2 (1841) 120
96. *The Chemist* 3 (1842) 88
97. *The Chemist* 2 (1841) 218
98. P.S. Brown, *Med. Hist.* 26 (1982) 414, 418; *C. & D.* 5 (1864) 196
99. P.S. Brown, *Med. Hist.* 24 (1980) 309
100. A.M. Carr-Saunders and P.A. Wilson, *The Professions* (1933) 71
101. *P.J.* 4 (1844–5) 248
102. *P.J.* 18 (1858–9) 600
103. *P.J.* 4 (1844–5) 4

CHAPTER THREE

The Foundation of the Pharmaceutical Society

Fiat emulsio—Make an emulsion

Medical reform and the general practitioner—The opposition to Benjamin Hawes'
Bill, 1841—The founding of the Pharmaceutical Society—The origins of the
Pharmaceutical Journal, the School of Pharmacy and the examination system—The
strategy of professionalism—Maintaining prices and reducing hours—The
benevolent fund—Education and collective social mobility—The origins of
scientific pharmacy—The Chemical Society, the Royal College of Chemistry and
the professionalisation of chemistry—The founders of the Pharmaceutical
Society—The Pharmaceutical Society as a professional association and its place in
the development of professions in Britain

In 1843 Jacob Bell wrote "a concise historical sketch of the progress of pharmacy in Great
Britain, from the time of its partial separation from the practice of medicine until the
establishment of the Pharmaceutical Society". The period covered was from the beginning
of the sixteenth century to the incorporation of the Pharmaceutical Society by Royal Charter
in 1843. The aim was to locate the creation of the Society within the history and the present
structure of the medical profession. Belying its title, the booklet is about retardation. The
absence of any significant British contribution to the evolution of pharmaceutical science is
seen as the consequence of the failure to develop the professional regulation of its
practitioners.

The gradual evolution of the science of pharmacy, from an amalgam of astrology and
alchemy towards an applied science, rooted in chemistry and botany, is charted with
reference to the successive editions of the London Pharmacopoeia from 1618 to 1836. The
paradox that a work, full of practical instructions for dispensing, should be produced by a
body, the College of Physicians, whose members publicly renounced the practice of
pharmacy, was a symptom of the organisational malaise of the chemist and druggist. The
co-existence of three discrepant Pharmacopoeias within the United Kingdom reflected the
continuing enmity between the Colleges of Physicians in London, Edinburgh and Dublin.
Bell presents the history of the medical profession as a story, not of the steady improvement
of medical education and health care, but rather of bitter conflict and struggle between
various groups of medical men. From the first medical act of 1511, the medical profession
has been a battleground. Physicians, surgeons, apothecaries and druggists have been
engaged in a series of acrimonious disputes over occupational territory. In the sixteenth

century while the physicians sought to prevent surgeons from practising physic, their own domain was being invaded by the apothecaries. Having separated from the grocers and set up, in 1617, their own Company, the apothecaries first established themselves as compounders and vendors of medicines and then began to claim the right to practise medicine. By the end of the seventeenth century physicians and apothecaries were locked in conflict. As the apothecary consolidated his position as a general practitioner in physic, surgery, pharmacy and midwifery, a gap appeared and was filled by a new class of compounders of medicines: the chemists and druggists. Jacob Bell discerns their genesis at the start of the eighteenth century. By 1730 the recriminations between them and the apothecaries were in full flood. Growing competition from the chemist and druggist led the apothecaries to seek protection from parliament: fighting a losing battle in the open market, they appealed to the legislature to create a monopoly in their favour. In 1794 the General Pharmaceutical Association of Great Britain was formed. The name is perhaps misleading: it was not an organisation of chemists and druggists but an association of apothecaries designed to resist the "encroachment which chemists and druggists have, of late years, made on the profession of the apothecary, by vending pharmaceutical preparations, and compounding the prescriptions of physicians". The General Pharmaceutical Association was short-lived and ineffective. The result of the apothecaries' exertions was not as anticipated: instead of a death-blow, their attack made the chemists and druggists unite to protect their interests. The position of chemists and druggists as suppliers of drugs and dispensers of medicines was strengthened. "The practising apothecaries justly complained that the dispensing chemist and druggists had greatly deteriorated the profits of their business", wrote Dr. G.M. Burrows (1776–1846), "but the practice had existed so long, that it had acquired from custom the force of law, and it was impossible by sudden violent means to suppress it".

Dr. Burrows was the chairman and driving force behind the Association of Apothecaries and Surgeon-Apothecaries, a body formed in 1812 to revive the programme of the General Pharmaceutical Association. In March 1813 a Bill prepared by the Associated Apothecaries was introduced in the House of Commons. "The chemists and druggists, against whom some of the most important provisions in the bill were levelled", reported Jacob Bell, "spontaneously took the alarm". A general meeting of chemists and druggists was held at the Freemasons' Tavern, Lincoln's Inn Fields and resolutions condemning the Bill were passed. A committee consisting of the leading chemists and druggists of the day including William Allen, John Savory, W.B. Hudson, Richard Phillips, Frederick Smith and John Bell was set up to organise opposition to the Bill. The campaign was co-ordinated to secure the maximum impact. An address urging the provincial chemists to support the movement was published immediately in seven of the leading newspapers. The brilliant young advocate, Henry Peter Brougham (1778–1868), who was later to secure renown as a legal reformer and Lord Chancellor, was retained as counsel. Model petitions were drawn up for various groups to present to parliament. An address, which analysed the Bill clause by clause and elaborated the objections to each, was printed and distributed, with an accompanying letter, to chemists and druggists throughout the country. They were urged to solicit their local M.P. to oppose the Bill. A circular letter was distributed to all members of the House of Commons. Those M.P.s already known to be favourable to the cause were contacted and briefed. George Canning, a former foreign secretary and a future prime minister, was interviewed and agreed to present the petition of the metropolitan druggists against the Bill. In many towns local associations were formed to consolidate the opposition and liberal subscriptions to the central fund were collected. A permanent fund of over £500 was established. Finally a delegation waited upon John Calcraft, the mover of the Bill, who agreed to its withdrawal.

The London Committee remained vigilant, and was able successfully to reapply the pressure when the Society of Apothecaries brought in its Bill in 1815 to regulate the practice of apothecaries. Section 28 of the Apothecaries Act exempted chemists and druggists from its operation. "The chemists and druggists", observed Jacob Bell, "by uniting their strength on the occasion, secured to themselves a continuance of all their former privileges". Clause 28 became a charter for the chemist and druggist, protecting him for over twenty five years from prosecution by the Society of Apothecaries.

The Apothecaries Act of 1815 was the abortive outcome of over twenty years of agitation by general practitioners who, in addition to claiming that their livelihoods were being undermined by the unfair competition of the druggist, also complained that their interests were not protected by any of the London medical corporations. The Act specified that in future apothecaries must be licensed by the London Society of Apothecaries, but it did nothing to improve the general practitioner's economic and social status.[1] The aftermath of the 1815 Act was recrimination rather than reconciliation. The divisions within the medical profession remained and were soon to be exacerbated by the arrival, in 1823, of Thomas Wakley's radical medical journal, the *Lancet*. In its pioneering days, the *Lancet* depicted the medical world as rotten with corruption and ineptitude. The London hospitals were rife with nepotism: patients suffered neglect, mistreatment and hamfisted surgery. Institutions created to protect the public damaged its health. The three medical corporations, the Royal College of Physicians, the Royal College of Surgeons and the Society of Apothecaries neglected their duties but abused their powers. Wakley believed that the medical profession would never attain its rightful place in society while it remained fragmented into the antagonistic and obsolescent branches of physic, surgery and pharmacy, each controlled by a self-perpetuating clique, utterly unrepresentative of the rank-and-file. Wakley's original solution was to turn the College of Surgeons into a democratically organised society of "surgeons in general practice", but, after a decade of unsuccessful struggle, the idea of uniting all general practitioners—whether physicians, surgeons or apothecaries—within a single organization gained ground. During the years 1845 to 1848 the attempt to establish a College of General Practitioners came near to fruition, but the scheme was finally abandoned in the face of the unrelenting opposition of the College of Surgeons.

Medical reform was intended to increase the corporate power of the medical profession within society. From one perspective we have seen that the professionalisation of medicine was an attempt to fix the patient more firmly under the control of the doctor. From another perspective it has all the appearance of an intra-professional struggle. Three general issues tended to recur in one form or another in virtually all aspects of the movement for medical reform. The first was the issue of occupational closure. Two approaches to licensure can be discerned in nineteenth century Britain. The restrictive approach, adopted in the 1815 Apothecaries Act, sought to restrict practice to qualified licentiates and make it an offence to practise without a licence. The definitional approach, adopted in the 1852 Pharmacy Act and the 1858 Medical Act, made it an offence to use a title for which one had not qualified, but otherwise left one free to practise. It was a characteristic Victorian compromise between regulation and free trade. Jacob Bell described it thus:

> the public were to be furnished with qualified practitioners in every department, and ample means provided for distinguishing between those who possessed the requisite proficiency and others; but no penalties were to be inflicted on persons who presumed to practise without a qualification, it being considered that the public are responsible for the results of patronizing such persons.

Instead of attempting to restrain the quack, inducements were offered to the qualified. Only the registered were eligible for such privileges as exemption from jury service, the right to recover fees in courts of law and appointment to public office.

Of crucial importance in the initiation of the medical reform movement was the attempt to eliminate the competition of the chemist and druggist and to create a monopoly for the licensed practitioner. In this the Apothecaries Act proved useless: unlicensed practice flourished with as much impunity after 1815 as before. The way the Society of Apothecaries used its powers gave restrictive licensure a bad name: instead of protecting the public from quacks, the Society sought to enhance its monopoly by harassing the more highly educated practitioners. "Men of rank and medical education were prosecuted by the Company", the *Lancet* observed, "while the uneducated pretender revelled in success and luxury".[2] The later campaign for medical registration was designed both to restrict entry into the profession and to suppress unqualified practice. Although there was no serious disagreement within the profession on the desirability of registration, there was a major division of opinion between the general practitioners and the Royal Colleges on the precise form the Register should take. As part of their attempt to break down the traditional barriers within the profession, the general practitioners wanted a single register, simply listing in alphabetical order all qualified practitioners, according them the same legal status and giving them the right to practise generally. The Royal Colleges, however, insisted that there should be three separate registers, one for physicians, one for surgeons, and one for apothecaries, thus maintaining the three "estates", each with its own exclusive, legally defined sphere of practice.[3]

The second issue was that of political representation. One of the most persistent demands of the general practitioner was for some form of participation in the affairs of the medical corporations. During the eighteenth century, the Royal College of Physicians successfully resisted all attempts to undermine its oligarchic structure. All political offices and decision-taking functions within the College were monopolised by the fellows, almost all of whom were graduates of Oxford and Cambridge and members of the Church of England. Neither the licentiates nor the extra-licentiates were allowed to vote in College elections or take part in formulating College policy. In the 1820s the members of the Royal College of Surgeons mounted an attack on the Council of twenty-one "pure" surgeons which ran the college and renewed itself by co-optation. They demanded that the officers of the College should be elected annually by the whole membership so that each member "may have a voice in the election of those persons who are to regulate the proceedings of the College". William Gaitskell put the matter succinctly in a letter to the *Lancet* in 1830:

> Various branches of the medical profession have colleges, charters, and corporations, from which the general practitioner is either altogether excluded, or

86

attached as an appendage only; he is not admitted to a participation in their councils, or to a share in their honours; as a general practitioner, he belongs exclusively to no one branch, and is, therefore, virtually excluded from all.[4]

The plans to establish new institutions to license practitioners, such as the London College of Medicine (1831–40) and the College of General Practitioners (1845–50), included provision for the effective participation of general practitioners in their government. The fact that the interests of the rank and file were unrepresented in the governing bodies of the profession was one of their most deeply-felt grievances: the enfranchisement of the general practitioner held a prominent place on the agenda for reform.

The third, related, issue was that of education and examination for general practice. General practitioners had special educational needs which were not being met by the existing medical corporations. The general practitioner was not a physician, nor a surgeon, nor an apothecary: his practice was based on the integration of all three branches. It was precisely this fact that led the medical corporations to disown him and deny him representation within them. None of them was willing to provide an appropriate examination and licence for general practice or even to recognise its importance. Thus, within the proposed College of General Practitioners, the intention was to examine "not in medicine alone, not in surgery alone, not in midwifery alone, or pharmacy alone, but in all those branches that are essential to constitute an efficient general practitioner". Radical reformers wanted to sweep away the existing nineteen licensing bodies with their geographical limits to practice and substitute a single national board to grant registrable qualifications valid throughout the United Kingdom. The more cautious believed that educational standards could be maintained by simply establishing a central supervisory council.

A central component of the process of medical reform was the struggle of the self-assertive general practitioner to achieve professional status. From 1794 to 1858 he became the protagonist in a protracted and often bitter conflict with the medical corporations and the chemist and druggist. Although the general practitioner's demands were closely inter-related, different aspects tended to come to the fore at different times. Moreover, the leadership of the campaign tended, especially during the 1830s and 40s, to pass rapidly from one short-lived organisation to another. The picture is further complicated by the fact that, although general practitioners were generally united in their opposition to both the chemist and druggist and the policies of the Royal Colleges, they were, on occasion, deeply divided as to the precise nature of the reforms they wished to bring about. Within parliament, the situation became at times particularly confused: between 1840 and 1858 there were no less than seventeen different medical reforms bills introduced into the House of Commons and, on one occasion, there were three separate Bills before the House at the same time.[5]

From 1834 the House of Commons became an increasingly important focus for the activities of medical reformers. In that year the Commons appointed a Select Committee, under the chairmanship of Henry Warburton, M.P. for Bridport, a timber merchant in Lambeth, to inquire into the state of the medical profession.

> The object of this Committee was to revise all the laws relating to the medical profession, to obtain authentic and satisfactory evidence in every department of the subject, and to reform any abuses which might be found to exist. Every person who was supposed to be likely to possess information of any importance was examined, and the mass of evidence thus collected was, as might have been expected, very voluminous.

The papers of the Warburton Committee were stored in a room in the old House of Commons at the time of the great fire in October 1834 and most of the material relating to pharmacy was destroyed.[6] In the end the Committee produced neither report nor recommendations but the surviving evidence was printed in full in 1835. Sufficient material was preserved to enable Henry Warburton, assisted by Thomas Wakley and Benjamin Hawes, to prepare "A Bill for the Registration of Medical Practitioners, and for establishing a College of Medicine, and for enabling the Fellows of that College to practise Medicine in all or any of its branches, and hold any Medical Appointments whatsoever, in any part whatsoever of the United Kingdom". The Bill, which was introduced on 11 August 1840, amounted to little more than an attempt to use legislation to set up one of Wakley's favourite projects, the London College of Medicine. Originally launched in 1831, the College of Medicine was designed to be a single, perfect corporation, democratically organised, with an impartial, efficient examining system, licensing all types of medical men as "doctors". It would have met all the general practitioner's requirements both in terms of providing a suitable education and licence and in terms of giving him effective political control over his own affairs. The new College possessed every virtue the existing corporations so conspicuously lacked. Warburton's Bill was withdrawn at an early stage. The absence of any penal provisions against the unqualified and the sheer complexity of the registration machinery were the principal objections raised.[7]

On 5 February 1841 a new Bill "to amend the Laws relating to the Medical Profession in Great Britain and Ireland" was introduced in the Commons by Benjamin Hawes (1792–1862), M.P. for Lambeth, a wealthy soap-boiler who married the sister of the great Victorian engineer, Isambard Kingdom Brunel. In introducing his Bill, Hawes made it clear that it embodied the general practitioners' programme of reform. "The profession at present was governed by nineteen self-elected medical bodies; it would, if his bill passed, be placed under the control of a council in each of the three kingdoms—the members of which would be elected by the whole body of the medical profession". Hawes argued "that there was no uniformity in the education of medical students, that there was no body to which they could look up, and that the medical profession generally had no confidence in the existing bodies". The licentiates of the Royal College of Physicians were excluded from all its privileges and the Fellows had employed their powers not for the benefit of the profession but for their own exclusive advantage. The Royal College of Surgeons was "a voluntary body, conferring diplomas, but without the power of giving legislative protection to its members—neither obtaining the confidence of nor conferring advantages upon the profession". "With regard to the Apothecaries' Company", he added, "it was so constituted, that it was impossible that it could obtain the confidence of the profession at large". His Bill would secure "uniformity of education, an authentic registration of the medical practitioners, and the establishment of a superintending body elected by the profession, to whom should be entrusted its general management".[8]

The Bill was an attempt to reform the whole medical profession, including chemists and druggists.[9] After the Bill was printed, Hawes claimed that he had no desire to injure or oppress the chemists; that while he proposed to restrict them, he also proposed to raise their character, to make them an educated body and to give them rank and privileges. He considered that the position he had assigned them was a boon rather than an injury.[10] Certainly the fact that his medical reform Bill included provisions for the education and regulation of chemists and druggists acknowledged their importance in health care. The Bill gave especial attention to the publication of a national Pharmacopoeia and the need to ensure strict adherence to its authority in dispensing. Moreover, chemists and druggists, together with other medical practitioners, were to be privileged by exemption from holding parochial offices, performing militia and constable duties, and serving on juries and inquests. It is possible that Hawes was naive and had been hoodwinked by Thomas Wakley and other spokesmen for the general practitioners, for, in the last analysis, the effect of his Bill would have been to make counter prescribing illegal and to place the chemists and druggists under the control of their arch-rivals and competitors, the apothecaries.

On 10 February 1841 a small group of London chemists and druggists met at 40 Westminster Road, the home of Robert Adolph Farmar. They came together to examine the implications for chemists and druggists of the recently printed medical reform Bill introduced in the House of Commons by Benjamin Hawes. Anxiety permeated the gathering. Although the Bill seemed to presage a disaster for chemists and druggists, no sign of opposition to the measure had yet emerged. If the Bill became law, their business would be ruined. Any chemist who recommended ten grains of rhubarb, or strapped a cut finger, or explained to a customer the usual mode of taking a medicine would be liable to a penalty of £20 and to summary imprisonment (or a ruinous law-suit) for non-payment. Chemists and druggists would be placed under the jurisdiction of a governing body, in which they were not represented, but, in the election of which, their chief competitors, the apothecaries or general practitioners, would have the largest number of votes. George Walter Smith, an assistant to Baiss Brothers & Co., the wholesale druggists, and George Baxter, who owned the shop at 244 High Holborn, suggested that a public meeting of the members of the trade should be called for Monday 15 February at the Crown and Anchor tavern in the Strand. The group readily agreed and a decision was taken to advertise the meeting in the *Times* and *Morning Chronicle* and by circulars to the trade. Farmar, Smith, Baxter and their friends lost no time in visiting as many chemists and druggists as possible to obtain signatures to the requisition for a public meeting. Although the response from retailers was discouraging, they succeeded in gaining the support of the principal wholesaling and manufacturing chemists and druggists. Their names were listed in the circular inviting the members of the trade to the Crown and Anchor and they constitute, in effect, a directory of the chief drug and chemical wholesalers and manufacturers in London during the 1840s.[11] It was very much in the interests of these firms to maintain as many retail outlets as possible. They could be expected to oppose any attempt to restrict the free trade in drugs and chemicals.

The meeting on Monday 15 February was well attended. The chemists and druggists were determined to

> defend themselves against the perpetual and unfair encroachments and aggressions
> of general practitioners, who, both privately and publicly, are constantly seeking
> to oppress them and detract from their rights.

The focus of the meeting was on the need to protect the right of the chemist and druggist to prescribe, give medical advice and perform minor surgery. Charles James Payne, who was to become the first vice-president of the Pharmaceutical Society, declared:

> If they were not allowed to prescribe, it would be necessary for them to shut up their
> shops. Look at the druggists' shops in poor neighbourhoods, and see the advantages

which they conferred. They were the physicians to the poor … No legislative
interference could point out where the line of demarcation should be drawn, but
they should leave it to the public to judge for themseves in whom they could repose
their confidence.

Thomas Keating, of St. Paul's Churchyard and flea-powder fame, pointed out that, while
the apothecary's pursuits "led him from home a great portion of his time", the chemist
"was there constantly at home to attend the wants of the poor". Jacob Bell argued that the
proposed Act would seriously damage the trade and "materially affect the comforts and
resources of the poorer classes of society". He believed that

> It ought to be left to the public to decide whether they would go to the physician
> or apothecary, or be content with the aid of the chemist and druggist.

A committee, "composed of representatives of the leading wholesale houses and the
leading retail chemists of the metropolis" was formed "for the purpose of watching and
opposing the progress of this Bill".[12]

Immediately after the meeting, the committee met and resolved to circulate 3,000 printed
copies of the proceedings. An appeal for subscriptions was launched and petitions to
Parliament were drawn up. A small deputation waited upon Benjamin Hawes to detail the
objections to his Bill. On 19 February he withdrew the Bill and told the House of Commons
that he intended to bring in a new Bill which would exclude all reference to chemists and
druggists. Thomas Wakley made the angry ripost that, in that case, the new Bill "would
not be satisfactory to any portion of the medical profession".[13] Hawes, nonetheless,
persisted and brought in his new Bill "for the better Government of the Medical Profession
in Great Britain and Ireland" on 26 February.[14] But Wakley was right: even the chemists
and druggists found the second attempt no less objectionable than the first. On 17 March
a petition from the metropolitan chemists and druggists, with 604 signatures, was presented
to the House of Commons. It pointed out that, if the new Bill passed into law, the
apothecaries, "who though dealing in drugs and in the habit of compounding prescriptions,
also practise medicine by visiting patients" would acquire the power to harass chemists and
druggists

> and eventually to suppress their trade altogether, thereby establishing a monopoly
> of the sale and dispensing of drugs in their own body to the detriment of the public
> interest in general, but especially to the prejudice of the poorer classes who would
> be severely taxed by the higher prices which they would have to pay for drugs in
> ordinary use.

The petitioners trusted that

> your Honourable House will never sanction a measure which would violate the first
> principles of just and sound legislation by placing the interests and even the very
> existence of an important branch of trade throughout the whole United Kingdom
> dependent upon the arbitrary control of a class of persons having an interest in its
> discouragement and suppression.

When the speaker of the House of Commons inquired whether any members had
petitions to present against Hawes' Bill, over half the House rose simultaneously, and a
shower of petitions covered the table. The House was counted out.

The chemists and druggists had won a major battle but the war was not yet over. The reform of the medical profession was now firmly established on the political agenda. The editors of *The Chemist* warned of bills which "will have the effect of giving such advantages to apothecaries as may at once prove the destruction of the interests and rights of chemists".[15] Medical reform is a mere blind; the real object is further infringement of the rights of chemists and druggists. There were well-founded reports that the Society of Apothecaries, anticipating, perhaps, its demise as the main licensing authority for general practitioners, was seeking new powers to compel chemists and druggists to undergo a qualifying examination in the Latin Pharmacopoeia, pharmaceutical chemistry and materia medica at Apothecaries Hall. In March, the College of Physicians revealed its plan to institute, with the help of the Apothecaries' Company, an examination for chemists and druggists.[16] Only the College of Surgeons, with problems enough of its own, had no intention of interfering with pharmacy. In their official capacity as pure surgeons, "they did not pretend to be able to distinguish one drug from another, and trusted to those whose duty it was to prepare their prescriptions".[17] The recently formed General Committee of metropolitan druggists wisely decided to remain *in situ* to await the next moves.

At this point, proceedings take a novel turn. On 20 March, the General Committee met as usual at 31 Throgmorton Street, the home of the treasurer, Richard Hotham Pigeon to hear the chairman, Joseph Gifford, report the recent triumph in the House of Commons. Once again the chemists and druggists had come together to ward off an attack on their privileges. The victory of 17 March was the latest in a struggle that had already spanned fifty years. But new developments were in the air. When the official meeting ended, a carefully selected group of committee members met for tea at 338, Oxford Street, the home of one of their number, Jacob Bell. He had set his mind on transforming the informal, ad-hoc committee of London druggists into a permanent professional organisation. When the idea of such a body was first mooted, "the most experienced members of the trade maintained that it would be impossible to form an association of chemists and druggists under any circumstances". "A few days occupied in personal communication with chemists in different parts of London", reported Jacob Bell, "tended at first rather to confirm this impression". There was no doubt that "they were resolved and determined in resisting any interference, and especially the endeavour to place them under the jurisdiction of the apothecaries". But "this, in fact, was the only subject on which any union whatever existed among them".[18] Bell decided to strike while the iron was hot: the opportunity might not speedily occur again.

> A correspondence had been opened with the chemists in all parts of the country on a subject in which all their interests were concerned; in the excitement occasioned by the threatened blow at their independence, minor considerations were forgotten; and all appeared disposed cordially to unite in promoting the general welfare . . . in the present crisis, jealousy seemed to be forgotten.

Bell decided to concentrate his efforts on the members of the General Committee. Among them, the idea of establishing a society was by now common property. It had frequently surfaced in their discussions only to sink under the weight of divergent blue-prints.

> The members of the Committee saw plainly that nothing short of a permanent Association could secure the trade against a recurrence of the inconveniences and

annoyances which it had from time to time experienced during the last half century ... But the task was one which required the most mature deliberation and unwearied perseverance. The members of the Committee were not unanimous either as to the details of the plan or the mode of accomplishing it, and there was every reason to anticipate still greater difficulty in amalgamating the various opinions of the body at large on so intricate and momentous a question.

Jacob Bell was astute enough to realise that no agreement would be reached in open committee: members needed to be taken on one side until a majority for the new initiative had been forged. The first "pharmaceutical tea-party" brought together those members of the committee who had already indicated their support for Bell's proposals. After a friendly discussion, they "agreed to a few resolution as the basis to the new society".

> Several other meetings of this unofficial character took place, at each of which other members were added to the number, until twenty-four of the Committee were unanimous on the general principles of the Association.

With a majority secured, Bell now referred the matter to the General Committee on 5 April, when the following resolutions were unanimously carried:

> 1st. That the permanent interests of Chemists and Druggists require that they shall immediately form themselves into a society.
>
> 2nd. That this Society be forthwith formed under the title of the PHARMACEUTICAL SOCIETY OF GREAT BRITAIN.
>
> 3rd. That the Society consist, in the first instance, of such established Chemists and Druggists as shall voluntarily come forward in aid of its objects and intentions.
>
> 4th. That the object of the Society be,—To benefit the public, and elevate the profession of Pharmacy, by furnishing the means of proper instruction; to protect the collective and individual interests and privileges of all its members, in the event of any hostile attack in Parliament or otherwise; to establish a club for the relief of decayed or distressed members.
>
> 5th. That at a general meeting of Chemists and Druggists, to be convened for the purpose of forming an outline of the Society, a Committee be appointed to frame such laws and regulations as may appear desirable for the attainment of the objects intended, which laws, etc., shall be afterwards discussed and completed at another general meeting of the members.

In accordance with these resolutions a public meeting was convened at the Crown and Anchor Tavern in the Strand on Thursday 15 April 1841. On that occasion the General Committee presented its report on the successful campaign against Hawes' Bill and urged the immediate formation of a permanent association, "having for its object the union of the members of the trade into one body, the protection of the general interests, and the improvement and advancement of scientific knowledge". Education, examination, registration, and representation were to be the watchwords of the new society. The historic resolution, "that for the purpose of protecting the permanent interests, and increasing the respectability of Chemists and Druggists, an Association be now formed under the title of the PHARMACEUTICAL SOCIETY OF GREAT BRITAIN", moved by William Allen and seconded by John Bell, was unanimously adopted. The existing committee was then requested to frame laws and regulations for the government of the society. At a subsequent general meeting, held at the Crown and Anchor on Tuesday 1 June, "the fundamental laws" were submitted and adopted. The society was to be governed by a council, consisting of twenty-one members, to be elected every year in May. A special resolution, however, was passed allowing the forty members of the General Committee to become the society's first council, with authority to act as such until the following May. William Allen was elected president; Charles James Payne, vice-president; Richard Hotham Pigeon, treasurer; and George Walter Smith and Robert Adolph Farmar, joint honorary secretaries. At the same time as the provisional committee was engaged in preparing the laws and constitution of the new society, Jacob Bell instituted a series of monthly scientific meetings at his house,

> for the purpose of diverting the minds of the members from political contentions to scientific pursuits, and of counteracting the petty jealousies of the *trade* by promoting an interest in the advancement of the *profession*.[19]

Theophilus Redwood recalled these early gatherings:

> ... as the new society had now been founded, these were ostensibly meetings of the society, to which the members, together with medical and other scientific men ... were invited for the purpose of reading and discussing papers relating to the practice of pharmacy. Although instituted and conducted by Mr. Bell on his sole responsibility and at his expense, these meetings were designed ... for the purpose of illustrating the advantage of scientific discussion, and as a starting point for meetings of a similar description which it was hoped the Pharmaceutical Society would carry out ... Mr. Bell's rooms were crowded, and men pursuing the same occupation in the same street or neighbourhood, who had never before exchanged a friendly greeting, were here hustled together, brought face to face and warmed into recognition ...

Jacob Bell was quick to realise that provincial chemists and druggists would need to be won over to the idea of a permanent professional association. In the absence of a national register, the best way of compiling a list of their names and addresses was from the information held by the wholesale druggists and the Society of Friends.[20] Bell's access to these sources, combined with his wealth and literary skill, placed him in a unique position to carry out this task. In June, he had 2,000 free copies of his pamphlet, *Observations addressed to the Chemists and Druggists of Great Britain on the Pharmaceutical Society*, distributed throughout the country. In July, he published, on his own initiative and at his own expense, the papers read at the first two scientific meetings held at his house as *The Transactions of the Pharmaceutical Meetings*. In the second number, which appeared on 1 August, the contents were widened to give the appearance of a scientific journal and the title changed to *Pharmaceutical Transactions*. The first six issues were printed for free distribution to chemists and druggists throughout Britain to make known the nature, objectives and constitution of the newly formed Pharmaceutical Society. As well as reports of meetings and scientific papers, the early numbers contain the prospectus of the Society, with an account of its origin; a comparison of the disunited and undervalued condition of pharmacy in Britain with the superior scientific and professional status of its practitioners on the Continent and even in America; and Jacob Bell's replies to a series of criticisms of and inquiries about the new Society. By September some members of the Society felt that it should undertake to publish its own transactions. No one, however, came forward with any definite proposals. Instead the Council agreed to purchase, each month, a sufficient number of Bell's periodical to be furnished, free of charge, to each member and associate. Bell readily agreed to the condition that the Society's transactions should be kept apart from other material and he adopted the new, more comprehensive, title, the *Pharmaceutical Journal*, to avoid the implication that it was an official publication of the Society.

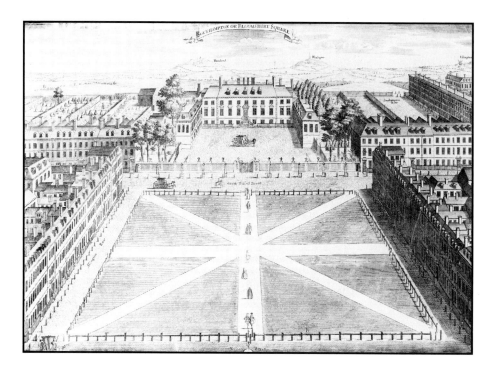

19   *Topographical view of Bloomsbury Square, by Sutton Nicholls published for a 1754 edition of* Stow's Survey, *looking north towards Bedford House. It shows the original appearance of 17 Bloomsbury Square before it was remodelled by John Nash in 1778.*

In September 1841 the Council began looking for suitable premises to serve as the Society's headquarters. In December, the house at 17 Bloomsbury Square was acquired, on a year to year basis, at a rent of £240: the agreement provided that the Council could relinquish it "when it may be desirable to do so". The first meeting, a meeting of council, was held there on 6 January 1842 and arrangements were immediately made for holding an evening meeting of the Society there on 12 January. The acquisition of permanent accommodation led to other changes. In place of two honorary secretaries, George Walter Smith was appointed resident secretary at an annual salary of £150 "with coals and candles". The appointing committee already had evidence of Smith's "industry, zeal and ability" and his employers, Baiss Brothers & Co., spoke handsomely of him. Moreover, the Committee have had an opportunity of learning that it is his anxious desire to promote the general objects of the Society and to give every satisfaction to the Council by sedulous attention to his duties, and courteous and consistent deportment.

A policeman and his wife were re-engaged to keep the rooms clean.

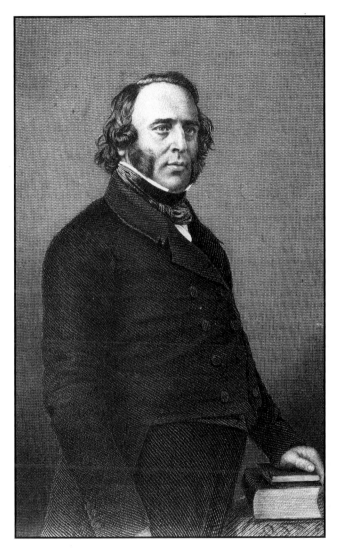

20   *Jonathan Pereira (1804–1853). Engraving by D.J. Pound from a daguerreotype by J.E. Mayall. Author of* The Elements of Materia Medica. *In 1843 Pereira was appointed Professor of Materia Medica at the Society's School of Pharmacy.*

The attention of the Council was concentrated from the beginning on establishing an examination system and a school of pharmacy. A series of evening lectures was immediately started as the forerunner of systematic courses of instruction. On 16 February Dr. Anthony Todd Thomson delivered an introductory lecture on materia medica, which was followed by lectures: on 2 March by Dr. Andrew Ure on chemistry; 16 March by Theophilus Redwood on pharmacy; 30 March by Jonathan Pereira on recent discoveries in materia medica; 20 April by George Fownes on organic chemistry; and on 11 May by Dr. A.T. Thomson on botany. During this period, arrangements were made to start the school of pharmacy and professors were appointed in the relevant subjects: Dr. Thomson in botany, Dr. Pereira in materia medica, Mr. Fownes in chemistry and Mr. Redwood in pharmacy. Dr. Thomson started his course on 17 May, the others in the following October. A board of examiners, consisting of the president and vice-president and eight "dispensing chemists", was appointed and regulations for the examinations were adopted. There was to be a minor examination for associates and a major examination for members. Every person presenting himself for examination was required to produce testimonials of having been apprenticed to or regularly educated by a vendor of drugs or dispenser of medicines. The text book was to be the London Pharmacopoeia and questions on the chemistry, materia medica, botany and pharmacy embodied in that work, would be asked. Candidates were required to translate prescriptions and to demonstrate an acquaintance with practical pharmacy: they were also required to know the antidotes for common poisons.

> The Pharmaceutical Society is instituted, for the purpose of uniting the chemists and druggists into one ostensible, recognised, and independent body—for protecting their general interests—and for the advancement of Pharmacy, by furnishing such a uniform system of education, as shall secure to the profession and the public the safest and most efficient administration of medicine.

This declaration of the Society's objectives was included in the fundamental laws adopted by the general meeting of 1 June 1841. The Society, as constituted by those laws, consisted of members and associates. Full membership was restricted to chemists and druggists who were, or had been, established in business on their own account. A chemist and druggist was defined as "a person who has been apprenticed to or regularly educated by a vendor of drugs or dispenser of medicines and who does not profess to act as a visiting apothecary or surgeon". Assistants, even those who passed the major examination, were not eligible for membership, but could become associates. Associates were not entitled to attend general meetings, vote, or hold any office in the Society. The primary qualification for membership was thus not educational or scientific attainment, but ownership of property. Only masters could become members; employees were considered journeymen. During the first year all bona-fide chemists and druggists and their assistants were to be admitted to the Society on payment of the annual subscription of two guineas for members and one guinea for associates: but, at a future date, none would be admitted without examination.

The Society was to be governed by a Council of 21 members, elected by and from the members. Two-thirds of the Council would be elected each year. Although choosing to follow the example of the Royal College of Surgeons and the Society of Apothecaries in determining the size of its governing body, the founders of the Pharmaceutical Society were careful to guard against their unrepresentative nature. "While they have vested in the

Council sufficient powers to render their services effective, they have made them entirely responsible to, and to be elected by, the members at large". The President, Vice-President and Treasurer were to be chosen from and by the Council, which also had the task of appointing the Secretary. The Council was to meet monthly: it was to make bye-laws, appoint examiners and lecturers, and run the library, museum and laboratory.

As the foundations of the Society were being laid in London, Jacob Bell was out and about drumming up support. No matter how splendid the Society might appear on paper, it would, without members, have neither the financial nor moral resources to carry out its objectives. A sizeable membership was required to "obtain the looked-for assistance from Government and the legislature. The object sought, however, was not easily to be accomplished among a class of men hitherto unorganized and unaccustomed to combined action". In starting the *Pharmaceutical Journal*, Bell had hoped to mobilise nation-wide support for his conception of a professional and scientific association of chemists and druggists.

> But it was necessary also to communicate personally with the members of the trade, many of whom never attended meetings, others seldom read pamphlets, and very few had ever bestowed a thought on the subject, or felt the want of scientific improvement. Still less could they understand what connexion could possibly exist between their personal interests, as chemists and druggists, and a pharmaceutical society, with school of pharmacy, board of examiners, and other arrangements for instructing the rising generation ... The chief difficulty consisted in inducing the parties concerned to give their attention to the subject. Being men of retired habits, generally at home, and seldom interfering with public business, something like a house to house visitation was necessary to bring the merits of the question fully and fairly before each and all of those whose co-operation was desired.[21]

The successful establishment of the Pharmaceutical Society became Jacob Bell's personal mission. In all his work for the Society the effects of his Quaker upbringing can be seen. The relentless drive, the single-mindedness, the discipline, the unremitting effort spring from deep inner sources. The silent dignity that enabled him to endure personal verbal abuse and repeated setbacks without recrimination and remorse is characteristic of Friends. The Quaker conviction that all differences can be settled by patient discussion and mutual respect led him to believe in the practice of bringing chemists and druggists together to discuss frankly the issues affecting them. On a more superficial level, the tactics he used and the style of his leadership were clearly based on Quaker foundations. His decision to visit, at his own cost, different parts of the country to make a personal appeal to chemists and druggists to support the Society has its parallel in the Quaker practice of travelling in the ministry. Soon after the foundation of the Society, he visited Bath, Bristol, Clifton, Exeter, Plymouth and Devonport. Later he went to Birmingham, Liverpool, Manchester, Newcastle, Leeds, Nottingham, Norwich, Dover and Brighton:

> for the purpose of bringing the members of the trade together, in towns where such meetings had rarely or never before occurred, and where, as in London, druggists were accustomed to look upon each other with jealousy and distrust. The mere act of bringing them together ... was an important step towards the social improvement of the body.

Theophilus Redwood adds that

> the unostentatious and disinterested zeal he manifested on these occasions gained for him a cordial welcome and attentive consideration of the subject of his mission.[22]

The Quaker tradition of inner strength to cope with the assaults and temptations of the external world, and the deep conviction of the ultimate triumph of the cause, are reflected in the way Jacob Bell set out to win converts:

> Starting on the hypothesis that the Society must sooner or later maintain its ground, the following rules of action were found essential in the preliminary labour of breaking the ice:- 1. Never to take offence at any reception, however cool, abrupt, or even rude. 2. Not to be discouraged at a cold shoulder. 3. Not to look down on a man because he has a small shop or lives in a back street. 4. Never lose sight of the main object, from a mistaken notion of dignity and self-respect. 5. Never be goaded into a quarrel or loss of temper. Experience fully demonstrated the efficacy of this line of policy . . .
>
> One of the most delicate matters to deal with at this early period was the alleged personal differences between members of the trade. It was a common remark, "Be careful not to ask A to meet B, they are not on good terms," or "C and D have not spoken to each other for years," etc. My answer in such cases was, "Then it is quite time to begin speaking to each other, and, as for feuds and differences, it is not our business to see them. Of course all were invited, they shook hands, and the clouds vanished . . .
>
> I was sometimes blamed by members of the Committee for "wasting my time" in "dancing attendance on men who were of no consequence". Here, again, I took the liberty of differing, my theory being that every man is of consequence. One who can argue cleverly on the wrong side could argue better on the right, his ability would then be available FOR instead of AGAINST the Society; he may also have a circle of friends over whom he has influence.[23]

In September 1841 the number of members and associates was 450: by the end of the year, it was about 800 and by May 1842, it had risen to just under 2,000.

In November 1841 a public meeting took place which was important, both financially and symbolically, to the newly formed society. During the years 1813–15 chemists and druggists had successfully repelled the attempts to control them by both the Association of Apothecaries and Surgeon-Apothecaries and the Society of Apothecaries. At the end of the campaign, the surplus of the fighting fund that had been created by nation-wide subscription, remained invested in the names of the trustees. On Monday 1 November 1841, the subscribers decided to present the balance to the Pharmaceutical Society. The resolution declared

> That the original object of this fund being the protection and advancement of the interests of chemists and druggists, this meeting . . . desires to recognise in the establishment of the Pharmaceutical Society of Great Britain a permanent and legitimate means of accomplishing such object; namely, by a general union and organization for the protection of present privileges and the education and improvement of the future members of the trade.

Jacob Bell's comments on this meeting are very instructive. The transfer of £862 18s. 2d. connected the Pharmaceutical Society with the chemists and druggists who, twenty-five years earlier, had won a major victory over the apothecaries. Yet it was the differences rather than the similarities that were more important:

> On the former occasion the proceedings of the trade were directed to a defensive resistance of threatened encroachments, and contemplated merely the preservation of accustomed rights and privileges by legal means and parliamentary influence. In the establishment of the Pharmaceutical Society ... the extension of pharmaceutical knowledge and the further improvements in the qualifications of the trade, individually and collectively, became the basis of the defence which was set up against future innovations or restraint.[24]

* * *

From the beginning of the nineteenth century short-lived associations of chemists and druggists were formed whenever attempts were made to impose restrictions or taxes upon them. In 1802 a small group of metropolitan apothecaries and chemists and druggists secured a modification in the new Medicine Act. In 1829 the threat arising from the exaction of new penalties under the Medicine Stamp Acts led to the formation of "The General Association of Chemists and Druggists of Great Britain". It survived little longer than it took for the grievance to be met by the Commissioners of Stamps. In 1819 a committee of metropolitan chemists and druggists helped to secure the withdrawal of a bill to regulate the sale of poisons. In 1838 "The Druggists' Provident Association", with the aims "of affording relief and assistance to its members in cases of sickness and distress, and of giving information to persons seeking to obtain situations in the trade", was formed with G.W. Smith as secretary and Francis Fisher as treasurer. Its life was brief: in 1841 it transferred its funds (a mere £15) to the Pharmaceutical Society's benevolent fund. Finally, the introduction of Benjamin Hawes' Medical Reform Bill, which revived the proposal to put the control of chemists and druggists in the hands of the apothecaries, precipitated the events that led to the formation of the Pharmaceutical Society.

These ephemeral, *ad hoc* associations represent the emergence of the chemist and druggist on the political scene. But they should not be interpreted as expressions of an incipient occupational consciousness, nor as stepping stones towards the establishment of a permanent professional organisation. Obvious features of these gatherings militate against such a view. They were protest meetings, reactions against interference, designed to restore the status quo. There were no calls for change, no list of radical demands, no programmes of reform, no desire for permanent organisation. All that there was, was a plea to be left alone, not to be unfairly taxed, not to be placed under grievous restrictions. Whenever their immediate interests were threatened, the London druggists would come together to stave off the attack: but there was no enthusiasm for projects of reform and regulation. When two of the most highly regarded London wholesale druggists, John Savory and W.B. Hudson, tried, in 1830, to interest "a considerable number of the chemists and druggists in London" in such a programme, they received "so little encouragement ... that the project fell to the ground". Their proposal had been to petition the government to introduce a bill to regulate the practice of pharmacy.

> The memorial which was prepared contained a brief and appropriate exposition of the importance of pharmacy to the health and life of His Majesty's subjects; the necessity of education and integrity in those whose duty it is to carry into effect the instructions of medical men; the prevalence of ignorant and incompetent persons

calling themselves chemists and druggists, and the frequency of injury to the public from this source; the difficulty of detecting adulterations and the necessity of proper qualification in pharmaceutists, in order to enable them to perform their duty in this respect; the advantages resulting from pharmaceutical education in foreign countries; the danger arising from the uncontrolled sale of poisons by ignorant persons; and, finally, the absolute necessity of some sanitary regulations for the elevation of this department in the profession, and the protection of the public.

This petition represents a summary of the grievances and solutions which reformers were to repeat for the remainder of the century. In 1830, however, the memorial proved abortive, "on account of the want of unanimity in the trade", and "because the parties concerned ... were not disposed ... to coalesce and embark in an undertaking which would have involved a departure from the strictly *defensive* policy hitherto adopted ...[25]

It is tempting, but quite wrong, to see the Pharmaceutical Society as a form of permanent organisation crystallising out of the series of public protest meetings which preceded it. There was nothing inevitable about the establishment of the Society. All the evidence suggests that, without the intervention of Jacob Bell, the struggle against Benjamin Hawes' Bill would have ended, like all previous struggles, with the chemists and druggists securing their privileges, but without the setting up of any form of permanent organisation. The fundamental divisions within the trade would have ruined any attempt to create an association based solely on political and commercial interests.

> Contentions with the apothecaries, defensive struggles against the Legislature or the Board of Excise, projects for equalising prices, or the early closing of shops, had agitated at intervals the Pharmaceutical body. These commotions, like the waves of the sea, had succeeded each other, each in turn producing a due proportion of foam, and then disappearing.[26]

The only bond of union among chemists and druggists was their determination to resist interference. The pharmaceutical body was not a tightly-knit band of brothers, awaiting formal recognition of their unity, but a number of disparate segments, pursuing different objectives, in different ways. The statement that "the time had become ripe for an organization devoted entirely to the interests of pharmacy" is either tautological or incorrect. The foundation of the Pharmaceutical Society was not the logical culmination of any growth in professional consciousness or solidarity

> Prior to the establishment of the Pharmaceutical Society there was no social or professional intercourse among chemists and druggists,—no medium of communication,—no common principle of action, or bond of union. Trade jealousies, suspicion and distrust, prevailed to such an extent as to render it difficult to bring the members of the trade together or to induce them to join in any common object. It required a man of independent means, disinterestedly devoted to the work, with tact, temper, and powers of persuasion, to overcome the difficulties of the undertaking, and such a man was Jacob Bell.[27]

It would be difficult to improve upon Theophilus Redwood's assessment. Jacob Bell's great achievement was to seize the opportunity presented by the proceedings against the 1841 Medical Reform Bill to set up the Pharmaceutical Society. It involved transforming an occasional, informal committee of London druggists into a permanent professional organisation. It entailed persuading the metropolitan elite to move from a defensive, laissez-faire position to one which sought actively to regulate and control the occupation. It meant the adoption of an aggressive professionalising strategy in place of the former protective trading policy.

When the Pharmaceutical Society was first established, there was little support from the majority of chemists and druggists for a permanent occupational association. Most of them believed, with good reason, that a British government, committed to free trade and open competition, was unlikely to impose restrictions and regulations on them. Present arrangements worked well. Each class of society was provided with the practitioners it could afford and the sale of patent medicines helped fill the Treasury's coffers. It was, therefore, more than fortunate for the survival of the Pharmaceutical Society during its first decade, that the radical medical reformers and the Society of Apothecaries both maintained their open hostility towards chemists and druggists, and that Sir James Graham, the Home Secretary in Sir Robert Peel's administration of 1841 to 1846, decided to promote a government bill for the regulation of the medical profession. In its early days the main attraction of the Pharmaceutical Society for most chemists and druggists was as a political organisation to protect their rights and privileges against attack by the apothecaries.

The fear aroused by medical reform bills was increased by the rearguard action of the Apothecaries' Company. By the 1840s their influence was already on the wane. Repeatedly snubbed by the College of Physicians and treated with contempt by Sir James Graham, the Society of Apothecaries sought to curry favour with the general practitioner by harassing the chemist and druggist. They made no attempt to conceal their hostility towards the newly-formed Pharmaceutical Society. In their view, it was not only unnecessary, "but in many respects highly objectionable". The chemist and druggist should not be elevated at the expense of the legally qualified apothecary: there was no need for any new body to examine and regulate chemists and druggists: the Apothecaries' Company was ready to do that themselves.[28] In the Spring of 1841, when the foundations of the Pharmaceutical Society were being laid, the Society of Apothecaries decided it was an appropriate moment to take its first case, under the 1815 Act, against a chemist and druggist for practising as an apothecary without their licence. Although Mr. Greenough of Liverpool, the chemist in question, admitted attending, advising and furnishing medicines to patients, the Lower Court held that he was protected by clause 28 of the Apothecaries Act. However, on appeal by the Society of Apothecaries, the Court of Queen's Bench ruled that if a chemist not only sold, but also administered medicines in the course of attending patients, he was practising as an apothecary and was not protected by clause 28.[29] The *Lancet*, the self-appointed spokesman of the general practitioner, lost little time in ramming home its interpretation of this decision. From September to November it went through the case, week by week, exalting in this victory of the apothecaries over their rivals, and vividly exaggerating the dangers to the public of unqualified prescribing. The Pharmaceutical Society handled the matter calmly and with due attention to the facts of the case. The Council made a decision, at the outset, not to support Greenough

> as he had been in the habit of acting professedly as a surgeon, designating himself
> as such in his bills, and charging for attendance as a medical practitioner ... By
> this course they consider that he had exceeded the legitimate function of a chemist

101

and druggist and had, in fact, made himself ineligible as a member of the Pharmaceutical Society.

In spite of all the fuss made by Thomas Wakley and the Society of Apothecaries, the Greenough decision was of little consequence: it had no bearing on the vital question of counter prescribing. "We cannot consider the case of Mr. Greenough at all applicable to chemists and druggists in general", wrote Jacob Bell, "and consequently the Pharmaceutical Society could not interfere in it in any way". Moreover, the legal judgment "cannot be considered a precedent which affects materially, if at all, the interests of chemists and druggists".[30] It was true that many chemists and druggists, particularly those in working-class areas, practised as apothecaries: but prohibiting them from visiting the poor would not help the general practitioner. Visiting patients was a loss leader: a way of maintaining good will but not of making money. The real bone of contention was counter prescribing. It was not the chemist visiting patients that riled the general practitioner but patients visiting the chemist.

In his efforts to drum up support for the infant Pharmaceutical Society, Jacob Bell was not averse to exploiting the anxiety and sense of foreboding among chemists and druggists. "The 'Medical Reformers' have not abandoned their design. They are only waiting for an opportunity to carry it into execution, and they are likely to persevere until an alteration of some kind is effected". Since "Chemists must and will be included in the scheme of 'reform', it remains for them to decide whether they will allow measures . . . to be forced upon them by persons who are indifferent or opposed to their interest, or whether they will maintain their independence under such regulations as shall conduce to their own welfare". The setting-up of the Pharmaceutical Society is "the only step which . . . can remedy existing evils and prevent the crisis of a destructive revolution by promoting a wholesome and desirable reform". "The daily papers and medical periodicals teem with gross and offensive attacks on chemists and druggists, which they are *not in a position* to refute; and charges are made against them which they are unable to controvert or to obviate". "They must in their present position, submit to any indignity because they have no power to resist it". Hence, "the chemists have no safe alternative but to take the government of their body into their own hands".[31]

Jacob Bell and his small coterie of London druggists intended to do exactly that; "to take the government of their body into their own hands". They used familiar arguments to justify their action. Unless we set our own house in order, others, much less benevolently disposed, will intervene. The public image of the profession can only be improved if the ignorant and unscrupulous members are rooted out. It is this "minority of the worst" which is dragging down the whole body, destroying the profession's credibility, undermining public confidence by its disreputable, unethical behaviour. The strictures of outsiders are made plausible by the actions of this small minority

> As long as chemists and druggists *collectively* neglect to take those means which are within their reach for rectifying these evils, the stigma, which ought to be confined to some individuals among them, is extended to all—as long as they continue to be subject to no educational regulations, they are exposed to the imputation of ignorance—as long as they are disjointed, unrecognized, and indifferent, the influence which they would possess as an organized body, is lost in the confusion of inoperative individual efforts.

The Pharmaceutical Society, under the leadership of the leading London chemists and druggists, would transform group disgrace into collective virtue. Instead of the tone of the profession being determined by the minority of the worst, it would be set up by the minority of the best. Jacob Bell and his band of followers set themselves up as exemplars of good practice, as men "solicitous of maintaining an unblemished reputation". To them it was peculiarly galling that

> the want of a uniform education among druggists, and the variable quality of the drugs which are found in the market (whether from adulteration, defects in the preparation, or the loss of their properties from keeping), are continually brought before the public.

There must be "a systematic regulation" of chemists and druggists: the righteous must supervise the wicked:

> The difficulty which exists in a majority of cases in estimating, with any degree of precision, the qualities of drugs, increases very much the responsibility of the druggist by placing the public in a great measure at his mercy. The chief ground, therefore, on which he can hope for success in his business is, *the confidence of the public in his integrity and experience*; and any circumstance which could tend to increase that confidence must necessarily be of great importance.

The fundamental objective of the Pharmaceutical Society was to take the amorphous, inchoate mass of individual chemists and druggists and mould it, by the leadership of the metropolitan elite, into a self-respecting profession which commanded the confidence of the public. The leading chemists and druggists saw themselves not as mere shopkeepers retailing goods at competitive prices but as skilled practitioners selling their services. The public relied upon their knowledge and skill in the manufacture, compounding and dispensing of drugs and chemicals. Their specialist knowledge of drugs and chemicals was required to provide the basis for determining their freshness and purity, for recommending them for their efficacy in treating disease, for furnishing advice on their dosage and mode of administration, and for warning of their dangers. Since the customer placed his health and even his life in the chemist's hands, honesty, reliability and integrity were of vital importance. It was both a duty and a necessity for *bona fide* chemists and druggists to maintain the demand for their services by a continuous demonstration that they are more expert, proficient and trustworthy than any private individual or any uneducated practitioner.

The elite pharmaceutists in London and the provincial cities relied on their individual reputations to build up their practice. But individual reputations were an insecure foundation for professional life in an increasingly mobile and anonymous urban society and, in any case, were not proof against tarnish by association with the unscrupulous. The task of the Pharmaceutical Society was to substitute the corporate reputation of a professional organisation for the individual reputations of practitioners, as the basis of public trust. The Society would achieve this by rooting out the charlatans and the incompetent, by exercising surveillance over the activities of its members, by drawing up a code of ethics, and by controlling the entry, education, examination and registration of future members.

> The organisation of a body of chemists into a society, the chief objects of which are avowedly to raise the character of the profession of pharmacy, and to ensure a

uniform and efficient administration of medicine, will confer upon every member that public confidence to which he is entitled. It will be in the power of the society to inculcate the impolicy of adulterations, to enlighten the public mind as to the mischief of cheap medicines, and thus to overcome to a great extent the prejudice which exists amongst too many of us in favour of a mistaken economy, and also to disseminate the advantages of that scientific knowledge which every druggist ought to possess.[32]

The society would have a moral influence on its members which would enhance professional status, for "there is, perhaps, no avocation in which *character* is of more importance than that of a chemist and druggist".

That which the law of the land or the laws of an association cannot effect, may be brought about by the moral influence of a code of ethics voluntarily subscribed to, and recommended for general adoption. The chemists having until lately been disunited, and ranked rather with the trades than the professions, have not had the advantage of that discipline which is the natural result of organization and professional intercourse.[33]

* * *

In the early days of the Pharmaceutical Society, three fundamentally different conceptions of its nature and purpose were espoused. The majority of members believed that they had set up a national trade association and a benevolent society. A small group of scientific chemists wanted the project "confined to the advancement of philosophy and useful discoveries". They were hoping to establish an exclusive scientific society. The third view was that the Pharmaceutical Society was to be the engine by which the trade of chemist and druggist was to be elevated to the profession of pharmaceutical chemist. This was the long-term goal for Jacob Bell. He was deeply committed to the conception of the Pharmaceutical Society as a professionalising organisation. He realised, however, that the infant society would need all the support it could muster: he decided to cast his nets wide. The lack of cohesion within the pharmaceutical body was reflected in and reinforced by the absence of any other formal organisation of chemists and druggists. The Pharmaceutical Society inherited an unploughed field: it was free to take on whatever tasks seemed worthwhile. From the outset the Society was multi-faceted: it performed a wider range of functions than any other occupational association. From the beginning the Society meant different things to different people: it was a *tabula rasa* on to which various groups projected their own images of its nature and future. Jacob Bell saw this as a strength rather than a weakness: the wide spectrum of its functions enlarged the constituency to which it appealed.

The infant Pharmaceutical Society, with its inescapable double-facing stance, drew upon all Jacob Bell's diplomatic skills. On the one hand, the Society had to endeavour to protect its members and advance their interests or it risked having no members at all. On the other hand, it had to make itself acceptable to powerful groups in the medical profession and in government. It first needed sufficient members to establish itself as a financially viable, permanent and representative organisation. It wanted to make good its claim to speak for the pharmaceutical body as a whole. To its potential members it offered protection and progress: to its putative sponsors it spoke of regulation and control. Protection of the current privileges of chemists and druggists appealed neither to the medical profession nor to government administrators: regulations to enforce educational and ethical standards were ineffective recruiting sergeants. The Pharmaceutical Society had been constructed out of a movement to safeguard the chemist's unrestricted right to prescribe over the counter. Yet, as soon as the Society was set up, it made public its intention to confine counter prescribing within narrow bounds.

"In an institution which is designed for the benefit of so numerous a body as the chemists and druggists of this nation", wrote Jacob Bell, "the peculiar circumstances and position of every class, comprised in that body, must be considered, and the inducements to unite in the common cause must be varied accordingly, for the purpose of securing the greatest possible amount of co-operation and support".[34]

In the long-run only the highest standards would be acceptable: in the short-run compromise was essential. Jacob Bell readily admitted that the difference between town and country business inevitably led to "some difference of opinion ... as to the precise boundary within which are included our normal and legitimate functions". He thought that the sale of oils and colours was acceptable in the provinces but that conspicuous displays of perfumery could not be recommended anywhere. The chemist could not be expected to ignore customer demand for patent and proprietary medicines and, "if the business of the chemist be creditably conducted, the sale of grocery ought not to be considered to detract from the respectability of the establishment". He urged chemists and druggists to be more active in the production and sale of horse and cattle medicines: they could do much to improve their quality. The Pharmaceutical Society, he insisted, would continue to protect the trade in all its accustomed privileges, including that of recommending medicines across the counter in simple cases, but chemists should not go so far as to advertise "medical advice gratis". Bleeding, cupping, applying leeches and drawing teeth, being surgical operations and therefore outside the jurisdiction of the Apothecaries Act, may be carried out by chemists without any valid objection from medical men. Nonetheless, "it is our duty to make our customers fully understand that we act as chemists and not as medical men". The aim of the Pharmaceutical Society is to overcome the hosility which exists between general practitioners and chemists by discouraging medical practice among its members. Although the chemist, wrote Jacob Bell, may be

> called upon occasionally to perform functions which approximate to those of medical men, he should not delude himself into the belief that his standing in society will be elevated in proportion as he induces the public to consider him a Doctor.[35]

Although Jacob Bell convinced himself he was following a Broad Church approach, his views must have seemed a betrayal to many of his followers. The great mass of chemists and druggists had no desire to become "professional men". They were not eager to acquire commercially irrelevant educational qualifications, nor to pay an annual levy to a remote London corporation. Above all, they did not welcome the prospect of having their work subjected to inspection and surveillance. They simply wanted to be left alone. Even the majority of those who joined the new Society were not attracted by its educational and scientific programme. Most of the early supporters wanted a society of chemists and druggists "simply for the purpose of supporting 'the interests of the trade' and opposing any Acts of Parliament which might be likely to interfere with those interests".[36] Jacob Bell opposed this on two grounds. First, such an association would not only heighten conflict between them and the apothecaries but also arouse the suspicions of the legislature. He publicly endorsed the advice given to the young Society by the editor of the *Medical Gazette* that "the words union, protection, independent privileges, unjust restrictions" ought not to be put forward too prominently. Tactically "it would have been well if circumstances had allowed of their being omitted altogether".[37] Secondly, trade issues were divisive. All the attempts which had previously been made to unite chemists and druggists had foundered on trade questions:

> ... the abortive efforts ... have all had reference to the pecuniary regulations of "the Trade"—the prices of drugs, the closing of shops, the limitations of the hours of business, and other restrictive arrangements, which, instead of cementing us in the bond of good fellowship, have appeared to foster and augment that reciprocal jealousy and distrust which is fatal to every kind of improvement.[38]

Yet, inevitably, the Pharmaceutical Society acted as both a defence and trade association. The Council kept a close watch on the medical reform bills which appeared in rapid succession during the 1840s. At one point, during the summer of 1845, the heady days of 1841 were recalled. The Council mobilised the membership to oppose a revised version of Sir James Graham's bill: the historic events of Spring 1841 were re-enacted. A public meeting was held at the Crown and Anchor, local secretaries organized petitions from the provinces, M.P.s were lobbied and a delegation was dispatched to the Home Office. Another medical bill bit the dust! Hostile medical bills were useful: they gave the Society an opportunity to demonstrate its relevance to the ordinary chemist and druggist.

> The occasional appearance of obnoxious or absurd Bills in Parliament afforded a favourable opportunity for demonstrating the connecting link between the personal interests of the members and their identification with a Society established for educational purposes and profession advancement.[39]

In 1847 a chemist and druggist from Dudley defended the Society in the *Pharmaceutical Times*, singling out its work in protecting chemists for special commendation:

> By its organization and timely remonstrance, we have escaped the impost of vexatious restrictions upon our calling (by the excise); we have to thank that body for its prompt resistance to the numerous medical bills prejudicial to our interests which have been proposed and abandoned ...[40]

The extent to which chemists should be allowed to produce and sell alcohol without acquiring a licence from and paying duty to the Inland Revenue was a contentious issue in the early nineteenth century. In 1843 several chemists and druggists were put on trial for selling spirits of wine without a licence: in 1846 the Government introduced a Spirit Licences and Duties Bill which would have extended the control of the Board of Excise. On both occasions the Pharmaceutical Society appeared as the accredited spokesman for the retail chemist. In December 1843 a deputation from the Society's Council met the Chancellor of the Exchequer and the Chairman of the Board of Excise to iron out the differences between chemists and excisemen. During the discussion the deputation tried to use the situation to further the interests of the Society. It was suggested that, instead of extending privileges to the trade generally, the government might find it more acceptable to restrict them to members of the Pharmaceutical Society alone. The Government would not bite, but the chemists had their penalties mitigated.

It was not unusual for chemists and druggists in different parts of the country to fall foul of the Excise. At one time it might be for evading the payment of stamp duty on medicines;

at other times for selling without licence spirit of wine for other than medicinal purposes. The Pharmaceutical Society, by furnishing legal advice and aid to the delinquent chemists did much to justify its claim for support from the rank and file. During the early 1840s the excise officers stepped up their investigations into the extent to which unlicensed chemists sold alcohol. The Council of the Society complained to Somerset House of the unnecessary interference with activities which had hitherto passed unnoticed and were looked upon by most chemists as tacitly sanctioned, if not strictly legal. The Inland Revenue Board replied by pointing out that a chemist made himself liable to penalty by selling spirit of wine for whatever purpose: the Excise did not generally institute proceedings when only small quantities were sold, or when it was sold for strictly medical purposes, but, if there were grounds for suspecting the indulgence was being abused, it was their duty to act. In July 1845 the excise detective officers discovered an extensive illicit distillery in a London suburb where large quantities of spirit had been produced for years, most, if not all, of which was sold by chemists and druggists in the form of sweet spirit of nitre. Seizures of large quantities of spirit in all its stages of production and conversion into spirit of nitre were made in various parts of the country. The Government decided it was time to staunch this loss of public revenue. In 1846 the Spirit Licences and Duties Bill was introduced which, if enacted, would have placed chemists and druggists as completely under the surveillance of the excise as publicans were. The Pharmaceutical Society regarded this as degrading and intolerable and joined forces with Thomas Wakley to mount opposition to the bill. The Government gave way and the bill was cut down to one for licensing the use of stills and retorts for distilling spirit mixtures: the authority for excise officers to enter and inspect premises was omitted. To make such a dramatic impact on legislation and administration was one of the most striking ways in which the Pharmaceutical Society could acquire prestige and demonstrate its usefulness to the profession it aspired to represent.

Jacob Bell identified two trade questions which could be guaranteed to split chemists and druggists into hostile camps: the fixing of prices and the regulation of opening hours. Both issues were important: both were highly contentious: both depended for their resolution on solidarity and unanimity. Jacob Bell did his utmost to steer the Pharmaceutical Society clear of any involvement in them. He knew that the Society could only harm itself by intervening: it lacked the power to have any beneficial effect. Bell argued that these issues were best dealt with at the local level. He approved of chemists and druggists forming local trade associations to regulate prices. In 1846 he praised the Leicestershire Association of Chemists and Druggists for setting up a scheme whereby retail drug prices were fixed by its committee and fines were imposed on those who deviated from the prescribed rate. "It cannot be denied that the 'cutting system' is highly injurious, and the interests of the public are best secured by a fair and uniform charge", he wrote.[41] From the mid-1830s onwards short-lived associations of chemists and druggists appeared in several towns with the object of restricting price competition: everywhere they collapsed from lack of solidarity and failure to exclude outsiders. Membership of such associations usually overlapped with that of the Pharmaceutical Society but the organizations remained distinct.

Attempts were also made at the local level to get chemists and druggists to agree on the limitation of business hours. There was widespread agreement that even the public gained little from chemists' shops staying open seven days a week from seven in the morning to eleven at night. But every attempt to restrict opening hours by voluntary agreements failed. In 1847 "Alpha" of Liverpool, in a letter to the *Pharmaceutical Times*, observed that:

> ... the cause of late hours is to be looked for, not in the requirements of the public, but in the want of union and in the spirit of rivalry existing among the druggists. They have no common ground on which they can meet and hold friendly intercourse; they feel no community of interests; each studies what he considers to be his own interest, to the exclusion of every other consideration.[42]

Even if every chemist in the land had agreed to a reduction in opening hours, the Pharmaceutical Society would have been powerless to prevent apothecaries, grocers and oilmen from selling drugs whenever they pleased. Jacob Bell was anxious not to have the Society drawn into the controversy. Not only did the matter divide retailer from retailer it also divided master and assistant. During the 1840s an early closing movement was formed by a sizeable group of London assistants, with the support of several retailers, to publicize the assistants' case for shorter hours of work. Their attempt to persuade the Council of the Pharmaceutical Society to both assist their efforts and endorse their objectives led to bitter conflict. The issue divided the Council, the membership and the whole pharmaceutical body. The assistants' case was taken up by both *The Chemist* and the *Pharmaceutical Times* in an attempt to discredit the Society and to increase the circulation of those journals. If assistants are obliged to work from dawn to dusk every day of the week, it was argued, how can they benefit from the Pharmaceutical Society's School of Pharmacy and Laboratory? Is it not sheer hypocrisy for Jacob Bell to urge young men to take advantage of the educational facilities provided by the Society, when he does nothing to give them the opportunity to do so? Reducing the hours of labour would do more to advance the scientific attainments of the rising generation than any amount of expenditure on the Society's pretentious lectures and meetings. Whatever truth there might be in these accusations, Jacob Bell knew that there was no effective action the Pharmaceutical Society could take to reduce business hours. The editors of *The Chemist* and the *Pharmaceutical Times* also knew it.[43]

Before the foundation of the Pharmaceutical Society, chemists and druggists were "almost the only class of the community" without "an efficient Benevolent Fund". "This is an extraordinary fact", observed Jacob Bell, "and the want of unity among our members, which has so often been commented upon, is the only circumstance which can account for it". Chemists and druggists and their dependents were certainly not less liable to misfortune than others. "The influence of competition, the depression of trade, the changes of fashion, and the caprice of the public, may, within a short period of time ... reduce a man from ... affluence to ... absolute want". Other occupations had well-established benevolent funds. In 1841–42 the Society for the Relief of Widows and Orphans of Medical Men had a capital of £41,000 and expended £1,300 in relief during the year. The Linen-drapers', Silk Mercers', Lacemen's, Haberdashers' and Hosiers' Institution, established in 1831, had funds of over £20,000 in 1842. The Tailors' Benevolent Society, established in 1837, obtained income of £1,200 per annum from its permanent fund and had built almshouses at a cost of £11,000. The Royal Society of Musicians had a benevolent fund which provided monthly allowances of 4 guineas (or 5 guineas if married) as well as allowances for widows and orphans. Each member of the Artists' Benevolent Institution received, when ill, £6 a month and their widows received life annuities.[44] In the absence of any state welfare provision, voluntary provident associations flourished in early Victorian England. By far the most important class of such associations were the friendly societies, but many trades had benevolent funds and mutual assurance schemes. They developed because of the need to provide succour against poverty caused by misfortune, sickness and death. The alternative was the degrading pauperism of the workhouse. Yet fear of destitution and the humiliation of the Poor Law were not enough to overcome the lack of fraternity among chemists and druggists. An earlier attempt to establish a benevolent society failed and soon the Pharmaceutical Society's efforts flagged. In spite of its potential as a recruiting sergeant, the Benevolent Fund was neglected by both Council and members during the Society's early decades. Nothing illustrates more clearly the priorities of Jacob Bell and the early Council members than the way in which the Benevolent Fund was starved of resources while the Journal, the School of Pharmacy and the Laboratory received first call on the Society's finances. In the first three years the Council annually allocated £500 from the Society's income to the Benevolent Fund; but when the Society's early prosperity faded, the contribution to the fund was the first victim of financial stringency. Robert Farmar voiced the feelings of many members when he expressed his unease and belief that "the work of retrenchment had been begun at the wrong end". There were other items of expenditure— the cost of the journal, the fees paid to the professors—"which might with much greater propriety had been reduced". "When the Society was founded", he reminded the members, "the Benevolent Fund was stated to be one of the leading objects, and was said to be a bond of union". Farmar might have added that the recently acquired Royal Charter of Incorporation included the Benevolent Fund as one of the principal objects of the Society.

Jacob Bell begged to differ. "The first and most important object of the Society was education", he said, "and the accommodation in the laboratory, not being at present adequate to the demand, it was absolutely necessary immediately to expend several hundred pounds in enlarging the premises". The Pharmaceutical Society was established to raise the status of chemists and druggists throughout the land. If that is the objective, argued Jacob Bell, education is the necessary starting point.

> The first thing to be done, and the most important consideration, was the establishment of the Society on a firm and permanent foundation, and the only foundation which could be relied upon was education. It was this which had already gained for the Society the influence and respect which it now enjoyed.

By steadily persevering in its "scientific and education proceedings", the Society "had gradually assumed a position which entitled it to respect and consideration from the government and the public".[45]

During the early years the setting up of a formal system of education took precedence over all other activities. The prestige and respectability of the Society were seen to depend upon it projecting an image of itself as a scientific and educational institution. A perusal of the balance sheet reveals that three items of expenditure absorbed the bulk of the Society's income; the fees of the professors in the School of Pharmacy, the equipping and running of the Laboratory, and the cost of the journal. Expenditure on the library, museum and the benevolent fund was sacrificed to the maintenance of the Society's educational activity. Yet, in the early decades, the function of the School and the Laboratory was more symbolic than practical. With some 3,000 young men below the age of twenty in the profession, fewer than eighty attended the lectures at the School each year and not more than twenty five could be accommodated in the Laboratory. Local branches of the Pharmaceutical Society in Bath, Bristol, Exeter, Norwich, Manchester, Liverpool, Birmingham and Newcastle made arrangements to provide lectures for students: the Council in London gave them much advice and, occasionally, a little money to encourage them. An excellent example was set but the immediate educational outcome was negligible.

None of these considerations deterred Jacob Bell from his mission. At every opportunity he reiterated his message: education is the means by which the trade of chemist and druggist will be transformed into the profession of pharmaceutical chemist. The "establishment of a system of education ... will give professional character, influence, and respectability to the body". "When every member of the pharmaceutical body has been equally educated and examined, everyone will be equally worthy of the confidence of the medical profession and the public". The School of Pharmacy was at the centre of Bell's strategy. "The existence of the School of Pharmacy ... will confer a degree of credit and character upon every individual connected with it". "Much of the usefulness of the Society depends upon the prosperity of the School of Pharmacy". "The School of Pharmacy is the ladder by which we may hope to ascend to our proper place in the [medical] profession".[46]

Education involved both intellectual and moral training. On the one hand, it implied the acquisition of a body of theoretical knowledge or a set of general principles to guide and supplement the practical training acquired by apprenticeship. The possession of a body of theoretical or esoteric knowledge most clearly separated the professions from manual occupations or mere trades. On the other hand, education was as much moral as intellectual. "The more you educate a man, the more like a gentleman he will always act", declared Emil Richter, the analytical chemist who worked for Savory and Moore, in 1856.[47] Education civilised man, raising him above the level of the brutish, unfeeling masses. It provided him with judgment and gave him a sense of moral responsibility. It endowed him with the capacity for rational behaviour. The aim of education was to produce scientists and gentlemen: men of integrity as well as knowledge. "Professional character *prima facie* is supposed to result from liberal and scientific education".

The promotion of education and science, moreover, argued Bell, is the best means of protection.

> ... the constitution of the Society provides, in the first instance, for the protection and welfare of its members; but the prominent means by which they are to secure these privileges consist in the promotion of the requisite education and scientific knowledge which will shield them from extraneous control and interference ... The scientific arrangements which we propose will become in great measure our means of defence ... the two grand objects of our society, protection and improvement are mutually dependent on each other ... The terms, improvement and protection are synonymous.[48]

Education was to be the basis for claiming government approval and support.

> The Society was established for the purpose of ... raising the character of those who practise pharmacy in Great Britain. It is proposed to attain this end, first, by uniting all the chemists and druggists into one body; secondly, by introducing a

system of pharmaceutical education; thirdly, by claiming for the body thus organized and educated, such protection and privileges as the qualification of the members would entitle them to possess.[49]

Chemists and druggists repeatedly objected to "the encroachments of grocers, oilmen, and others, who retail drugs in a manner which materially injures" their business. While acknowledging that, "this practice is obviously an evil which demands a remedy", Jacob Bell pointed out that, in the absence of a uniform system of education, the Society was powerless to act:

> If we were to petition Parliament to prohibit the sale of drugs by unqualified persons, we might expect to be answered with ... "Prove that you are qualified yourselves. You undergo no specific and uniform education; you can show no test of your proficiency; you are under no regulations whatever, and, therefore, possess no more claim to be recognised as a scientific body—a branch of the medical profession—than the grocers and oilmen."

But,

> The educational regulations, adopted by ourselves, our school of pharmacy, our board of examiners, our certificates of qualification, and the records of our scientific proceedings, would at once be received as a guarantee of the justice of our claims.[50]

If the Pharmaceutical Society allowed itself to become a mere trade protection association, dissension, conflict and disintegration would follow. Commerce divides, science unites. The relationship between protection, enhanced status and educational advance was clearly stated by Jacob Bell in 1842:

> ... the most effectual method which any class of men can adopt for securing their political rights, and advancing their professional standing, consists ... in a steady and persevering attention to intellectual improvement, and the establishment of such regulations as are calculated to ensure collective privileges by increasing the amount of individual merit.

Behind the educational activities of the Pharmaceutical Society lay the aim of making pharmacy a distinctive branch of the medical profession. In 1842 Jacob Bell wrote a historical survey of the healing arts which led him "to the consideration of the position which pharmacy occupies, or ought to occupy, as a branch of the medical profession". He gave lengthy consideration to the way in which the traditional pharmaceutical practitioners—the apothecaries—had become general medical practitioners, while retaining their right to dispense and sell drugs. Meanwhile, the art and science of pharmacy in Britain had been degraded "to the level of mere trade". This had led to the idea that a necessary consequence of improving the character and education of the chemist and druggist would be to convert him into a medical practitioner. The apothecaries adopted a system of education which was medical and surgical rather than pharmaceutical: "the odium which rested on Pharmacy as a *trade*, induced them to aspire to medical practice as a *profession*". But pharmacy was now "deserving of a separate and distinct place in the arrangement of the medical profession". A need had emerged for specialist practitioners of pharmacy to assimilate and put into practice the changes in materia medica and improvements in dispensing which had been created by the advances in chemistry and botany.

111

Pharmacy in the present day embraces so many sciences, and has become so complicated from the discoveries which have recently been made, especially in Chemistry, that a complete knowledge of the subject can only be acquired by those who devote their exclusive attention to the pursuit. The science of Chemistry is alone sufficiently comprehensive to engage the whole time of those who are desirous of becoming acquainted with all its details ... These revolutions in chemical science give rise to changes in nomenclature, and improvements in the processes of the laboratory, which innovations involve the study of Pharmacy in increasing difficulty, and confer on the pursuit the character of a philosophical profession. It is the province of the Pharmaceutical Chemist to apply the various discoveries which are made in this science to his own peculiar department ... the principles of Chemistry should be understood by every person who undertakes to prepare a prescription, and in many of the daily operations of Pharmacy a profound knowledge of the science is indispensable.

The range of the Materia Medica is too extensive to be embraced in the mind without a systematic study of all its minutiae in the first instance, followed up by constant application. The variations in the quality of drugs, and the sophistications to which they are liable, increase the responsibility of the Druggist, and demand the utmost vigilance ... The detection of adulterations is, therefore, one of the most onerous duties of the Pharmaceutical Chemist, and it is one which requires, beside chemical knowledge, a practical acquaintance with the sensible properties of all the substances used in medicine.

The science of Botany, although to a great extent comprised in the Materia Medica, alone affords occupation for the whole life of those who are ambitious of attaining proficiency; and even that amount of knowledge which every Chemist ought to possess of the plants which are used in medicine cannot be acquired without many years of study ...

Pharmacy ... is not likely to advance as a science, and keep pace with other sciences, unless it be followed by a class of persons who devote themselves exclusively to it ...

But if proper encouragement were given to the followers of pure Pharmacy; if this pursuit were held in the estimation which it deserves, and which it enjoys in other countries; if the same professional credit were attainable in this field of labour which is within the reach of the members of other professions, the inducement which now exists to encroach on the medical practitioner would be greatly diminished, or cease altogether, and the science of Pharmacy might be expected to flourish.[51]

Jacob Bell's vision of the future emerges in these passages. A scientific revolution is creating a new division of labour within the medical profession. The Pharmaceutical Society is required to organise the practice of pharmacy in the way the Royal Colleges already organise the practice of physic and surgery. The Fellows of the Royal College of Physicians confine themselves to the practice of "pure" medicine: membership of the council of the Royal College of Surgeons is restricted to those who practise "pure" surgery. The founder of the Pharmaceutical Society proclaims the virtues of "pure" pharmacy. Although justified by reference to innovations in knowledge, Jacob Bell's vision is securely tethered to the past. The medical profession is seen as having its ranks and orders, each with its own function and sphere of usefulness, and each regulated by its own corporate body. The time has come for pharmacy to take its place, separate but equal, alongside the other orders. On the first anniversary of the foundation of the Pharmaceutical Society, Jacob Bell declared:

> We have taken the first step towards placing ourselves on a permanent and sound basis, as a body independent in ourselves, and yet constituting a section of the medical profession.[52]

A year later he welcomed the grant of the Royal Charter as

> a step, and a very important step, towards the accomplishment of the object which we have in view—namely, the establishment of Pharmacy on a safe and creditable foundation as a branch of the medical profession.[53]

The key to professionalism is greater specialisation. A medical profession founded on a rational division of scientific labour would be characterised by interdependence and co-operation instead of the present antagonism and competition. Strong fences make good neighbours. Jacob Bell concluded his survey of the progress of pharmacy with these words:

> Those who are sincere in the desire for the advancement of our own legitimate profession, which is pure Pharmacy, will perceive the importance of confining our attention as much as possible to that pursuit, by which course we shall not only be more likely to attain the object in view, but shall also conciliate the other branches of the profession, and establish an amicable and harmonious relation among all parties.[54]

Pure pharmacy meant scientific pharmacy. Selling drugs was still to be the legitimate occupation of the new pharmaceutical chemist, but the addition of scientific research to his responsibilities would augment his role in new directions. With the co-operation of the physician, he would help to advance the theory and practice of medicine by assisting in studies of the mode of action of medicines, developing more efficient techniques for obtaining already known remedies, and even by discovering and manufacturing new medicines. The elite group of London chemists and druggists who founded the Pharmaceutical Society saw themselves as the carriers of the seeds of a new scientific discipline. Their belief in the authenticity and utility of science informed their plans for the reform of the profession. The emphasis on education, examination, qualification and registration coincided with their commitment to the canons of orthodox science. The 1840s were a time of great excitement and opportunity: the work of Magendie, Pelletier and Liebig were transforming the practice and prospects of scientific pharmacy.

* * *

The beginning of modern pharmacy can be traced to the work of Francois Magendie (1783–1855) and Pierre-Joseph Pelletier (1788-1842). In 1809 Magendie carried out a series of ingenious experiments on various animals to study the toxic action of several drugs of vegetable origin, such as upas and nux vomica. For the first time an experimental comparison was made of the similar effects produced by drugs of different botanical origin. Magendie held that the toxic or medicinal action of natural drugs depends on the chemical substances they contain, and that it should be possible to obtain these substances in the pure state. As early as 1809 he suspected the existence of strychnine, isolated ten years later, in accord with Magendie's predictions, by Pelletier. Pelletier, who spent his life investigating drugs at the École de Pharmacie in Paris, achieved his first major success in 1817 when he discovered the emetic substance in ipecacuanha root, which he named emetine. By

113

pioneering the use of mild solvents, Pelletier successfully isolated a whole range of important biologically active compounds from plants, thus founding the chemistry of the alkaloids. For over twenty years Pelletier continued his alkaloid and phytochemical research. He discovered brucine, caffeine, cinchonine, colchicine, narceine, strychnine, veratrine and, most important of all, quinine. Quinine, the chief alkaloid in cinchona bark, became for the next hundred years the only effective treatment for malaria and represents the first successful use of a chemical compound in combating an infectious disease. Pelletier's isolation of active constituents from crude drugs was a major development in pharmacy, but it was Magendie who was responsible for introducing the recently discovered alkaloids into medical practice. In 1821 he published the first edition of his *Formulaire pour la préparation et l'emploi de plusieurs nouveaux médicaments*, a revolutionary therapeutic manual which led to the use of strychnine, morphine, brucine, codeine, veratrine and quinine by physicians. Magendie also generalised the therapeutic applications of iodine and bromine salts, and indicated the use of hydrocyanic acid in therapeutics.[55]

The work of Magendie and Pelletier not only introduced a new level of precision into the practice of pharmacy but created a need for educated and skilful practitioners. An end could be seen to the days of crude drugs of unknown and variable composition, of imprecise plant extracts and mixtures. If pure compounds were used, accurate dosage could be prescribed and the toxic effects due to impurities in crude drugs could be eliminated. The growing use of experiments to investigate the action of such substances on the animal body led to the determination of doses and detailed descriptions of the properties of drugs. With the entry into medicine of pure, toxic chemical substances, a premium was placed on their standardisation and purity and the administration of precise doses. This, in turn, required practitioners whose integrity and reliability, technical skill, and knowledge of the theory and practice of chemistry, could be guaranteed. Not all those who sold drugs in England were enthusiastic about the exactness of dosage made possible by the isolation of these new alkaloids (or "alcalis" as they were then termed) or about their increasing use, to the exclusion of the long-accepted powdered roots, barks and leaves. A typical reaction is found in the seventeenth edition of the *Medicine Chest Guide*, issued by Reece and Co., Chemists, Piccadilly, London, just prior to 1840:

> If the atropine of the deadly nightshade . . . be mixed with a conserve or dissolved in a fluid, to render it safe for the human stomach, surely it cannot differ from a carefully made extract. As to solution of alcalis in alcohol, termed tinctures, they have no advantage over common tinctures of the drugs from which the alcalis have been derived.

In spite of such resistance, physicians made increasing use of these new alkaloids.

The other great influence on mid-nineteenth century pharmacy was Justus Liebig (1803–73), who "was unquestionably the greatest chemist of his time".[56] Liebig was the person primarily responsible for the emergence during the 1830s and early 1840s of organic chemistry as a new frontier of scientific endeavour. The new specialty developed on the continent out of chemical studies of the constituent parts of animals and plants. Though there was a great deal of well-publicized controversy over his fundamental theories of organic chemistry, the analytical methods for its investigation, which he developed in his laboratory at Giessen, were accepted as sound and accurate.

The opening of Liebig's chemistry laboratory at the University of Giessen in 1824 was a critical event in the history of nineteenth century science. Liebig's was the first institutional laboratory in which students underwent systematic preparation for chemical research. After an initial course of qualitative and quantitative analysis using known compounds, each student was required to produce pure substances in good yield from raw materials. Once this preliminary training had been satisfactorily completed, the student was allowed to pursue original research under Liebig's general supervision. The combination of the most rigorous practical training and its incredibly low cost proved irresistible to students from all over Europe. The success of Liebig's laboratory depended on his invention of relatively simple, fast and reliable experimental techniques. With practice, any determined student could obtain reliable results using Liebig's combustion apparatus for analysing organic compounds. The use of this apparatus and its relatives permitted both brilliant and mediocre students to produce knowledge in the emerging field of organic chemistry in a systematic way and on a large scale. Liebig codified and systematised both the research techniques employed and the preliminary training he gave his students. Two of his pupils, H. Will (1812–1890) and C.R. Fresenius (1818–1897), published books on the methods of qualitative and quantitative analysis used at Giessen, and these were rapidly translated into English.[57]

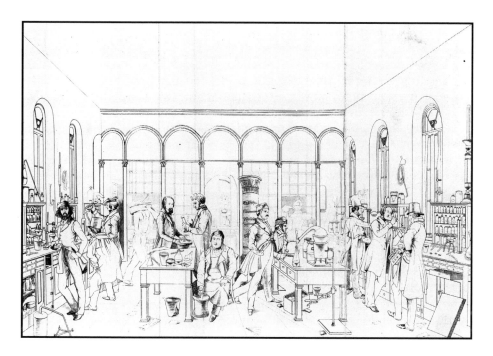

21   *The laboratory at Giessen in 1842.*

The new analytical methods developed in the Giessen laboratory began to be used systematically to study the processes through which organic constituents were produced in both healthy and diseased living systems. Organic chemistry came to be viewed as the key to the study of the physiology and pathology of both plants and animals. This was argued most forcefully by Liebig in his widely read volumes, *Organic Chemistry in its Applications to Agriculture and Physiology* (1840) and *Animal Chemistry or Organic Chemistry in its Applications to Physiology and Pathology* (1842).

During the early nineteenth century the study of physiology and pathology became recognised routes to the improvement of medical practice. It was now argued that the study of organic chemistry, as the key to these subjects, should be viewed in the same light. Future medical progress would be achieved through chemical knowledge of how the body worked. The editors of *The Chemist* put it this way in 1842:

> Any alteration or change in the chemical relations of organic bodies, must be accompanied by corresponding ones in their functions and actions, which it is the duty of medical men to note and ascertain, in order to trace their causes, and thereby prevent or relieve the diseases which they are calculated to induce. Neglect of these subjects can now no longer be excused, since ignorance of their importance, and immediate connection with the states and actions of health and disease, cannot be pleaded; it has, however, been reserved to this eminent individual [Liebig] to show them its necessity, as a branch of medical science . . . [58]

This was seen to be important not only to the physician, surgeon, and general practitioner but to the pharmaceutical chemist as well. Since the action of internal medicines was chemical, chemical knowledge of bodily processes would help elucidate the mode of operation of medicines and lead to the development of improved ones. Leibig's work implied a reversal of the traditional relationship of chemistry to medicine. Not only was chemistry emerging from its former position of dependency on medicine and claiming to be a science in its own right, it was even threatening to usurp the leading role. Not surprisingly, physicians' reactions to Liebig's ideas reveal a marked concern for professional prerogatives. They resented any attempt to derive principles of treatment from his laws. They claimed that chemistry had nothing to say of the vital functions of the organised issues. Chemists should stick to nutrition: vital laws were the province of the physiologist. Although the *Lancet* published Henry Ancell's exposition of Liebig's views and declared that "there is far more chemistry in medicine, . . . there is far more of exact science in medicine, than physicians are inclined to believe", the medical press generally was hostile. Dr. A.P. Wilson Philip claimed to see no value at all in efforts to apply chemical methods to physiological problems; and Dr. Golding Bird expressed the prevalent view that "a more melancholy error can scarcely be committed than that of explaining the phenomena of the animal organism too exclusively on chemical principles".[59]

From its foundation the Pharmaceutical Society placed great emphasis on practical chemistry. Its promotion as an academic subject was motivated by the Society's efforts to upgrade the trade of chemist and druggist by emulating what was best in the much praised European systems of pharmaceutical education. The early volumes of the *Pharmaceutical Journal* contain many articles on pharmaceutical chemistry: Richard Phillips, the editor and translator of the 1836 edition of the *Pharmacopoeia Londinensis*, and curator of the Museum of Economic Geology, contributed a series of reports on pharmacopoeial preparations, incorporating tests for adulteration.[60] An attempt was made to keep journal readers abreast of the most important continental research. A knowledge of chemistry was expected of examinees for both the minor and major examinations. The Society's laboratory was modelled on that at Giessen, and when Liebig visited it "two or three of the processes usually conducted by students in the laboratory were modified at his suggestion".[61] The case for training pharmacists in chemistry was eloquently stated by the first vice-president of the Society, Charles James Payne, in 1842:

> Without some knowledge of chemistry a man is working in the dark, he can know nothing correctly of the results of, or the reasons for the operations he constantly performs—he can never properly judge the accuracy and quality of his preparation, he can neither detect any error that may occur nor rectify any untoward circumstance that may arise—he has no established data to reason upon— no fixed principles to guide him; but is like a mariner without a compass, exposed to endless confusion and mishap.[62]

* * *

By 1841 London was well served by learned societies. During the first four decades of the nineteenth century, leaders in many sciences had created large specialised associations. In 1839 the Inventors Advocate listed 41 scientific, literary and similar societies in London with a total membership of 17,000. Many of them were dedicated to particular sciences: two societies served astronomy and seven represented natural history. Yet it was 1841 before an enduring association of chemists was established. The Chemical Society was founded only a few weeks before the Pharmaceutical Society.[63] On 23 February 1841 twenty five men met at the Society of Arts in London and agreed to form an organisation called the Chemical Society of London. At another meeting on 30 March the Society was formally inaugurated and an executive council of sixteen was elected. At the founding meeting on 23 February, Robert Warington, who became the Society's first secretary, suggested four facilities that the Society would offer its members:

> The reading of notes and papers on chemical science (in the most extensive meaning of the term), and the discussion of the same. The formation of a laboratory, in which might be carried out the more abstruse and disputed points connected with the science. The establishment of a collection of standard chemical preparations, of as varied a nature as possible, for reference and comparison, and thus to supply a very great desideratum in the metropolis; the formation also of a library, to include particularly the works and publications of continental authors.

By 30 March Warington's proposals had been articulated to form a vision of a scholarly forum. At the inaugural meeting it was declared:

> That this Society is instituted for the advancement of Chemistry and those branches of science immediately connected with it.
>
> For this purpose periodical meetings of its members shall be held for the communication and discussion of discoveries and observations relating to such subjects, an account of which shall be published by the Society in the form of Proceedings or Transactions.
>
> That the formation of a Library of works relating to its proper subjects, of a Museum of Chemical Preparations and Standard Instruments, and the establishment of a Laboratory of Research, are also ulterior objects of the Society.

The aims of the Chemical Society were much more clearly focused than those of the Pharmaceutical Society: the Chemical Society was strictly a forum to advance the science of chemistry. Like the Pharmaceutical Society, it had two grades of members. Members "properly so called" would ideally be "high" chemists, i.e. those men "who have prosecuted the science with zeal and research". Associates, who would be without voting rights but would not pay a subscription, would consist of "a large number of young gentlemen pursuing chemistry as a science, such as pupils, managers of manufactories etc . . ." The Chemical Society was an exclusive and select society. Members were admitted in two ways. The seventy-seven "original members" had been personally invited in February 1841 to become members by the Preliminary Committee. All other members had to be elected. The aspirant's application form, signed by three members, was hung outside the Society's meeting room for three successive meetings; a vote was taken during the fourth and a two-thirds majority was required for election. In contrast, the Pharmaceutical Society opened its doors to all chemists and druggists in business on their own account. "Every Society must have a beginning", explained Jacob Bell,

> and reformation must in all cases be a work of time. We must take our brethren as we find them. We have no power to restrain those who are already in business, even though they may be less qualified than could be desired; nor would it be fair to exclude them while they evince a desire for improvement by a willingness to join us . . . it is more becoming to exercise charity and forbearance than to judge harshly of the imperfections of one another.

Such laxity, however, will be shortlived. In the early stages,

> we cannot be so strict in this respect as we shall hereafter. The leading druggists in each town are generally the first to become members, and it is their duty to ascertain, to the best of their ability, the claims of future candidates.

By 1842, with a membership of 2,000, the Pharmaceutical Society saw the need

> to maintain the respectability of our institution . . . by inquiring rather more narrowly into the merits or claims of those who apply for admission . . . we consider it right to expect a satisfactory introduction or recommendation as a guarantee that every person admitted comes within our definition. It has been found necessary to use a discretionary power in this particular in London. . .[64]

In 1848 Jacob Bell claimed that "precautions were taken from the beginning to exclude all persons known to be disreputable or unworthy of being classed with the general body of chemists and druggists"; but the need to increase the membership ensured that the gates remained wide open.[65]

The Chemical Society developed more slowly than the Pharmaceutical Society. The membership grew from 77 at the outset to 185 after five years, reached 221 in 1850 and 323 in 1860. Meetings were held every two weeks from April 1841 and a museum and library were soon started, although as late as 1848, were described as only "in course of preparation". Memoirs and proceedings were at first published irregularly: the quarterly journal did not appear until November 1847. Nonetheless, the success of the enterprise in surviving its infancy was recognised by a Royal Charter granted in 1848. The Society, hitherto known as the Chemical Society of London, was retitled "The Chemical Society" and its members redesignated "Fellows". The Charter proclaimed the identity of the Society with its science.

The simultaneous foundation of the Pharmaceutical Society and the Chemical Society was a decisive event in the establishment of pharmacy and chemistry as distinct academic disciplines. The Pharmaceutical Society created an autonomous profession of pharmaceutical chemists whose interests were defined by the problems of pharmacy rather than those of chemistry. The Chemical Society played a major part in freeing chemistry from its connexion with the practice of medicine and pharmacy and establishing it as an independent discipline. The creation of the Pharmaceutical Society was a significant turning point in the organisation of science in this country. Three levels of organisation in science can be distinguished; research areas, specialties and disciplines. Research areas are the short-lived conjunctures of problems and investigations that are the immediate context of advancing knowledge. Specialties are more enduring: they are characterised by special skills, traditions and often charismatic leaders. Disciplines are inherently large and complex institutions. They have none of the intellectual coherence of specialties. Their institutional importance is complemented by a diversity of approaches. They bring together under one umbrella a range of different programmes and methods. Consequently they raise a series of intriguing questions for the historian of science. How have disciplines been constructed? What has held them together? How and why have their boundaries changed? The year 1841 witnessed a major regrouping of the chemical community in England on the basis of a clear separation between chemistry as a scientific discipline and pharmacy as a branch of medicine. The Pharmaceutical Society and the Chemical Society constituted the institutional framework for the social construction of a division of labour which has been so successful and so enduring that today it seems both "inevitable" and "natural". Yet both Societies were founded at a time of profound disagreement over the definition of categories and the membership of groups within the scientific community. Alternative scenarios for the classification and arrangement of the members of the chemical community were vigorously advocated and defended. There is nothing inevitable or natural about the present day division between "chemistry chemists" and "pharmacy chemists". The differences which now exist are the result of the earlier establishment of social and institutional boundaries. Once the boundaries were delineated and the territories marked out, processes of differentiation and integration occurred. The differences between the groups became accentuated and the similarities within the groups became reinforced.

The Chemical Society became the basic institutional framework through which a profession based on the science of chemistry evolved in England. Formal professional activities focusing on chemistry began to develop from 1831 when, as Section B of the new British Association for the Advancement of Science, chemists came together within the wider context of the scientific fraternity. Chemists did not, however, emerge as a distinct group until the Chemical Society succeeded in welding together the elites created by new opportunities for chemical education, employment and innovation. The founders of the Chemical Society were consciously aiming to develop chemistry as a scientific discipline and to provide it with the prestige that Liebig claimed for it in Germany. In its early decades the Society was dominated by the still new but rapidly expanding classes of academic and consulting chemists and manufacturers in chemically related industries. Three quarters of the early members were manufacturers and professional and academic chemists.

During the 1830s and 1840s a host of positions, outside of the fields of medicine and pharmacy, were being created which gave men an opportunity of earning a living through their knowledge of chemistry. These posts were created as responses to problems created by rapid industrial and technological progress. There was increasing recognition of the relevance of chemical knowledge to the solution of technical problems in agriculture, mining, manufacturing industry and government. The growth of these posts was paralleled by an expansion of opportunities in teaching and research.

Agriculture was an important base for the employment of men as "chemists". In 1846 the *Pharmaceutical Times* declared:

> Agriculture is an art and science, no less than dyeing and bleaching and metallurgy, and must yield to the progressive impulse of an advancing chemistry.[66]

If agriculture was to withstand the impact of foreign competition, it must become more efficient. The chemist had important contributions to make. The future of agriculture, it was argued, rested in part on understanding the nature of soils and the mode of operation of chemical and other agents that altered soil conditions. The chemist, on the basis of soil analysis and his knowledge of plants' needs, could offer advice on what fertiliser was appropriate and in what quantities for particular soils and plants. Landowners were interested not only in the possibility of applying chemical knowledge to agricultural problems but also in consulting the chemist about the mineral resources of their estates.

During the early 1840s it was argued that Britain would lose its resource-based industrial lead over the rest of the world and become dependent on foreign products unless production was improved through the use of science. Manufacturers in several industries were faced by technical problems the solution to which demanded chemical expertise. Chemists acted as consultants in glass manufacture, gas engineering, calico-printing, metal refining, chemical manufacture, soap-making and brewing and distilling. Of 295 early members of the Chemical Society 105 could be classified as employed in manufacturing: they were chemists, engineers, managers and proprietors; categories that can be only loosely differentiated.

Government, too, offered employment opportunities to chemists during the 1840s. Its own establishment had to cope with technical problems, while attempts to grapple with crises like the mining disasters of 1842 and 1843 quickly involved chemists. Departments which made occasional use of chemists took them on permanently and some entirely new functions were created. During the 1840s the Customs and Excise sent men to University College London for intensive training in chemical analysis. By 1854 seventy-seven officers had been trained. New government laboratories were established at the Museum of Economic Geology (1839) and in the Geological Survey (1845). They provided general chemical services to the government. By 1847 they had examined the sanitary condition of Buckingham Palace, reported on graveyards, analysed urban water supplies, reported on coals for the navy, and conducted analyses for the Treasury. In 1840 David Boswell Reid, who had taught practical chemistry in Edinburgh, was employed to design the ventilation system of the new Houses of Parliament.

During the early nineteenth century the teaching of chemistry in England was closely allied to the study of medicine. The educational requirements of the medical profession determined chemical curricula and the lecturers themselves were invariably medical men. William Allen, the first president of the Pharmaceutical Society, who was appointed lecturer in chemistry at Guy's Hospital in 1802, was a notable exception to this rule. During the 1830s and 1840s medical education became a prominent issue in the general practitioner's search for professional status. For professional as well as scientific reasons, laboratory instruction in practical chemistry then became required of medical students. By 1850 practical chemistry courses were offered at ten London medical schools. However, lack of resources to pay for this new type of training led to large classes, superficially taught. There was little call for extra staff in the established medical schools. More important for chemical careers was the emergence of new institutions in which chemistry was taught. The first were colleges established for vocational training: the Royal Military Academy at Woolwich, the College for Civil Engineers at Putney, the East India College at Addiscombe and the Royal College of Agriculture at Circencester. The second variety were laboratories and colleges where chemistry was taught within a general educational framework: the Royal Cornwall Polytechnic Institution and the Queen's Colleges in Birmingham, Belfast, Galway and Cork. Between 1843 and 1848 chemistry teaching laboratories were opened at the Royal Manchester Institution, the Royal College of Chemistry, University College London, King's College London, and the Liverpool College of Chemistry. Chemistry was also introduced into the curriculum of progressive secondary schools during the 1840s. Several of the more ambitious institutions, Queenwood College, Belfast Academical Institution, Liverpool Royal Institution School and the Liverpool Mechanics Institute Boys' School taught practical chemistry and hired experienced chemists.

By the 1840s participation in the science of chemistry had acquired vocational significance for men in agriculture, manufacturing, government, teaching and research. The Chemical Society brought them together and provided a variety of ways in which their participation in chemistry could be enhanced and expressed. The Society strengthened the cohesion of this newly created chemical community and differentiated it from the medical and pharmaceutical professions. The Pharmaceutical Society and the Chemical Society were complementary organizations. They represented entirely compatible views of the appropriate boundaries of chemical communities. The professionalisation of pharmacy was strengthened by the simultaneous professionalisation of chemistry: growing specialisation furthered the mutual development of separate identities. A clear difference was established between practising chemistry in a pharmaceutical context and as a subject in its own right.

Chemistry was highly respected by the founders of the Pharmaceutical Society. It was seen as central to the education of the new class of "pharmaceutical chemists" and numerous papers on the subject were presented at its scientific meetings. Of twenty-three honorary members elected to the Pharmaceutical Society in 1841, six had been among the founders of the Chemical Society. Nonetheless, the pursuit of chemistry *per se* was not regarded as a professional activity. Jacob Bell saw the Chemical Society as the legitimate outlet for intellectual rather than vocational interests:

> Its objects being purely scientific, it numbers among its members men in many professions, who are devoted to the study of chemistry, and embrace within its sphere every department of that science.[67]

Jacob Bell, Theophilus Redwood and Jonathan Pereira joined the Chemical Society: but only five of the six hundred founder members of the Pharmaceutical Society had done so by 1850.

The birth of the Chemical Society was the outcome of the belief that practitioners of chemistry should be united and that chemistry as a science should be unified. It was a landmark in the evolution of chemistry from a pharmaceutical and medical specialty to an academic discipline. By encompassing teachers, researchers, and appliers of chemistry, the Chemical Society became the vehicle of the discipline. The existence of a chemical society with interests other than medical and pharmaceutical was entirely compatible with the Pharmaceutical Society's aim of creating an autonomous profession of pharmacy. But, although the Chemical and Pharmaceutical Societies offered authoritative and mutually consistent definitions of the chemist and the pharmaceutist, their categorisations did not go unchallenged. A quite different view of the appropriate boundaries of chemical communities was advocated by the journals, *The Chemist*, first published in 1840, and the *Pharmaceutical Times*, first published in 1846, and institutionalised by the Royal College of Chemistry, founded in 1845.

A symptom of the ebullient growth of chemistry as both a science and a vocation was the appearance in January 1840 of a new periodical. *The Chemist; or, Reporter of Chemical Discoveries and Improvements, and Protector of the Rights of the Chemist and Chemical Manufacturer*, edited by Charles Watt, "Lecturer on Chemistry" and John Watt, was intended to serve chemical manufacturers, chemical analysts and inventors, medical men and pharmaceutists. The journal was divided into three parts, dealing with chemistry, manufacturing and pharmacy; but certain fundamental objectives were seen to be in common. One, which was given great prominence at first but then less stridently pushed, was the reform of patent law. A more persistent issue was the improvement of chemical education. More than a year before the foundation of the Pharmaceutical Society, *The Chemist* was urging Parliament to insist on "the cultivation of chemistry by those engaged in dispensing medicine". The retail chemist, "the compounder and dispenser of the products of pharmacy", ought to be "a man of scientific attainments, who can at once detect the unchemical nature of any prescription". Yet, far "too often he can do little more than combine products purchased, at the cheapest possible rate, of some wholesale druggist, without being at all able to determine the goodness or badness of any one thing he is called upon to dispense".

> The retail chemist ought, therefore, to be compelled to undergo a strict examination as to his knowledge of the nature of drugs and their medical properties, so as to enable him to detect any error in prescription and insure his committing no mistake through ignorance.[68]

Urgent legislation was also required "to re-organize the profession of medicine, and to remedy the sad catalogue of abuses which have so long prevailed, and are so congenial to certain classes of its members". Education in chemistry is essential for the medical practitioner:

> Among other improvements which we hope soon to see made in the medical profession is the compulsion to obtain a far greater amount of chemical knowledge than is now done. It is easy to show its general importance to medical science and this is by no means confined to pharmaceutical chemistry. We contend that it is of infinitely greater importance than has generally been allowed by physicians, in relation to physiology and pathology. The chemical composition of the different parts of the body, and the actions by which they are affected and maintained, are, indeed, subjects of the highest importance to the medical practitioner . . .[69]

For different reasons, the manufacturer also needed chemical knowledge. By 1844, *The Chemist* was reporting that:

> The worthy manufacturers of the generation now passing away are having their
> sons instructed in chemistry, as affording the best means of competing with others,
> and of protecting themselves from the machinations of the fraudulent.[70]

The Chemist agglomerated chemical manufacturers, chemical analysts and inventors,
physicians, and chemists and druggists into a class of practitioners who shared a
competence in the application of scientific chemistry. This vision of a community of diverse
chemical practitioners inspired several other journalistic ventures. *Annals of Chemistry and
Pharmacy* appeared in 1842 but lasted only two years. The *Pharmaceutical Times: A Journal
of Chemistry Applied to the Arts, Agriculture and Manufactures* emerged in 1846 from the
pharmaceutical supplement to the *Medical Times*. In November 1848 the title was changed
to the *Chemical Times and Journal of Pharmacy, Manufactures, Agriculture and the Industrial Arts*,
marking a shift towards non-pharmaceutical chemistry. The readers of all these journals
were assumed to be users rather than creators of chemistry: the emphasis was on
application not research.

The idea that men with vocational interests in practical chemistry constituted a class who
could share a common territory found institutional embodiment in the Royal College of
Chemistry.[71] In November 1843 John Gardner (1804–1880), an apothecary, and John
Lloyd Bullock (1812–1905), a chemist and druggist, proposed the setting up of a "Practical
Chemical School" as an appendage to the Royal Institution. The school was to have two
departments: the first, devoted to pure science, would be, administratively and physically,
part of the Royal Institution; the second, devoted to applied chemistry, would occupy
separate premises (owned by Bullock) and be administered by Gardner as secretary and
Bullock as scientific director. The pure science department, like Liebig's university
laboratory, was to be a centre for training students in research methods through laboratory
practice in chemical analysis. Such a programme would equip students to follow any
subsequent chemical career.

> Whether the object of the student be to qualify himself as a teacher of chemistry,
> to learn the bearing of science on medicine and physiology, or to become a
> manufacturer, the same purely scientific education in the art of research is
> recommended to all ...

The applied science department, which was to be devoted to vocational training and
research on practical problems, would combine the functions of a department of technical
chemistry, a pharmaceutical institute, and an analytical practice.

> In order to meet the especial exigencies of this country and at once to adopt the
> mature improvements of the best continental schools ... a practical laboratory
> should be provided for the application of Chemistry to Medicine, Arts and
> Agriculture ... In this department, the course of manipulation required by the
> Apothecaries' Company; the analysis of soils or commercial articles for subscribers;
> the preparation of all the articles in the Pharmacopoeia in a consecutive course; and
> afterwards the application of chemistry to the Arts, as dyeing etc. might be taught
> ...

Gardner and Bullock initiated the movement from which the Royal College of Chemistry
emerged in October 1845. An independent, privately-funded institution, its objective was
the promotion of the science of chemistry and its application to agriculture, arts,

manufactures and medicine. Although the College did not develop in the way envisaged by its founders, it did train men in practical chemistry for a wide variety of industries and professions. The laboratory-centred educational programme instituted at the College subsequently formed the basic model for the professional training of specialist chemists in England. In 1853 the Government assumed financial responsibility for the Royal College of Chemistry and it was incorporated into the Metropolitan School of Mines and of Science Applied to the Arts.

In 1848 the *Pharmaceutical Times* observed:

> We are accustomed to societies distinguished, as if by the most scrupulous analysis, by only the finest shades of difference. Within half a mile of Trafalgar-square you shall find one science represented by three institutions; and a stranger will with difficulty understand the difference when you tell him that here chemistry is taught in its practical uses in pharmacy (School of Pharmacy), there its limits are extended by patient investigation of difficult and unexplained phenomena (Royal College of Chemistry), while a body of men (Chemical Society) are met in a third place to occupy themselves with the consolidation of both pure and mixed science.[72]

The visions of the leaders of the Pharmaceutical Society and the Chemical Society were mutually compatible. Far more problematic was the relationship between the Pharmaceutical Society and those who opposed the attempt to create a peculiarly pharmaceutical science. Jacob Bell took pains to distinguish the curriculum of the School of Pharmacy from that of the Royal College of Chemistry, where, he pointed out

> ... a wider field is taken and many of the researches, while they are highly interesting and improving to the chemist, are rather calculated to divert the mind of the druggist from his own legitimate sphere, leading him into more abstruse science unconnected with his particular business.[73]

The Chemist, the *Pharmaceutical Times* and Lloyd Bullock expressed the difference between their vision and that of Jacob Bell through personal abuse and repeated criticisms of his policies. *The Chemist* was the most vitriolic critic. The facilities of the Pharmaceutical Society, it asserted,

> are not for the benefit of the whole, but for the aggrandizement and profit of the select few—we might say, for one individual. The motives which have led to this fine piece of show-off cannot be too highly condemned ... The subscribers are justly indignant at being made to pay the exorbitant fee of two guineas per annum for the sole purpose of gratifying the ambitious cupidity and puerile vanity of Jacob Bell.

> The Society appears to be represented by one individual,—not the President, not the Vice- president, nor the Secretary,—but by a member of the Council,—restless, ambitious, and anxious to get all into his own hands ... he has already commenced making the Society a means of emolument and profit ... an individual is thus raising himself into notoriety—taking the whole business into his own hands, and his own house - and establishing a property for himself which he draws from the funds of the Society.

The Society was excessively dominated, and indeed used by, the metropolitan elite: neither the meetings nor the educational facilities were attuned to the needs of provincial members. Possessing the diploma of the Pharmaceutical Society, it was stated, did not raise the status of the chemist and druggist, because the examination for it carried no respect, nor did the examiners. It was no secret that the original members received their diplomas merely by paying the membership fee. "In the course of our experience it never has occurred to us to see any undertaking so badly carried out, so misconducted in every movement, in fact, so completely ruined, as this Society has been". Looking ahead, "we are but too sure of the speedy and total extinction of this Society, and that, like the British Association, the pit of oblivion awaits it". *The Chemist* ceased publication in 1858.[74]

Both *The Chemist* and the *Pharmaceutical Times* challenged the intellectual focus of the Society: neither had any sympathy for the attempt to create an independent pharmaceutical science. The *Pharmaceutical Journal*, they said, was an haphazard collection of low quality oddments; the promised laboratory course in practical chemistry had not materialised. In 1849 the *Chemical Times* lamented

> No perceptible progress has, in fact, been made by the chemist and druggist in the study and knowledge of the principal department of his calling, viz., *practical chemistry*, and more particularly, *chemical analysis* . . . the great majority of chemists and druggists in this country, highly educated though most of them are in other respects, are almost totally ignorant of the very rudiments of that science which forms the fundamental basis of their profession.[75]

On one level, the animus that the editors of *The Chemist* and the *Pharmaceutical Times* displayed towards Jacob Bell and the Pharmaceutical Society was motivated by jealousy and self-seeking. Smarting at the Society's success, they publicly denounced it as a failure. Jacob Bell's journal was a healthy rival to their own: the School of Pharmacy threatened to undermine their private teaching ventures. Both Charles Watt and John Scoffern, the editor of the *Pharmaceutical Times*, were involved in teaching chemistry in London private schools. On another level, however, important matters of principle were at stake. A small group of "operative" and "analytical" chemists in London, although initially supporters of the Pharmaceutical Society, soon formed an opposition. They differed from Jacob Bell on the broad lines on which the Society should develop. They wanted an exclusive scientific society "confined to the advancement of philosophy and useful discoveries". They objected to opening the floodgates to all and sundry: only chemists with scientific pretensions should be allowed in. The most articulate representative of this tiny core of metropolitan chemists was John Lloyd Bullock (1812–1905). He had studied with Liebig during the winter of 1839 and had spent some time studying with Dumas and Orfila in Paris. In May 1841 he set up shop as a chemist and druggist at 22, Conduit Street, Mayfair. In a lecture, delivered at these premises in June 1844, Bullock explained why he left the Pharmaceutical Society:

> . . . instead of advancing the profession of pharmacy, this society, by its very exceptionable practices, has rendered it the more difficult to effect any good, and will serve but to obstruct all attempts at future reform and improvement.

Bullock objected to the fact that the Society had opened its doors to persons "with no other qualification than the payment of its exorbitant annual demand". Fit and unfit were admitted. The timid join in great numbers because "an expectation has been studiously held out that members of this society only would be held legally qualified to pursue pharmacy". The grandiloquent diploma

> was designed especially to permit the less scrupulous persons, who were willing to pay for it, to impose upon the public, with a document which could not readily be distinguished from a legal licence to practise.

But the most respectable and the best qualified to advance pharmacy have been deterred from joining.

Besides making personal objections to the behaviour of Jacob Bell, Bullock was scathing in his assessment of the activities of the rest of Britain's chemists and druggists. Richard Phillips' articles in the *Pharmaceutical Journal* demonstrated, he said, how the efficacy of the physician's prescription was destroyed by the ignorant dispenser and the fraudulent wholesaler:

> ... the plain truth is, the majority of chemists and druggists in this country are totally ignorant of chemistry ... They undergo no examination—they are under no restriction. A grocer may displace his canisters any day he pleases, an oilman his casks, and supply their places with substances, single grains of which may consign to their graves their equally ignorant neighbours. The boy who has carried out the medicine of the general practitioner, learns to spell the names on the bottles in the dispensary, and he is forthwith qualified to be a Pharmacien; he takes a shop, writes up "Chemist", and the confiding public enjoys the precious boon.

The government has a duty to protect the public by enacting that the druggist "shall be qualified by a knowledge of chemistry, shall undergo an examination before a competent authority, and receive a sanction, in the shape of a licence, to practise pharmacy". But, "in this country any restraint upon the liberty of the subject is looked upon with jealousy, even the liberty to poison is esteemed too sacred to be abridged".

The Pharmaceutical Society was doing nothing to tackle the real reasons for the inferior professional standing of the chemist and druggist. The essential reform was "that every pharmacien must be a profound practical chemist". Bullock's use of the term "pharmacien" indicates the direction he believed the profession should take. He wanted the initiate to undergo a continental-style education. He shared with Jacob Bell an admiration for the system of professional education and regulation found in France and Germany, where the science of chemistry was pursued with a healthy vigour unknown to this country.

> Nothing can serve to display the unsatisfactory state of the practice of pharmacy in this country more than the reflection that all the vegetable alkaloids—those subtle principles which present to us the properties of medicinal plants, and now in constant use throughout the world—not one was discovered in this country. We are indebted to the French and German chemists and pharmaciens for this improvement, the benefit of which is really incalculable.

For Bullock, pharmacy was a branch of the science of chemistry. "Chemistry is our corner-stone", he asserted, "it is more to the pharmacien than anatomy is to the physician or surgeon".

> There is no longer any distinction between Galenical and chemical remedies. Such vegetable substances as are employed by the physician are as much under the dominion of chemistry as the metals. Nay, the dependence of their properties, in

relation to disease, upon subtle principles, which have been detected and separated by the chemist, shows us that a knowledge of chemistry is even more necessary in dealing with them in the operations of pharmacy than it is with mineral compounds.

Pharmacy must necessarily be separated from medicine. The medical practitioner ought, of course, to understand the processes employed in the manufacture of medicines but he cannot, in this era of scientific progress, occupy himself with their preparation. The pharmacien's education should include all the sciences on which the practice of pharmacy was based: Bullock specifically mentioned botany, mineralogy and natural philosophy. The study of languages was also necessary: Latin because it was the language of the physician, French and German because they were the languages of the leading chemists. But the chief study of the pharmacien was chemistry. Chemistry was to be studied in the laboratory where the qualitative and quantitative techniques of inorganic and organic chemistry were to be learnt. Finally, the undertaking of a laboratory research project would complete the acquisition of the principles of the science. Only after this thorough scientific training should the student apply himself specifically to pharmaceutical problems. For a pharmacien so trained, research would be a continuing concern:

> ... there is not one single agent in use as a remedy, there is not a plant, a mineral, a metal, about which there is not much still undetermined; and as chemists and physiologists are rapidly together advancing the knowledge of the human body, the nature of its elements, and the laws of their combination, so must the demand arise for improved forms of remedies, new substances which may meet the requirement of advanced science, and the most refined adjustments of those already known to the exigencies of disease, and disturbances of natural functions.

Chemistry was the scientific base which would give the practice of pharmacy the status of a profession rather than a trade. In discussing the differences between a trade and a profession, Bullock emphasized the public service function of the educated pharmacien. The sale of adulterated medicines would be eliminated. Through cooperative research with physicians, medical treatment would be improved: knowledge of chemical principles would provide an understanding of the healing properties of medicine. The contribution of the new pharmacien, however, would extend far beyond the sphere of medicine. In particular, the provincial practitioner, with his training in practical chemistry, would serve as the analytical adviser of the farmer and the manufacturer as well as the physician. To those who intended to take up the vocation of pharmacy, he gave this advice. Follow chemistry "until you have sufficient skill to perform a satisfactory analysis of inorganic and organic compounds". For, once this skill has been acquired,

> not only will it enable you ... to prepare the remedies of the physician—to manufacture the several ingredients as he usually prescribes them— to avoid the use of a spurious, adulterated, or deteriorated drug— any wrong chemical substance; but chemistry will enable you ... to discover new or improved forms of remedies; new, cheaper and better processes for preparing old ones; and thus you will, at the same time, and by the most honourable means, ensure your success in business ...

The study of practical chemistry would bring benefits to the community and greater profit to the pharmacien. In closing, Bullock mentioned that he was actively involved in trying to launch a school of practical chemistry.[76]

It is clear that Bullock agreed with much of Jacob Bell's analysis of the state of pharmacy in Britain and with many of his reform proposals. In the final analysis, however, there is a fundamental difference between them. Jacob Bell believed that pharmacy "should ... be considered, not as a distinct science, but a distinct branch of the science of medicine". In 1841 he made an unsuccessful attempt to get pharmacy admitted to the medical section of the British Association for the Advancement of Science. In that year he wrote a paper on the state of pharmacy in Britain, the object of which

> Was to show the connexion of pharmacy with medical practice in ancient times—the origin of a division of labour in the profession,— the beneficial result of the cultivation of the separate branches by different classes of men, and at the same time, the mutual dependence of each branch on the other ... Neglect and other circumstances ... have prevented pharmacy from keeping pace with the other branches and assuming that position which it enjoys in all civilized nations except our own ... Finally, the constitution and merits of the Pharmaceutical Society were detailed and advocated as being the most effectual remedy for existing evils and deficiences.[77]

In 1844 Jacob Bell claimed that the Pharmaceutical Society "has become a bond of union, means of defence, and medium of friendly intercourse amongst a previously scattered body of men, who are now a recognised part of the medical profession".[78]

Bullock, on the contrary, saw pharmacy as a branch of the science of chemistry. Pharmaciens would receive the same training as those who would later work as teachers, researchers, industrial consultants and analytical chemists. The status of the pharmaceutical chemist would be linked to that of other professional scientists: it would no longer be constrained by the medical hierarchy. The status system of the medical profession accorded him a position of inferiority. Freed from that, his real worth as a member of the chemical community would be recognised. Pharmacy would thus be separated from medical practice in a more radical way than Bell advocated. Within the British Association the place for the pharmacien was in Section B, the section devoted to chemistry and related sciences.

* * *

In 1837 Justus Liebig travelled to England to deliver an address to the British Association for the Advancement of Science. In it he urged English men of science to participate in advancing the frontiers of organic chemistry "and unite their efforts to those of the chemists of the Continent":

> We live in a time when the slightest exertion leads to valuable results, and, if we consider the immense influence which organic chemistry exercises over medicine, manufactures, and over common life, we must be sensible that there is no problem more important to mankind than the prosecution of the objects which organic chemistry contemplates.[79]

Although Liebig claimed to be "a man of science and not of commerce", he could not resist the temptation to be lured into business. In 1845 he discovered a process for using what was previously regarded as a waste product to make a cheap substitute for the very expensive drug, quinine. With Liebig's consent, the substance, amorphous quinine, was patented in England under Bullock's name since English patent law prohibited foreign patentees. While the patent was kept secret, the discovery was widely advertised as a scientific advance in the *Lancet* and at the Royal College of Chemistry. A lecture given at the College by its secretary, John Gardner, induced several manufacturing chemists to try to make it. Only then was it announced that the discovery had already been patented. This attempt by Liebig, Bullock and Gardner to use a scientific institution to promote their own personal gain was trenchantly exposed by Jacob Bell in the *Pharmaceutical Journal*. He presented it as a clear violation of the norms of both science and business:

> In cases of this kind, a departure from the usual straight-forward course, naturally gives rise to various conjectures, and, in this instance, it was currently reported, and generally believed, that several parties, beside the patentee, had an interest in the speculation; and that the plan ... had been resorted to for the purpose of ensuring its success by bringing the new remedy before the profession as a scientific discovery, eulogised in a widely circulated and influential journal, and in other quarters, in a manner which would have been indelicate had it been known to be a merely commercial transaction.[80]

After this expose, Liebig's reputation in England slumped considerably, not only because of his shady business dealings, but also because Theophilus Redwood proved that his great discovery was nothing more than the worthless product of slipshod work. At the same time, Jacob Bell revealed that John Gardner, Bullock's accomplice, was involved in other sharp business practice. Gardner, a self-styled surgeon who purchased a Giessen M.D. (making him one of that university's notorious "Doctors payable-at-sight") practised from his brother's pharmacy. Brother John prescribed, brother Thomas dispensed. In 1846 they jointly published *The Family Medicine Book*, which professed to be a guide to self-medication, but was really as Bell pointed out, a cheap druggist's price-list of items sold by Thomas Gardner. In the same year John Gardner's association with the Royal College of Chemistry ended in disgrace.

In later life, Liebig's commercial ventures were more successful. In 1866 he assumed the directorship of the scientific department of Liebig's Extract of Meat Company. The famous meat extract made use of the wasted meat of the Rio de la Plata cattle, slaughtered for their leather, to provide the "plastic food" required to produce blood, build organs and replenish muscles. Within a few years the successful company was supplying the British army in Abyssinia.

Liebig and his followers saw no contradiction between profit and *Wissenschaft*. The search for scientific truth is paramount, but since all knowledge is practical, it is science which gives nourishment to industry. One of Liebig's most striking phrases, "Intelligence in union with Capital", epitomises the chemists who founded the Pharmaceutical Society in 1841. They were a small band of the wealthiest and most enterprising chemists and druggists in London. They were men who had been quick to exploit the commercial opportunities presented by scientific progress. They combined scientific conviction with business acumen. Their attitude towards scientific research was decidedly entrepreneurial. Their main concern was to apply chemical knowledge to production in order to make a profit. They were not primarily concerned with advancing knowledge nor with contributing magnanimously to the health of the nation. Luke Howard FRS (1772–1864), a leading chemical manufacturer and once a partner of William Allen, applied himself assiduously to his hobby of meteorology but published nothing on chemistry. He explained himself in a letter to the poet Goethe:

> It may appear singular that with such opportunities, I should have published nothing *as a Chemist*. The reply to such a proposal would be short, and decided.

C'est notre *metier*—we have to *live* by the practice of Chemistry as an art, and not by exhibiting it as a science. The success of our endeavours, under the vigorous competition which every ingenious man has, here, to sustain, depends on *using*, while we can do it exclusively, the few new facts that turn up in the routine of practice.[81]

The men who created and controlled the Pharmaceutical Society in its early decades were, in the words of Theophilus Redwood, "the most influential members of the drug trade, representing every department of the business". One of the firms associated with the birth of the Society had been trading in drugs and chemicals since the seventeenth century and was still in business in the 1890s. Edward Horner, of Horner & Sons, was a member of the original committee of the Pharmaceutical Society. The connection between overseas trade and scientific pharmacy was recognised by the Society when it set up "a scientific committee for the promotion of pharmacological knowledge" in 1845. The idea came from Dr. Jonathan Pereira, the Society's professor of materia medica and a close friend of Jacob Bell. No country in the world, he argued, was as well placed as Great Britain for carrying out scientific inquiries into the properties of drugs: "her numerous and important colonies in all parts of the world, and her extensive commercial relations, particularly fit her for taking the lead in investigations of this kind".[82] William Allen, Hanburys & Barry was another old-established firm, with a continuous history at 2 Plough Court in the City of London since 1715. William Allen FRS was the first president of the Society, and both John Barry and Daniel Hanbury served on the first committee. William Allen (1770–1843) was a Quaker, scientist and philanthropist. He served an apprenticeship in the pharmaceutical establishment of Joseph Gurney Bevan in Plough Court and later succeeded to the business. Luke Howard was apprenticed to Ollive Sims, a fellow Quaker chemist and druggist, of Stockport in Cheshire and set up shop in London in 1790. He was not very successful and in 1796 became the junior partner of William Allen. The new firm of Allen and Howard "attempted to bring science, such as it then was, into connection with the preparation of medicines". In addition to the wholesale drug trade and the retail business, Allen and Howard established a laboratory at Plaistow for the manufacture of chemicals. In 1802 Allen became the first specialist outside the medical profession to be appointed to teach in an English medical school. From 1802 to 1826 he lectured on chemistry and experimental philosophy at Guy's Hospital and for several years he held the chair of experimental philosophy at the Royal Institution. His chemistry syllabus of 1802 reveals that his teaching was abreast of current developments: the new chemical nomenclature of Lavoisier and Guyton de Morveau was used, the oxygen theory was applied, and attention given to the analysis of chemical substances into their elements. Allen also encouraged the inclusion of practical work in the chemistry teaching. His syllabus states that lectures were to be illustrated by experiments and after 1816 the apparatus belonging to the teaching laboratory was illustrated on the title page. The syllabus also claims that students were to be given a closer acquaintance with practical chemical operations, for they were to have access to a laboratory where they would have an opportunity of seeing the various chemical processes conducted on a large-scale and of becoming "acquainted with every step necessary in the management of such operations". It is probable that Allen was offering his students the chance to visit the Plaistow chemical laboratory.[83]

In 1807 the partnership between Allen and Howard was wound up. Howard moved to

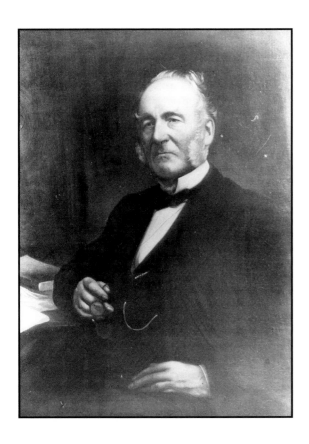

22 *Daniel Bell Hanbury (1794–1882) treasurer of the Society from 1852 to 1867. He was a nephew and business partner of William Allen.*

Stratford in the East End leaving Allen to concentrate upon galenical preparations. Howard's company became involved in the manufacture of a wide variety of chemicals. Between 1808 and 1817 the company regularly achieved net profit on sales of 16 to 25 per cent. During the next eight years, results were even better, mostly between 25 and 30 per cent. In 1830 peak sales of £37,000 were reached. However during the 1830s, competition developed and sales and profits fell. Howard's response to competition was to produce a steadily increasing range of products for both the pharmaceutical and industrial markets. In the early days the business was based on the refining of three natural products brought from India: nitre used in the manufacture of sulphuric acid, borax used for flux, and camphor for mothballs and medicines. Far more complex, but very profitable, was the manufacture from 1823 of the new substance quinine. During the 1830s the sale of iodine became important and the firm sold about 10,000 ounces a year. Although Howard demonstrated a flair for devising improved methods of producing pharmaceutical chemicals, a wide variety of mordants and inorganic dyes were also sold to the calico printing industry. By the 1860s the old corn mills that housed his works in the East End were known as Howard's Quinine, Borax and Tartaric Acid Works, and some 200 people were employed there.[84]

131

In the meanwhile, William Allen journeyed far in the cause of "promoting and extending religion, charity, education and civil liberty", wisely leaving his business interests in the hands of his confidential clerk, John Thomas Barry (1789–1864), who joined as a partner. Allen's activities fostered business with overseas customers, especially those in North America and the West Indies: Barry developed the manufacturing side. Once described as a "neat and exact experimentalist", Barry evolved, in 1819, a method of preparing extracts by evaporation *in vacuo*, using a temperature of 100°F instead of 212°F. By this means he obtained extracts three times as strong as those prepared by boiling in open pans. Not only were these extracts more uniform in strength but could also be produced at lower cost. When cod liver oil came into prominence in 1847 as a remedy for consumption, Allen, Hanburys & Barry began to process it in quantity, later setting up its own factories in Newfoundland and in the Lofoten Islands.

The wealth of the majority of the founders of the Pharmaceutical Society was of a more recent origin. The first half of the nineteenth century offered great opportunities for the medium-sized well-run retail business. The demand for drugs from the growing middle class and from the hospitals and dispensaries for the sick poor was the spur to the development of the wholesale trade and of chemical and drug production. The retail chemists in the City and West End of London developed laboratories and manufactories where they made up their own preparations for wider distribution. The names of two of the founding fathers of the Society became known to a wide public by their association with a proprietary medicine: Charles Dinneford (Fluid Magnesia) and Thomas Keating (Keating's Flea Powder). Many of the leading pharmaceutical manufacturing companies of the years following the Second World War trace their own origins back to the businesses set up by founding members of the Pharmaceutical Society. J.S. Lescher was a partner in the wholesale firm of Evans & Lescher, which specialised in supplying galenical and chemical preparations to hospitals and dispensaries. Evans & Lescher became Evans Medical Ltd. Barron, Harvey & Barron formed part of the group that became British Drug Houses Ltd. Samuel Foulger & Son of Wapping and Herring Brothers were later both absorbed by Willows Francis Ltd. Thomas Morson & Son was amalgamated in the late 1950s with Merck, Sharp & Dohme Ltd. Charles Barron, Samuel Foulger and J.S. Lescher were members of the first committee and both Thomas Herring and Thomas Morson served as presidents of the Society.

Thomas Herring (1785–1864) and his brother Thrower Buckle Herring were wholesale druggists who moved in 1815 to extensive premises at 40 Aldersgate Street. The firm produced on a large scale vegetable and other powders of superior quality by means of a powerful and efficient drug-mill which they installed on the premises. Such work had invariably been done in the past by a class of men called "drug-grinders" who were not noted for the production of good and genuine powders. Herring's vegetable powders—such as rhubarb, jalap and ipecacuanha—"were fine, soft, impalpable, bright-looking powders, such as could not be produced with the pestle and mortar". Thomas Newborn Robert Morson (1799–1874) acquired an interest in scientific chemistry during his apprenticeship to an apothecary in the old Fleet Market in the City. Morson succeeded to that business in 1821 but before doing so, he lived for three years in the establishment of M. Planche, a *pharmacien* of Paris. Here he came under the influence of Magendie and Pelletier and learned about the new processes being developed for manufacturing chemicals and the newly discovered alkaloids. Morson was quick to realise the commercial potential of the

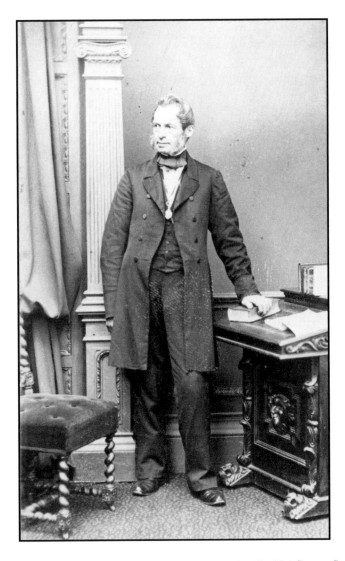

23 *Peter Squire (1798–1884) carte-de-visite by J.E. Mayall, 224 Regent Street, London, c. 1865. Squire, a prosperous high class London chemist and druggist, played a leading part in the formation of the Society and was three times President. He was the first chemist and druggist to be appointed to supply and dispense medicines to the Royal establishment.*

alkaloids: in his Fleet Market laboratory he made the first morphine and the first quinine sulphate produced in Britain. These premises proved to be too restrictive and he moved in 1826 to Southampton Row and two years later purchased premises in Hornsey Road to build a laboratory for the manufacture of drugs and chemicals. Creosote, another recent discovery, was produced there in large quantities. Morson's linguistic ability, scientific

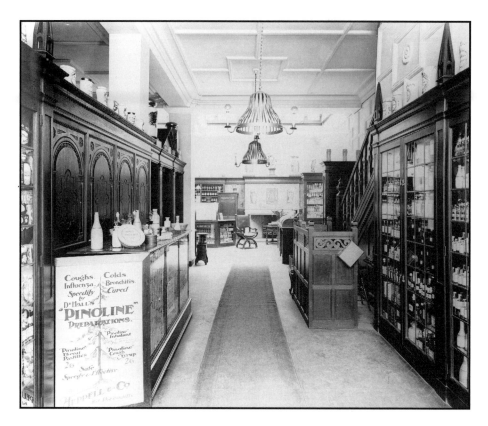

24   *Heppell & Co., 164 Piccadilly, London, in 1912. This business, with its original and fashionable fittings, offered a high class of service in the West End of London; bankrupt by 1922, it survived as Heppell's (1922) Ltd.*

interests and considerable wealth enabled him to develop contacts with distinguished European scientists. Among the many famous visitors to his "Science Sunday Evenings" was Baron Justus von Liebig.

Richard Hotham Pigeon (1789–1851) was the chairman of the inaugural meeting of the Pharmaceutical Society on 15 April 1841, and became the first treasurer of the Society. He was a prominent member of the Wholesale Druggists' Club, a commercial association established to discuss and regulate the trade in drugs and chemicals. Its members were men with influence in the City of London and at Westminster and with extensive contacts with retailers throughout the country. Pigeon ran a very prosperous business from the house in Throgmorton Street which he had first entered as a apprentice at the age of 16. In 1835 he was elected treasurer of Christs's Hospital and was instrumental in increasing the number of children educated there, widening the curriculum and persuading Queen Victoria, Prince Albert, the Prince of Wales and the Duke of Cambridge to become patrons. The early meetings of the Pharmaceutical Society took place in his house, and his status gave the infant Society an air of respectability. Another chemist whose standing was important in this respect was Peter Squire (1798–1884), the owner since 1831 of a notable pharmacy in Oxford Street. In 1837 he became the first chemist and druggist to replace an apothecary in supplying medicine to the Royal Family. He played a prominent part in the founding of the Society and was made president in 1849–50 and again during the years 1861–3. By his many papers on the practice of pharmacy and the publication of *The Three Pharmacopoeias* (1851), *The Pharmacopoeias of the London Hospitals* (1863) and *A Companion to the British Pharmacopoeia* (1864) he greatly improved the processes for making pharmaceutical preparations and stressed the need for uniformity in formulas. He retained his connexion with the Oxford Street pharmacy for almost fifty years.

Robert Alsop (1803–76), like so many of the leading lights in the Pharmaceutical Society, was a Quaker. After an apprenticeship and assistantship with John Bell, he established himself in 1826 as a chemist and druggist in an "old-fashioned shop at the corner of Sloane Square, Chelsea, with its palms, ferns, and tree-frogs in the window". He made several important contributions to practical pharmacy: he introduced an infusion jug and a minim measure. His methods for preparing mercuric nitrate ointment and spirit of nitrous ether were used for many years. But it was the production of soda and mineral water which brought the prosperity that enabled him to give up the practice of pharmacy in 1855 to devote himself to philanthropic and religious causes. Richard Battley (1770–1856) was a very active and zealous supporter of the Pharmaceutical Society and first in a line of distinguished pharmacognosists. About 1800, after serving as an assistant surgeon in the navy, he bought an apothecary's business in St. Paul's Churchyard. In 1812 he moved to Fore Street, where he carried out many improvements in pharmaceutical processing. Like Alsop, he made significant contributions to pharmaceutical practice. He has a good claim to introducing the cold-water process for making infusion and extracts, particularly of opium and cinchona. His liquor cinchonae was made official in the *London Pharmacopoeia*. He became a highly regarded lecturer in materia medica at several London hospitals, as well as holding classes at his own materia medica museum. His wealth, however, was created by the wholesale business he established under the name of Battley & Watts.

Jacob Bell controlled the Pharmaceutical Society for the first eighteen years of its existence. Throughout that time he was a member of the Council and the proprietor and editor of the *Pharmaceutical Journal*: but he held no other office until elected President in 1856. His influence stemmed from the crucial part he played in the creation of the Society and from the unstinted commitment of his time and energy to its growth. He was an assiduous member of every committee and delegation. He became the articulate, thoughtful and well-informed spokesman for the cause. In 1859 the Vice-president attributed the thriving state of the Society "in a great degree" to "the exertions and energy" of Jacob Bell "who had taken a prominent part in originating, rearing and upholding the Society". It is no disparagement of his achievement to be reminded of the strength of bonds which existed among the leading London chemists and druggists. Prior to 1841 they were enmeshed in a network of cross-cutting ties: the Quaker faith, mutual involvement in business endeavour and a decidedly entrepreneurial view of science united them. Above all, they were linked by the experience of success: the combination of enterprise and expertise had made them wealthy men. Yet trade jealousies, suspicion and distrust prevailed, inspite of the bedrock of common interests. The foundation of the Pharmaceutical Society provided a rich variety of ways in which the metropolitan elite could express its participation in the common enterprise of pharmacy. The holding of office, membership of committees, contributions to the scientific meetings, the writing of articles, and even the reading of the journal furthered professional as well as personal interests. Once formed, the Pharmaceutical Society took on the character of a crusade, a drive for higher standards of performance and greater recognition by other professions, the government and the public. The professionalising strategy of the society was designed to make the extraordinary occupational activities of the metropolitan elite the criterion for evaluating the work of the ordinary, common or garden variety chemist and druggist. The programme of reform was a reflection of the behaviour of wholesale, manufacturing and dispensing chemists: it was not calculated to meet the needs of the great majority of British chemists and druggists. The Pharmaceutical Society was not created in response to their demands. Jacob Bell and his friends in London were not bombarded with *cahiers* and lists of grievances from their colleagues in the provinces. No attempt was made to make the Society reflect the hopes and aspirations of Britain's chemists and druggists. A series of articles in the *Pharmaceutical Journal*, entitled "Illustrations of the Present State of Pharmacy in England', was not an inquiry into the profession's requirements, but an exposé of its shortcomings. The founding fathers developed a strong sense of mission: the sinners to be converted were the potential members of the Society. The foundation of the Pharmaceutical Society was an attempt by the metropolitan elite to regulate and control the rest of the profession. Rooted in the economic and status concerns of the leading London chemists and druggists, the Society was bound to promote their interests when it sought to further the interests of the profession as a whole. When the Society tried to persuade its members to place professional responsibility and public service above self-interest, when it inveighed against price competition and short-sighted profiteering, when it condemned chemists and druggists for their ignorance and incompetence and disowned them for practising as apothecaries, it was promoting the interests of the metropolitan elite against the immediate interests of other sections of the trade. It is not surprising that many chemists and druggists, regarding the Society as a futile and unwarrantable interference with their individual liberty, declined to join. The realisation that a fully developed professional association involved many restrictions on the activities of individuals and that the promotion of the interests of an elite many prove the long-term salvation of the many, was a pill not easily swallowed by nineteenth century chemists and druggists.

From the very start of his involvement in the Pharmaceutical Society Jacob Bell saw it as a professional association. Proposals to restrict it to either a trade association or a scientific society he rejected unequivocally. A trade association implied a mean and narrow spirit: a scientific society would be exclusive and ineffective. Denied room to breathe, it would soon die. Bell's vision was of a multi-faceted, multi-purpose body. The Pharmaceutical Society that he envisaged would unite under its auspices all the chemists and druggists in Britain; it would be active in promoting the solidarity and professional consciousness of it members; it would represent its members to the public, to other occupations, and to the government. It would protect the interests of the profession and guard it against interference and encroachment. It would ensure that the profession was self-governing and self-regulating: it would secure its members' professional autonomy. The ignorant, incompetent, and unscrupulous would be excluded by a system of education, examination, qualification and registration. Educated practitioners would be protected against unfair and unethical competition and their status and remuneration would be enhanced. The progress of chemistry and pharmacy would be promoted. The victims of circumstance would be relieved by an occupational welfare scheme.

*   *   *

The Pharmaceutical Society has a special place in the history of professions in Britain.[85] It was unique in the wide range of functions it set out to perform and a pioneer in developing the strategy of professionalisation and the concept of a modern professional association. The Society took upon itself a wide range of functions: it was, at one and the same time, a qualifying authority, an educational institution, a scientific society, an occupational and trade association and a benevolent society.

In the preliminary discussions which culminated in the Society's foundation, the title "College of Pharmacy" was suggested. It was rejected, not as being inappropriate to the Society's aspirations, but as too presumptuous at the beginning.[86] The phrase did not imply an educational institute but a community of persons devoted to common pursuits. The founders had in mind the College of Physicians and the College of Surgeons. They, together with the Society of Apothecaries, were the examining and qualifying authorities for the medical profession. The Pharmaceutical Society was to be the new link in the chain, the examining and qualifying body for chemists and druggists. From the outset it sought to establish itself as the portal through which all intending chemists and druggists would need to pass. It soon established examinations for those at the start and end of their apprenticeship and for those about to commence in business. "The Pharmaceutical Society was designed as a means of raising the qualifications of pharmaceutical chemists and placing between them and unqualified persons a line of demarcation".[87] The list of members and associates was intended to serve as a register of those considered competent and qualified. The fact that chemists and druggists both worked as isolated individuals and were directly concerned with matters of life and death made Jacob Bell appreciate the need for a written code of ethics to promote a uniform standard of conduct and practice. It would, however, have been merely self-defeating for the Society, still weak in membership and prestige, to ride the horse of professional integrity with tight reins from the start. Instead all available resources were poured into the School of Pharmacy and the laboratory to buttress the Society's credentials as an educational institution. Yet the idea of combining teaching and examining was widely regarded in England as undesirable and unacceptable. Neither the Royal Colleges nor the Society of Apothecaries organised their own teaching but recognised instead teaching within other independent institutions. Using the University of Cambridge as a precedent, London University had been specifically set up as the examining board for University College and King's College. Only in the Scottish Universities were the functions of teaching, examining and qualifying to be found under the same roof.

Within the medical profession, the qualifying associations resisted the attempts of their licentiates to turn them into occupational associations. Those who obtained qualifications from the Royal Colleges and the Apothecaries' Society were not bound to the qualifying body by subscriptions or the use of facilities: above all, they had no say in the government. During the 1830s and 1840s new voluntary associations were formed to act as occupational associations for the medical profession. An occupational association is a political organization. Its aim is to create a power base for the protection and improvement of the working conditions, job security and monetary rewards of the individual professional. Its primary function is to organize, to gather together all those within a particular occupation and thus to promote solidarity and group consciousness. The organizing function is a continuous process extending beyond the period of formation: an ungrateful and apathetic membership has to be made continually aware of its obligations to one another and of the benefits derived from union. The first British Medical Association, founded 1836, and the National Association of General Practitioners, founded 1844, were both failures. Much more enduring was the Provincial Medical and Surgical Association, founded in Worcester in 1832, which adopted the name British Medical Association in 1855. The Pharmaceutical Society was for chemists and druggists what the Royal Colleges and the BMA combined became for medical practitioners, a qualifying association and a representative organization of the whole profession.

The Pharmaceutical Society experienced difficulties from the outset in acting as an occupational association since it comprised both employers (as members) and employees (as associates). The division between master and servant was built into the original constitution. As long as assistants (associates) had reasonable prospects of setting up in business on their own account, their inferior status could be regarded as merely temporary. They could be regarded as journeymen rather than as employees. But this justification of the division between members and associates was dubious even in 1841 and became more so as the years passed by. Once the examination system became established, the qualification for membership became both financial (having capital to set up in business) and educational (having passed the major examination). Pharmaceutical chemists who were not their own masters were denied the privileges of full membership. Instead of a trade union of professionally qualified members, the Pharmaceutical Society was, at one level, a traders' association, a union of retail proprietors. Indeed, it required a great deal of effort by Jacob Bell to make it more than that. Most chemists and druggists would have preferred an organisation to restrict unwanted competition than a "highfalutin" professional association. There was resentment that the contents of the *Pharmaceutical Journal* were scientific rather than commercial and that subscriptions were used to underwrite the School of Pharmacy rather than boost the benevolent fund.

The Pharmaceutical Society incorporated features found in other institutions and movements. The idea of promoting excellence in "pure" pharmacy and the size of the Council (21 members) were derived from the Royal College of Surgeons. Many of the Society's activities were characteristic of the host of scientific and medical study societies which flourished in London during the first half of the nineteenth century. The museum, the library, the scientific meetings and the published transactions were used to promote pharmacy as a scientific discipline and to enhance the Society's status in the eyes of the medical and scientific communities. The Society's founders had the good sense to incorporate the leading ideas of the medical reform movement into their new organisation. They rejected the conservative and exclusive model of the existing medical corporations. The Council was elected by the members, who were given free access to the museum, library, lectures and meetings and provided *gratis* with detailed accounts of proceedings in a regularly published journal. The Pharmaceutical Society was the first medical corporation to adopt the idea of democratic and representative government, uniformity of education, and the publication of a register of qualified practitioners.

When the Pharmaceutical Society was founded there was no established pattern of professional development. The Society set out on an uncharted journey: there were no way-marked paths to follow. Today there exists a recognised trajectory of professional development which occupations seek to follow in their search for professional status. Organisation and certification are seen as essential foundations. Speed of development may be faster now because the stages of professionalisation are believed to be known. In 1841 the situation was quite different. When Jacob Bell insisted on the crucial importance of education and qualifications, he was relying more on faith and intuition than on historical precedents. When he urged chemists and druggists to forget the narrow and divisive issues of the trade of pharmacy to unite in promoting the science of pharmacy, he had to turn to the continent of Europe to find instructive illustrations. When the Pharmaceutical Society was founded only three other modern professional associations existed; the Institution of Civil Engineers, founded in 1818, the Law Society, founded in 1825, and the Institute of British Architects, founded in 1834. The energies of the Law Society were at first directed toward "facilitating the acquisition of legal knowledge". Not until 1877 did it acquire the "entire management and control" of solicitors' examinations and not until 1888 was any substantial advance made in the fight for self-government in matters of discipline. Both the Institution of Civil Engineers and the Institute of British Architects introduced qualifying examinations much later than the Pharmaceutical Society. The architects introduced an unsuccessful voluntary examination system in 1862; compulsory examinations were delayed until 1882. The civil engineers had no examination until 1897. Both the architects and civil engineers relied on pupilage as the method of training, assuming it was sufficient if the principal vouched for his pupil's competence at the end of training. Chemists and druggists likewise underwent apprenticeship but the Pharmaceutical Society sought to encourage a more uniform, theoretical and modern mode of education by insisting on public examinations as the test of qualification.

The Pharmaceutical Society of Great Britain was incorporated by Royal Charter on 18 February 1843. At the beginning of the previous November, Sir James Graham, the Home Secretary, had intimated that, if the Council of the Society petitioned the Queen in Council, a charter might well be forthcoming. Graham had already begun work on his medical reform bill and the establishment of a body to regulate chemists and druggists was an important part of his strategy. He was keen to recognise the Pharmaceutical Society as the representative association of chemists and druggists with the task of providing the public with duly qualified practitioners in pharmacy. This would leave the rest of the medical profession to be regulated by the Colleges of Physicians and Surgeons. The Society of Apothecaries would be put out to grass. The repeal of the 1815 Act would deprive them of their power to license and their role as examiners would be reduced to assisting the College of Physicians examine general practitioners. Their pharmaceutical escape route would be blocked by the incorporation of the Pharmaceutical Society. Sir James Graham was firmly opposed to medical monopolies; he believed government had no right to restrict public choice; an individual should be at liberty to select whomsoever he wished as his health adviser. Nonetheless, the state had to satisfy itself that public appointments were filled by reliable, responsible and adequately trained persons. It also had a wider obligation to ensure a general supply of educated practitioners. The new medical register, therefore, would enable the general public and the state to distinguish the qualified from the unqualified. The register would have three divisions reflecting the three distinct orders of physicians,

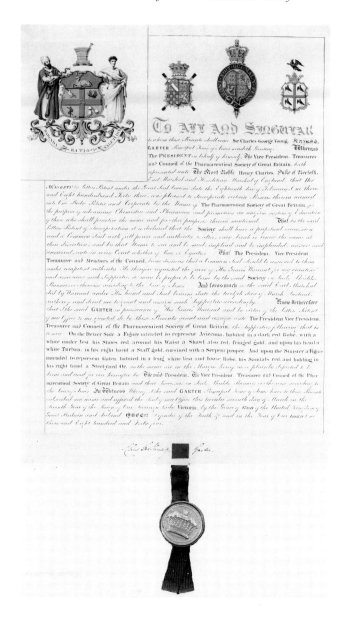

25 *Grant of Arms dated 1844. This was the second grant of arms issued by the College of Heralds and was marked by the addition of Galen and Avicenna as supporters to the arms.*

surgeons, and licentiates in medicine and surgery. The Royal Colleges would become the examining and qualifying authorities for all medical practitioners. To enable the Colleges to fulfil their new role, Graham suggested they seek new charters. He wanted them to broaden the constituency from which their governing bodies were selected and to make provision for examining general practitioners. The Surgeons responded by accepting a new charter in September 1843 which introduced the fellowship, abolished life appointments to the Council and Board of Examiners, and renamed the body the Royal College of Surgeons of England. The Physicians, believing they had more to lose than gain, refused to co-operate. The only substantive outcome of Sir James Graham's attempt to reform the medical profession was the Royal Charters of 1843, the first to the Pharmaceutical Society, the second to the Royal College of Surgeons.

In 1843 the only effective way to achieve legal incorporation was by obtaining a Royal Charter. At that time, incorporation could only be achieved via Statute or Royal Charter. Incorporation by Act of Parliament was a lengthy, expensive and troublesome process. The procedure is complex and uncertain: since the bill can be blocked at any of several stages, much depends on the existence and development of opposition. The Royal College of Physicians' charter of 1518 was revised and ratified by Act of Parliament in 1522 and in 1815 the Apothecaries Act enlarged and confirmed the Society of Apothecaries' charter of 1617. But the Company of Surgeons in 1797, the Institute of Accountants in 1878 and the Institute of Chemistry in 1883 attempted, but failed, to secure incorporation by private Act. From 1862, the Companies Act provided an easier route to acquiring the advantages of a legal corporate existence; and many professional and other non-commercial societies have remained content with the simpler, cheaper and more convenient expedient of registering themselves as limited companies. Incorporation by the Companies Act ensured maximum legal protection with a minimum of outside interference. But, in 1843, incorporation for the Pharmaceutical Society meant obtaining a Royal Charter.

There was no compelling reason for the Society to acquire corporate status. The Institution of Surveyors survived for thirteen years between 1868 and 1881 in an unincorporated state.[88] There are, however, a few minor disadvantages in such an existence. Without incorporation, a society cannot sue or be sued in its own name; property can only be held by "Deed of Trust", entailing the selection of individual trustees; and officers of the society, having no legal protection, may be held individually liable. Incorporation was, therefore, administratively convenient, but not vital. The Society's charter conferred no exclusive legal privileges and led to no augmentation of its powers. Indeed, a charter could prove a hindrance if subsequent events made a change in powers or purposes necessary and such alteration required the expense of petitioning for a supplemental charter. In 1901 the Society was granted a supplementary Charter when it was discovered that the value of its property exceeded the limit laid down in the Charter of 1843.

In the preamble the Charter defined and limited the Society's objectives by declaring that it was established

> for the purpose of advancing chemistry and pharmacy, and promoting an uniform system of education of those who should practise the same; and also for the protection of those who carry on the business of chemists and druggists; and that it is intended also to provide a fund for the relief of the distressed members and associates of the society, and of their widows and orphans.

Theophilus Redwood pointed out that

> although the charter gave no legal power to the society that was not previously possessed, it greatly increased its influence by showing that its objects, and the

141

means by which they were proposed to be attained, were approved of and sanctioned by the Government.

Jacob Bell saw the grant of a Royal Charter as an important step towards the establishment of the Society as a medical corporation on a par with the Royal Colleges. With a glance over his shoulder at the sinking Apothecaries' Company, he remarked

> This event is important—being the first public recognition of the chemists and druggists as the representatives of pharmacy. It cannot henceforth be said that the chemists and druggists have no political existence; and, consequently in the event of any legislative enactments being proposed in which their interests are concerned, they may now claim not only to be heard, but to be consulted. By virtue of their charter, they possess the power of regulating the education and admission of members, and thus of providing the public with qualified practitioners in pharmacy, while they establish an ostensible distinction between the members of their body and unqualified persons ... and it may be supposed that the Council of an incorporated society, representing so large a body as the chemists and druggists of the United Kingdom, would possess the advantage of an amount of influence which might on a great variety of occasions, be beneficially exerted.[89]

Incorporation by Royal Charter was rightly regarded by the Pharmaceutical Society as a highly prized privilege, a mark of its authority and public standing. It was accepted that applications were not automatically granted and that the law officers of the Crown guarded the exclusive character of charters. The grant of a charter was considered proof that the Society had undergone a careful scrutiny of its *bona fides*, its objectives and capacity to fulfil them, its representative character, and its general worthiness. The charter conferred on the Society moral authority over all chemists and druggists, moral responsibility for supervising their activities, and a moral, but not a legal, monopoly of regulating entry into the profession. In short the charter was a laying on of hands which converted an unofficial collection of individuals into a pillar of society. Its possession made membership of the Society seem more attractive or at least more advisable, for those chemists and druggists who had hitherto hung back. *The Chemist*, realising the importance of the charter for the Pharmaceutical Society's success, renewed its campaign of denigration. It accused the Society of trying to frighten chemists and druggists into becoming members with the erroneous claim

> that if they did not join the Society, and pay their money, after a certain time, a Charter would be granted, and then they must belong to it, or be stopped in their practice.

But, it hastened to add, the Society

> never will possess an atom of power to compel chemists to become members. The Charter does not confer on it any power beyond that of a trading company. A chemist and druggist who is a member of the Society possesses no advantage over one who is not, ... this Society ... cannot stand ... there is every prospect of its speedy extinction.[90]

The Pharmaceutical Society's charter remains, however, a legitimate source of institutional pride. By the end of the nineteenth century, a Royal Charter had become established as the status symbol of professional associations. Even after 1862, when the Companies Act provided less demanding paths, the charter was regarded as the dignified route for professional bodies to achieve incorporation. The full implications of chartered status were not revealed, let alone grasped, in 1843, for the very good reason that they did not then all exist. The functions and responsibilities which chartered professional bodies were expected to perform were by no means cut and dried or crystallised by the 1840s. The Pharmaceutical Society was not a mere novice with nothing to do except conform to the norms established by his seniors. No rules and regulations had yet been established: there was no consensus about the functions of chartered bodies and the methods they should use in their performance. The Pharmaceutical Society was one of the founding fathers of modern professionalism. From 1843 to the end of the century a steady stream of newly chartered bodies emerged: the chemists and druggists were followed by veterinary surgeons (1844), private schoolmasters (1849), accountants (1880), chartered surveyors (1881), actuaries (1884), chemists (1885), patent agents (1891) and librarians (1898). In the present century the stream became a flood. The establishment and nurturing of a professional body is a difficult task and knowledge of how to do it was inevitably taken from those who had already performed the feat successfully. The Pharmaceutical Society was one of the pioneers in establishing a pattern of development which later institutions could adapt to their own needs.

NOTES AND REFERENCES TO CHAPTER THREE

1. S.W.F. Holloway, "The Apothecaries' Act 1815: a reinterpretation" *Med.Hist.* 10 (1966) 107–129, 221–236
2. *P.J.* 6 (1846–7) 341–3, 347–8
3. S.W.F. Holloway, "Medical education in England, 1830–1858" *History* 49 (1964) 299–324
4. *Lancet* 1830 (2) 451
5. Ivan Waddington, *The Medical Profession in the Industrial Revolution* (1984) 77–95
6. Bell and Redwood 77
7. Charles Newman, *The Evolution of Medical Education in the Nineteenth Century* (1957) chapter 4
8. *Hansard*, 57 (3rd series), 17 March 1841, 331–3
9. 1841 (19) II 573
10. *P.J.* 5 (1845–6) 10, 244.
11. Bell and Redwood 86–91, 146–7
12. *The Chemist* 2 (1841) 81–83
13. *Hansard*, 56 (3rd series), 19 February 1841, 742
14. 1841 (84) II 607
15. *The Chemist* 2 (1841) 85
16. C.R.B. Barrett, *The History of the Society of Apothecaries of London* (1905) 221–3
17. Bell and Redwood 94–5
18. *P.J.* 18 (1858–9) 599–600
19. *P.J.* 10 (1850–1) 162
20. *P.J.* 13 (1853–4) 348
21. *P.J.* 18 (1858–9) 600–1
22. Bell and Redwood 154–5
23. *P.J.* 18 (1858–9) 601–2

24. Bell and Redwood 110–11
25. Bell and Redwood 73–4
26. *P.J.* 10 (1851–2) 161–2
27. Bell and Redwood 148–9
28. C.R.B. Barrett, *Society of Apothecaries* (1905) 223, 226
29. *Apothecaries' Company v. Greenough* 11 L.J.Q.B. 156 and 1 Q.B. 799
30. *P.J.* 1 (1841–2) 176–8
31. Jacob Bell, *Observations addressed to the chemists and druggists of Great Britain on the Pharmaceutical Society* (1841) 4–6
32. Jacob Bell, *Observations* (1841) 5–8
33. *P.J.* 12 (1852–3) 369
34. *P.J.* 1 (1841–2) 37
35. *P.J.* 2 (1842–3) 1–7
36. *P.J.* 1 (1841–2) 36
37. *P.J.* 1 (1841–2) 78
38. *P.J.* 1 (1841–2) 41
39. *P.J.* 18 (1858–9) 586
40. *Pharmaceutical Times* 2 (1847) 406
41. *P.J.* 5 (1845–6) 389–90
42. *Pharmaceutical Times* 3 (1847–8) 124
43. *The Chemist* new series 3 (1845) 272–3; new series 5 (1847) 308–10. *Pharmaceutical Times* 1 (1846–7) 138–9, 155–6, 169- 70, 238–9; 2 (1847) 143–4, 195–6, 271, 289
44. *P.J.* 3 (1843–4) 1–4
45. *P.J.* 4 (1844–45) 549–50
46. *P.J.* 1 (1841–2) 85, 640; *P.J.* 3 (1843–4) 97, 145
47. *Select Committee on the adulteration of food, drink and drugs* 1856 (379) VIII Q. 3783
48. *P.J.* 1 (1841–2) 37–9, 78
49. *P.J.* 2 (1842–3) 741
50. *P.J.* 1 (1841–2) 38–9
51. Bell and Redwood 115–9
52. *P.J.* 1 (1841–2) 564
53. *P.J.* 2 (1842–3) 615
54. Bell and Redwood 143
55. J.M.D. Olmsted, *Francois Magendie: Pioneer in Experimental Physiology and Scientific Medicine in XIX Century France* (New York 1944); M.P.Earles, "Early theories of mode of action of drugs and poisons" *Annals of Science* 17 (1961) 97 – 110
56. J. R. Partington, *A History of Chemistry* (1963) 4, 300
57. J.B. Morrell, "The chemist breeders: the research schools of Liebig and Thomas Thomson", *Ambix* 19 (1972) 1–46
58. *The Chemist* 3 (1842) iv
59. Margaret Pelling, *Cholera, Fever and English Medicine 1825-1865* (Oxford 1978) chapter 4, 113–45
60. Richard Phillips, "Illustrations of the present state of pharmacy in England", *P.J.* 2 (1842–3) 315–20, 396–9, 528–32, 651–2 and *P.J.* 3 (1843–4) 108–11, 244–7
61. Bell and Redwood 193
62. *P.J.* 2 (1842–3) 323
63. The following section is based on Robert Franklin Bud, *The Discipline of Chemistry, the Origins and Early Years of the Chemical Society of London*, Ph.D. thesis, University of Pennsylvania, 1980
64. *P.J.* 1 (1841–2) 83, 87, 510
65. *P.J.* 7 (1847–8) 156

66. *Pharmaceutical Times* 1 (1846–7) 50
67. Bell and Redwood 81
68. *The Chemist* 1 (1840) 2
69. *The Chemist* 2 (1841) vi
70. *The Chemist* new series 2 (1844) 2
71. The following section is based on Gerrylynn K. Roberts, *The Royal College of Chemistry (1845–1853): A Social History of Chemistry in Early Victorian England*, Ph.D. thesis, The John Hopkins University 1973 and her article, "The establishment of the Royal College of Chemistry: an investigation of the social context of early Victorian chemistry", *Historical Studies in the Physical Sciences* 7 (1976) 437–485
72. *Pharmaceutical Times* 3 (1847–8) 711
73. *P.J.* 6 (1846–7) 197; 8 (1848–9) 110–11
74. *The Chemist* 3 (1842) 3, 25
75. *The Chemical Times* 4 (1848–9) 406
76. *The Chemist*, new series 2, (1844) 277–282. J. Lloyd Bullock, "A lecture on the state of pharmacy in England, and its importance to the public; with remarks on the Pharmaceutical Society".
77. *P.J.* 4 (1844–5) 113–4
78. *P.J.* 3 (1843–4) 572
79. Quoted in Robert H. Kargon, *Science in Victorian Manchester* (Manchester 1977) 103, 105–6
80. *P.J.* 6 (1846–7) 160–72
81. D.F.S. Scott (ed.) *Luke Howard (1772–1864): His Correspondence with Goethe and his Continental Journey of 1818* (York, 1976) 4
82. Bell and Redwood 148, 170–1
83. Noel G. Coley, "Medical chemistry at Guy's Hospital (1770-1850)" *Ambix* 35 (1988) 157–8
84. A. W. Slater, *Howards, Chemical Manufacturers, 1797–1837, A Study in Business History* M.A. thesis University of London 1956
85. A. M. Carr-Saunders and P.A. Wilson, *The Professions* (1933) and Geoffrey Millerson, *The Qualifying Associations* (1964)
86. *P.J.* 1 (1841–2) 36
87. *P.J.* 7 (1847–8) 156
88. F.M.L. Thompson, *Chartered Surveyors, The Growth of a Profession* (1968)
89. Bell and Redwood 141–2, 159
90. *The Chemist* 4 (1843) 175

CHAPTER FOUR

The 1852 Pharmacy Act

Dosis augeatur—Increase the dose

The Pharmaceutical Society and medical reform—The St. Albans by-election, 1850—The Pharmacy Bill, 1851—The Select Committee on the pharmacy bill, 1852—Dispensing doctors and prescribing chemists—The consequences of the 1852 Pharmacy Act

The sense of urgency that inspired the foundation of the Pharmaceutical Society was based on the belief that a comprehensive reorganisation of the medical profession was at hand. It was widely assumed that the regulation of chemists and druggists would form part of any measure of medical reform. From the druggists' point of view the problem with the campaign for medical reform was that its driving force was the discontents of the general practitioner. The energies of the radical reformers were directed more to the suppression of chemists and druggists as medical practitioners than to their elevation and protection as practitioners of pharmacy. Benjamin Hawes' bill in 1841 proposed a governing and examining board for chemists and druggists in which they were to take no part. The establishment of the Pharmaceutical Society was intended to change all that. The Society was intended to become the body corporate of the chemists and druggists, managing its own affairs and setting up its own plan of education and examination. "In advocating a distinct system of education and examination, and desiring to superintend and manage the same, we are claiming no more than is enjoyed by other bodies", Jacob Bell pointed out. "We must be united among ourselves ... in the attainment of the one grand object, which involves our professional character and independence".[1] The first task of the Pharmaceutical Society was to provide the public with qualified practitioners in pharmacy. Once this had been achieved, "we may fairly claim for such practitioners an adequate remuneration for their labour and skill, which involves, in some degree, the restraint of ignorant pretenders". It is not unreasonable to call upon the state to protect qualified practitioners "against the encroachments of illiterate persons". "Unless some adequate advantages be granted to qualified persons, the inducement to qualify will not exist".[2]

For Jacob Bell, the objects to be attained by medical reform were threefold:

> First, to provide the public with qualified practitioners in every department; secondly, to secure to such persons a fair and proportionate amount of remuneration for their labour and skill; thirdly, to restrain ignorant pretenders from doing mischief.[3]

In the early years, Bell insisted that chemists and druggists must be included in any medical legislation.

We have always maintained that our body is and must be considered a branch of the medical profession, and that whatever regulations, respecting education, registration or protection, may be considered necessary for medical practitioners, the same or similar enactments are no less requisite in our department.[4]

It would be absurd to lay great stress on the importance of science and skill in writing the prescription, and at the same time to leave the preparation of it to chance. We may, therefore, conclude that some provisions, with reference to chemists and druggists, will be comprised in the Medical Bill ...[5]

It is obvious that the arguments in favour of restrictions in the profession apply equally to all departments of it, and that the safety of the public is as much concerned in the suppression of unqualified dispensers of medicine as it is in the suppression of unqualified medical practitioners. If restrictions are to be established, the chemists are quite as much interested in them as any other class of the profession, and have as much right to be protected by them; but the difficulty in the arrangement consists in defining the boundary line between the medical practitioners and the chemists on one side, and between the chemists and the grocers etc. on the other.[6]

Boundary lines were the central issue in the struggle. How was the field of pharmacy to be divided up? Who was to be installed in what territory? Could the state be persuaded to guarantee and patrol the borders? To chemists and druggists the phrase "unqualified practice" meant grocers and oilmen; to general practitioners, it meant chemists and druggists. Could the Pharmaceutical Society construct a wall against the incursions of grocers without conceding ground to general practitioners?

"At the time that the Pharmaceutical Society was founded", claimed Jacob Bell in 1844, "an Act of Parliament was the ulterior object to which the chemists aspired".[7] The Royal Charter of Incorporation was not regarded in any other light than as a precursory measure which would place the Society in a recognised position and pave the way for an Act. Bell's expectation that Sir James Graham would include the regulation of chemists and druggists in his long-awaited medical reform bill was shattered in August 1844. The Home Secretary decided that his task of devising acceptable and effective regulations for physicians, surgeons and general practitioners was complex enough without adding chemists and druggists to the list. So long as his medical bill was before parliament, there was an expectation that a government pharmacy bill would follow. By 1846, however, all chance of such an outcome had vanished. It was at this point that the Council of the Pharmaceutical Society turned its attention to the task of preparing its own bill.

The first proposal was simply a bill to oblige all dispensing chemists to pass a qualifying examination. The Pharmaceutical Society would be given powers to enforce the requirement. This bill soon ran into difficulties. The Society comprised less than a third of all retail chemists. In 1845 there were only 1,691 members when the total number of chemists in business on their own account was in excess of 5,000. Lack of support was an incentive to gain legislative protection but an hindrance to its attainment. Parliament would be reluctant to recognise as the regulatory authority so unrepresentative a body. The idea took root within the Council that it was

inconsistent with the principles of modern legislation that the same corporate body should be an educating and an examining body, with the power of granting degrees or diplomas giving legal authority for the performance of professional duties.[8]

This view was founded on a (dubious) interpretation of the history of University College

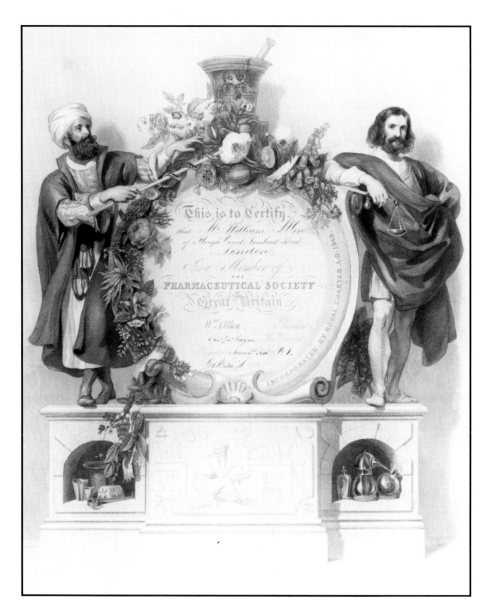

26   *Certificate of William Allen (1770–1843), the first issued by the Pharmaceutical Society of Great Britain, dated 1 June, 1841. The certificate was designed by H.P. Briggs RA, a close friend of Jacob Bell. The garland surrounding the central medallion incorporates a variety of medicinal plants, flanked by the figures of Galen and Avicenna who also appear as supporters on the Society's coat of arms. The original steel plate is in the Society's museum collection.*

London. Founded as the London University in Gower Street, the institution was intended as both an educational establishment and a degree awarding body. However, when application was made for a charter, it was held that one of those functions must be relinquished, and the founders accepted a charter for it as an educational body, resigning the power to grant degrees to the University of London, which was created specifically for that purpose. All the authorities, both legal and parliamentary, consulted by the Pharmaceutical Society, advised that the objection sustained in the London University case would apply equally to the Society if it attempted to obtain legal authority to combine the functions of education and examination.

Since the Society's charter already defined it as an educational body, it was proposed, in a newly drafted bill, to create a College of Pharmacy, entirely disconnected with the Society, to take over the job of examining and registration. The Pharmaceutical Society in this arrangement would remain a purely voluntary society concerned with education, the promotion of the science of pharmacy, protection from legislative interference and the maintenance of the benevolent fund. This half-baked scheme was approved by the annual general meeting of the Society in 1846. Although wise and loyal members, like Robert Farmar and Mr. Edwards of Dartford, protested that the proposals would "reduce the Pharmaceutical Society to insignificance", and although Jacob Bell publicly endorsed their misgivings, the Council were determined to proceed. Fortunately, the opposition of the Royal College of Physicians to the very idea of a "College of Pharmacy", saved the Society from its sudden impulse to commit *hara-kiri*.[9]

The publication in 1847 and 1848 of the reports of two parliamentary select committees on the state of medical education and qualification revived interest in the subject of medical reform after the collapse of Sir James Graham's efforts. The Council of the Pharmaceutical Society, recovered from its bout of collective insanity, abandoned the idea of an independent college of pharmacy, and drafted a new bill. This provided for the registration of all persons already engaged in business as chemists and druggists and for the examination and regulation of future entrants to the profession. Unregistered persons would be prohibited from preparing, compounding or dispensing any medicine for sale or gain. The Act would be implemented by the Pharmaceutical Society, unaided by any other institution. The members of the Society were much less enthusiastic about this bill than the Council had anticipated. Many members

> considered themselves entitled to some privileges or distinction as the founders of
> an improved system and questioned the justice of admitting to an equal status those
> who had not united in the movement, and had contributed nothing towards the
> expenses of the Society.

It took all Jacob Bell's powers of persuasion to convince them that "the public utility of the measure was a more important consideration than the personal or exclusive privileges of the founders of the Society".[10]

There was, in any case, little immediate prospect of this bill being brought before parliament, "for although attempts had been made to interest members of parliament in its favour, no one had been found who seemed disposed to take it up".[11] The Council exerted all the pressure it could. The local secretaries in the provinces were set to work getting members of the public to sign petitions urging the legislature to ensure that those who dispensed medicines and handled dangerous drugs were properly educated. These petitions were soon pouring into parliament, joining those already presented from the president and council of the Royal Colleges of Physicians and Surgeons. At the same time the Society achieved widespread publicity for accounts of the carefree manner in which poisons were supplied to the public and for reports of deaths caused by the incompetent administration of medicines. In November 1847 a deputation from the Council of the Society, in an attempt to get government backing for its bill, had an interview with Sir George Grey, the Home Secretary. He made encouraging noises but reiterated the view that pharmaceutical legislation should follow, not precede, medical reform.

From the day the Pharmaceutical Society was created, Jacob Bell realised that an Act of Parliament would be needed to achieve its objectives. Although he devoted his best efforts to persuading the nation's chemists and druggists to join together voluntarily to regulate and control the profession, he knew, from the outset, that compulsion would be quicker and more effective. The Pharmaceutical Society, unlike the Royal College of Surgeons, could confer no aura of prestige upon those who passed its examinations. Like the Apothecaries' Company, it needed an Act of Parliament to secure its authority and status. After the collapse of Sir James Graham's attempts to reform the medical profession, the prospect of a comprehensive act to regulate the practice of medicine, surgery and pharmacy dimmed. By the late 1840s, falling membership and income gave urgency to the Pharmaceutical Society's search for legislative backing. The Society could not afford to wait until the rest of the medical profession settled its differences: the self-inflicted wounds would take too long to heal. From 1847 the Society's strategy became centred on the attainment of an act to regulate the activities of chemists and druggists, independent of the rest of the medical profession. The profound implications of the decision for the future development of the practise of both medicine and pharmacy were neither anticipated nor discussed.

Jacob Bell, with the help of his solicitor George Brace, drafted a suitable bill.[12] Then, with his customary doggedness, he arranged a series of "interviews with official persons and with members of parliament in the hopes of being able to get the Bill" introduced. But no one could be persuaded to undertake the task. Neither a government nor a private member's bill was forthcoming. In desperation and with considerable misgiving, Jacob Bell began the search for a seat in the House of Commons: the only way to secure a pharmacy act, he decided, was to introduce it himself. Bell was not an obvious candidate for parliament. He had no family connexions; he had no personal influence in any constituency; he had no political reputation. He had little to offer the electorate in return for their support; his election would not bring business or industry to the borough that returned him. His objective was to represent the Pharmaceutical Society rather than his constituents. Being a shopkeeper was not an advantage. "It would be next to impossible to apply to a well dressed man in the street a more offensive appellation than 'shopman'", it was said in 1843. An unfriendly observer remarked, "Mr. Bell, however respectable he might be, ... was not in that position in society or sufficiently known to command a majority of the votes". Even his friend and solicitor, George Brace, confessed, "I did not think he was a person of sufficient political importance to get in, unconnected as he was, from local circumstances". But Bell had one indispensable asset: he was a man of some wealth and was prepared to use his money to gain a seat. In such circumstances, no better constituency could have been found than the parliamentary borough of St. Albans.

The parliamentary borough of St. Albans returned two members of parliament and was co-extensive with the municipal borough, which had, in 1850, a population of about 7,000. The right to vote, however, was restricted to resident freemen by birth, servitude or redemption, to inhabitants paying scot and lot, as defined in 1714, (i.e. paying parochial taxes), and to £10 householders, enfranchised by the 1832 Reform Act. The total number of registered voters in 1850 was only 483, of which 354 were £10 householders, 66 were scot and lot payers and 63 were freemen. The borough was, like all others, nominally divided into political parties. The Conservative party, under the auspices of the Earl of Verulam, whose family had for many years returned one of its members as the representative of the borough, embraced most of the Anglican clergy and resident gentry. The Liberals, formerly under the influence of the Spencer family, were headed by a few of the gentry and most of the respectable tradesmen who dissented from the Established Church. "But these distinctions were not always observed, nor was any very strict party discipline maintained. Attached to both parties was a large number of electors obeying their respective leaders, whose allegiance, however, mainly depended upon the distribution of money". It was not unusual for the electors of St. Albans motivated, with few exceptions, solely by pecuniary considerations, to split their votes between candidates of opposite political opinions.

The acknowledged agent for the Conservative party in St. Albans was Thomas Ward Blagg; the agent for the Liberal party was Henry Edwards. Blagg was the town clerk of St. Albans and clerk to the magistrate for the Watford division. Edwards had once been a clerk and manager of Musketts' bank in St. Albans, but, by 1850 was, and had been for some years, a farmer at Bricket Wood, about four miles from the town. Since 1832 Blagg and Edwards had come increasingly to work together to manage the elections and share the spoils among their supporters. Their task was to bribe the electors on the one hand and recompense themselves at the expense of the candidates on the other. But, in addition to the two recognised parties, there was another of no fixed politics who called themselves "the Third party" but who were often called "the Contest party". Their aim was to prevent the unopposed return of members selected by the other two parties. It was their practice, at all elections in which a contest seemed improbable, to hang up a key in different parts of the town as a sign to the electors that a candidate would be forthcoming "to open the borough".

Elections in St. Albans had little to do with politics. "We talk about parties", said one election agent, "but they are so amalgamated and shifted about by the money that has been spent ... that I must confess I am lost in parties ... the party in St. Albans ... has been for years moved by money". "A man's politics in St. Albans", observed a defeated candidate, "is his breeches pocket". "The great majority of the people here ... have always been known to be bought and sold without regard to principle or anything else". Two thirds of the electorate regularly sold their vote. In the 1841 election all the electors took the bribery oath, swearing that they had not been tampered with, yet over £4,000 was distributed in bribes. One voter, with a particularly tender conscience, returned his bribe before the oath was administered, only to claim it back after the oath had been taken! In the course of the eight elections fought since 1832, over £24,600 was spent in bribing an electorate comprising fewer than 500 persons.

For Jacob Bell, the road to St. Albans began at 40, Parliament Street. It was there that, in 1849, he first met James Coppock, the Liberal party's national agent. Coppock was by profession a solicitor, but, from his office in Parliament Street and from the Reform Club in Pall Mall, he spent his time watching over and attempting to control the electoral situation in the constituencies. He had his agents in all of them. His business was to ensure the registration of Liberal voters and to find candidates for vacant seats and seats for aspiring politicians. Coppock was recognised as the Liberal party authority on electoral intelligence.[13] When he met Bell "he made inquiries as to his (Mr. Bell's) politics, and as to the expense he was willing to incur, because it was as absolutely necessary to know the depth of a member of parliament's pockets as his politics"; and then they parted. At about the same time, George Brace, who kept his ear to the ground in the hope of finding a suitable constituency for his client, was in touch with William Balcomb Simpson, a fellow solicitor and clerk to the County Court of St. Albans, about an anticipated vacancy in the representation of that borough.

The news was a little premature: it was not until the second week of November 1850 that Mr. Raphael, the Liberal M.P. for St. Albans, died. Brace, on hearing the sad news, wrote to Simpson to come up to London and see him, which Simpson did. Their meeting on 19 November was inconclusive. Simpson, who aspired to oust Edwards as the patron of St. Albans, pressed Brace to let Bell came forward immediately, but Brace was not convinced that Simpson was a person of sufficient influence to ensure victory and, moreover, rightly suspected that he was in touch with other interested parties. Brace put Simpson off by saying that there was no danger in two or three days delay. When, later that day, Bell was informed of what had transpired, he agreed that Brace should go down to St. Albans to make inquiries.

The next day, while Brace was on his way to St. Albans, Simpson, accompanied by a fellow conspirator, Aubrey Bowen, went to London to see Bell at his home in Langham Place. In the early morning post Bell had received a letter from Coppock inviting Bell to call on him "about a vacancy in Parliament". Bell had this letter in his hand when Messrs. Simpson and Bowen were introduced. The object of their visit was to get Bell to announce his candidature at once: £2,000 or £2,500 was mentioned as the probable cost. Bell was assured that everyone in St. Albans was determined to put down the system of bribery which had prevailed there in previous elections. Bell listened to what Simpson and Bowen had to say but dismissed them without coming to any arrangement.

In the meantime, Brace was in St. Albans where the first person he saw was Langley, a printer, who told him that the person of the greatest influence in the borough was Henry Edwards. Brace then visited a Mr. Dorant, whom he had known previously, and who not only confirmed what Langley had said about Edwards, but offered to introduce Brace to him. On their way to see Edwards, Brace popped into Langley's and, without having consulted Bell, ordered the printing of a hand bill, calling upon the electors to reserve their votes, as a gentleman would appear "of moderate Whig principles, who was neither a Roman Catholic nor a chartist". Edwards later described his meeting with Brace:

> He was a great deal like a dumb man; he was afraid of me, and I was afraid of him.
> He would not tell me his name. It was all dumb motions.

The result, however, was that Brace ultimately mentioned the name of Jacob Bell as the candidate and asked what would be the probable expense. Edwards said about £2,700; and, in answer to Brace's remark that this might lead to an investigation before the House of Commons, said "No one need be apprehensive of that; there will be no bribery". Edwards, who was awaiting instructions from Coppock, made it clear that he was not at that moment in a position to take up Bell but made an arrangement to meet Brace again at Watford station the following day. When Bell heard this, he decided to accompany Brace.

Accordingly Bell and Brace, accompanied by Colt, Brace's partner, went down on the morning of 21 November to Watford Station. On their alighting on the platform, Aubrey Bowen stepped forward with a letter from Simpson. In this letter Simpson said that Brace had done mischief by going down to St. Albans and seeing Edwards the previous day; that Edwards had assumed to himself the entire control and management of the intended election and that he would allow none to interfere; that the electors were very dissatisfied with Edwards' conduct; and that he, Simpson, could not consent to act with Edwards in any way. He concluded by strongly urging Brace to bring Bell into the borough and make a canvass at once. Bowen pressed the same case. "It is impossible", replied Brace, "I have come down to see Mr. Edwards". He crossed the railway bridge and greeted Edwards, who immediately declared that he was ready to commit himself to Bell. Brace did not reciprocate the enthusiasm, but said, "he must pause before he put the case into his hands, for it appeared to him that there was a split altogether in the borough, and he did not know anything about a conservative candidate coming forward". Edwards replied, "I can satisfy you at once about that. No conservative candidate can come forward. There is Mr. Blagg; I will introduce you to him". Blagg was in Edward's debt for help received in seating Mr. Repton, the Conservative candidate, at the last election and had agreed to use his influence with his party to return anyone whom Edwards might bring forward. Blagg assured Brace that "there would be no conservative candidate and no opposition on the part of a conservative candidate". Edwards then urged Brace to let Bell come forward, and pointing to a gentleman who was walking about, said, "Is that Mr. Bell walking up and down the platform?" Brace replied, "Yes, it is", but added that he could not introduce him as he did not feel it was safe to let him proceed. No introduction took place. Instead Brace crossed the line and told Bell

> that there was a disagreement between the two liberal parties; that there was no difficulty in reference to the conservative party, because the conservatives were not likely to contest the borough at the ensuing election; but there was a split in the liberal party, under which circumstances he had been unable to effect any arrangement, or to obtain any information which would justify him in recommending him to proceed.

Brace left for Yorkshire on business by the next train, under the impression that Bell would follow his advice. Bell, indeed, intended to do so, but was keen to see Coppock first.

On that or the following day, Bell called on Coppock, who began by saying "that Mr. Raphael was dead, and that there was a vacancy". He did not let on that he had already in vain approached Mr. Craven, who had unsuccessfully fought the seat in 1847, and Serjeant William Shee. After some inquiries about Bell's political opinions, the subject of money was discussed. Coppock explained

> that the borough of St. Albans had been reputed to be similar to a good many other boroughs, that was to say, that there had been some corruption in it; that there were three parties in the borough, one conservative and two liberal parties; that they were all desirous of retrieving the character of the borough; that the usual expense of elections there had been on average from £2,000 to £3,000.

154

Coppock asked Bell how far he was prepared to go. Bell replied that "it was not a pecuniary question with him", but asked what he thought the expense would be. When Coppock said "from £2,000 to £2,500", Bell indicated that he would not come forward on such terms; and so, for the time, they separated. Bell, however, saw Coppock again on several occasions but no definite agreement was reached until 28 November, on which day he was at last introduced to Henry Edwards at Coppock's office in Parliament Street. On this occasion Bell insisted: "First, that there should be bribery; secondly, no treating; and thirdly, no intimidation". Edwards reassured him: "With regard to bribery, you may be perfectly satisfied about that; if I have anything to do with it, I will take care there is no bribery". Coppock assured Bell that he "need not be at all uneasy upon that subject".

Thus Jacob Bell placed himself in the hands of James Coppock and Henry Edwards and agreed to stand as the Liberal candidate for St. Albans. The question of expenses was purposely left in the dark: no sum of money was ever mentioned to Bell by Edwards. But it was perfectly understood between them that money to the extent of £2,500 would be forthcoming, if required. Coppock later admitted that £200 was more than any election in St. Albans ought to cost. "£200", he said, "would leave fifty guineas for the person who managed the election". Bell explained to Coppock that he wanted nothing to do with money matters, "he would rather leave that in the hands of his friends, and settle it afterwards". It transpired that these "friends" were Thomas Hyde Hills, who ran Bell's shop in Oxford Street and lived with him in Langham Place.

As soon as Bell had left, Edwards told Coppock "that expenses were beginning to be incurred and that it was necessary he should make payment on account and the best way would be to advance £500". Coppock asked him how he would like it. "In sovereigns", was the reply. Coppock told him to go to the offices of Brace and Colt in Surrey Street. Edwards went there and, after several delays, a packet containing 500 sovereigns was delivered to him that evening at an hotel in Euston Square, by a man using the name of Jenkins, but whose real name was Thomas Elam. This packet came from Hills, who instructed Elam to convey it to its destination "without asking any questions". Thomas Elam was a woollen-draper of Sackville Street and the brother of Benjamin Elam, a chemist and druggist of 196 Oxford Street, who was elected a member of the Pharmaceutical Society in 1853.

The packet containing 500 sovereigns was taken down to St. Albans that evening by Edwards and locked up in a house taken as a committee-room in a street which was soon to receive the name of Sovereign Alley. "At the time when I got back to St. Albans", said Edwards, "a contest was imminent. The town was all in a ferment,—Mr. Simpson's party and other parties,—for a contest. I seemed more convinced there would be a contest when I got back than before. They said they were determined to have a man, no matter whom".

On 30 November Ebenezar Randell, a solicitor who had been appointed Bell's election agent, wrote to Edwards to tell him that Bell planned to come down to St. Albans the following Monday with some friends to canvass and added that:

> he has charged me as his solicitor emphatically to protest against all treating, bribery, and corruption of voters in any form, and distinctly to assure you that he will not be answerable for or pay any bills or accounts, except such are are strictly legal.

Both Bell and Hills were anxious to cover their tracks in the event of a bribery petition being filed after the election. Hills admitted that he deliberately complicated the affair as much as possible "so that if any inquiry was to be made about it, if he could prevent it, it might not be found out whom the money came from". Bell was perfectly aware that Hills was passing money on his account to Coppock and Edwards for the purposes of the election. Hills admitted that at different periods he advanced sums in packets of 500 sovereigns each, amounting to £2,500 and that he would have advanced to the extent of £3,000, if necessary.

The apparent canvass began on Monday 2 December when Bell made his entry into St. Albans: but Edwards had already begun to see electors in the house in Sovereign Alley. The house consisted of three rooms below and two above. In one of the downstairs rooms there was always refreshment and there the voters attended in great numbers in the evening and waited until they were introduced to Edwards. One of Edwards' sons was stationed as doorkeeper at the head of the stairs: his duty was to admit the voters, one by one, into the room where Edwards sat alone. Edwards began to see the electors in this room on 29 or 30 November, and on the evening of the first day he saw and secured from 40 to 50 voters, to each of whom he gave a sum varying from £5 to £8. The voters thus secured were afterwards canvassed at their own homes by Jacob Bell and his party when they formally promised their votes. The course adopted and pursued up to the day of the election was of such systematic and unblushing bribery that, in the words of William Payne, a local watercress grower, "they gave money the name of Bell-metal in St. Albans; they do not call it silver or gold".

The first sum of 500 sovereigns was distributed within a week, and Edwards applied to Messrs. Brace and Colt for another advance. He wrote them a letter, stating that his son was coming to London and would take any packet that was ready for him. George Colt dealt with the letter and gave the signal to Hills who arranged for Elam to carry the packet of 500 sovereigns to Coppock's offices in Parliament Street. Young Edwards then took the parcel to his father in St. Albans. In this manner, at intervals of about a week, a further sum of £1,500, in three separate packets, was passed along the line.

All seemed to be going according to plan; but the better things went for Bell and Edwards, the more Simpson and the Third party became enraged. Simpson's ambition was to replace Edwards as the borough-monger of St. Albans. He had served an excellent apprenticeship, having been clerk in turn to Blagg and Edwards; and his efforts had been appreciated. His post as clerk to the County Court at St. Albans had been acquired, through the patronage of Coppock, on the recommendation of Edwards, as a reward for his work in the 1847 election. But Simpson over-reached himself: he quarrelled and finally broke with Edwards, yet failed to induce Brace to put Jacob Bell in his hands. In the end, George Colt told him firmly that "unless he united himself with Mr. Blagg and Mr. Edwards, he certainly could not be entertained in the character of an agent". This made Simpson determined to find a candidate of his own, and he lost no time in visiting Mr. Chambers, a gentleman resident in Hertford, who was not, however, interested. Undeterred, Simpson, Bowen and other members of the Contest party set off to London in search of a candidate. Coppock, of course, was fully informed of their activities:

> I found that the third party were determined to have a man. I heard of their going
> to this person and to that. It was brought to me regularly if they went to a person,
> and I knew almost every person they went to. They were using every effort they
> could to get a candidate, without regard to politics or anything else, simply for
> expenditure.

156

On their arrival in London, Messrs. Simpson, Bowen , Blanks, and others called upon Mr. Norton, a barrister, of liberal politics, and proposed to him to become a candidate, with an intimation that £2,500 would be required. Norton declined on the ground that he had learned from Coppock that "there was somebody down at St. Albans canvassing". They then went to the National Reform Association in Cheapside and asked "if anybody wished for a seat in Parliament, as St. Albans was vacant". When no response was forthcoming, they called at the office of Messrs. Stevenson and Tucker, solicitors, of Sun Chambers in the city. They saw Mr. Tucker and inquired if he knew anyone who wanted a seat in Parliament. He asked them what the price of the borough was, as he understood it was "rather an expensive concern". Blanks protested:

> He did not know that; he knew what other boroughs were, and he considered St. Albans was a milk score to a good many other boroughs.

Tucker called on Alderman and Sheriff Sir R. W. Carden and asked him if he wanted a seat in Parliament: "he knew of a place which he thought would just suit him; and stated that £2,000 or £2,500 was about the sum which would be required". Carden replied that "although he had a desire to enter Parliament, he certainly had no desire to pay for entering it". "You know you cannot get into any place unless you do pay", said Tucker. Prophetically Carden replied, "Then I never shall get into any place".

Later, however, Carden agreed to see "a deputation" from St. Albans: the Third party were becoming desperate. He told them he would "not spend one shilling in anything like bribery". They replied that they were all of one mind about the degradation in which the borough had been placed and that there was a determination by the most respectable electors to support any gentleman who would come forward on "purity principles" with a pledge that no money should be expended, directly or indirectly, in influencing a vote. They produced a requisition to him signed by forty-five electors. Carden replied that it was a small document and not enough to induce him to stand. The Contest party returned to St. Albans and called a public meeting at which over a hundred signatures were added to the requisition. In the end, Carden was persuaded to come down to St. Albans on 6 December, and, after canvassing the town, published an address in which he pledged himself to observe to the last the principle of purity of election.

Alderman Carden's reception in the town was most flattering. "It gave me", he said, "inducement to believe that all the hopes and expectations held out by the party who came to me would be fully realised".

> Out of sixteen town councillors ten did me the honour of walking arm-in-arm by my carriage into St. Albans; and out of the sixteen twelve voted for me, two against me, and two stood neuter. I had five clergymen voted for me; in fact I believe that the whole of the respectability of St. Albans, with few exceptions, was on my side, and I really believed that I was going to achieve a triumph, and that I should amend the borough of St. Albans, and emancipate it from the thraldom that existed.

But one man's thraldom is another man's happy hour. Elections were regarded by most voters in St. Albans as an irregularly occurring Christmas. Alderman Carden's sanguine expectations were soon at an end. Very early he discovered that the majority of the electorate had been secured by bribery, and that he had no chance unless he chose to pursue the same practices. It was no fault of his committee that he did not do so: his friends in St.

Albans showered him with hints that voters could "be bribed and the election won". The Third party repeatedly asked him whether he seriously intended to stick to the purity principle. He later recalled his reply and the effect it had:

> I said . . . "I would not give you a shilling if you would bring me a hundred votes". Within half an hour from making that declaration, they flocked to the polls in shoals—To vote for Mr. Bell!

The election took place on Christmas eve, 1850. Jacob Bell topped the poll with 276 votes (198 of which had been obtained by bribery). Sir Robert Carden received 147 votes. The Bell-metal may not have been pure but it did the trick. The operation of the purity principle does not account for all Alderman Carden's support. He spent over £500 on the election,

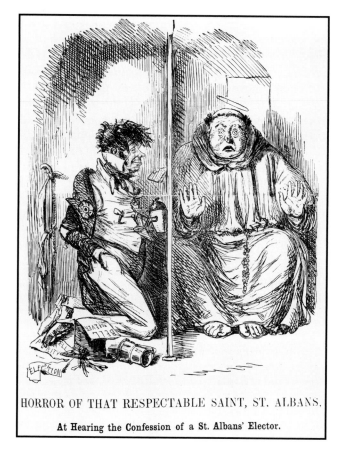

HORROR OF THAT RESPECTABLE SAINT, ST. ALBANS,

At Hearing the Confession of a St. Albans' Elector.

27   Horror of that Respectable Saint, St Albans, At Hearing the Confession of a St Albans' Elector. *Cartoon from* Punch *1851* **21** *225, to illustrate the satire on the investigation into Bell's election victory at St Albans, "Newe Lives of the English Saintes. By A. Newman".*

a good part of which was used by his agent, Richard Lowe, in buying votes. It is possible that this was done without Carden's knowledge and against his wishes. At the end of the day, mused the Earl of Derby,

> The Alderman returned to town a poorer man, but with enlarged experience as to election matters; and Mr. Bell never contributed so much to the depletion of a patient by any drugs he sold, as he suffered by the drastic experiments tried upon his purse by the electors of St. Albans.[14]

Alderman Carden was neither a saint nor a fool. He knew that although St. Albans could be won, before the poll, only by bribery, after the poll, it could be won by petition. His purity campaign had been conducted in the hope of thus securing the seat. Jacob Bell's side had committed such gross and notorious bribery that Carden was convinced he must succeed upon petition. "A spiteful Alderman", wrote Bell to a friend, "is trying to skin me alive". But if Bell lost his seat, Henry Edwards would lose his influence in St. Albans. Farmers know how to protect their lambs. While the House of Commons was setting up a Select Committee to investigate the petition, Edwards was making arrangements for the crucial witnesses to go absent-without-leave. George Sealey Waggett, "who is declared by the Counsel for the Petitioners to be a most essential witness for the elucidation of their case", was entrusted to the care of John Hayward, one of Edwards' most reliable henchmen. James Skegg and Thomas Burchmore, both described as "vital witnesses", were watched over by Edwards' 26-year-old son, Frederick. All attempts to secure their attendance before the Select Committee failed. A reward was offered for their discovery in the *Times* and *Hue-and-Cry*; the police were instructed to search for them; and a now taciturn Henry Edwards was arrested and locked-up in Newgate prison.[15] A month after the Select Committee issued its report, the missing persons were located in Boulogne, enjoying, at Mr. Bell's expense, an unexpected Spring holiday.[16]

The attempt to unseat Jacob Bell collapsed. In April 1851 the House of Commons Select Committee declared that he was duly elected the member of parliament for the Borough of St. Albans. Inspite of successive adjournments, the petitioners had been unable to proceed with their case, having failed to procure "the attendance of persons whose evidence was proved to be most material to the prosecution of the case". Moreover, "although all diligence had been used for the purpose of securing the attendance of the parties required, such endeavours had been unsuccessful". Nonetheless, the general tenor of the evidence that had been collected, "leads the Committee to believe that a system of gross corruption prevailed at the last election ... and also on former similar occasions". It was, therefore, suggested that a Commission with legislative authority should be appointed to inquire "into the corrupt practices alleged to be customary at elections for the Borough of St. Albans".

The House of Commons took up the Select Committee's recommendations and passed, in August 1851, a Bill establishing a Commission, with very extensive powers, consisting of three lawyers, Frederick Slade, William Forsyth, and Thomas Phinn, who were empowered to make such inquiries as they thought fit, not only into the 1850 election, but also into preceding elections. The Commissioners established themselves in the Town Hall at St. Albans on Monday 27 October 1851 and continued their work until the beginning of December. Their report was issued on 2 February 1852. The Commission had the powers not only to force witnesses to testify but also to protect them from the legal consequences of self-crimination. Hence, "the disclosures before the Commissioners were as frank and open as it was possible to conceive". Jacob Bell, who had every reason to remember his own cross-examination, bore "testimony to the excellent manner in which the St. Albans Commissioners conducted that inquiry . . . A mouse was not more helpless before three bull terriers, than a witness was before those learned Commissioners. If one missed him, the next was sure to trip him up, and the third swallowed him".[17] The Commissioners' Report revealed, in the words of the Earl of Derby,

> that there had been a system of corruption long and steadily continued from election to election—that two-thirds of the electors had been implicated in notorious bribery—and that as long as St. Albans was gifted with the privilege of returning members to parliament, so long its constituency would consent, without reference to politics or principles, to be driven like sheep to the poll under the direction of those individuals from whom they received the price of their corruption.[18]

On 3 May 1852 the borough of St. Albans was disfranchised and the electorate incorporated into the county constituency of Herfordshire. Jacob Bell remained in the Commons until July, when parliament was dissolved. In the ensuing general election, held in July 1852, he fought the small decaying borough of Great Marlow in Buckinghamshire (electorate 354) and came bottom of the poll. In the same election, his brother James, the architect, was returned for Guildford and remained its M.P. until defeated in March 1857. In 1854, Jacob Bell fought another by-election, this time in his home constituency of Marylebone (electorate 19,892). He polled over 4,000 votes but was defeated by a Liberal candidate with all the right connexions, Viscount Ebrington.

The stench of hypocrisy pervaded the St. Albans affair from beginning to end. The hypocrisy and cynicism of those actively engaged in the election, of Coppock and Edwards, of Simpson and the "purity party", of Carden and Bell, were mercilessly laid bare by the three Commissioners in the autumn of 1851. But the exposure was itself an act of hypocrisy. The Government, which set the Commission up and brought about the disfranchisement, was deeply involved in electoral bribery and corruption. Coppock dispensed government appointments to reward his supporters. Few members of parliament reached Westminster with unsullied hands. "There could not be a doubt of the downright corruption of the House", declared John Roebuck, the radical M.P. "Elections costing from £5,000 to £10,000 were as plentiful as blackberries", said Jacob Bell, and some were reputed to cost as much as £40,000 to £60,000. "A man who had spent £20,000 in the most unblushing bribery and was not petitioned against because his opponent had bribed as much as himself, walked into the House as bold as brass and inveighed against the corruption of St. Albans". James Coppock, in his evidence before the St. Albans Commission, revealed:

> I know something of most places in England; and if, instead of going through the register of voters, as I see by the papers Mr. Edwards has done here, and marking down "sold his vote", I were to go through the list of boroughs, beginning with the first in the list, say Abingdon, to Stafford, and to the last letter of the alphabet, and put opposite the names of members "bought his seat", I should make quite as extraordinary a list as Mr. Edwards has made of this borough.

The system of bribery "was not confined to St. Albans", Jacob Bell pointed out, "but prevailed in many boroughs throughout the kingdom". If the House of Commons were to be content with making St. Albans the scapegoat, and grafting upon it the sins of every member of that House, upon the supposition that by exterminating that one borough the House would be left perfectly pure, that such a course would be a complete delusion, and not only a delusion, but an injustice.

It was easy to disfranchise St. Albans because it was a small and insignificant place. In 1852 its voters were punished, not because they were corrupt, but because they were independent. Freed from the coercion of landlords and employers, and true to the spirit of nascent capitalism, they treated their votes as commodities, as "a private property to be sold—not as a public trust to be exercised". John Roebuck spoke eloquently in their defence:

> He very much wished to ask what difference there was between the man who sold his vote for £5 and the man who sold his borough for £2,000? . . . a poor man sold his vote for £5, and he was branded . . . a corrupt voter. Yet, at the same time, a rich man was in the habit of selling what he called influence, and was allowed to do so with impunity . . . they came forward to disfranchise St. Albans, because 200 people in that case had done no worse than one rich man did in another borough.

The disfranchisement of boroughs like Sudbury in 1844 and St. Albans in 1852 was not enough to deter others from similar practices. It was the whole system which needed reforming: bribery was deeply rooted in the electoral practices of the age. In March 1852 Jacob Bell argued that the disfranchisement of St. Albans "would be holding up a cloak to screen not only acts which had been committed, but those which were in course of preparation at this moment". He warned that:

> The Blaggs and Edwardses were in a state of activity in every borough in the Kingdom. Instead of stopping the system of corruption, they were rather encouraged by seeing that Government were determined to wreak their vengeance on St. Albans alone . . . it was generally expected that the coming election would be the most corrupt that had taken place for years. They would find that the opinion of Parliamentary agents and of the press. A large number of boroughs were in the market at various prices.[19]

Disfranchisement was a token gesture, intended to prolong, rather than terminate, the system of corruption. It was not until the Ballot Act of 1872 and the Corrupt Practices Act of 1883 that any effective action was taken to change the system.[20]

In his own lifetime, Jacob Bell had to endure much moral censure for his behaviour during the 1850 by-election. In a letter, written in January 1852, he defended himself to a Manchester Quaker, chemist and druggist, George Dawson, in these terms:

> I am aware that I made a mistake in going to St. Albans. I found this out when it was too late to retract—I have never from that time had any opportunity of doing so—as I was like a person who had taken his seat in a train and is unable to stop it.
>
> I dare say the affair will injure me in many ways and it may probably injure the cause in which I have been engaged for many years—If this should be the case I cannot help it. I must grin and bear it. There has been a great deal of noise about that Borough—but if I wished to stand another election I should not know where to find a better. I believe they are all alike in principle with the exception of a few where local circumstances give the representative an influence which enables them

to walk over the course. But I believe there never was and never will be a contest without bribery or corruption in some form or other. I observe the same principles to operate in parish matters and in every case in which human nature and public duty are placed in competition with each other. Of course I do not in any degree defend these proceedings, but I know more about it now since I have tasted of the tree of knowledge of good and evil and passed through the fiery ordeal of a Parliamentary Commission.

It is difficult to believe Bell's story of the innocent corrupted. Bribery at St. Albans was "as notorious as the sun at noonday". The evidence shows that he declined to commit himself to St. Albans, until he had gained detailed information about the borough from several sources. By that time, he had already devised a covert system of transferring to Henry Edwards money which he must have known would be used to bribe voters. Nonetheless, we must guard against judging Jacob Bell by inappropriate moral standards. The Ballot Act of 1872 and the Corrupt Practices Act of 1883 have changed the meaning of legitimate political behaviour. It is not that political behaviour is more moral now than it was in Jacob Bell's day; it is merely that the criteria by which forms of political behaviour are adjudged acceptable or unacceptable have changed. The meaning of legitimate political behaviour has been transformed, not the legitimacy of political behaviour. Electoral reform should not be seen as the constitutional expression of the growing moralisation of English society, but rather as the result of attempts by the political elite to retain or enhance its powers at a time when the social structure of England was rapidly changing. Acts to eliminate corruption are signs of a change in strategy, not of an increase in morality.[21]

Whatever the relative moralities of Englishmen in the 1850s and the 1980s, the exchange of money or other favours has scarcely been rooted out of the electoral system. If tangible political rewards did not exist, political activity would be inconceivable. Rarely today do candidates bribe voters individually: but the practice is now general by which parties promise rewards to whole groups of voters to gain their support. In the debate on the Corrupt Practices Act of 1883, one M.P. pointed out that "the Bill . . . left untouched one great source of corruption—that gigantic kind of corruption attempted by the Premier, in 1874, when he promised the total abolition of Income Tax".[22] In a pamphlet, published in 1858, the third Earl Grey argued:

> To give money bribes to electors is not worse, or rather is not nearly so bad, as to court their favour by flattering their passions and prejudices, and by encouraging them knowingly in mischievous political errors. More real guilt is incurred because greater injury is done to the Nation, by having recourse to the arts of the demagogue, than by the illicit use of money for the purpose of carrying an election.[23]

The view, that the type of electioneering regarded as legitimate today is nothing but a more virulent form of the corruption practised by Jacob Bell, was stated, with prophetic insight, by William Greg, in an article entitled "Parliamentary Purification", published in the *Edinburgh Review*, shortly after the disfranchisement of St. Albans.

> When plain and simple bribery has been cured or reduced within the scantiest limits, we should have to be on our guard against the increase of a different, and a subtler, and perhaps in effect a more noxious species of corruption. If corrupt and

low-minded voters still retain the franchise, they will still seek to sell their votes, though they will have to look for payment in a different coin. If candidates are not more stern and lofty in their integrity than heretofore, they will be exposed to temptations of another sort, even more difficult to resist, more easy to conceal from the world, and more easy to palliate to their own consciences. If they may not any longer open their purses to gratify the inferior class of electors, they will be expected to warp their principles to suit them. They will be urged to purchase votes as before,—and to purchase them at a far higher and more fatal price. They will be pressed, and often, we fear, induced, to lower their political creed, to modify and impair their genuine opinions, to "file their mind" (as Shakespeare hath it), to profess views they do not hold, to give pledges they cannot redeem, in order to obtain the suffrages of men to whom the suffrage ought never to have been vouchsafed.[24]

* * *

On 12 June 1851 Jacob Bell moved in the House of Commons for leave to introduce "a bill for regulating the qualifications of pharmaceutical chemists, and for other purposes in connexion with the practice of pharmacy". It was read for the first time the following day. The bill was intended to give the Pharmaceutical Society the powers to regulate the practice of pharmacy in Great Britain. The Society was to be given the duty of compiling a register, of "pharmaceutical chemists, chemists and druggists, and dispensing chemists", comprising all its members and associates and any other persons who produced, within a year, evidence of their being already in practice. From twelve months after the passing of the Act, no person would be admitted to the register without first passing the Society's examinations in Latin language and classical knowledge, botany, materia medica, pharmaceutical and general chemistry, and toxicology. Thereafter, it would be illegal for an unregistered person "to exercise the business or calling of a pharmaceutical chemist, chemist or druggist, or dispensing chemist, in any part of Great Britain, or to use the name or title ... or any other name, title, sign, token or emblem implying that he is registered under this Act". For every offence a penalty not exceeding £20 was specified. Qualified medical practitioners would suffer no abridgement of their privileges provided they did not use the titles of pharmaceutical chemist, chemist and druggist, and dispensing chemist.[25]

In moving the second reading of the bill on 2 July, Bell explained that

> the object of the measure was to improve the qualifications of pharmaceutical chemists, and to establish the principle, that all those who were to compound the prescriptions of physicians and surgeons ought to receive a certain amount of education, and pass an examination, as a test of their fitness for the performance of their important and responsible duties.

In support of the view that professional examinations needed to be compulsory to be of any value to the public, Bell quoted Sir Astley Cooper, the eminent surgeon, and referred to the unsatisfactory state of affairs in pharmacy:

> According to the present arrangements, the examination of candidates by the Society was a voluntary matter; and accordingly, if a person presented himself for examination, and he was found to be incompetent and unfit to receive a certificate, he might commence business without one, ignorant though he were, and could snap his fingers at the examiners ... It was the object of the Pharmaceutical Society, in introducing the Bill, to make the examination obligatory.

Improvements would be gradual. Those already in business would not be affected but as they left the stage their place would be taken by educated persons: "it was not for 1851 but for 1870 that they were now to legislate".

Mr. Ralph Bernal, the Whig M.P. for Rochester, supported the bill. Some chemists, he said, were very ignorant and did not know the difference between oxalic acid and Epsom salts or between iodine and aconite. Others, however, were well informed: the best chemists in London were members of the Pharmaceutical Society.

> All that the Bill proposed was, that a certain society, which was already incorporated, should have the power of examining parties and giving certificates, and without these certificates persons should not be allowed to enter the profession ... the Bill would prove highly beneficial to the public at large ...

The bill was not allowed to proceed without opposition. Joseph Hume, F.R.S., a member of the Royal Colleges of Surgeons of Edinburgh and London, was the radical M.P. for Montrose. During the last twenty years, he argued, the House had had one bill after another dealing with the medical profession. This and preceding governments had found difficulty enough handling the three medical bodies already in existence and now it was proposed to add another one. The responsibilities proposed to be devolved upon this pharmaceutical society should be the duty of the Apothecaries' Company. The addition of a fourth body, invested with a monopoly in its particular business, would only complicate matters and interfere with that general measure which it was so essential to have enacted for the regulation of the medical and surgical profession. Hume's opposition was reinforced by that of the Tory member for Oxfordshire, Joseph Henley. As a magistrate and graduate from Magdalen College Oxford, he could be expected to see through any humbug:

> The real state of the case was, that a society set up about seven years ago by Royal Charter, induced many chemists to pay two guineas a year for a fine label, which they put in their window, with the hard words "Pharmaceutical Chemists" upon it; but he believed the bubble had burst, and that the same importance was not attached to the richly-framed label as the poor and ignorant were at first inclined to bestow. People now went for their drugs to some honest respectable tradesman whom they were accustomed to trust, and had lost all faith in these gaudy labels, which were nothing better than show advertisements.

With impeccable logic, he went on to complain that the bill did not "interfere with patent or proprietary medicines, however injurious they might be".

The Home Secretary, Sir George Grey, pointed out that there was no chance of the bill passing at this late stage of the session.

> It was a bill that ought to be before the public a considerable time ... He thought also this branch of the subject ought not to be considered except in connexion with the medical question generally; and he felt very strong objections to creating in this body a monopoly, giving them an exclusive right to determine who should, and who should not, be dispensing chemists.

Jacob Bell accepted the Home Secretary's proposition "that the bill should be read a second time *pro forma*, in order that it should be printed with amendments, and circulated throughout the country". Two days later, Thomas Wakley, speaking strongly in favour of the bill, tried to induce the House to alter the arrangement and proceed with the appointment of a select committee, to which the bill would be referred, so as to permit its passing that session. This tactic was not successful: the amended bill was printed and left to stand over until the following session.[26]

The amendments ensured the appointment of a Board of Examiners for Scotland, to meet in Edinburgh; enabled provincial members of the Pharmaceutical Society to vote by proxy or by post; exempted assistants and apprentices already in the trade from the necessity of passing the qualifying examination; and made registration permissive instead of compulsory for those already in business.

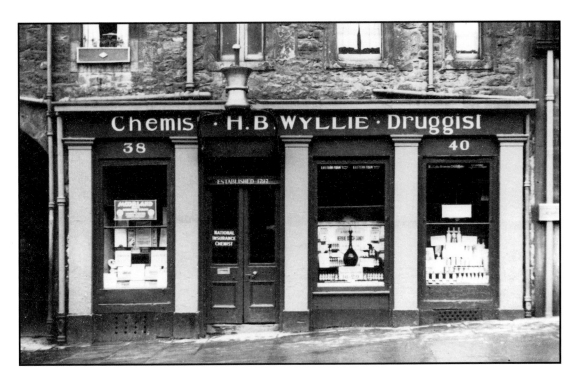

28   *H.B. Wyllie, Chemist Druggist, 38–40 Grassmarket, Edinburgh, was one of the oldest established pharmacies in the capital.*

While the proceedings were taking place in the Commons, 558 petitions with 15,264 signatures were presented in favour of the bill and two petitions were presented against it, one from the Royal College of Surgeons of Edinburgh and one from the Faculty of Physicians and Surgeons of Glasgow. These Scottish corporations opposed the bill under the impression that it would interfere with the right of their members to practise pharmacy: amendments were made to conciliate them. The Society of Apothecaries remained implacably hostile to the Pharmaceutical Society and mounted a broad-based assault on the bill. One of their objections was easily overcome by the removal of toxicology from the list

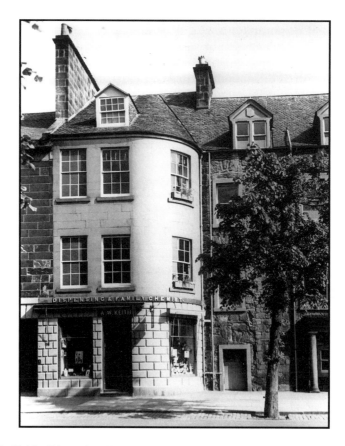

29 *A.W. Keith, Dispensing & Family Chemist, 73 South Street, St. Andrews, Fife. This imposing shop front forms part of an old tenement building.*

of examination subjects. The Apothecaries' Company argued that as a knowledge of toxicology involved the medical treatment of cases of poisoning it was out-of-bounds for chemists and druggists. The fact that the public interest might be served by having chemists tested in their knowledge of the chemical nature and the appropriate antidotes of poisons was of less importance to the Master and Wardens of the Society of Apothecaries than the assertion of their petty privileges.

Jacob Bell introduced the amended pharmacy bill on 12 February 1852 in unpromising circumstances. Ten days earlier the St. Albans Bribery Commission had published its damaging report: the fall of the Liberal government raised the prospect of a speedy dissolution of parliament. Nonetheless, the second reading took place on 17 March and the bill was referred to a select committee. Bell began by presenting petitions in favour of the bill from the President and Censors of the Royal College of Physicians, the President and Council of the Royal College of Surgeons, one signed by 150 eminent medical practitioners resident in London and numerous petitions from medical practititoners, chemists and druggists, and members of the public in various parts of the country. In his speech on the second reading, Bell pointed out that the Pharmaceutical Society had been founded "as the institution which should regulate the education of and examine future chemists".

> This Society was entirely of a voluntary character; its powers did not extend beyond its own members ... consequently the influence of the society numerically on those entering the business was small ... It was, therefore, necessary, in order to extend that beneficial influence, to increase the powers of the society, and for this purpose the pharmacy bill was introduced.

The bill established a standard of qualification for pharmaceutical chemists.

> He felt assured that if the bill should pass, it would, in a few years, raise the character of pharmaceutical chemists. It would oblige all those who regularly follow the business to learn the rudiments of chemistry and the collateral sciences. Among the number some would be found who, by their natural talent and industry, aided by the fundamental education rendered necessary by the bill, would turn their attention to the higher branches of science, and reflect credit on the country. The majority, however, would confer a benefit on the public in another way, by performing in a more safe and efficient manner the duties of pharmaceutical chemists in the preparation of medicines, many of which are powerful poisons, and ought not to be entrusted in the hands of ignorant and inexperienced persons.

The new Home Secretary, Spencer Walpole, was no more enthusiastic about the bill than his predecessor. Considering the great powers given by the bill to the Pharmaceutical Society, he was not prepared to give his assent before the bill had been examined by a select committee.

> The second clause gave very great and irresponsible powers to the Pharmaceutical Society in making by-laws and regulations; and the fifteenth clause subjected persons to serious penalties for assuming the business of a chemist and druggist ...

Edward Bouverie, an under-secretary at the Home Office in the previous Liberal government, also opposed the bill:

> Very grave objections could be stated to the bill as it now stood. In fact it would give a trading monopoly to a chartered body, of which that House knew very little indeed. So far as he could understand the object of the bill, it was intended to turn chemists and druggists into apothecaries, and to derive a revenue for the society by levying large contributions from chemists already in business ... unless great care were taken they would find a fresh crop of medical practitioners springing up among the chemists.

Jacob Bell protested that the aim of the bill was diametrically opposed to that stated and was about to explain further when called to order. He sat down. The bill went to the select committee.[27]

The select committee gathered evidence from physicians and surgeons representing the medical corporations in London and Edinburgh, from the clerk and solicitor to the Apothecaries' Society, from general practitioners and from representatives of the Pharmaceutical Society. Evidence was also taken on the laws relating to pharmacy in France (from Professor Kopp of Strasburg), in Germany (from Professor Hofmann of the Royal

College of Chemistry), in Sweden (from Dr. Hamberg of Stockholm) and in Mauritius (from M. Baschet). From the evidence presented it is possible to summarise the arguments for and against the pharmacy bill.

Those who supported the bill attempted to show that pharmaceutical knowledge had been much neglected in this country until promoted by the Pharmaceutical Society; that the success of medical treatment depends to a great extent on the knowledge, skill and judgment of those engaged in the dispensing of medicines; and that the adoption of regulations to ensure a supply of educated pharmaceutical chemists was in the public interest. "The object is not merely to raise the position of chemists and druggists", pointed out J.F. South, President of the Royal College of Surgeons, "but it is to protect the public from medicines being improperly supplied and being improperly prepared and made up by ignorant persons".[28] On the continent, it was claimed, chemists are all highly educated men. Governments provide schools of pharmacy where students "have the opportunity of obtaining all the information which the present age of discovery can afford; and they are compelled to undergo a strict examination before they can establish themselves in business".[29] "In France the laws", wrote Jacob Bell, "are so stringent that no person is permitted to give medical advice in the most trivial cases, without possessing a qualification and a licence. A chemist is prohibited from preparing any recipe or prescription for a patient, unless written by a medical man; and no person can carry on the business of a chemist and druggist without having undergone an examination, neither can he employ an assistant who is not qualified". In Norway, Sweden, Denmark, Finland, Russia and Germany "not only are unqualified persons prohibited from practising in any department of the profession but the number of regular practitioners is limited by law; only so many being licensed as are considered to be required by the population in their respective districts ... The course of education is definite and complete; and the examinations, through which each candidate must pass, are very severe ... the profession enjoys a monopoly which is rigidly maintained".[30] In Sweden, Germany, Mauritius and France, there is strict legal separation of medicine and pharmacy: physicians do not sell medicines and chemists do not prescribe. It is not mere coincidence that all the important pharmaceutical discoveries have been made by continental chemists; morphia and chloroform by Germans, quinine and strychine by the French. "It is to the want of a proper standard of qualification", said Douglas MacLagan, Fellow of the Edinburgh College Surgeons and lecturer in materia medica, "that we must in a great measure attribute the smallness of the amount of pharmaceutical invention or discovery which has emanated from Great Britain".[31]

The purpose of the pharmacy bill was to define by law the boundary between chemists and druggists and other retailers. The act would not have interfered with the right of grocers and oilmen to sell a few simple drugs or patent medicines, but it would have made it impossible for newcomers to set up as chemists and druggists, without first undergoing training and passing an examination in London or Edinburgh. After the passing of the act only registered persons would be permitted to carry on the business or calling of chemist and druggist. The register, by defining the membership of the profession, would have reserved the rewards of the pharmaceutical business to qualified practitioners alone. Competition in the sale of drugs from outside the ranks would have been dramatically reduced. The act would not only have reduced competition from other tradesmen, it would also have reduced competition within the profession. The act would have imposed an educational restriction on entry to the occupation. By adding this new educational burden to the existing requirement for capital, it was hoped to regulate internal competition through the mechanism of the Pharmaceutical Society's board of examiners. The basic idea was to enhance the remuneration and status of chemists and druggists by reducing their numbers. The act implied a contract between the Pharmaceutical Society and the community. In return for granting the Society its monopoly powers, the community would be supplied with educated and responsible pharmaceutical chemists. Both the chemist and druggist and the public at large would be protected.

Jacob Bell faced two difficulties in arguing this case. The first was that the pharmacy bill proposed to qualify the very people that leaders of the Pharmaceutical Society denounced as ignorant and unscrupulous. Although the act would, in the long run, guarantee the qualification of all pharmaceutical chemists, it would, in the short run, admit to the register, with the minimum of scrutiny, the motley ranks of practising chemists and druggists. If it was indispensable to public safety that nobody should be allowed to practise as a chemist and druggist without undergoing a test of competence, was it possible to justify the proposal to permit unqualified persons to practise with impunity, simply because they were already doing so? Jacob Bell replied that all great reforms must have a beginning, that legislation must not be seen to act retrospectively, and that the Apothecaries' Act had established the precedent in 1815.

The second difficulty was that the pharmacy act seemed to run counter to the dominant ideology of the day, the doctrine of free trade. A nation that had only recently abandoned protectionism by repealing the Corn Laws and the Navigation Acts and drastically reducing the number and level of import duties, might be thought unlikely to favour the creation of new monopolies and restrictive practices. "The present is an unfavourable time for attempting to introduce legislation with reference to pharmacy", wrote Jacob Bell, "because the tendency of the age is rather to remove restrictions than to interfere with 'the liberty of the subject' in commercial matters". As a Liberal member of parliament, he had declared himself in favour of free trade. His defence of the pharmacy act as a restriction on ignorance rather than on trade seems as unconvincing now as it must have been at the time.

> It is not our object to create a monopoly, and to limit the number of pharmaceutical chemists but to oblige those who embark in the business to possess the needful qualification ... the necessity of education would shut out incompetent persons from the privilege of commencing business. But it would not limit the number of competent chemists ... The sale of drugs would be as free and unlimited under the new system as it is at present; but it would be in more competent hands.[32]

The free trade case was more effectively presented. In his evidence before the select committee, Dr. John Gairdner, Fellow of the Edinburgh College of Surgeons argued that competition is the public's security against ignorant chemists.

> This ignorance of which so much talk is made ... is now in the course of being remedied, and ... has been for many years in a progressive state of remedy, by causes which are in operation. Every man who embarks his capital in a drug trade, does so under the influence of competition in his own circle; he does so even in the small villages and hamlets in the country ... this principle of competition, which

may at any time rob him of his business, operates as a penalty on his ignorance at every instant of time, and in every corner of the country. If you introduce a system of penalty, which in point of fact excludes competitors with those who are now in the field ... you will destroy the security the public at present enjoy, and substitute a species of security which is altogether illusory, or at least greatly inferior.

"The same amount of science, the same knowledge of chemistry, which is essential in one place, is by no means essential in another", continued Gairdner. "A small village will never be able to support a highly trained chemist".

> They can get a man now who will serve their purpose, but if you force them to take a man who has been examined under this bill, and who had gone to the expense of going to Edinburgh or London, and going through a course of lectures there, they probably would lose the advantage of having a useful man among them altogether. I think the public are quite safe if they will trust to this system of competition, and to the penalty which the loss of capital embarked in an unsuccessful trade necessarily imposes upon those who fail ... if you abolish in any degree this species of natural protection, and substitute for it an artificial system of penalty, my opinion is that you will fail in your object.[33]

Jacob Bell thought Gairdner mistaken. But he did not attempt to demonstrate in detail the dangers to the public of unlicensed practice, nor did he challenge the idea that the operation of the market was "natural" and that any interference with it was "artificial". Although he was convinced that the competition of the ignorant and unscrupulous was destructive of all attempts to raise educational and ethical standards, he knew his bill would qualify the very people he wanted to drive out of the profession.

Paradoxically the major objection to the pharmacy bill was that it would increase rather than decrease competition. The most obstinate and co-ordinated opposition to the bill came from the general practitioners.[34] Licentiates of the Society of Apothecaries, who fervently approved of their own Society's use of its monopolistic powers, acquired in 1815, to exclude from competition the better educated Scottish graduates, resented the Pharmaceutical Society's attempt to gain from the legislature similar powers against the encroachments of grocers and oilmen. Representatives of the Scottish medical corporations, who boldly recommended the invigorating discipline of the free market to Jacob Bell's chemists and druggists, deplored the effects of unregulated counter prescribing on the incomes of their alumni in general practice. The pharmacy bill had the singular effect of uniting the traditionally hostile camps of English apothecaries and Scottish medical graduates. Both feared that the act would give the new pharmaceutical chemist a competitive advantage over the humbler class of general practitioners.

"I have no doubt", declared Dr. John Rose Cormack, F.R.C.P. (Edinburgh), "that by the enactment of this bill, the chemists will obtain greater prestige and influence with the public and that their counter practice will increase in consequence of it". The bill, he continued,

> would bring into greater competition than at present the humbler class of general practitioners with the chemists and druggists, and that it would in that way cause in a number of localities the medical practitioners to be really superseded ... in the poorer localities the chief profit is derived from consultations which take place

170

in the shop, and ... those who have a larger poor practice, and who go out to visit their patients, cannot subsist; whereas a man who confines himself to counter practice may make a good income. Now, I think, that this measure, by giving a greater prestige and status to the chemists, would operate very severely upon the humbler class of medical practitioners ... I think that the display in shops of the diploma of the Pharmaceutical Society has led a number of the less informed part of the public to suppose it is the diploma of a medical practitioner.[35]

Dr. Edward Crisp thought the bill would just as effectively undermine the livelihood of medical men who kept open shop.

A young man now beginning practice labours under this disadvantage, which would be greatly increased under this bill: he is often compelled, contrary to his inclination and much against his pride, to keep an open shop; to put bottles in his window, and to sell drugs, because he finds that the little property he has must soon be expended if he does not pursue this course, which it is necessary for him to pursue in order to compete with the chemist and druggist, whose chief profit in many places in populous districts arises from counter practice. The very practice which I think young practitioners ought to obtain is obtained by chemists and druggists, and I think this bill would greatly increase that evil, because the chemist and druggist would take a title superior to that of the apothecary. I hold that the title "pharmaceutical chemist" is far superior to that of an "apothecary", the name with which the College of Physicians and Surgeons up to this time brand a general practitioner.[36]

Dr. George Webster, once president of the original British Medical Association, developed the same theme.

It is notorious that counter practice is carried on to a great extent by the great majority of chemists, and that not a few even visit patients at their own houses. With more education, I believe that such persons would consider themselves better qualified to give advice, and treat diseases, though utterly ignorant of the nature and treatment of such diseases; and the public, seeing a showy diploma exhibited in chemists' shops and windows, will be deceived into a belief that it is proof of medical qualification. This has already happened with the present flashy, so-called diploma of the Pharmaceutical Society.[37]

The general practitioners' main objection to the bill was that it gave chemists and druggists the opportunity to become a new class of medical practitioners. "This new body to be constituted", warned Dr. James Watson, president of the Faculty of Physicians and Surgeons of Glasgow, "will, I think, grow up like the Apothecaries' Company into a body of medical men".[38] Henry Ancell, a leading spokesman for the general practitioners, asserted that it was perfectly well known that "a very large proportion" of "the general body of chemists and druggists" desire to practise physic; "the aim and object of a great many of them is to practise physic".[39]

I may state that the bill draws a distinction, no doubt, between the medical practitioner and the pharmaceutical chemist; but I do not think that the mere drawing of that distinction will be sufficient to prevent a pharmaceutical chemist from becoming a medical practitioner. We all know that the designation "apothecary" has become almost obsolete; that is to say, the public and the medical profession have both got disgusted with the word "apothecary"; if you want to institute a new class of practitioners, one of the most efficient means of doing so is to create a new name; and I think that you will be facilitating an establishment of a new class of medical practitioners if you render current the term "pharmaceutical chemist".[40]

Jacob Bell rejected these arguments. He insisted that the purpose of the bill was "to produce a distinct class of pharmaceutical chemists, not at all connected with the medical profession".

This is a bill, the object of which is to qualify men in pharmacy and chemistry, to prohibit them from being medical men and to exclude medical men from being pharmaceutical chemists.

This bill, he pointed out, draws "a positive line of demarcation between the functions of the medical practitioner and the functions of the chemist". Indeed, "this bill tends to draw a more distinct line between medical practice and the business of chemists and druggists than was ever drawn before by any statute".

The object of the bill is to check the prescribing activities of chemists by separating the practice of pharmacy from that of medicine, making them distinct bodies.[41]

Thomas Wakley, in his enthusiasm for the bill, tried to allay the fears of general practitioners in language which mocked the pharmaceutical chemist's claim to professional status.

This bill does not refer to the medical profession; this bill does not constitute a medical corporation; it constitutes a corporation composed of chemists and druggists; it is only a bill for increasing the powers of an existing trading corporation.[42]

Even trusted friends of the Pharmaceutical Society used strange arguments to defend the bill. George Walter Smith, the Society's secretary, opened his evidence by accurately recalling the objections to Hawes' bill in 1841, but went on to declare that,

the intention has been, that the Society should consist solely and entirely of chemists and druggists, and the great desire was to prevent the chemists and druggists from trenching on the medical profession.[43]

Why a society, founded to protect the interests of chemists and druggists, should try to stop them carrying on their traditional counter prescribing, was not made clear. Supporters of the bill argued that, with improved education and higher status, chemists would be less inclined to act as medical men. Dr. James Arthur Wilson, the senior physician of St. George's Hospital, expressed his view that the bill, by establishing the authority of the Pharmaceutical Society, would be more effective than any other measure in stopping counter practice by chemists and druggists.

I believe that they would become less and less practitioners over the counter . . . They are practitioners now to a great extent in many instances, and very reprehensible the practice is; and by none, I believe, is it more deprecated than by the leading numbers of the Pharmaceutical Society. But I believe if their station was raised as pharmaceutical chemists, if they were recognised under an Act of

Parliament as a scientific body, with a real chartered and Parliamentary existence, they would be less and less inclined to meddle with the practice of physic, to tamper with what they know little or nothing about.[44]

The most perceptive and cogent defence of the pharmacy bill was made by Dr. Garrett Dillon, of Spanish Place, Manchester Square, London, in a letter written in April 1852 and published in the *Lancet*. In response to a blistering attack by Dr. George Webster, that doughty defender of the down-trodden doctor, Dillon ventured the view that the bill "promises to the public, and to the profession also, great benefits".

> And now, with respect to the "counter practice" of the chemist and druggist, about which Dr. Webster so loudly complains. That such a practice is carried, to a limited extent, as incidental to the business of the chemist and druggist, cannot be doubted; but I question whether it is so dangerous to the public, or so injurious to the interests of the profession, as Dr. Webster seems to imagine. I am pretty sure that, on the contrary, it is a great convenience to the humbler classes, who cannot afford to call in a qualified practitioner upon every little alarm or derangement of health ... of a temporary nature, and easily corrected by a dose or two of simple medicine. I am equally certain that this "counter practice" of the chemist relieves medical men of a great deal of profitless trouble; for though the class of patients who resort to it pay their three pence or sixpence to the chemist over the counter, they are but rarely in circumstances to pay a "doctor's bill"; and it would be grievous to the profession to see any of its members dragging such persons into the county courts for payment.
>
> Dr. Webster says that it is his firm conviction that, by the passing of this bill, *"counter practice" will increase ten-fold*, for the chemists and druggists will, as he imagines, hold up their flaring diplomas to decoy and cheat the public into the belief that they are perfectly qualified to cure disease.
>
> Now, this is all, to say the least of it, but assumption, partaking, truly, a good deal of morbid apprehension ... I entertain hopes of better results from the passing of the bill, for I foresee that, instead of making knaves and imposters of the chemists and druggists ... it will elevate their position, and make their trade a scientific pursuit ... And more, it will secure to the public, at the humblest shop, accuracy and safety in the preparation of medicines, upon the efficacy of which life itself may be depending.
>
> Of domiciliary visits to patients by chemists to treat disease, I have no apprehension. Such a practice is known to be incompatible with success in the trade of the chemist and druggist, and ... none of those who are prosperous in that business attempt it. "Counter practice" is quite a different thing; it is but temporary, and never extends to the regular and continuous treatment of any disease involving danger to life and limb; and, upon reconsideration, I hope that Dr. Webster will see that it would be beneath the dignity of the profession to notice it with the hostility of the restrictive clause that he suggests. The doctor points to the restriction upon the French *pharmaciens* as a model for us to follow in restraining the chemist and druggist from carrying on *counter practice*. But it should be recollected that in France medical men are not allowed to supply medicines to their patients, nor to derive, directly or indirectly, any profit from the sale of the medicines they prescribe.[45]

The contrast in the relationship between medicine and pharmacy in France and Britain was a constant point of reference in the debates on the bill. The dispensing doctor was a peculiarity of the British; there was no French equivalent to the English apothecary. "From choice or necessity", explained Dr. John Rose Cormack, "many medical men supply medicines to their own patients, and others, in addition to that, sell medicines just as a chemist and druggist would do, and in some neighbourhoods, we cannot conceal the fact, the medical practitioners and the chemists are rivals in counter practice".[46] Both general practitioners and chemists and druggists kept establishments seen by the public as "doctors' shops". "In the same street", wrote Jacob Bell, "may be seen two shops, fitted up exactly alike. The windows of each are adorned with coloured show-bottles, cut smelling-bottles, medicine chests, tooth brushes, and perchance a few proprietary medicines". One shop belongs to a general practitioner, the other to a chemist and druggist.[47] Douglas MacLagan thought this gave rise to much confusion. "The pubic are very apt to suppose that a person who has a druggist's shop is a doctor; it is a very common thing to call a druggist 'doctor'".[48] General practitioners feared that educating, examining and licensing the chemist and druggist would make him a more formidable rival. The more proficient he became in pharmaceutical chemistry and the more his shop specialised in dispensing and the sale of medicines, the more the public would see him as a doctor and his shop as a health centre. As long as self-medication was widespread, as long as physicians' prescriptions belonged to the patient and could be repeatedly presented to the chemist for dispensing, general practitioners had good reason to fear that registered pharmaceutical chemists would be more effective competitors than the present assortment of druggists, whose shops were not easily distinguished from those of grocers and oilmen.

The general practitioner wanted to both have his cake and eat it. He wanted to claim the status and income of a professional man but retain the right to supply medicines to his patients and even to keep open shop for the sale of drugs. However much he might aspire to the titles of physician or surgeon in general practice, as long as he continued to deal in drugs, he would be regarded as "a mere poacher on the manor of the physician, the surgeon and the druggist".[49] If apothecaries were to be transformed into general medical practitioners and obtain recognition as members of a learned profession, their association with the sale of drugs had to be brought to an end. The general practitioner's task was to build up public confidence in his role as a trusted counsellor, unequivocally committed to his patients' welfare. The roles of fiduciary and vendor do not fit easily together. Doctors who dispense drugs at a profit leave themselves open to the temptation to over prescribe or to prescribe the drug they have in their necessarily limited stock, regardless of whether it is the most appropriate treatment. In 1845 *The Times* argued that, to counter accusations of over-prescribing, general practitioners should charge only for medical and surgical attendance rather than for items of medicine supplied. It should be made "an absolute disqualification for the standing of a surgeon" to use "the tradesman's style of charging". *The Times* went on:

> Apothecaries may properly prescribe and charge for medicines, but then they should be merely and avowedly apothecaries—scientific tradesmen. The man who is both a surgeon and an apothecary, has no right to engross the repute of a professional man and the sordid profits of a trade. If he insists on his professional status, he must sink the counter and the till.[50]

In the same year, the Shropshire and North Wales Medical and Surgical Association urged that every semblance of trade should be done away with in the medical profession, and the keeping of retail drug shops by medical men (a practice so common in London, and so degrading to the profession) should be especially prohibited.[51]

As early as 1840 Richard Carmichael, an eminent Irish surgeon, had argued that the prescriber of medicines, save in remote rural districts, should be forbidden to sell them.

Practitioners cannot be prevented, for obvious reasons, from supplying their patients with medicines, if they please, but they should not be entitled to charge for them; it being one of those important and leading objects of medical reform to separate pharmacy from the practice of physic.[52]

The simplest and most effective way of separating pharmacy from the practice of physic would have been for general practitioners to give up selling drugs. In 1849 the *Medical Times* pointed out that if the "medical man persists in identifying himself with the tradesman, he cannot expect the public to draw a distinction".[53] The obstacle in the path of the general practitioner's rise to professional status was his own counter practice not that of the chemist and druggist. The remedy was in his own hands: abandon the drug trade, send his prescriptions to the pharmaceutical chemist, and charge only for visits and advice. There really was no other way to create a clear mark of distinction between the profession of medicine and the business of the chemist and druggist. It was, however, a solution few general practitioners were willing to contemplate. Selling drugs for profit was essential to his livelihood. It accounted in most cases for three-quarter of his income; sometimes even more.[54] As late as 1888, Walter Rivington, surgeon to the London Hospital, found it necessary to classify general practitioners into the dispensing and non-dispensing orders. The dispensing order he sub-divided into "surgeon chemists" and "surgeon apothecaries". The "surgeon chemists" kept open shop, "with glass cases containing tooth brushes, nail brushes, patent medicines, seidlitz powders, Eno's fruit salt, soap, scents, delectable lozenges, chest protectors, and feeding bottles". The retail business was the great source of income and could not be given up without serious damage to the enterprise. The "surgeon apothecary" did no retail trade, but charged for advice and medicine. Dispensing prevailed but "as the scale is ascended the surgery retires more and more into the background, until it reaches the interior of the dwelling where it is no longer exposed to the vulgar gaze ..." Eventually the non-dispensing order is reached. Here general practitioners prescribe medicines made up by chemists and perform the minor operations of surgery, charging lower fees than those of the physicians and surgeons.[55]

The general practitioner's reluctance to give up the sale of drugs was paralleled by the chemist and druggist's attachment to counter prescribing. In the eyes of the great majority of chemists and druggists, counter practice was not an incursion into the professional territory of the physician but the routine performance of the shopkeeper's role. In early Victorian Britain retailing was still a skilled occupation. Before the development of factory production and the transformation of the processing of most consumer goods, the producer/retailer survived in many trades. Shopcraft skills and specialist knowledge of products retained considerable importance. Grocers carried out the preliminary tasks of cleaning, sorting and grading goods before blending, labelling and weighing them for sale. Butchers slaughtered and dressed their own meat. Bakers and confectioners produced their particular kinds of bread, pastries and sweet stuffs from a wide variety of ingredients, relying on the special features and quality of their merchandise rather than its price to attract sales. Competition in the retail trades was based on service and product differentiation rather than on price. Grocers prided themselves on the special flavour of their teas, butchers boasted of the unique quality of their meats. Boot and shoe makers, cabinet makers and upholsterers, milliners and dressmakers, saddlers and curriers staked their reputations on the attractiveness and durability of their distinctive products. Their goods were far from standardised but varied in quality and style. Retailers were expected to have special skills and knowledge, to offer information, advice and guidance on the goods and services they provided, and even to produce goods to meet the peculiar requirements of individual customers. Counter prescribing was charateristic of all specialist retailing: it was not a peculiarity of the chemist and druggist. Like other retailers, the chemist prepared his own products, had his particular specialties, prided himself on the purity and freshness of

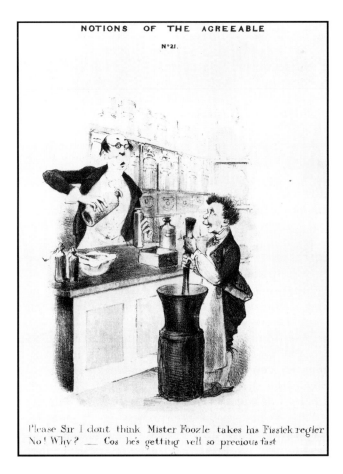

30 Notions of the Agreeable No 21. *Anon. Coloured lithograph published by W. Spooner, 377 Strand, London. c. 1830–40.*

his goods, and extemporaneously made up medicines to his customers' instructions. Most counter prescribing was initiated by the customer. It was an aspect of self-medication. All chemists and druggists engaged in it: refusal to do so would have met with the client's incomprehension and loss of confidence. "Although you may declare it to be illegal to give advice, you will not prevent the public from going to the dispenser of drugs and asking his advice", said Robert Renton, a Scottish physician, "nor will you be able to prevent the dispenser of drugs from giving that advice, by any Act you can pass".[56] R.B. Upton, the clerk and solicitor to the Apothecaries' Society, in attempting to locate the boundary between legitimate and illegitimate practice, unwittingly revealed the absurdity of the attempt. In his idiosyncratic view:

> The business of a chemist and druggist is to sell medicines which he is asked for; but the moment a chemist and druggist applies his skill to symptoms, and recommends a remedy, that moment he steps beyond the line to which the law has confined his practice .... if a patient comes to him and describes the kind of medicine he wants, the chemist is at liberty to give it to him; but if he puts out his tongue and gets him to feel his pulse, the chemist is not at liberty to supply the medicine ... I think that a chemist and druggist who professes to treat disease in any way, and who suggests a remedy appropriate to a disease, is trenching upon the province of the medical practitioner.[57]

Upton was more concerned to protect the province of the apothecary than to promote the welfare of the patient. As the *Pharmaceutical Journal* pointed out in 1862,

> in some localities, the principal part of the business of the chemist consists in prescribing for the poor, who, if deprived of this cheap means of obtaining remedies for their ailments, would ... be deprived of all medical relief.[58]

"The chemist can very easily refer a wealthy person to a medical man", observed Richard William Giles, a leading Bristol chemist, "but it would be simply a farce to recommend a servant to go to a medical man".[59]

Masters as well as servants sought advice from the chemist. Self-diagnosis and self-treatment kept the doctor from the door. The idea of calling in an expert to discover whether and to what extent a person was ill and to have the illness defined and categorised appealed more to the doctor than to the patient. Sick people preferred to visit the chemist's shop to have their own diagnoses confirmed, to gain information about the type and range of remedies available and to get some advice about dosages and modes of administering them. The general practitioner's attack on counter practice was an attack on the rights of the patient as much as on the activities of the chemist. Counter practice was little more than standard retailing practice. What doctors objected to was self-medication. The professionalisation of medicine involved not only the suppression of unlicensed practice and the control of the chemist and druggist but also the restriction of public access to drugs, the commodities of medicine. Henry Ancell prepared, at Thomas Wakley's request, a clause for "the restriction of irregular practice" to be inserted in the pharmacy bill. Its wording neatly illustrates the connexion between counter practice and self medication and how restrictions on the chemist were also restrictions on the public. Ancell's proposed clause read:

It shall not be lawful for any individual registered under this Act ... to prescribe, administer, dispense or sell for medical use any virulent poison or poisonous medicine or compound, unless prescribed by a medical practitioner.[60]

Fortunately, the select committee could not be persuaded to hand over the control of all powerful remedies to the medical profession. In 1862 the *Pharmaceutical Journal* reminded its readers that pharmaceutical chemists had the right, in supplying the public with medicines,

> to advise with their customers as to the best selection and mode of application of such domestic remedies. The qualified pharmaceutist is capable of affording important assistance to his customers in this respect, and unless the public are to be restricted from prescribing for themselves, they cannot surely be prevented from seeking information with reference to the action of the remedies they employ from those who are able and willing to give it them.

In November 1861 the editor of the *Chemist and Druggist* obtained counsel's opinion on the right of chemists to prescribe. Tompson Chitty took the view that counter practice was no different in law from any other retailer's advice to his customers.

> A chemist may, in his shop, so far prescribe for a customer as to advise with him as to the nature and quality and mode of application of the medicines which he is about to sell and also as to which of his commodities will best suit the requirements of his customer. He may listen to his customer's statements as to the reasons for his wishing to become a purchaser and may suggest to and advise him as to which of his commodities will be most suitable and beneficial to the customer or may dissuade him from purchasing or taking that which a customer in his ignorance may have applied for. This advice is merely incidental to the sale and dispensation of the chemist's wares and drugs, and cannot, of course, be made the subject of a charge.

In no case can a chemist attend upon a patient at the patient's house to advise or see the patient to prescribe; but

> a chemist may go to his customer's house to take an order for specific goods from the customer, ... he being too unwell to go out, just as any other tradesman may do.
>   In either case, a chemist may, of course, recover goods sold by him on credit; he is no more compelled to deal for ready money only than is any other tradesman.
> But in all cases the chemist must be simply a "vendor of his goods".

He must not seek to make profit by giving advice. In short, a chemist who makes no professions, does not hold himself out in a false position, and acts bona fide with ordinary skill and ability, not being guilty of gross negligence, is no more liable to criminal proceedings than any other practitioner. "It seems to me", concluded Tompson Chitty, "that the system which is called 'counter practice' is perfectly legal".[61]

Important implications emerge from this. Tradesmen deal in commodities; the principle of *caveat emptor* applies. Professional men sell advice; their integrity must be guaranteed. Chemists and druggists are responsible for the quality of the drugs they sell; physicians and lawyers for the objectivity of their advice. The apothecary destroys the purity of these categories by claiming the right to sell both goods and advice. He muddies the water and threatens the established order. The general practitioner, not the chemist and druggist, was the real danger to the stability of the medical profession.

The House of Commons select committee fundamentally revised Jacob Bell's bill. The exclusive powers sought, by which only examined and registered persons would be allowed to exercise the business or calling of chemist and druggist, were held to be incompatible with the principles of free trade and at variance with the Government's views on the regulation of medical practice. No trace of monopoly survived the select committee's revision. The proposal to prohibit unqualified practice was rescinded. All mention of "chemists and druggists" and "dispensing chemists" was removed. The main restriction imposed by the bill was to the use of the title of pharmaceutical chemist or pharmaceutist. The maximum penalty for offenders was a mere £5. "The select committee of the House of Commons", reported *Annals of Pharmacy and Practical Chemistry* in 1852, "has so thoroughly mutilated the chief provisions of the pharmacy bill, that it has become nothing but a bill confirmatory of the charter of the Pharmaceutical Society, with a few slight amendments".

> The bill, as amended by the committee, confers no exclusive privileges on the Pharmaceutical Society, further than the one that no persons except its members can call themselves pharmaceutists or pharmaceutical chemists. It leaves to anybody the privilege of assuming the title of chemist and druggist, or any other except the two named, and of practising all or any departments of the business as at present.[62]

Although the select committee had been unimpressed by the case for prohibiting unqualified practice, it had been convinced of the need to prevent educated pharmaceutists developing, as the apothecaries had done in the past, into a new class of medical practitioner. Already toxicology had been removed from the list of examination subjects. Now, at the suggestion of Thomas Wakley, a clause was inserted forbidding the Pharmaceutical Society from conducting examinations in the theory and practice of medicine, surgery and midwifery. The eleventh section of the bill decreed that no member of the medical profession could be registered under this act and that the name of any pharmaceutical chemist who obtained a medical or surgical qualification would be removed from the register.

With these and some other minor modifications, the bill received the royal assent on 30 June 1852, Jacob Bell's last day as a member of parliament. "An Act for Regulating the Qualifications of Pharmaceutical Chemists" confirmed and extended the powers previously conferred on the Pharmaceutical Society by its charter. From the passing of the act, the title of pharmaceutical chemist or pharmaceutist was reserved for members of the Society and those who passed its major examination. It became an offence "to assume, use, or exhibit any name, title, or sign" implying registration under the act or membership of the Pharmaceutical Society. Instead of becoming "a powerful lever in the hands of the Pharmaceutical Society for promoting the advancement of pharmacy and the interests of those engaged in its pursuit", the act merely secured to registered pharmaceutical chemists a title by which they might be recognised.[63] "We have never disguised our disappointments at the mutilations to which the original bill was subjected", wrote Jacob Bell.[64] "Something was gained", added Theophilus Redwood, "although much less than had been looked for".

William Bastick and William Dickinson, the editors of *Annals of Pharmacy and Practical Chemistry* held Jacob Bell partly responsible for the failure of the bill. "We must say that had its advocacy been in less feeble hands, the issue would not have been so near a total defeat".

Bastick and Dickinson were inveterate opponents of Bell and seized any opportunity to belittle his efforts. In this instance, however, they may have had a point. The parliament that passed the emasculated pharmacy bill had earlier, on 5 June 1851, passed the Arsenic Act. Bell made no attempt to link the sale of poisons to the regulation of chemists and druggists. He let slip the opportunity to press the view that the education and registration of pharmaceutists were the public's surest guarantee of the responsible sale of arsenic. Considerable publicity had brought the subject of poisoning to the attention of both the public and the government. The Registrar General's reports highlighted the large number of deaths, both accidental and criminal, occurring each year from poisoning. During the years 1839 to 1849 70 persons in England and Wales had been convicted of murder by poisoning and it was a favoured method of committing suicide. As early as 1849 the Pharmaceutical Society had conducted a questionnaire survey of its members' experience of selling arsenic, and, in March 1850, in conjunction with the Provincial Medical and Surgical Association, it sent the Home Secretary a memorial recommending, in the interests of public safety, that only medical men and pharmaceutists should have the right to sell arsenic. It should not have been difficult for Jacob Bell to argue that regulation of chemists and druggists would be the most effective constraint on the indiscriminate sale of poisons. Instead he persisted in emphasizing the need for pharmaceutical chemists to be educated and examined to perform the task of dispensing physicians' prescriptions. In general, Bell does not seem to have appreciated the necessity of convincing parliament that increased powers for the Pharmaceutical Society would contribute to the containment of a growing social problem.

The consequences of the 1852 Pharmacy Act were far removed from the aims and intentions of Jacob Bell. Instead of enlarging the powers of the Pharmaceutical Society, the Act imposed new restrictions upon it. The Council could no longer add to or amend the by-laws without the approval of the Secretary of State and a special general meeting of members. Licentiates of the Society of Apothecaries were excluded from membership: if enacted earlier, this would have deprived the Pharmaceutical Society of the services of its second president and first vice-president, Charles James Payne. The scope of its examinations was now specifically limited by statute. The original bill made provision for the registration of all existing chemists and druggists and the examination of all future entrants into business. Had it been enacted, chemists and druggists would gradually have been transformed into pharmaceutical chemists: they would have been educated, examined, registered and licensed to practise. In the short term, a clear line of demarcation would have been established between the chemist and druggist and such tradesmen as grocers and oilmen. At the stroke of a pen, the register would have realised the distinctive unity of the whole body of chemists and druggists. Alas, it was not to be. The 1852 Pharmacy Act certainly drew a line of demarcation, but it was a line which created a deep division within the pharmaceutical body. A fissure opened up between pharmaceutical chemists and the rest; between, on one hand, members of the Pharmaceutical Society and non-members who had passed the major examination, and, on the other, the unincorporated mass of chemists and druggists. The Pharmaceutical Society, which had always claimed to speak for the whole profession, became, after 1852, the organization of a minority, representing less than a third of all retail chemists.

Immediately after the Act was passed, the Pharmaceutical Society did its utmost to limit the damage. A special general meeting held at the Society's headquarters in Bloomsbury Square on 4 August 1852 recommended the Council "to adopt a liberal construction of the terms of the Act in regard to the admission of chemists in business on their own account before the passing of the Act". The meeting expressed its belief that "the Pharmaceutical Society should include among its members all duly qualified dispensing chemists throughout the United Kingdom". Meetings held in Liverpool, Manchester, Newcastle, Nottingham, Norwich, Bristol, Glasgow, Aberdeen and Edinburgh endorsed these views. The Council agreed to admit to membership all chemists who had commenced business before the passing of the Act, on production of testimonials of their respectability, without requiring them to pass an examination, provided they made application before 1 May 1853. Nearly 800 chemists were admitted as members under this special dispensation.

It was not, therefore, the policies of the Pharmaceutical Society but the reluctance of the majority of chemists and druggists to join that created the institutionalised rift between pharmaceutical chemists and chemists and druggists. The Council, far from being exclusive, had thrown open the doors to new members. However, once the gates had been closed again, the Society set about the task of strictly enforcing the legal distinction between pharmaceutical chemists and the rest. The 1852 Act gave the Society the power to prosecute those who fraudulently claimed to be connected with it. This was a power not possessed by any other medical corporation. The Royal College of Physicians and the Society of Apothecaries had the authority to prosecute those who practised illegally, but proof of practice was not easily obtained. The illegal assumption of a title and the display of an unauthorised sign were very conspicuous offences, admitting of easy proof and liable to summary punishment.

Many chemists and druggists, although reluctant to join the Society and pay the requisite dues, were happy to take commercial advantage of the prestige attached to membership and to the title "pharmaceutical chemist". The sole surviving letter book of the Society's secretary and registrar, covering the years 1856 to 1862, is full of letters threatening legal proceedings against retailers who trespassed against the provisions of the 1852 Act. Unscrupulous chemists would use the Society's coat of arms and describe themselves as pharmaceutical chemists on prescription envelopes, on bills and letter heads, in newspaper advertisements, and on their shop fronts, without having any connexion with the Society. In such ways the criminal makes his perverted obeisance to respectable society.

The 1852 Pharmacy Act marks the beginning of the legislative process which led to the present division between the medical and pharmaceutical professions. Immediately before the passing of the 1852 Act, it was still possible to regard chemists and druggists as an integral part of the medical profession, as one of its four branches, together with physicians, surgeons and apothecaries. Witnesses before the 1852 select committee testified to this fact and argued the case for an act to regulate the profession as a whole, rather than one dealing, in isolation, with just one part of it. "We cannot help regarding pharmacy as being part of the profession", remarked Dr. James Watson, president of the Faculty of Physicians and Surgeons of Glasgow, "and I believe that if there were any general bill brought forward it must include *pharmaciens* as well as others; it should be a thing to regulate the whole body of the profession in all its departments".[65] Today the medical profession and the pharmaceutical profession are two distinct bodies, their membership defined by two separate registers. The members of these professions are differentiated by modes of recruitment, education, fields of study, qualification, career patterns, and levels of remuneration, prestige and power. Physicians, surgeons and general practitioners are now all part of a unitary profession, both legally and institutionally. Pharmacists, the descendants of the nineteenth century chemist and druggist, are not part of that profession and are quite clearly separate from it. The nineteenth century apothecary has disappeared, or, perhaps, survives in the anomalous form of the so-called rural, dispensing doctor. Yet there is nothing inevitable about the present division between the practice of medicine and that of pharmacy. This division of labour does not represent a natural process of specialization of function. It was socially and politically constructed by three acts of parliament, the 1858 Medical Act and the Pharmacy Acts of 1852 and 1868. The 1852 Pharmacy Act started that process. It defined the registered pharmaceutical chemist as someone who had never been examined in medicine, surgery and midwifery and who did not possess a qualification to practice medicine or surgery. The 1858 Medical Act, by drawing a sharp line of demarcation between those practitioners who were qualified and entitled to register, and those who were not, clearly established the legal and institutional boundaries of the medical profession. The three grades of physician, surgeon and apothecary were drawn together into one fold and a legal fence was set up between them and the chemist and druggist. It may be too much to say that the 1852 Pharmacy Act made the exclusion of pharmaceutists from the medical profession inevitable, but it obviously made its achievement much easier. Without the 1852 Act, the 1859 Medical Register might well have been published in four sections, one of which would have contained the names of the pharmaceutical chemists.

NOTES AND REFERENCES TO CHAPTER FOUR

1. *P. J.* 2 (1842–3) 678
2. *P. J.* 3 (1843–4) 509
3. *P. J.* 2 (1842–3) 677
4. *P. J.* 4 (1844–5) 101
5. *P. J.* 2 (1842–3) 678
6. *P. J.* 3 (1843–4) 511
7. *P. J.* 4 (1844–5) 295
8. Bell and Redwood 179
9. *P. J.* 5 (1845–6) 387–9, 529–32, 557–63
10. *P. J.* 12 (1852–3) 1
11. Bell and Redwood 188–9
12. This section is based on the *Report of the St. Albans Bribery Commission*, 1852 (1431) XXVII
13. Norman Gash, *Politics in the Age of Peel* (1953) 422–7
14. *Hansard* CXX 1852, 974
15. *Hansard* CXV 1851, 1117–21, 1207, 1226–8, 1357–64.
    Hansard CXVI 1851, 22–6, 148–66, 217–26, 308–9
    Report of Select Committee on St. Albans Election Petition, 1851 (193) XII and 1851 (220) XII
16. 1851 (381) XLVII 214–2
17. *Hansard* CXIX 1852 , 982
18. *Hansard* CXX 1852, 976
19. *Hansard* CXIX 1852, 609, 617, 980, 616, 610, 1475, 1473

20. Charles Seymour, *Electoral Reform in England and Wales* (New Haven, 1915)
    Cornelius O'Leary, *The Elimination of Corrupt Practices in British Elections 1868–1911* (Oxford, 1962)
21. D.C. Moore, "Political morality in mid-nineteenth-century England: concepts, norms, violations", *Victorian Studies* XIII (1969–70) 5–36.
22. *Hansard* CCLXXIX 1883, 1652
23. Earl Grey, *Parliamentary government considered with reference to a reform of parliament* (1858) 120
24. [William Greg] "Parliamentary purification", *Edinburgh Review* XCVIII (October 1853) 586
25. For successive versions of the pharmacy bill see
    1851(395) V 321, 1851(517) V 329, 1852(51) IV 73, 1852(370) IV 83
26. *Hansard* CXVIII 1851, 111–18, 849–50
27. *Hansard* CXIX 1852, 467–8, 1218–22.
28. *Select Committee on the Pharmacy Bill*, 1852(387) XIII Q.227
    Hereinafter referred to as *S.C.P.B.*
29. *P.J.* 1 (1841–2) 4
30. *P.J.* 3 (1843–4) 509–10
31. *S.C.P.B.* Q 1806, 1919–21
32. *P.J.* 5 (1845–6) 385–6
33. *S.C.P.B.* Q 1449
34. *Annals of Pharmacy and Practical Chemistry* 1 (1852) 177
35. *S.C.P.B.* Q 2404, 2376
36. *S.C.P.B.* Q 2299
37. *S.C.P.B.* Q 2130
38. *S.C.P.B.* Q 1635
39. *S.C.P.B.* Q 2518
40. *S.C.P.B.* Q 2532
41. *S.C.P.B.* Q 1439, 1512, 2836, 2172, 1562
42. *S.C.P.B.* Q 2290
43. *S.C.P.B.* Q 1391
44. *S.C.P.B.* Q 175
45. *Lancet* 1852 (1) 482–3
46. *S.C.P.B.* Q 2427
47. *P.J.* 4 (1844–5) 248
48. *S.C.P.B.* Q 1844
49. *Lancet* 1836–7 (1) 647–8
50. *Times*, 17 October, 1845
51. *P.J.* 5 (1845–6) 340
52. *S.C.P.B.* Q 2579
53. *Medical Times* 19 (1848–9) 594
54. Irvine Loudon, "The vile race of quacks with which this country is infested", in W. F. Bynum and Roy Porter, *Medical Fringe and Medical Orthodoxy, 1750–1850* (1987) 120–22
55. Walter Rivington, *The Medical Profession* (Dublin, 1888)
56. *S.C.P.B.* Q 1966
57. *S.C.P.B.* Q 345, 346, 348
58. *P.J.* 3 [2] (1861–2) 297
59. *S.C.P.B.* Q 1331
60. *S.C.P.B.* Q 2520
61. *P.J.* 3 [2] (1861–2) 297–8

62. *Annals of Pharmacy and Practical Chemistry* 1 (1852) 177
63. Bell and Redwood 218
64. *P.J.* 12 (1852–3) 49
65. *S.C.P.B.* Q 1660

CHAPTER FIVE

The 1868 Pharmacy Act

Misce et fiat mistura—Mix and make a mixture

Consolidation and financial crisis—The United Society of Chemists and Druggists—Free trade *versus* regulation—Exemption from jury service—The G.M.C. plans to regulate pharmacy—The Chemists and Druggists Bills, No. 1 and No. 2—The collapse of the United Society—The origin of the British Pharmaceutical Conference—The demand for legislative regulation of the sale of poisons—The Arsenic Act 1851—The Poisons Bills of 1857/8—The Select Committee on the Poisons Bill of 1857—The Bradford disaster and the Poisons Bill of 1859—John Simon's report to the Privy Council on poisons and pharmacy, 1863—The passage of the Pharmacy and Poisons Act of 1868 through the Lords and the Commons.

When Jacob Bell first began thinking about an act to regulate the practice of pharmacy in Great Britain, his idea was to secure for all chemists and druggists a monopoly of the right to sell medicines. This is made explicit in the original draft of the bill. It was proposed to compile a register of chemists already in practice and to make it illegal henceforth for unregistered persons to engage in "the business or calling" of chemist and druggist and "to prepare, compound or dispense for sale . . . any medicines or medicinal substances". After Sir James Graham made clear the free trade principles on which medical reform would be based, Bell realised there was no prospect of his own pharmacy bill being enacted. Parliament might be persuaded to restrict the use of titles but not the right to practise: the public must remain free to patronise the unqualified. In view of this, Bell made the clauses of his 1851 bill deliberately ambiguous. All the chemists and druggists in Great Britain were to be registered as "pharmaceutical chemists" and that title alone was to be reserved for their use. The sting was in the tail; a final clause provided:

> That the term and expression "pharmaceutical chemist" used and employed in this Act shall be construed to mean, and shall comprise and and include, chemists and druggists, dispensing chemists, and every other name denoting a vendor and dispenser of medicines.

The intention was to create a *de facto* monopoly by preventing the unregistered from assuming any and every title which would indicate to the public that medicines were on sale. As we have seen, the bill received so great a mauling and was so drastically altered during its passage through the Commons, that chemists and druggists as a whole gained nothing by its enactment. The 1852 Pharmacy Act left the business and title of chemist and druggist open to anyone without restriction. Nonetheless, the position of the Pharmaceutical Society as a voluntary association was considerably strengthened. The Act gave legislative authority to its examinations and other proceedings, and made the titles "pharmaceutical chemist" and "pharmaceutist" the property of its members and those who passed its major examination. For Jacob Bell the outcome was deeply disappointing. From the first his object had been to incorporate and define the entire body of chemists and druggists: what he achieved was the legal recognition of a select group from among that body.

The immediate reaction of the Council and members of the Pharmaceutical Society was to behave in a generous way. All *bona fide* and respectable chemists and druggists were encouraged to join the Society without being examined. Nearly 800 of them seized the opportunity, but the short-sighted and pinch-penny majority could not be dislodged from their apathy. One source of new recruits was Scotland. The 1852 Act, by granting Scotland a separate Board of Examiners, did much to swell the ranks of the North British Branch. Although a committee with president, vice-president, treasurer and secretary had been formed in Edinburgh in the early days, the Pharmaceutical Society had made little progress north of the border, despite the zeal of John Mackay, the secretary and close friend of Jacob Bell. In 1852 Bell went on a tour of Edinburgh, Glasgow and Aberdeen to drum up support. The Society of Chemists and Druggists, which had existed in Aberdeen since 1839, agreed to align itself with the Pharmaceutical Society.

The majority of British chemists and druggists were decidedly unclubbable. Their lukewarm response to the Pharmaceutical Society's magnanimity was probably unaffected by the hostile reception it received from the editors of the *Annals of Pharmacy and Practical Chemistry*. William Bastick and William Dickinson warned their fellow chemists against accepting such gifts:

> No, Gentlemen, it is not that the Council are anxious for you to be registered: it is Mr. Jacob Bell who requires your assistance as members, so that his Journal may have 650 more subscribers, and his remuneration be *pro tanto* increased.[1]

They argued that

> . . . had there been no such monstrosity connected with the Pharmaceutical Society as the "Pharmaceutical Journal", there would have been no attempt to enact unjust and illegal bye-laws by the Council of that Society. This fact will be fully established when it is recollected that every member added to the Pharmaceutical Society becomes an involuntary subscriber to the Journal . . . As we have hinted before, the editor of the "Pharmaceutical Journal", through the undue power which that Journal confers, is the Great Mogul of the Pharmaceutical Society. His will is the law of the Society.[2]

Those "unjust and illegal bye-laws" had been drawn up by the Council of the Pharmaceutical Society to put into effect the unanimous decision of a special general meeting, held in December 1852, to admit to membership, without examination, respectable chemists already in practice. On that occasion the motion had been moved by Jacob Bell and seconded by William Dickinson. Six months later, at the meeting held to confirm this policy, Dickinson performed a complete *volte-face* and became its chief opponent. He now declared himself strongly against the registration of persons as pharmaceutical chemists who had not passed the Major examination and accordingly opposed the by-laws made under the 1852 Act which effected that object. Only two other members of the Society were prepared to join Dickinson and Bastick in voting against the Council's policy at the May meeting. Undeterred, the dissentients commenced legal proceedings against the Society, and persuaded Lord Palmerston, the Home Secretary, to give only a qualified approval of the new by-laws, pending the hearing of the case. The by-laws were confirmed for one year only, subject to their legality being established in a court of law. On 24 November 1853 legal proceedings began in the Court of Queen's Bench. After very lengthy argument, Lord Campbell delivered his judgment on 26 January 1855. When the decision went against Dickinson, he immediately declared his intention of carrying the case to a Court of Appeal. The Pharmaceutical Society was dragged unwillingly into another round of expensive and needless litigation. On 30 May 1855 a Court of Error, consisting of eight judges, unanimously confirmed Lord Campbell's judgment. Sir George Grey, the new Home Secretary, confirmed the by-laws, without reserve, a few weeks later. The Dickinson-Bastick litigation cost the Pharmaceutical Society at least seven hundred pounds and at times threatened to bring the work of the Society to a halt. All that Dickinson and Bastick managed to achieve was the diversion of precious resources from the Pharmaceutical Society to the legal profession: not for the first, nor for the last time, the poor were made to subsidise the rich.

William Bastick and William Dickinson, the instigators of this distressing and useless litigation, were intelligent and successful London chemists. Both were early members of the Pharmaceutical Society and were welcomed into its leading circle. Both were elected members of the Council. Bastick also served as an examiner for several years. Dickinson, after a varied experience learning the trade in Birmingham, Liverpool, Manchester, Cheltenham and Leamington, worked as an assistant for five years with Savory and Moore in Bond Street and in due course set up his own very profitable establishment near Marble Arch. Bastick built up a thriving business at his Brooke Street pharmacy near Grosvenor Square, using the knowledge he had acquired studying under Liebig at Giessen to improve the quality of pharmaceutical preparations. Although Dickinson and Bastick were highly successful businessmen, their contribution to the Pharmaceutical Society was wholly negative. They developed an obsessive antagonism to Jacob Bell and his circle whom they depicted as using the Pharmaceutical Society for their own personal and commercial advantage. Dickinson and Bastick were maverick saboteurs, envious of Jacob Bell's success and eager to wound him. They were utterly unprincipled and entirely destructive. Although purporting to speak for the majority against a self-serving elite, they had no following and were never able to create an opposition party. Their attacks gathered support neither from within nor from without the walls of the Pharmaceutical Society.

From the day they were elected to the Council, Bastick and Dickinson brought to its business rancour and obstruction. In 1851 the work of the School of Pharmacy was disrupted by their underhand treatment of Professor Pereira. They arranged the unauthorised publication of garbled accounts of his lectures on materia medica and drove him to resign his chair prematurely. In their eyes, Pereira had the misfortune to be both an intimate friend of Jacob Bell and a warm supporter of the Pharmaceutical Society. In the following year, Dickinson and Bastick started a monthly periodical, the *Annals of Pharmacy and Practical Chemistry*. It had a meteoric and unsavoury career of less than three years duration. In a reminiscence, published in 1880, Joseph Ince recalled that it was, in many ways, "an excellent periodical".

It was printed in a bold and beautiful type. It contained a good resume of foreign chemistry and pharmacy; its translations from the French and German, specially the latter, were executed with great skill, and it furnished, monthly, valuable papers bearing upon trade interests. But ... its leading articles were loaded with a continuous personal abuse of Mr. Jacob Bell, his public and private actions, and the whole tenour of his career. These strictures went beyond the limits of fair criticism.[3]

While claiming to be supporters of the Pharmaceutical Society, the editors of the *Annals* made vicious and unwarranted attacks on the Council, the *Pharmaceutical Journal* and the School of Pharmacy. It was typical of the duplicity of Dickinson and Bastick that, at the very time they were challenging the Pharmaceutical Society's right to widen its membership base, they published a leading article welcoming a new organisation, whose sole *raison d'être* was the alleged exclusiveness of the Pharmaceutical Society. The British Association of Chemists and Druggists will become, it was asserted, "the most extensive organization ever effected by chemists and druggists". Members will not be burdened with annual subscriptions and the upkeep of a journal and educational establishment. On payment of a guinea, each member will receive a certificate "which will proclaim to the world that the possessor is a duly qualified chemist and druggist". A newly created Royal College of Pharmacy will then effect "a complete registration of all duly qualified chemists and druggists". Dickinson and Bastick predicted that "before many years have elapsed, the Pharmaceutical Society will be classed with the dodo and other extinct animals".[4]

Unlike the dodo, the British Association of Chemists and Druggists was never hatched. This ill-conceived brainchild of two London chemists, Charles Linder of the Strand and John Rossiter of Notting Hill, was founded on two erroneous assumptions. The first was that the Pharmaceutical Society was thwarting the "general disposition" of chemists and druggists "to combine for the protection of their interests"; the second was that professional status could be achieved "without any efforts to promote education, to advance the art and science of pharmacy, and to deserve the confidence of the public".[5] Linder and Rossiter blamed the Pharmaceutical Society for not incorporating "the ten thousand chemists and druggists established in business in Great Britain". "Imperfect and partial legislation" had closed the Society's doors against them: becoming a member had been made "unnecessarily expensive and troublesome". The Society had failed "to secure to chemists and druggists their proper position and legitimate rights".[6] Linder and Rossiter found it easier to criticise the Pharmaceutical Society's efforts than to improve upon them. There was no stampede to join their association: after its inaugural meeting, it sank without trace.

The task of establishing the Pharmaceutical Society as the foundation of a profession of pharmacy was a long, uphill struggle. Without any external financial support and little encouragement from the state, the Society was gradually building a reputation as the national authority for pharmaceutical knowledge, professional standards and education. The test of an organisation's status within the community is found, not in the claims that it makes for itself, but in the recognition of the validity of those claims by those best fitted to judge.

When the General Council of Medical Education and Registration was established by the 1858 Medical Act, it was assigned the task of publishing a book containing a list of medicines and compounds and the manner of preparing them, together with the true weights and measures by which they are to be prepared and mixed ... to be called the *British Pharmacopoeia*.

By a subsequent Act it was provided that this book should supersede the Pharmacopoeias of London, Edinburgh and Dublin.

For five years previously, the Royal College of Physicians in London had been in the process of preparing a new edition of their own pharmacopoeia and in doing so had requested the assistance of the Pharmaceutical Society. The pharmacopoeia committees of the College and the Society had worked closely together. In November 1858 it was resolved by the inaugural meeting of the General Medical Council, as it came to be called, to request the co-operation of the Pharmaceutical Society in the preparation of the first *British Pharmacopoeia*. This was an honour not less gratifying for being thoroughly deserved. There were not many of the members who were capable at that time of doing such research as was required but all those who were so qualified readily entered into the work. One of the most important questions to be answered was the system of weights and measures to be recognised in the *Pharmacopoeia*, and this subject had already been discussed at Pharmaceutical Society meetings. Various systems were proposed: all more or less ingenious. So many were, in fact, offered to the Pharmacopoeia Committee that it was perplexed rather than enlightened and none of the propositions was accepted. It was at first thought that the Pharmacopoeia would be ready in 1861 but it was not until the early part of 1864 that the first *British Pharmacopoeia* was published. Its appearance attracted much attention and much was expected of it: but the task of combining all the best features of the three Pharmacopoeias already in use and adapting them to the requirements of prescribers and dispensers in England, Scotland and Ireland proved to be an impossible one. The work was acceptable to no one and instead of superseding the existing pharmacopoeias was itself superseded by them. The G.M.C. decided to bring out a new edition as soon as possible, and appointed Robert Warington of the Chemical Society and Professor Theophilus Redwood of the Pharmaceutical Society as joint editors. The work was reconstructed in accordance with a plan drawn up by Professor Redwood.

The Pharmaceutical Society had received further public recognition in 1862. In that year the Director-General of the Army Medical Department issued a new regulation by which a person seeking appointment as a dispenser in the army was required to furnish evidence of having passed the Society's major examination and of being registered as a pharmaceutical chemist. In the past serious accidents had occurred as a result of employing sergeants and other men without qualifications to dispense. This endorsement of the value of the Society's scrutiny of the knowledge and skills of young men trained in pharmacy testified to the integrity and thoroughness of the examiners. It implied state recognition of the Society's attempts to raise the standards of British pharmaceutical education.

The history of the first eighteen years of the Pharmaceutical Society is the history of the later part of Jacob Bell's life. His death on Sunday 12 June 1859 would have proved an even greater loss, had he not constructed the Society on such sure foundations. By the time he became president in May 1856, an office he held until his death, Jacob Bell combined a clear vision of the Society's future with a firm grasp of political reality. "Pharmacy has had few such leaders", wrote W.J. Uglow Woolcock in 1906. "The advent of such a leader is required to shake the world of pharmacy from the heavy slumber of indifference into which it tends to fall, and to stir into action those whose one cry is for protection, but who will not protect themselves".[7]

As a memorial to Jacob Bell, the Council of the Pharmaceutical Society appropriately decided to launch an appeal for funds to establish scholarships for young men, "less favoured by fortune than by industry", to enable them to study in the School of Pharmacy. The outcome was the creation of the Jacob Bell memorial scholarships. Scientific work requires scientific training. By 1859, the first generation of pharmaceutical chemists, the product of the Society's own system of education, was beginning to make its own contribution to the progress of pharmacy. At his death, Jacob Bell left his own proofs of his commitment to the work of the Society. He bequeathed £2,000 to the trustees of the Society to be applied to the furtherance of pharmaceutical education and transferred the ownership of the *Pharmaceutical Journal* to the Society.

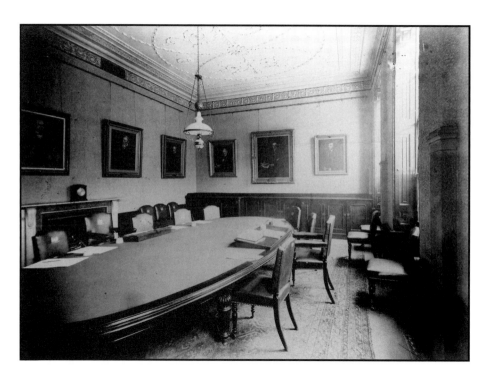

31 *The appearance of the newly re-located Council Chamber at 17 Bloomsbury Square, in 1883/4. The walls are hung with a selection of portraits of the founders and early members of the Society.*

After the passing of the Pharmacy Act in 1852, Bell had declared his conviction that pharmaceutical chemists now had the opportunity of becoming the third estate in the medical profession, and that "they ought to possess an establishment not inferior in scale and importance" to the Colleges of Physicians and Surgeons.[8] In 1857 the Society's headquarters at 17, Bloomsbury Square were significantly enlarged. The lease of the two

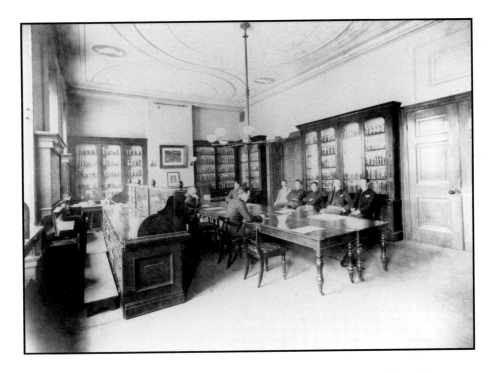

32 *A group of examiners seated in a first floor examination room of 17 Bloomsbury Square, 1883/4. Previously used as the lecture room it later became the histological laboratory.*

adjoining houses, 72 and 73 Great Russell Street, was first acquired. These houses together formed a block of buildings which had originally been united as a nobleman's mansion and the whole was now secured by the Society for a period of 90 years. The library and museum, the lecture theatre, the examination rooms, the secretary's offices, and the council and committee rooms were all re-arranged and extended at considerable cost. In 1859 the Council decided to use Bell's legacy of £2,000 to enlarge the premises by adding an extra storey to house new chemical laboratories. The cost of improving the premises in Bloomsbury Square proved much higher than the original estimates. Although an excellent long-term investment, the unanticipated expenditure contributed to the Society's financial crisis in 1861. Nonetheless, in 1862, with the suite of well-lighted and ventilated laboratories now fully in use, Dr. (then Mr.) John Attfield was appointed, under the title of Director and Demonstrator of Chemistry and Pharmacy, to take over from Professor Redwood the entire management of the practical classes. Later his title was changed to that of Professor of Practical Chemistry. This appointment was one that gave a great deal of satisfaction especially because Attfield was trained in the Society's own school and had been medallist in chemistry and pharmacy as well as in botany and materia medica in 1854.

Under Jacob Bell's ownership, the *Pharmaceutical Journal* had two main objectives: first, to win the support of chemists and druggists for his strategy of professionalisation, and,

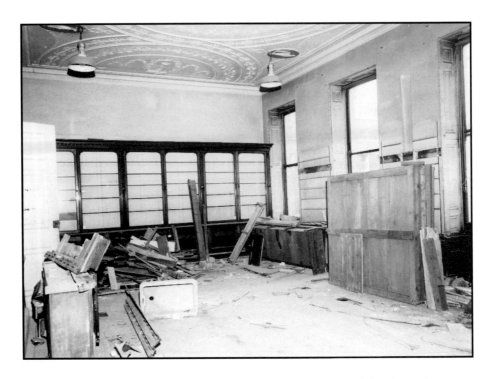

33 *Histological laboratory, 17 Bloomsbury Square. The removal of the nineteenth century fittings prior to its re-furbishment as the new Council Chamber in June 1960.*

secondly, to present to the outside world, the image of a scientific and responsible Society. The difficulty of reconciling these aims made the editor an easy target for criticism. The usual line of attack was well stated in a member's letter published in October 1853. From the point of view of the ordinary chemist and druggist,

> there is too large a proportion of the purely scientific in it, as if the wants of the trader were of inferior importance to those of the man of science ... while providing food for his brain, it must not be forgotten that his daily bread is the ultimate aim of his mental exertions.[9]

In 1859 three editors were appointed to take over the journal, each taking a special department. Professor Redwood became responsible for chemistry and pharmacy; Professor Bentley for botany and materia medica; and John Barnard for commerce. Under its new editors, the *Pharmaceutical Journal* maintained and enhanced its reputation as a scientific periodical and played its part in furthering the professional status of the Society. But, in the year that Jacob Bell died, a new journal appeared that soon became a formidable competitor. The *Chemist and Druggist* began in a small way as a monthly trade circular, its first number appearing on 15 September 1859, under the editorship of Major William Vaughan Morgan.[10] At the beginning it was little more than an advertising medium for Morgan Brothers of Bow Lane, London, the principal suppliers of chemists' sundries. It

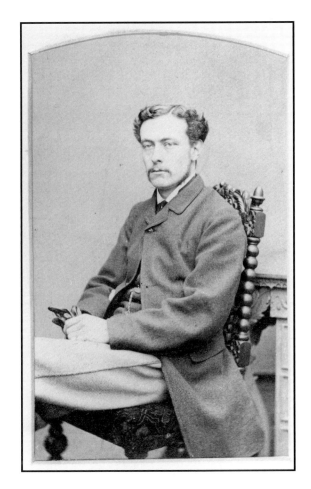

34   *Carte-de-visite portrait photograph of (Sir) W.A. Tilden (1842–1926). Awarded one of the first two Jacob Bell Memorial Scholarships in 1861 and later Professor of Chemistry at the Royal College of Science. These awards by examination were established to commemorate Jacob Bell and his interest in pharmaceutical education.*

rapidly grew in size and circulation and became established as an influential and widely read publication. The *Chemist and Druggist* filled a special niche. It concentrated on trade and political issues, adopted a critical stance towards the Pharmaceutical Society and deliberately angled its material to appeal to the unincorporated chemist and druggist. It was fortunate to be founded at a time when the disadvantages of being outside the Pharmaceutical Society were suddenly brought home to a considerable number of potential readers. It became their medium of communication.

For the first eighteen years of its existence the Pharmaceutical Society was controlled by Jacob Bell. For a time after his death, Bell's contemporaries, Thomas Morson and Peter Squire, and his younger colleagues, Thomas Hyde Hills and Daniel Bell Hanbury, made their influence felt. But increasingly the direction of the Society came into the hands of the Secretary and Registrar, the only full-time salaried official. Elias Bremridge, who was appointed to that office in 1857, was fortunate to have the chance of learning the ropes for two years while Bell was president. Bremridge was responsible for the day-to-day

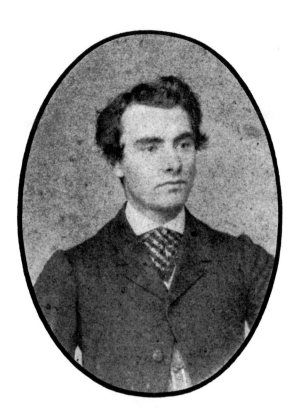

35 Carte-de-visite portrait of T.W.H. Tolbort, Bell Scholar, 1861. Portrait photographs of the recipients of this award were mounted in an album kept by the Society, a tradition maintained for nearly 100 years.

administration of the Society: his job was to keep the ship afloat and in good working order. Inevitably he came to have an increasingly important part to play in guiding the ship as well. Even though the turnover of membership of the Council in the nineteenth century was sluggish, no elected member was able to accumulate as much knowledge and experience of policy making as the Secretary and Registrar. Elias Bremridge was always the servant of the Council; but a wise servant anticipates his master's needs, looks for dangers on the horizon, and humbly suggests appropriate courses of action. Elias Bremridge's power was acquired by a process of slow accretion.

It is not possible to discover who first alerted the Council to the growing financial crisis of the Society, but, at the annual general meeting in May 1861, the president, T.N.R. Morson, made the situation clear to the members. There was an urgent need to ensure a permanent income adequate to maintain the Society in an efficient state. The heavy costs of the Dickinson litigation and of the expansion and refurbishment of 17 Bloomsbury Square had been met. But the future income of the Society had been imperilled by the by-laws enacted in 1853. Since that time members who entered the Society by examination were not required to pay the annual subscription: the admission fee of five guineas entitled them to the privileges of membership for life. "A more suicidal arrangement could not have been devised", lamented the president.[11] The ranks of members admitted before 1853, who paid each year a guinea subscription, were annually thinned by death and withdrawal.

194

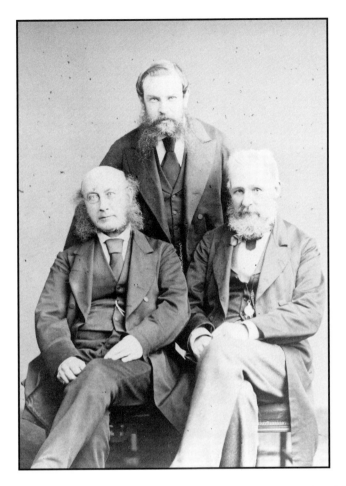

36 *Group photograph of Professors Attfield (1835–1911), Bentley (1821–94) and Redwood (1806–92) of the Society's School of Pharmacy. This photograph was preserved as a memento by one of their students.*

Inevitably the income of the Society, under the existing by-laws, would decline year by year, and, at no distant period, the Society's activities would have to be destructively curtailed. The Society would be left with an unviable income derived from the interest on capital and the small number of fees paid on admission.[12]

In the discussion on how the financial crisis might be resolved, there was general agreement that some alteration was needed in the terms on which members, associates and apprentices should in future be admitted to the Society. Several Council members, including T.N.R. Morson, the president, Thomas Herring and George Edwards, founding members, suggested that a further attempt should be made to enlarge the boundaries of the Society by recruiting chemists and druggists, whose age, respectability and long connexion with the trade, merited membership but who, for various reasons, had not previously

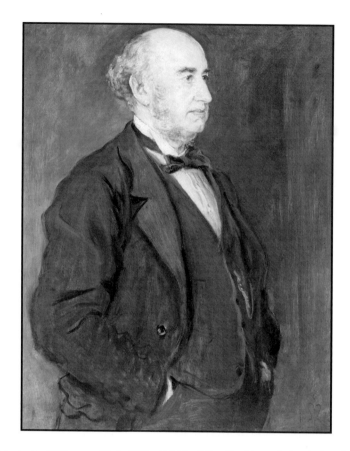

37   Oil portrait of Thomas Hyde Hills (1815–91), President of the Society from 1873 to 1876, by Sir John Everett Millais PRA (1842–1896). Painted "in three hours" and presented by the artist to his friend Hyde Hills in 1873, who eventually bequeathed it to the Society.

joined.[13] They would, of course, be required to pay an entrance fee and the traditional annual subscription. A lively discussion followed. Strong objections were raised against relaxing the terms of admission. Had not all established chemists been given ample opportunity to join the Society on three separate occasions, in 1841, in 1843, and again, more recently, at the passing of the Pharmacy Act? Why should the efforts of those who had taken the trouble to qualify by examination be set at nought in this way? Between May and the end of the year pains were taken to ascertain the views of members throughout the country. The situation was complicated by the concurrent emergence of a new society, the United Society of Chemists and Druggists. The creation, in January 1861, of an alternative society did not have the effect of encouraging the Pharmaceutical Society to open its gates in a competitive drive for members. The *Chemist and Druggist*, which supported the new society, made its own strident analysis of the Pharmaceutical Society's dilemma and, in doing so, must have helped to consolidate opposition to any relaxation in the terms of

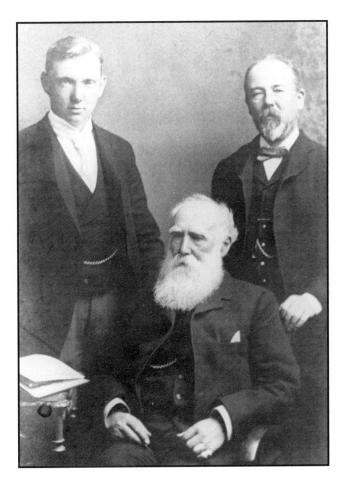

38   *Three generations of Bremridges: Elias aged 81, Richard Bremridge aged 51, and Richard Harding Bremridge aged 21. Elias, appointed in 1857, was the third Secretary of the Society and was succeeded by his son Richard in 1884. The Society's telegraphic address of "Bremridge" recalls their family name.*

admission. In its brash way, the *Chemist and Druggist* explained exactly what the problem was. "The Pharmaceutical Society needs money, money cannot be got without members, and members do not come forward for examinations". The Society needs to become "a practical institution, sufficiently broad in its rules, objects and regulations to admit and benefit the whole trade". "Nothing is to be gained by exclusion and isolation", it continued, "the time has gone by when any body of intelligent men can really hope to benefit by future special parliamentary enactments". The Society's managers should realise that there is no longer any possibility of "some grand compulsory enactment . . . that would make it a felony to deal in drugs without the ornamental diploma of the Society". The Society, if it is to survive, must become "more tolerant of 'tradesman'-like views". It concluded

197

> The United Society has only sprung into existence because two-thirds of the trade are excluded from the advantages of a central organization; and any straight-forward honest attempt on the part of the old Association to meet the new one half way would be hailed by all sensible chemists and druggists as a hopeful movement.[14]

The members of the Pharmaceutical Society were in no mood to be "sensible", if that implied abandoning the struggle for a new pharmacy act and swallowing the crude notions and strident tones of the United Society. The proposal to open the gates was firmly rejected. But the alteration of the by-laws to substitute annual subscriptions for admission fees was approved. The annual subscription was fixed at one guinea for members and half a guinea for associates and apprentices. The new by-laws, by which these changes were made, were passed at a specially convened meeting on 15 January 1862 and confirmed by the Home Secretary on 23 June 1862. "Those laws", declared the *Pharmaceutical Journal* defiantly, "clearly set forth that nothing but examination can admit our future members ... the terms of registration and of admission into the Pharmaceutical Society are definitely and permanently settled by these bye-laws ... no one can henceforth be placed on the Register of Pharmaceutical Chemists without previously passing the required examination".[15]

Yet some members still longed to unite all chemists and druggists within the Society's fold. In June 1864 the Council instituted a special examination for chemists of thirty years and above, who had been engaged in business on their own account for at least five years. This examination, of a more practical nature than that usually offered, enabled established chemists to qualify without having to go through a special course of study and without undergoing the ordeal of being examined in the company of young assistants and apprentices.

* * *

A year after Jacob Bell's death, an organisation was set up which, within a few years, was able to mount a serious challenge to the Pharmaceutical Society's position as the representative body of British chemists and druggists. During its short life of less than eight years, the United Society of Chemists and Druggists revealed both the strength and weakness of the Pharmaceutical Society. The strength lay in the structures and strategy established by Jacob Bell: the weakness lay in the deep divisions within the pharmaceutical constituency. The inherent tensions characteristic of the social relationships of pharmacy practitioners were the force which gave the United Society birth, supplied its energy, and finally tore it apart. In the early days of the Pharmaceutical Society Jacob Bell fought hard and successfully to ensure that the Society did not become cast as a mere trade protection association. During its first eighteen years the Society was able to hold in check the public expression of unmitigated, self-serving, trade concerns. The setting-up of the United Society burst the dam. A public platform was provided for those who not only wanted to promote narrow, sectional, commercial interests, but also believed that the way to do so was to advocate them loudly and pugnaciously.

The preliminary prospectus of the United Society of Chemists and Druggists appeared in the *Chemist and Druggist* on 15 August 1860 and its inaugural meeting was held at the London Coffee House on Ludgate Hill on Wednesday 23 January 1861, with Alderman Dakin, a London wholesale druggist, in the chair. At that meeting Dakin was elected president, Cyrus Buott, the driving force behind the new society, was confirmed as secretary, and Charles Linder, an old opponent of the Pharmaceutical Society, was made

Treasurer. Like the earlier British Association of Chemists and Druggists, the new society sprang from dissatisfaction with the Pharmaceutical Society.

> Whatever may be the virtues of the Pharmaceutical Society, it only partially represents one-third of the Chemists and Druggists' trade, and its constitution is not of a popular, unexclusive, homely character. Its memberships are based upon election and examination; its subscriptions are evidently too high, and its regulations too stringent to attract more than a small proportion of the trade; its "benevolent fund" . . . is surrounded by restrictions such as no effective charity can work under. Its charter compels it to refuse relief to any persons who are not members and associates of not less than four years standing . . . a corporation of this kind, whatever may be its educational value, is not adapted to satisfy the pressing wants of the trade *as they at present exist*.[16]

In short, the Pharmaceutical Society lacks "that plain practical organization required to meet the business exigencies of the trade".

The British Association of Chemists and Druggists had sought to improve the "social position and professional status" of dispensing chemists. The United Society, however, described itself as "a general trade union" and "a broad, open benefit society", formed "for plain, business-like, trade-benefit purposes", to represent the interests of chemists and druggists "as a trading community". The emphasis of the declared objectives of the new society seemed to indicate a society complementary to rather than competing with the Pharmaceutical Society. At various times the objectives were stated to be: (1) the establishment of a mutual benefit fund for the assistance of members in sickness, destitution, old age and death, (2) to carry out, by district meetings and combined action, any improvement for the welfare of the trade, such as early and Sunday closing, (3) to answer any legal questions relating to the trade rights of members, free of cost, (4) to enable members to have an analysis made, by duly appointed trade analysts, of any article at a nominal fixed rate of charges, (5) to keep a register of the transfer of businesses, required partnerships, and situations for assistants, (6) to establish a reference library and a reading room furnished with trade periodicals and works of scientific interest, (7) to establish a school for members' children and an asylum for decayed members of the trade, and, finally, (8) to watch the progress of, and support or oppose any legislative enactment that may affect the interests of chemists and druggists as a trading community. It was this last objective that brought the United Society into head-on conflict with the Pharmaceutical Society.

Repeated claims were made at its inaugural meeting that the United Society was antagonistic neither to the Pharmaceutical Society nor to the ideals of Jacob Bell. The president, in his opening remarks, spoke of Jacob Bell "who had done so much, whose absence they all felt, and whose loss they all deeply deplored;" one speaker declared that "all chemists and druggists recognised Jacob Bell as their worthy and lamented friend". The United Society, said another, "would aid and assist the Pharmaceutical Society . . . they had no desire in any way to interfere with the objects for which the Pharmaceutical Society was instituted". Nothing could have been further from the truth.[17] From its start, the United Society adopted an anti-professional stance. The admission fee was fixed at five shillings to be within the means of the poorest members of the trade, and payment of this fee was the only condition of membership. "There must be no false pride in defining what proposed member is really a chemist and druggist". "The purchase and sale of drugs and chemicals or of anything connected with a chemist and druggist's business must be ample qualification for membership". The Pharmaceutical Society's emphasis on the dispensing of prescriptions, on education, and on science was rejected as elitist.[18]

> The Pharmaceutical Society had the ennobling idea—although rather visionary— that chemists and druggists should be merely dispensers of prescriptions and that they should not condescend to sell ... sundries ... Now that could never be done, seeing that in many districts prescriptions were very rare, and that poverty drove the poor man to the chemist as his friend and doctor.

The members of the Pharmaceutical Society were portrayed as "pharmaceutical snobs". They "look with contempt on the trade side of a druggist's business", and see themselves as "dispensers of chemicals with the highest possible knowledge of pharmacy". But they are merely deluded "traders who wish to be raised to the more showy rank of 'professional men'".

> If the whole trade—calling—profession—or occupation of drug-selling could be detached from the trade in fancy hardware, and scented confectionery, the ideal of many a discontented pharmaceutist would be realised. A shop would not then be a shop ... but a temple of science,—a fountain of health—a something half-way between a "surgery" and a "laboratory". [The proprietor] relieved from an enforced attention to all those mean and contemptible—though profit-making articles—which go by the general name of "Druggists' Sundries" [would become a scientist]. "He would not be a mere buyer and seller of drugs, with just sufficient knowledge to avoid poisoning his customers, but an authority upon analysis, a contributor to scientific journals ... His customers would not then be called by so humble and shop-keeping a title, but would only be recognised in the form of "patients" or "clients" ... This fancy picture of what a chemist and druggist might be is the day dream of many a worthy trader".

Day dream it will always remain: it can never become reality.

> In some few favoured neighbourhoods, with the prestige of an historical reputation, a chemist and druggist may maintain his establishment by the sale of medicines alone, but in ninety-nine hundredths of the general trade the traffic in drugs must be joined to a traffic in "sundries" ... the bulk of the trade, whether members of the Pharmaceutical Society or not, are compelled to deal in "all things and many others".[19]

"In hundreds of villages, districts of towns, corners of cities", declared the *Chemist and Druggist*, "it would be starvation and bankruptcy to sell nothing but medicines".[20]

The Pharmaceutical Society's relationship with the medical profession aroused the deep suspicion of the United Society. The Pharmaceutical Society, it was alleged, is "so closely allied to the medical profession on whom it depends, that it forgets the majority of us have no dealings with the physician or surgeon; and we find that institution which was established to protect the general interests of the chemist and druggist is exclusively devoted to those whose lot is to dispense prescriptions and retail perfumery".[21] The United Society was openly hostile to the medical profession, which it saw as a major threat to the livelihood of chemists and druggists. Government bills to regulate the sale of poisons were seen as attempts by the medical profession to eliminate counter practice and to give medical practitioners control of dangerous drugs.

It is useless for the followers of the late Jacob Bell to play fast and loose with the medical profession; there is no real sympathy—nothing but a hollow mockery of artificial courtesy between them. The prescribing lion will never lie down with the dispensing lamb ... (except to swallow him). The medical profession have long ago thrown down the gauntlet of the whole trade and it is high time that the challenge was taken up.

Unlike the Pharmaceutical Society, the general public have "no general desire to strengthen the medical profession at the expense of the chemist and druggist ... the poor and needy look upon us as friends and advisers in their hour of trouble. The medical profession know this too, and not being strong enough, with all their class feeling and class organisation, to alter this state of things, they wish an unthinking Government to step forward and help them". The Government, however, would be advised to "let the demand come from the public first for legislative interference and not from a body of interested professionals".

The real crime of what is called "illegal practice" in the eyes of doctors is the remuneration which it produces. It is not the public good—the safety of life, the principles of medical science, or any fine- sounding phrase—which doctors really care about; it is the dirty money. They are not contented with the guineas of the rich, but they covet the humble shillings and pence of the poor ... It is only the chemist and druggist that they tilt against, simply because he is often their rival in the dispensing part of their business. They want the bodies of the public handed over to them by Act of Parliament for unconditional physicing, and would be very indignant if a counter-movement took place among the chemists and druggists to prevent them selling drugs. A medical education very seldom includes the practical knowledge of drugs which the most humble trader often possesses.[22]

The United Society proclaimed its commitment to free trade and opposition to all legislative interference. "Not only does Free Trade secure the public the best at the lowest cost, but by the same law of operation it provides and encourages the best talent, the highest skill, and the greatest experience". There should be no interference with "that self-adjusting meter of demand and supply which at present enables even the poorest and most remote districts throughout the country to be provided according to their wants". Some sections of business can always be found to argue that, however advantageous free trade is in its general application, protection is justified in their case: but this is to deny the "generally known truth, that whatever is required to be propped up by legislative protection, must be extremely rotten at the foundation, and that the weakness of the dealer must be strengthened at the cost of the consumer".

The safe basis of operation is non-interference. Do not legislate. When a restrictive privilege is given, a penalty is somewhere inflicted; open the doors of opportunity and Free Trade will provide you with the best fitted men for the position. In a free and open competition the support of the public is taken away from the ignorant and incompetent, and infallibly rests with the industrious and experienced.

The medical profession, with the connivance of the Pharmaceutical Society, seeks legislation to suppress counter practice on the ground that it is unqualified practice and that the supply of medicine to the public is fundamentally different from the supply of other goods. The supply of medicine must be restricted and under the control of educated and certified practitioners, it is argued. But the United Society,

> have now an organisation which can bid defiance to compulsory legislation, and they are determined, with the co-operation of the trade, to protect the right of a chemist and druggist to prescribe—a right which common sense, long-continued custom, experience, and the wants of the poorer classes, thoroughly justify.

The effect of compulsory examination, as advocated by the Pharmaceutical Society, would be that

> the trade, confined to the richer and exclusive few, would in time become a monopoly, producive of gross injustice, and while ostensibly seeking to elevate the professional character of chemists and druggists, would entirely destroy their usefulness to suffering humanity as the "poor man's doctor".

The distinction that is drawn between the vending of physic and the sale of any other article, if it has any validity at all, makes the case for free trade even stronger: no obstacle should be allowed to

> prevent the public having the best men in it—men whose special ability would be shown by results, who could not falsely assume a position of great responsibility under the cover of a certificate of mere legal qualification . . . Free Trade, even in physic, provides more checks for its safe and skilful practice than the most rigid system of examination; indeed, there is grave doubt whether the system of examination tests is not after all a very delusive protection from ignorant incapacity—failing to provide against the very evil for which it is considered the greatest safeguard. A certain amount of formal routine knowledge is sufficient to pass the barrier, and having once obtained the legal qualification, the stimulus is withdrawn— the daily opportunities for acquiring experience may be disregarded, and professional carelessness follows a release from a sense of responsibility. Yet the chartered privilege remains that enables in too many cases the ignorant pretender to stand in the place of a really qualified man.

"The fatal error" of the Pharmaceutical Society is that "they have ignored the fact that the best of all knowledge is gained by experience, open and free to every sincere inquirer, and not packed up in a box, the key to which is only to be found at Bloomsbury Square".[23]

The leaders of the Pharmaceutical Society found the public expression of such views by chemists and druggists depressing and disappointing and sought to counter them in a dignified and thoughtful manner. For them the issue was one of pharmaceutical responsibility. Free trade in physic "means that any man, however ignorant, is justified in carrying on the business of a chemist and druggist, supplying the public with dangerous substances the properties of which he may be unacquainted with, and dispensing medicines for the sick". His experience is acquired at the fatal expense of the public. The Pharmaceutical Society has, from its beginning, exposed the evils of free trade in physic and poisons; it has opposed the unrestrained liberty to supply the public with dangerous drugs; and has urged the need for a thorough practical and scientific qualification for all chemists and druggists. The regret is that the Pharmaceutical Society has failed to convince chemists and druggists "to recognise the necessity or importance of requiring from those who deal in dangerous medicines or poisonous substances, that they should prove by the test of examination, that they are qualified for such a responsible duty".[24]

It was, however, the success rather than the failure of the Pharmaceutical Society that led to the creation of the United Society. Jealousy and resentment were the main recruiting sergeants of the new society. During the 1850s and 1860s membership of the Pharmaceutical Society began to bring valued privileges. The 1852 Act reserved to members and to those who passed the major examination the titles "pharmaceutical chemist" and "pharmaceutist". Although the latter term was widely used in journals in the 1850s to describe qualified practitioners, it was the title "pharmaceutical chemist" which carried most weight with the general public. As the Pharmaceutical Society's scientific and professional status rose, so the right to claim membership increased in value. Commercial advantage as well as social status accrued to those who called themselves "pharmaceutical chemists". The Secretary and Registrar was vigilant in protecting the use of the diploma and titles of the Society to preserve and enhance the privileges of its members. On 21 August 1861, in an important and well-publicised case, a chemist named Mikisch was fined £5 at the Bloomsbury County Court for displaying the title "pharmaceutical chemist" over the door of his shop without being registered.[25] Many other errant chemists and druggists were threatened with legal proceedings for similar offences.

By far the greatest prize the Pharmaceutical Society gained for its members was exemption from jury service. All those who had belittled the efforts of the Society and had steadfastly refused to join were suddenly faced with the fact that membership brought with it a highly valued privilege and legal recognition of the professional status of pharmaceutical chemists. The leaders of the United Society were consumed with rage.

In 1862 a bill was introduced into the House of Commons dealing with the mode of summoning juries. The Council of the Pharmaceutical Society needed little persuasion to seize the opportunity thus provided for extending its members' privileges. Exemption from the duty of serving on juries had become the hallmark of the professions. The privilege had long been conceded to medical men on the ground that to take them away from their professional duties might inflict unnecessary inconvenience and injury on their patients. On similar grounds exemption was now claimed for pharmaceutical chemists. The Pharmaceutical Society prepared a clause which was introduced at the committee stage into the new bill by J.J. Powell, M.P. for Glasgow. There was every prospect of the clause being incorporated into the bill without opposition: the Pharmaceutical Society's canvass of support among M.P.s had been uniformly encouraging. Unfortunately, the United Society of Chemists and Druggists had been alerted to the Pharmaceutical Society's manoeuvre and hastily arranged for Western Wood, M.P. for Marylebone, to move for a similar exemption for all chemists and druggists.

This altered the entire complexion of the proposal. Whereas pharmaceutical chemists could be identified by reference to a legally authorised register, there was no means of defining who was a chemist and druggist. The United Society was hoist with its own petard. To demonstrate the unrepresentativeness of the Pharmaceutical Society's membership of 2,500, the United Society claimed that there were 40,000 chemists and druggists in the country. This tactic of issuing statements grossly inflating the total gave unintended strength to the view that exempting so many would add to the difficulty already experienced of getting the duty of juryman properly performed. Thus the United Society gave Sir George

Grey, the Home Secretary, the excuse he sought to oppose both proposals. Since the bill dealt with the mode of summoning juries, he said, it was not the appropriate occasion for exempting persons from serving on them. A special bill should be drawn up for that purpose though he added that he would oppose such a bill as the exemption would remove too many intelligent men from the jury lists. In the face of this opposition, both Powell and Wood withdrew their motions. When the bill came out of the Commons, however, it was discovered that, notwithstanding what had been said, a clause had been agreed to, without opposition, exempting from jury service "managing clerks to attorneys, solicitors and proctors . . . and all subordinate officers in goals and houses of correction".

When the bill went to the House of Lords, the Council of the Pharmaceutical Society petitioned them to grant to pharmaceutical chemists the privilege requested earlier. A clause similar to that proposed in the Lower House was passed by the Lords without opposition. The exemption, however, was now made to include veterinary surgeons as well. The bill came back to the Commons and Sir George Grey opposed the exemptions. On the division the numbers were equal—53 votes on each side—but the Speaker gave his casting vote for rejection of the Lord's amendment. When the bill went back to the Lords for their reconsideration, Lord Wensleydale moved that the amendment in respect of the exemption of pharmaceutical chemists be insisted upon. Physicians and surgeons, he pointed out, had, in consequence of their being often required in cases of great emergency, been exempted from serving on juries: and he could see no reason why the members of the Pharmaceutical Society, which comprised only some 2,000 members, should not be placed in the same category. Their duties in making up prescriptions were responsible and delicate and it was desirable that they should not be called away to attend at distant places as jurymen. It was not suggested that all 40,000 chemists and druggists should be exempt, for they "did not undergo any examination nor were they members of a registered society". The House of Lords were persuaded to maintain their position with regard to pharmaceutical chemists but to abandon the exemption for veterinary surgeons.

While the Lords debated the bill, Elias Bremridge organised a vigorous canvass of members of parliament by the Council in London and by local secretaries and members in the provinces. When the bill came back to the Commons, Sir George Grey at first intimated that he would not offer any further opposition, but a private member, Edward Craufurd, intervened and moved the rejection of the Lords' amendment. Sir George Grey and Sir G.C. Lewis supported him, arguing that if pharmaceutical chemists were to be exempt there were stronger grounds for exempting chemists and druggists generally. Although government ministers, including Lord Palmerston and W.E. Gladstone, supported Craufurd's motion, the Lords' amendment was adopted by 45 votes to 12. Pharmaceutical chemists obtained exemption from liability to serve on all juries and inquests.

Elias Bremridge's vigilance, energy and political flair had galvanised the Pharmaceutical Society into action and secured a bonus built upon the foundations established by the 1852 Act. The *Pharmaceutical Journal* justifiably claimed the result as a triumph for organisation, registration and qualification. The exemption is a highly regarded privilege, it declared, and asked, what better means could have been devised for advertising the qualifications of pharmaceutical chemists and directing public attention to the points of difference between them and those who use only the title of chemist and druggist?[26]

The effect of the Pharmaceutical Society's triumph on the United Society was devastating. The meaning of education, examination, qualification and registration was suddenly changed. They were not mere words in a game of professional charades but, as Jacob Bell had always insisted they were, the stepping stones to public recognition and privilege. The leaders of the United Society reacted predictably. The Pharmaceutical Society was denounced for feathering its own nest. The appropriately named Mr. Slugg "characterised the Pharmaceutical Society as a small body of men, . . . who by intrigue, . . . contrived to obtain a privilege not extended to the trade in general".[27] The leadership of the United Society suddenly jettisoned deeply-held and widely-publicised beliefs: the ordinary chemist and druggist was invested with a new persona. The principles of free trade and laissez-faire were denounced. The third annual report of the United Society concluded that "the great and increasing number of unqualified persons in the trade was an evil which must be met by some legislative measure". The time had come for parliament to recognise "the peculiar responsibility attaching to the sale of poisons and other dangerous drugs". The run-of-the-mill chemist and druggist was now portrayed, not as the poor man's doctor, but as the dispenser of physician's prescription. "The fact that the making up of a large proportion of prescriptions cannot be delegated without risk and disadvantage to the public has been thoroughly set aside" by the legislature. Spokesmen for the United Society began to sound like men reading Jacob Bell's speeches. The public interest demands that chemists and druggists should be regarded as different from other traders. Medicines are not like other commodities. "Pharmacy at the present time, in reference to dispensing especially, has become a very grave and responsible duty". Alderman Bowker, a leading member of the United Society in Manchester, said "that some definition was necessary in styling the trade. At present anybody who chose to vend drugs with his other wares might call himself a druggist; but he was hardly a man competent to fill the responsible duties behind a druggist's counter". What was needed was an act of incorporation for the whole trade. Chemists and druggists, to be properly recognised, must become a registered body. Qualification was necessary for the performance of responsible and difficult duties. New entrants should be required to serve a five years apprenticeship and pass an examination. The United Society should set up local examining boards throughout the country. Overnight, the United Society of Chemists and Druggists had become the poor man's Pharmaceutical Society.[28]

In 1863 a scheme was put forward by a committee of the General Medical Council to bring pharmaceutical "education, examination and practice" under the control of the G.M.C. The committee drafted a bill which proposed: (1) a general system of pharmaceutical education and examination regulated by the G.M.C., (2) the registration of all persons qualified to practise pharmacy by such examinations, (3) the restriction to such persons of the right to compound prescriptions of physicians and surgeons, (4) the appointment by the G.M.C. of pharmaceutical inspectors to enforce the Act, (5) the prohibition of the sale of all secret remedies and the imposition of a penalty for selling any proprietary medicine unless a sworn certificate of its composition was displayed in the shop where it was sold. The bill, which was never introduced into parliament, and, was, indeed, never adopted even by the G.M.C., kept the hostility between the Pharmaceutical Society and the United Society on the boil.

The Council of the Pharmaceutical Society, on the whole, approved of the proposals. "We hail the principle of the proposed measure as correct", reported the *Pharmaceutical*

Journal, "it aims at the production of a comprehensive, complete, and consistent system of education and examination which shall tend to ensure a sufficient qualification among practitioners in every department of medicine, and thus contribute to the safety and welfare of the public". "The principles of the proposed measure are the principles of the Pharmaceutical Society", it continued, "the Medical Council are pursuing the same course with us as that originally taken with regard to the physicians, surgeons and apothecaries. If the proposed bill be carried into effect, it will necessarily cause a complete revolution in the state and practice of pharmacy in this country".[29] Daniel Hanbury thought it an opportune moment to support a medical bill which would transform pharmacy into "a responsible and important profession". "That medicine, surgery, and pharmacy should be regulated by one comprehensive act of parliament appears to me highly advantageous", he wrote. "I entertain no fear of the Medical Council wishing to act in any way to the prejudice of pharmacy. I believe it is the public good that that body has at heart".[30]

The leadership of the United Society needed more convincing. The threat of medical interference with the drug trade threw them into a state of frenzied activity. Cyrus Buott, "an active secretary who appeared to be almost ubiquitous", ran around organising protest meetings throughout the length and breadth of the land. In every large town—and many smaller ones—"the unincorporated, unregistered, and unrecognised members of the drug trade" came together to express their opposition to the G.M.C. proposals. The *Chemist and Druggist* reported that "the chemists and druggists have met and decreed and recorded that neither the Medical Council nor the Pharmaceutical Council shall reign over them". The Central Committee of the United Society declared, with an understandable degree of exaggeration, "that the proposal of the Medical Council to forcibly dispossess upwards of 30,000 chemists and druggists of their practice to dispense medicine is an unwarrantable interference with their civil rights and trade interests, and would be attended with danger and injustice to the entire community". The G.M.C. bill was "unjust in principle and an unwarrantable attempt to interfere with their rights as independent citizens". The issues were clearly stated by Cyrus Buott at a meeting in Birmingham in March 1864. "The question . . . was this, whether chemists and druggists in this country should be subject to the control of, and render tribute to, the Medical Council, without having a voice or representation in that council". The jurisdiction of the G.M.C. meant control by doctors and "doctors were opposed to, and had no interests in common with the chemists and druggists. They claimed both sides of the druggist's counter". If the doctors' proposals were carried "it would deprive one-half of the population of the country of medical aid, and would leave the other half to the mercies of the doctors". This theme had been taken up earlier in a letter to the *Daily Telegraph* in January 1864:

> How would the poor fare under a medical despotism? . . . They who have witnessed medical abuse of power, as the law now stands, will shudder to think how our virtuous and industrious masses, who are too poor to go to the doctor and too proud to go to the dispensary, would fare if forced to seek relief from suffering at the hands of doctors by law provided.

The activities of the Pharmaceutical Society confirmed the deepest suspicions of the United Society. The Juries exemption had demonstrated that the Pharmaceutical Society promoted its own members' interests without regard for the rest of the trade. Its support for the G.M.C. bill was prompted by the same motives.

First, let us ask who would be the losers supposing the proposed bill became law? Not the pharmaceutists but the chemists and druggists. And who would be the gainers? The pharmaceutists alone, and no one else. And yet these disinterested people say they are going to fight for us, and ask us to trust them, with the Jury bill treachery fresh in our minds![31]

"The Pharmaceutical Society only represent themselves, and are, therefore, unfitted alone to represent the majority of the trade". But how fitted was the United Society to represent the majority of the trade? The answer must be rather less fitted than the Pharmaceutical Society. In 1862 there were about 7,000 proprietor chemists and druggists in Britain of whom 2,000 were members of the Pharmaceutical Society. These were *bona fide* members, whose names and addresses were published, and who paid a guinea a year each in subscription. The United Society made many claims about its membership but produced no evidence to substantiate them. It was prone to make wildly inaccurate statements about the total number of chemists and druggists in the country: its highest estimate was 40,000, its lowest 18,000. In 1861 the Census could discover no more than 16,026, of whom 3,388 were under the age of 20. The United Society gave the impression that it represented all the chemists and druggists outside the Pharmaceutical Society, but it is doubtful whether it ever had as many as a thousand members. Although the agents of the Society were very active in hunting over the country for recruits, enlisting all and sundry on any terms, the sole condition of membership being a single payment of five shillings, the largest amount collected in any year in "subscriptions, donations and members' fees" was considerably less than £500. The United Society had an office in New Ormond Street in London and a paid agent, Cyrus Buott, "who is most active in his vocation, and is very badly paid out of the two or three hundred a year he is able to collect in subscriptions", but it had no library, museum, lecture room, laboratory, nor any board of examiners. Essentially the United Society was an organisation of chiefs without indians. Its relationship with the new journal the *Chemist and Druggist* was not entirely harmonious. Although the journal was used to send out warning signals and to rally provincial chemists to attend meetings and pass resolutions, the reporting of the Society's activities was more objective than the leadership could tolerate. There were plans to set up the Society's own periodical but they came to nothing. The history of the United Society shows how easy it was to get chemists and druggists to attend protest meetings and how difficult it was to get them to sustain their involvement. "The limited success of the United and the Pharmaceutical Societies, and their consequent want of power to carry out any really useful legislation", observed the editor of the *Chemist and Druggist*, "is caused by the apathy of the trade, . . . want of organisation, want of public spirit, want of mutual confidence; . . . the chemists and druggists of this kingdom prefer blindly trusting in providence to putting their own shoulders to the wheel".[32]

The Council of the Pharmaceutical Society adopted a very laid-back approach to the G.M.C. bill. While the United Society worked itself into a frenzy, the Pharmaceutical Society remained calm, awaiting events. It was felt that the proposals which were creating so much alarm among chemists and druggists were merely exploratory and were unlikely to pass into law in the form in which they had been introduced. Was it likely that the British parliament would happily "deprive thousands of respectable tradesmen of the right to exercise their trade to which they had been educated, to which they had devoted the greater part of their lives, and in which was invested their only means of support"?[33] The wisdom of the Pharmaceutical Society's approach soon became manifest. Although the General Medical Council was agreed that the practice of pharmacy should be restricted to qualified men, there was little support for the idea that the G.M.C. itself should undertake the regulation of the required system of education and examination. Dr. Storrar, the representative of the University of London on the G.M.C., said:

> Nothing could certainly be more unsatisfactory than the state of pharmacy in this country; but it would be an unfortunate act of the Council to embroil itself with the druggists. The Council should drop pharmacy and encourage the Pharmaceutical Society to go on with an independent measure.

Dr. Sharpey, one of the secretaries of the Royal Society, and a member of the G.M.C. nominated by the Government, also favoured independent legislation for pharmacy. Professor Robert Christison of Edinburgh University

> disapproved of any attempt to introduce pharmacy into the Medical Act. The present state of the practice of pharmacy was a disgrace to the country and to the Legislature. He hoped, however, that the Council would not meddle with the subject, except by offering its aid and influence to any body which should take up the subject of legislation in regard to pharmacy; and he thought that this could be entrusted to no better persons than the pharmaceutical chemists.

The result was that the G.M.C. wrote to the Home Secretary

> drawing his attention to the present defective state of the law regarding the practice of pharmacy, under which any person, however ignorant, might undertake it, and expressing the opinion . . . that some legislative enactment was urgently called for to ensure competency in persons keeping open shops for dispensing medicines and for the compounding of physicians' and surgeons' prescriptions.[34]

The Medical Council's decision to leave pharmaceutical legislation to be worked out by the pharmacists themselves left the ball very obviously in the Pharmaceutical Society's court. On 17 March 1864 a special general meeting was convened to consider the possible introduction of a new pharmacy bill. The president, G.W. Sandford, thought the time had come to make the Society's examinations compulsory: "the medical profession, the public, the legislature, and the chemists themselves, all agree in acknowledging the necessity for compulsory powers". The subject was discussed at length by members from various parts of the country. Those in favour of new legislation argued that the voluntary system had failed; the educated were exposed to the unlimited competition of ignorant and stupid persons. "By making the examination compulsory, they would greatly benefit the public and give prosperity and permanence to the Society". Mr. Hollier of Dudley advised the Society "to open the door so wide as to meet all the requirements of the profession and by so doing hold . . . the front position in the foremost rank, and not allow the United Society . . . to cut the ground under their feet". The opposition case was thoughtfully presented by a small but articulate group. J.S. Lescher was for waiting. "Every effort had been made to induce the chemists and druggists to join the Society . . . but they had stood aloof . . . he believed that it was owing to the Jury Act which gave to pharmaceutical chemists a tangible benefit they must attribute the present movement". John Abraham of Liverpool was against protection. The Pharmaceutical Society was progressing, it was becoming more and more a body to be looked up to and respected: they must not lower its character by admitting less qualified and less respectable persons. He supported free trade: promoting sectional interests was robbery of one's neighbours. "They had no right to prevent a man from taking medicines . . . prescribed by any one he chose". "Had it occurred to them", he asked, "why it was that the Medical Council wished for such powers? Was it not one of their grievances that chemists and druggists interfered with their profession by prescribing medicines? . . . They complained exceedingly of the encroachment on their rights by prescribing chemists and druggists". William Dickinson's support for the opposition cause dealt it the *coup de grace*. The standing of pharmaceutical chemists was high and rising, he said. The Jury Act had given them a privilege they should hang onto. "What they had to do was to watch over their own interests . . . The Medical Council, the United Society, or any other body going to Parliament, would find in the Pharmaceutical Society a body capable of taking care of themselves". It was the wrong time to amend the Pharmacy Act: they should leave well alone. Such advice from William Dickinson must have been enough to ensure a large majority for the resolution that

> it is highly expedient that the Pharmaceutical Society make early application to Parliament for an amended Pharmacy Act, by which the legitimate interests of persons already in business (whether as principals or assistant) should be protected, and proper provision made for the compulsory examination of those who intend to commence hereafter.[35]

At a meeting of Council on 19 April 1864 the new Pharmacy bill was considered and ordered to be printed in the *Pharmaceutical Journal*. It was again fully discussed at the annual general meeting in May 1864 and unanimously adopted. In the meanwhile, the executive of the United Society had produced its own bill designed to incorporate the whole body of chemists and druggists. The two bills, when submitted to parliament, became known as "the Chemists and Druggists' Bills", that from the Pharmaceutical Society being No.1, and that from the United Society No.2.

The No.1 bill, which was introduced by Sir Fitzroy Kelly, had two essential features: it augmented the powers of the Pharmaceutical Society and restricted the dispensing of doctors' prescriptions to qualified persons. The bill provided that, after a certain date,

> It shall not be lawful for any person to carry on the business of a chemist and druggist in the keeping of open shop for the compounding of prescriptions of duly qualified medical practitioners in any part of Great Britain unless such person shall be a pharmaceutical chemist . . . or shall be duly registered as a chemist and druggist under this Act.

All persons in business as chemists and druggists before the chosen date were entitled to registration, but in future passing the Minor examination of the Society was to be the essential requirement for registration. Registered chemists and druggists were to be eligible for election as associates of the Pharmaceutical Society, with the right to attend meetings and to vote, but could not become members or serve on Council without first passing the Major examination and becoming registered as "pharmaceutical chemists". Keeping open shop for the compounding of doctors' prescriptions and the use of the titles, "pharmaceutical chemist", "chemist and druggist", "chemist", and "druggist" would render an unregistered person liable to a penalty of £5. The benefits of the Pharmaceutical Society's benevolent fund were to be made available to all registered chemists, their widows and orphans.[36]

The No.2 bill, which emanated from the United Society and was piloted by Sir John Shelley, M.P. for Westminster, was a much more elaborate measure. Its promoters sought to by-pass the authority of the Pharmaceutical Society but the United Society itself lacked the necessary organisation and educational arrangements. A new corporate body had to be erected by legislation. The bill proposed that the Government should appoint a Commissioner who would, by public advertisements, call a meeting in London of "the chemists and druggists of England and Wales". Those answering the summons would, without further inquiry, proceed to elect the president, vice-president and twenty-one members of the first Council of the Chemists and Druggists' Society. The Commissioner, with the approval of the Secretary of State, had the power, if dissatisfied with the proceedings, to annul them and order a new election, and of repeating this for an unlimited number of times—"a very necessary provision under the circumstances", observed the editor of the *Pharmaceutical Journal*. When at last elected, the new body would appoint a registrar, treasurer and examiners. Henceforth, all those keeping shop or store for the retailing of drugs, except registered medical practitioners and pharmaceutical chemists, would be required to (1) pass an examination in the knowledge of drugs and medicines in general use and of their ability to read physicians' prescriptions with ease and accuracy (2) register as chemists and druggists and (3) employ none but registered assistants. However, all persons, who, at the time of the passing of the Act, were engaged in business as chemists and druggists, or who were their assistants and apprentices, might register without examination on payment of a guinea. In future only registered persons would be entitled to recover charges accruing from the sale of dangerous drugs or "active poisons" (named

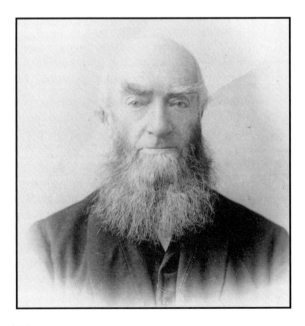

39 *John Jones of Caernarvon, a past local Secretary of the Pharmaceutical Society and Annuitant of the Benevolent Fund in 1901. From an intriguing collection of carte-de-visite portraits of the fund's beneficiaries that were assembled between the 1880s and 1930s.*

40 *Two early receipts, one for donations made to the Society's Benevolent Fund by S.W. Wymondham in 1845, and one a receipt for the annual subscription as a country member of the Society.*

in appended schedules). Certain precautions were to be observed in the sale of "active poisons". All persons registered under the Act were to be exempt from jury service and service in the militia.[37]

The United Society's bill was seriously marred by its need to provide for the erection of an entirely new regulatory authority; but its strength lay in its proposal to impose some restriction on the sale of poisons.

The publication of the two bills inaugurated a period of feverish political activity and debate. On 22 November 1864 a deputation of the Council of the Pharmaceutical Society met Sir George Grey at the Home Office in an unavailing attempt to gain Government support for its bill.[38] Elias Bremridge prevailed upon local secretaries throughout the country to whip up support and in many provincial towns a high proportion of the local chemists signed petitions approving of the No.1 bill. The United Society was slow off the mark and less well organised. Its secretary was dismayed to find that many of its supporters had been induced to sign declarations in favour of the rival bill. At meetings up and down the land and in the correspondence columns of both trade journals, acrimony reared its ugly head. In March 1865 a grand deputation of more than twenty members of the United Society, aided and abetted by eight members of parliament, made tracks to the Home Office

211

and convinced Sir George Grey that British chemists and druggists were a divided, quarrelsome, devious and back-biting lot.[39]

The two bills came on for second reading in the House of Commons on 29 March 1865. In introducing the Pharmaceutical Society's bill, Sir Fitzroy Kelly pointed out that, as the law now stood, there was no qualification required for a man to start in business as a chemist and druggist, and, therefore, no protection whatever for the public from ignorant and incompetent persons making up medical prescriptions. By the present bill, chemists and druggists would be examined, registered and licensed by the Pharmaceutical Society. The Army medical board "had stamped their approval on the examination and the whole proceedings of the Pharmaceutical Society: no one could be an army dispenser without producing their certificate". The effect of this bill would be to protect the public in the way the army is now protected by prohibiting anybody from making up prescriptions unless he had passed an examination by the Pharmaceutical Society. Those already in practise would be entitled to be registered without examination but it would be necessary for them to produce the certificate of a medical practitioner stating that they had actually carried on the business of a chemist and druggist before the Act came into operation. Referring to the United Society's bill, Sir Fitzroy Kelly said that it had two aims, one identical with his bill. The other was "a much more extensive object—namely to prescribe the terms and conditions upon which the sale of poisons and drugs ... should hereafter be sold". Now that, he thought, was too complicated a matter to be introduced in a bill of this sort, for it would interfere with the freedom of many branches of the trade. The Government should deal with this subject in a separate measure. Both the No. 1 and the No. 2 bills "admitted the necessity of affording to the public some protection against incompetent and ignorant persons carrying on the trade of chemists and druggists; they agreed that some examination should be applied to all; and the only difference between them in this respect was by whom the examination should be conducted". His bill proposed that "it should be in the hands of the already recognised body—the Pharmaceutical Society—who had conducted their operations in that respect with great effect and success". The No. 2 bill proposed an elected Council of 21 members who were to appoint examiners, no provision being made for the qualification either of the Council members or of the examiners.

Sir John Shelley began his speech by insisting that, although the United Society had no intention of infringing the privileges of the Pharmaceutical Society, the limitations of the latter's bill required to be pointed out. The No.1 bill prescribed qualifying examinations for those who made up medical prescriptions "but there was a very large portion of the trade carrying on a lucrative business that did not see or make up a medical prescription once a week, and the bill as to these would be comparatively useless". "The trade", he continued, "was divided into two classes, namely, those who wished to become scientific chemists and those who carried on the trade of chemists and druggists who required little or no qualification for the branch of the trade in which they had embarked". The Pharmaceutical Society "was possessed of great privileges and wealth, and had done a great deal of good in towns but its benefits had not reached the agricultural districts". (i.e. the districts represented by the majority of M.P.s) It had once numbered 4,000 members but now had fallen to only 2,300. The United Society had over 3,000 members. (This number was plucked from the air). The examinations of the Pharmaceutical Society were too expensive: an outlay of between £30 and £40 was needed (a fee of 10 guineas and the expense of coming to and staying in London). "He could not assent to the principle of forcing the whole of the chemists and druggists to pay for that examination".

The two bills, however, were not "a mere squabble between two great societies" but "an important public question". The Pharmaceutical Society's bill "was not calculated to promote the interests of the trade at large, nor yet to reduce the danger to which the public were exposed in the sale of drugs". The United Society's bill dealt with a major public concern, the regulation of the sale of poisons. It was the duty of the House of Commons "to see, in the public interests, that some legislation should take place by which the sale of poisons should be efficiently regulated". It was a great pity that the Pharmaceutical and United Societies had not come together and mutually agreed upon the principles of a bill to give the public the protection it required in the sale of dangerous drugs, "but when they found that a Society that had been established so many years shirked it, and the Government did nothing, it was right that someone else should take steps to put the matter on a right footing".

In the discussion that followed it was generally admitted that there ought to be a compulsory examination for chemists and druggists and that such examinations, in the words of Sir George Grey, "might with safety be placed under the direction of the Council of the Pharmaceutical Society" which "was a very important and useful body". Dr. Brady said that the Pharmaceutical Society "was composed of men of the highest knowledge in chemistry and the examinations of the Society were formed upon a very high standard", and Mr. Kinglake agreed that the Society submitted its members to a very difficult examination. The United Society, on the other hand, had no examination and admitted clerks and apprentices who knew nothing whatever about chemistry. Lord Elcho pointed out that the Pharmaceutical Society "had a good library, laboratory, and lecture-room, and had expended £70,000 on the education of the chemists and druggists of the country". The United Society "was nothing more than a trading body, and a sort of benefit society". Sir George Grey, the Home Secretary, recalled that:

> he had seen the representatives of the Pharmaceutical Society and also of the general body of chemists and druggists, and his advice to them was that they should meet together, and agree upon a general outline of a bill. Unhappily, though, it was, perhaps, not a matter of surprise, there were jealousies existing among members of the same profession and it had not yet been possible to bring them together and induce them to agree to the principles of a bill.[40]

Both bills were read a second time, and referred to a Select Committee. The Committee held four sittings and heard only the evidence the Government wanted presented. Evidence was given by Professor Alfred Swaine Taylor, the leading toxicologist of his day, who for 34 years held the chair of medical jurisprudence and chemistry at Guy's Hospital; by Sir (then Dr.) John Simon, the medical officer of the Privy Council; by Sir (then Dr.) Richard Quain, F.R.C.P., physician at the Brompton Hospital and the Crown nominee on the General Medical Council; by Dr. James A. Wilson, F.R.C.P., physician and lecturer at St. George's Hospital and lecturer on materia medica at the Royal College of Physicians; and by John Mackay, the Edinburgh chemist who was secretary of the North British Branch of the Pharmaceutical Society. The evidence taken by the Committee was entirely in favour of some restriction being imposed by law on the sale of poisonous drugs. Professor Taylor argued the case at length. The sale of dangerous drugs needs to be restricted "to save life and prevent their use in murder or crime". "Probably there are 550 deaths every year in this country from poison. I think our lives require that these things should not circulate about as easily as they do". "I think the state in which the profession of pharmacy and the sale of drugs has been allowed to continue in England is a disgrace". The rule of *caveat emptor* is upheld at the cost of public safety. "People cannot judge about medicine, or what may be put into a bottle as they can in purchasing any other things ... no man would go to an ignorant and an uneducated person for the purpose of having a leg taken off ... No person should be licensed to make up a medical prescription except a person educated to the business". The legislature should interpose to protect the layman "against his own confidence and ignorance in a matter in which he would not be a good judge". The sale of poisonous drugs by chandlers, grocers, oilmen, drapers and small shopkeepers should be strictly prohibited: no one should be allowed to sell drugs except persons properly educated and examined in the nature of drugs and their properties.

The witnesses were also in agreement in commending the work of the Pharmaceutical Society. Dr. Richard Quain believed that "nothing could be better than all its arrangements ... The Pharmaceutical Society has sought, by the character of its arrangements, to obtain the high character it has succeeded in obtaining". The museum was "one of the best I have ever seen" and the Minor examination "was so admirably arranged and so perfect, that it might be very well accepted" as the basic qualification. Dr. J.A. Wilson added that the Pharmaceutical Society's examinations were "remarkably competent; more than the public had any right to expect". The Society had long ago secured "the confidence of the medical profession and the public".

While the Select Committee was sitting, the General Medical Council issued a report emphasising "the necessity of regulating by statute the practice of pharmacy by chemists and druggists throughout the kingdom". The G.M.C. indicated a strong preference for the Pharmaceutical Society's bill. "They think the bill promoted by the society well fitted to attain various important objects, and reasonable in its demands for powers and privileges". They thought its operation should be extended to Ireland and suggested a clause making it imperative on chemists to follow the formularies of the *British Pharmacopoeia*. They also insisted that provision should be made to prevent registered chemists from converting themselves into unqualified medical practitioners. They argued that the bill made the admission of existing chemists and druggists to the register too easy, and that the whole profession of pharmacy ought to be subject, as the medical profession was, to the control of the Privy Council.

In spite of this powerful expression of support by the G.M.C., the Pharmaceutical Society's bill did not prove acceptable to the Select Committee, which had become convinced that the restriction of the sale of poisons was a *sine qua non* of any act of parliament regulating pharmacy. The Select Committee arrived at only two definite conclusions: "First, that no compulsory examination or registration ... should be required of persons now carrying on the trade of chemists and druggists;" and, second, that no person shall "after a day to be fixed by the Bill, sell certain dangerous drugs, to be scheduled in the Bill, unless he be examined and registered".

The Committee rejected the proposal that persons compounding medicines from the prescriptions of medical men should be examined and objected to the organisational features of the United Society's bill. Ultimately they decided to abandon both bills and to recommend that the Government should, early in the new parliament, bring in its own bill on the subject.[41]

In the post-mortem on the two bills their strengths and weaknesses were laid bare. The bill of the United Society commended itself to both the Government and the public health lobby by addressing itself to the question of the sale of poisons; but it was ruined by the absurd organisational proposals designed merely to circumvent the Pharmaceutical Society. The Pharmaceutical Society's educational and examination system was the major asset of the No.1 bill. Although it was publicly endorsed by the G.M.C., the No.1 bill was not calculated to win widespread approval. It ignored the moral panic about poisons, and, by focusing upon the dispensing of physician's prescriptions, appeared to leave the great bulk of the drug trade untouched. Worst still, by rubbing in the distinction between pharmaceutical chemists and the rest, it seemed deliberately to provoke the opposition of the United Society.

There were deep ideological and structural divisions within the pharmaceutical constituency. For eighteen years the Pharmaceutical Society under Jacob Bell's leadership had papered over the cracks to give an appearance of common purpose and endeavour. But in the 1860s the tensions and conflicts which had lain dormant were brought to the surface. The theoretical debates—profession versus trade, science versus practical experience—were related, in complex ways, to the divisions between dispensing and prescribing chemists, between the well-established and the struggling, between proprietors and assistants, and between London and the provinces. The Pharmacy Act of 1852, by establishing the legal barrier between pharmaceutical chemists and chemists and druggists, a barrier reinforced ten years later by the Juries Act, enormously increased the difficulty of the Pharmaceutical Society's task of binding the pharmaceutical body together. The emergence of the United Society threatened to institutionalise pharmacy's internal divisions within a two-party system. That this was not the final outcome was due to two main factors. First, the British Pharmaceutical Conference, throughout the period of the most bitter conflict, brought together leading members of both societies in amicable scientific and social intercourse. Second, on both sides, leading members publicly expressed their reservations about their Society's policies. The lack of unity within each Society meant that the basis for compromise and realignment were kept alive: extremists on both sides were prevented from constructing insurmountable ramparts.

It was early in the life of the Pharmaceutical Society that Jacob Bell initiated the scientific meetings that were to play a large part in developing, first, an increased awareness of the lack of scientific knowledge among many of the members and, secondly, the desire to become better acquainted with the new discoveries in methods and their application to the widening field of pharmaceutical practice. George F. Schacht (1823–1896), a chemist of Bristol, suggested in 1852 that the Society should organise a series of annual meetings at which papers relating to the practice of pharmacy should be read and discussed and that these meetings should be held in a different town each year, somewhat on the model of the British Association for the Advancement of Science and the Provincial Medical and Surgical Association. He thought that meetings of this kind would encourage provincial members to take a more active role in the Society. Schacht intended that these peripatetic meetings should be organised and controlled by the Pharmaceutical Society, but the Council was reluctant to act on his suggestion. Ten years later, however, Richard Reynolds of Leeds and H.B. Brady of Newcastle, both members of the rising generation of scientific pharmaceutical chemists, revived Schacht's scheme but in a slightly modified form, proposing to establish an association independent of the Pharmaceutical Society. The inception of the British Pharmaceutical Conference, convened by a circular published in the *Pharmaceutical Journal*, took place on 2 September 1863 at Newcastle-upon-Tyne. Henry Deane, owner of a retail business in Clapham, was called to the chair. Deane became the first president and Dr. Attfield and Richard Reynolds joint general secretaries. The object of the Conference was the advancement of British pharmacy in a scientific direction. An important political decision was made at the outset: membership of the Conference was not confined to members of the Pharmaceutical Society. The participation of those who supported the United Society and those who supported no society was actively encouraged. From the small gathering which met on this occasion, the Conference grew rapidly in size and importance. By the time of the third meeting in Birmingham in September 1865 there were over 300 members.

Some of the leading members of the Pharmaceutical Society expressed, at an early stage, their dissatisfaction with the bill, which the Council had devised. Barnard S. Proctor, one of the leading pharmaceutical chemists in Newcastle-upon-Tyne and an enthusiastic supporter of the British Pharmaceutical Conference, made public his unease in a well-argued letter to the *Pharmaceutical Journal* in February 1865. "Something better than the proposed bill could be accomplished", he wrote, "and probably accomplished with less difficulty". Dispensing the prescriptions of legally qualified medical practitioners is a branch of business quite unimportant to nine-tenths of provincial druggists and, he might have added, to most metropolitan chemists as well. "There is not one country druggist in a hundred who could live by his dispensing. There is not one in a hundred who could not live almost as well as at present without it". The Pharmaceutical Society's bill "will leave the public unprotected and the practice of the drug trade almost unaltered . . . it will still leave the necessity for a Poison bill and the probability of our having to oppose poison bills of an impracticable or obnoxious character". "Nothing is so sure to deprive us of public sympathy and support", he continued, "as an apparent desire to pass a public bill for our own purposes". The present bill

> is felt to be unfair towards some of those who do not belong to our Society registering them on a list inferior to that occupied by the members of the Pharmaceutical Society,—the distinction being nominally, but not really, one of qualification, the inferior register containing many able and well-informed men and the superior containing, as it unavoidably will do for years to come, the names of some who, as far as regards qualifications, are unworthy of the position.

"A measure must be liberal towards existing interests", he concluded, "if it is to be stringent in its future action".[42]

Other well-established members of the Society echoed these views. W.B. Randall of Southampton pointed out that "he was a pharmaceutical chemist but not by examination and there were gentlemen in his town who were apparently quite as well qualified to act in every way as himself". Henry B. Brady, one of the founders of the British Pharmaceutical Conference, and another distinguished chemist from Newcastle-upon-Tyne, pointed out that

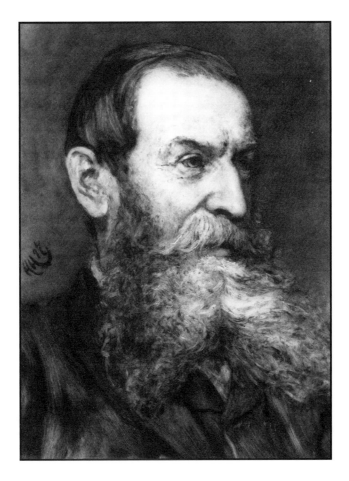

41 *Professor John Attfield FRS (1835–1911). A "Herkotype" from an oil portrait of 1897 by Sir Hubert von Herkomer RA. Attfield was appointed Professor of Practical Chemistry in 1862, a post he held until 1896. He was a founder member of the British Pharmaceutical Conference and the Institute of Chemistry.*

The Pharmaceutical Society was not held in so much estimation in the remote provinces as it was in the metropolis, and consequently its diploma was less valued. Of the leading men who practise pharmacy not more than three-fifths were members of the Society, and many of those who were not members were equal in social standing and influence to those who were.[43]

There were, however, powerful arguments against abandoning the distinction between pharmaceutical chemists and chemists and druggists, even though the majority of the members of the Pharmaceutical Society had never been examined. Since its foundation, 821 men had passed the Major and 923 the Minor examination: of 2,100 members in 1863 only 430 had passed the Major examination. Admitting all chemists and druggists on equal terms would have the effect of lowering the status of the pharmaceutical chemist without elevating that of the chemist and druggist. A leading Manchester chemist, W. Wilkinson, reminded readers of the *Pharmaceutical Journal*, in October 1865, that for nearly twenty-five years the Pharmaceutical Society had had to encounter a great deal of (at least passive) opposition from the trade generally. The non-examined pharmaceutical chemists were the men who founded the Society and for many years were its principal supporters: without their subscriptions there would be no school, no laboratory, no examinations. It is only the fact that membership now brought some privilege that those who previously scorned to join, wished to gain admission. In any case, a practical examination had been instituted for men established in business to provide a means of admission for well-qualified non-members. Surely this was a more honourable way of joining the Society than floating in with the "red-and-green bottle men, whose future admission to the trade it is considered by all parties desirable to prevent?" Wilkinson ended with a fine flourish:

> Let us, then, keep faith with the medical profession, the public, and our own examined members, by continuing to make examination the condition of admission to the Society, and all who are really qualified and desirous of joining us will find means of doing so, but let us not, by throwing open the Society to all in the trade, reduce all to the same level, and thus undo all that for the last twenty years we have been endeavouring to do.[44]

Nonetheless it was evident to all candid observers that the only chance of carrying a pharmacy bill through parliament was for the Pharmaceutical Society and the United Society to agree upon some measure and direct their united efforts towards getting it passed. Internal disagreements in both societies made progress easier. From the autumn of 1865 the United Society increasingly failed to justify its name. Unseemly disputes arose at public and committee meetings between its leading members and Cyrus Buott, the secretary. The president, Alderman Dakin resigned in anger, and Alderman Bowker of Manchester declined the invitation to succeed him. Eventually Henry Matthews of Gower Street, London, analytical chemist, unconnected with pharmacy, was elected to the difficult office of presiding over a disintegrating society. In certain provincial cities, such as Manchester, a nucleus of established chemists and druggists kept the United Society on its feet. By 1866 the *Chemist and Druggist* reported that the United Society had fallen into an "incoherent state" in which "deplorable dissension" prevailed at the committee and other meetings. Cyrus Buott, its forceful and persevering secretary, attempted to rule the proceedings in opposition to the president and a majority of the Executive Committee.

Backed by provincial members, Buott succeeded, at the annual meeting, in carrying his policies but at the cost of tearing the society apart and weakening its power for any effective work. Several of the most influential members resigned and either joined the Pharmaceutical Society or held themselves aloof from both societies. By 1866 there were very few chemists and druggists who failed to realise that the success of a new pharmacy bill depended upon its promotion by a well organised and incorporated association such as the Pharmaceutical Society.

Within the Pharmaceutical Society earlier disagreements about the strategy incorporated in the 1865 bill gave prominent members the mandate to point the way forward. Elements of the United Society's bill could be taken up without attracting the charge of either opportunism or inconsistency. "In going to Parliament", an editorial in the *Pharmaceutical Journal* explained , "it is necessary to study the feelings of the Legislature, to observe what principles are recognised in legislation, and to shape our course" accordingly. "The regulation of the sale of dangerous drugs will be made the ostensible object of any extension of pharmaceutical legislation that we may be able to obtain".[45] The Pharmaceutical Society's new strategy was to try to win Government support for legislation regulating the practice of pharmacy by including within it some restrictions on the sale of poisons. These restrictions, however, were to be kept to a minimum. George W. Sandford, the president, explained in a letter to Henry Matthews, that the Society remained opposed to "a mere poison bill, fettering us with registration of sales and attendance of witnesses, prescribing a particular form of bottle in which poisons might be kept and sold, and a particular corner of our shops in which they should be placed".[46]

As the United Society disintegrated, the Pharmaceutical Society took the initiative. Early in 1866 the Council submitted to the Home Office a memorandum in which the outlines of a measure were sketched which it was thought would meet the recommendations of the 1865 Select Committee and prove acceptable to chemists and druggists in general. On 16 January 1867 the Society's Parliamentary Committee discussed these proposals at the Home Office with Earl Belmore, the under-secretary. Eight days later the Executive Committee of the United Society presented the same proposals to a public meeting of the trade held at the London Coffee House on Ludgate Hill. The president, Henry Matthews, was in the chair and about sixty persons attended. After some discussion, it was decided to send a deputation consisting of the Executive Committee and any other gentlemen willing to join them to wait on the Council of the Pharmaceutical Society. The Council made arrangements to receive this deputation and another deputation of non-aligned members of the trade on 19 February. There were two items on the agenda: (1) the admission of chemists and druggists to membership of the Pharmaceutical Society and (2) the future constitution of the Council. On the first point, it was made clear that those in business at the time of the passing of the act, who became registered as chemists and druggists under the act, would have the right to be elected members of the Pharmaceutical Society without examination. They would become members but not pharmaceutical chemists, the higher and parliamentary title being reserved to the existing members and to those who passed the Major examination. With regard to the second issue, George Sandford explained that it was proposed to limit Council membership to pharmaceutical chemists. This was to maintain the Council at a high standard and retain public confidence in it; to hold out an inducement to pass the Major examination; to protect the accumulated property of the Society; and to respect the vested interest obtained by the expenditure of more than £100,000, collected over a quarter of a century, entirely from members' subscriptions. Nonetheless, remembering that the Pharmaceutical Society was established to embrace all chemists and druggists in Great Britain, the Council would be willing, in the event of obtaining an act of parliament requiring the examination of all men entering the trade in future, to agree that chemists and druggists should be eligible to be elected to the Council, provided always that two-thirds of the Council should always be pharmaceutical chemists. Both deputations expressed their satisfaction with these proposals.

The negotiations, however, were not yet over. The concessions made to outsiders met with resistance from within. A group of members who saw the indiscriminate admission of chemists and druggists as the thick edge of the wedge asked the Council to call a special general meeting. They argued that those who had taken no part in gaining for the Society the high reputation it enjoys had no claim to its honours; the test of examination "which has so long prevailed in the admission of members" should not be discarded so lightly. They considered the Council's new bill unfair to present members and against the public interest. Similar views were held by the General Medical Council and Dr. John Simon who were just as firmly opposed to the idea of qualifying without examination the serried ranks of chemists and druggists.

The publication of the requisition and notice of meeting produced its own reaction. Twenty-four of the leading pharmaceutical chemists by examination, all prominent members of the British Pharmaceutical Conference, drew up a manifesto, which was published, prior to the meeting, in the *Pharmaceutical Journal*. The manifesto group, which included H.B. Brady, M. Carteighe, H.S. Evans, R.W. Giles, Joseph Ince, Richard Reynolds, G.F. Schacht, and W. Smeeton, expressed their "cordial approval of the liberal policy adopted by the Council towards all chemists and druggists", which clears the way for carrying into effect the primary object of the founder of the Society, namely, "the amalgamation of the whole trade, and the compulsory examination of all persons entering it after a given time".

The general meeting of 15 May 1867, by a large majority, pledged its support for the Council's policy. At the same time, the United Society not only withdrew its opposition but began to co-operate actively with the Pharmaceutical Society in promoting the new bill. In November 1867 the Council instructed the Parliamentary Committee to take steps for introducing the new bill into parliament. A copy was sent to the Home Office and on 4 February 1868 the Home Secretary, Gathorne Hardy, received a deputation from the Pharmaceutical Society, who were accompanied by the president and two other members of the United Society. The Home Secretary said that he approved of all the propositions submitted to him; he entirely concurred in the necessity of an educational qualification for persons entrusted to compound medicines; he considered the prospects of the bill greatly improved by the unanimity of the delegation; but he could not say whether or not the Government would introduce a measure on the subject. The Home Secretary, however, continued to meet with George Sandford, the president of the Society, and on 18 February put his views in writing:

> To G.W. Sandford, Esq.
> Sir, I am not unwilling to support a Bill restricting the title of "Chemists and Druggists" to
> 1. Those now in business as such.
> 2. Those to be examined for the future and passed by proper examiners.
> 3. Pharmaceutical Chemists.
> 4. Medical practitioners under the Medical Act.
> No others to be allowed to sell certain drugs, etc., named. I think this will be sufficient.
> Yours faithfully,
> Gathorne Hardy.

In a later letter of clarification, the Home Office informed the president of the Pharmaceutical Society:

> that Mr. Hardy does intend the prohibition of selling dangerous drugs by

unauthorized persons to include also dispensing or compounding for payment such drugs as may be specified as "dangerous" or "poisonous".

The bill which was introduced in the House of Lords on 11 May 1868 was entitled "A bill to regulate the sale of poisons and alter and amend the Pharmacy Act, 1852". The title indicates that it was as much a poisons bill as a bill to regulate the practice of pharmacy. So far it has been considered as a development from the Pharmacy Act of 1852, but its evolution has also to be seen in the context of attempts to legislate about the sale of poisons. It has to be considered as a development from the Arsenic Act of 1851.

* * *

During the late 1840s public concern was generated about the ready availability of poisons. The public health lobby embarked on a campaign to restrict their sale. An alliance was forged between members of the medical profession agitating for reform and the, as yet, small sector of administration in government. Professional arguments about the need to control the sale of dangerous substances were supported by reference to official statistics. The Registrar General's office, established in 1837, as one of the first central government agencies, provided the scientific basis on which the public health case was based. Statistics of deaths by poisoning were used as public health propaganda. In the late 1840s the reports of the Registrar General drew attention to the large number of deaths occurring annually from poisoning, of which more than a third were caused by the use of arsenic. In 1849 statistics were supplemented by sensationalism. Several cases of murder came before the public and the newspapers created the impression that an epidemic of secret poisoning had broken out. In a letter to the *Times*, the Rev. Robert Montgomery, the minister of Percy Chapel, St. Pancras, whose religious poems were extravagantly praised in the press and derided by Macaulay in the *Edinburgh Review*, denounced chemists and druggists as "venal poison-mongers" who "traffic for pence in murder". Many solutions to the problem were forthcoming, some advocated that the retail sale of arsenic should be prohibited altogether, others that every sale should be reported at the nearest police-station.

Both the Provincial Medical and Surgical Association and the Pharmaceutical Society took the opportunity to make public their professional involvement in this area. The Pharmaceutical Society carried out a detailed investigation, through a questionnaire to its members, of the sale of poisons in Britain. The results of this survey were published in a report which established the Pharmaceutical Society's right to be regarded as an authority in this field. The Provincial Medical and Surgical Association and the Pharmaceutical Society together put forward recommendations to the Home Secretary which formed the basis of the Arsenic Act of 1851. By that Act, retailers of arsenic were required

(1) to enter in a book the name, address and occupation of the purchaser, the date of the sale, the quantity and the purpose for which the arsenic is required

(2) unless the purchaser is known, to sell only in the presence of a witness known to both parties

(3) to sell only to adults

(4) to mix the arsenic with soot or indigo in stated proportion

(5) to ensure that the entry is signed by the seller and the purchaser, and, where necessary, by the witness.

With no adequate provision for its enforcement, the Arsenic Act was more a declaration of intent than an effective piece of legislation. In 1854 Sir (then Dr.) John Simon

(1816–1904), who became the leading public health reformer of his day, indicated his growing interest in the regulation of pharmacy. Educated as a surgeon at St. Thomas's Hospital, Simon had been appointed in 1848 the first medical officer of health to the City of London. Simon was convinced that "comprehensive and scientific legislation" could solve all public health problems. He was an unswerving advocate of increasing government regulation in all fields of health. He wanted to establish himself as "the medical dictator" of Britain: he believed he possessed an unerring capacity to identify, articulate, and serve the public interest. The firmness of his aims was matched by the flexibility of his methods of attaining them. He was a very astute politician.[47] In May 1854, in the Preface to his *Reports relating to the Sanitary Condition of the City of London*, he argued that powers, and officers to enforce them, should be provided uniformly to all local authorities to prevent the adulteration of drugs. "It is notorious that some important medicines are so often falsified in the market, and others so often mis-made in the laboratory, that we are robbed of all certainty in their employment". Yet we acquiesce "in our present defencelessness against fraud and ignorance; in doses being sold—critical doses, for the strength of which we, who prescribe them, cannot answer within a margin of cent. per cent". And so also with the sale of poisons; how can we acquiesce "in pennyworths of poison being handed across the counter as nonchalantly as cakes of soap?"

> Again, with the promiscuous sale of poisons, what incredible laxity of government! One poison, indeed has its law . . . but why should arsenic alone receive this dab of legislation? Is the principle right, that means of murder and suicide should be rendered difficult of access for criminal purposes? Does any one question it? Then, why not legislate equally against all poisons?—against oxalic acid and opium, ergot and savin, prussic acid, corrosive sublimate, strychnine?[48]

John Simon's rhetoric was aimed at an educated and informed audience, but the demand for poisons legislation was soon to come from all sections of society. In the years 1855 and 1856 a succession of cases of criminal poisoning occurred, the press coverage of which "greatly agitated the public mind, and forcibly called attention to the unguarded manner in which poisons are supplied to those who desire to use them, whether legitimately or otherwise". The "slow poisoning case at Burdon", in June 1855, in which a Mr. Wooler was accused of murdering his invalid wife by long-continued administration of small doses of arsenic, was followed, in February 1856, by the death of John Sadlier, M.P. for Sligo, whose body was found on Hampstead Heath after he had committed suicide by swallowing essential oil of almonds. Public excitement was further increased by the trial and conviction of William Palmer of Rugely in 1856. Palmer, a qualified medical practitioner, was accused and convicted, entirely on circumstantial evidence, of poisoning, with strychnia, his wife, his brother, and his friend and gambling companion, John Parsons Cook. He was hanged at Stafford in June 1856. "Rarely if ever has a case of poisoning excited so intense and widespread an interest as was manifested in connection with Palmer's trial", wrote Theophilus Redwood. "The crime had become not only common, but . . . scientific". Strychnia was also the substance used by William Dove of Leeds to poison his wife. His trial in July 1856 encouraged the popular press to intensify the public sense of alarm. The question of legislation was raised by Lord Campbell in the House of Lords on 10 July.

Lord Campbell began by referring to the Palmer trial "which had occupied the attention of all Europe". He was shocked to say that for several years past the crime of poisoning had become remarkably common and in his opinion some new law was imperatively required for the regulation of the sale of poisons. The institution of burial societies led parents to poison their own children, and the system of life insurance encouraged people to take out insurance on the lives of others, with the premeditated intention of committing murder. He knew from his own experience that murder was frequently committed in this way. Until recently no restriction whatever had been placed upon the sale of poisons; it was possible to purchase arsenic as easily as Epsom Salts with the consequence that cases of poisoning by arsenic became alarmingly common, especially in Essex and Norfolk. A check had now been placed upon the sale of arsenic but another poison, nux vomica, had taken its place. Anyone might go to any chemist in England and buy a pennyworth of nux vomica by merely stating that he intended to use it for poisoning rats. Even strychnia could easily be obtained. There ought to be some restraint placed on the sale of poisons.

The fact that Lord Campbell's speech was taken seriously is a measure of the degree of moral panic that the press and the public health reformers managed to generate. There was now general agreement in the press that the situation was intolerable. All respectable citizens, and even some members of parliament, were agreed that it was the Government's duty to act. The Government sought for some reassuring measure, which would save it from defeat, and might even protect the public from criminal poisoning.

In May 1857 the Government's bill was introduced in the House of Lords by Earl Granville (1815–1891), Lord President of the Council and leader of the House of Lords. The thinking of John Simon, who in 1855 had been made medical officer to the General Board of Health, permeated the bill. The "Bill to Restrict and Regulate the Sale of Poisons" proposed to repeal the Arsenic Act and to apply its provisions generally to a large number of other dangerous substances. In deference to the Treasury, however, patent medicines, that important source of revenue, were to be exempt. No poison was to be sold to anyone other than an adult; a witness knowing both seller and purchaser was to be present; and the purchaser was to produce a certificate signed either by the local clergyman or a legally qualified medical practitioner or a justice of the peace justifying the use for which the poison was required. A full entry of the sale was to be made. Packets containing poisons were to be wrapped in tinfoil as well as in paper, and bottles were to have the word "Poison" moulded on them. Solid poisons were to be coloured with soot or indigo and liquid poisons with archil. Vendors of poisons were to keep them under lock and key, and in certain vessels; and if they should be convicted of any failure to carry out the provisions of the act, they were to be fined £20 and on a second offence were to be disqualified for ever from selling poisons or carrying on the business of a chemist and druggist. Sale to photographers, bird-stuffers, artists' colourmen and veterinary surgeons, as well as sales by wholesale to retailers were to be exempt, and so were sales of medicine compounded on the prescription of qualified medical practitioners.

The Council of the Pharmaceutical Society objected to practically the whole bill. The restrictions were so overbearing as to be ridiculous. Self-medication and the legitimate sale of poisons for everyday uses would be halted. A public meeting, held at Bloomsbury Square on 3 June, unanimously endorsed the view that the bill "would prove no protection to the public but on the contrary greatly augment existing evils and also throw needless obstacles on the legitimate sale of useful and necessary medicines". On 6 June a deputation from the Society waited on Earl Granville. Three days later its members gave evidence to the Select Committee to which the bill had been referred.

The Pharmaceutical Society's position was that the most effective safeguard in the supply of poisons to the public was the creation of a profession of pharmacy.

> As at present there is absolute free trade in poisons, and in medicines generally, we consider that the first step to be taken is to commence a register of all persons at present dealing in poisons and to enact a law that in future no unregistered person should be permitted to sell certain classes of medicines which might be enumerated in a schedule of poisons; and that, after a certain date, all persons dealing in these substances, and dispensing prescriptions for the sick, shall be required to pass an examination . . . That we consider would be the most efficient security to the public against accidents from poisons and against criminal poisoning also.

There was a great and increasing number of poisons used for a wide range of purposes, not only in medicine, but in arts, manufacture, and agriculture. People in many walks of life required access to these dangerous substances, not only for self-medication, but also in the household, workshop and field. The sale of poisons constituted a major part of the trade of the chemist and druggist. "Poisons, or medicines which, in certain quantities, would be poisonous, form so large a proportion of the stock of every chemist that a prohibition from selling all which may be considered as poisons would be an absolute prohibition from exercising the business of a chemist". The proposed government regulations were so detailed and so cumbersome that the chemist would be faced with the alternative of either allowing his business to grind to a halt or else exposing himself to penalties and disqualification. "The security of the public", argued Jacob Bell, "would be better effected by an attention to the intelligence and qualification of the vendor than by any arbitrary regulations with regard to the shape of the bottles, or to the obtaining of certificates from clergyman or justices of the peace or those various regulations which have been proposed in the bill before the House of Lords". If professional pharmaceutical chemists were given a monopoly of the sale of poisons, the public could rest assured that the sale would be in the hands of intelligent, educated, and responsible persons. The sale of poisons is an activity which requires the exercise of judgment and discretion. It cannot properly be carried out by routinely following regulations. Delicate inquiries may have to be made about the purchasers' intentions and judgments made about their state of mind. The seller cannot know too much about the poisons he supplies. He must be able to dispense them accurately: he must be familiar with their properties and uses. Instead of following inflexible, uniform procedures, the pharmaceutical chemist must use his discretion in a unique set of circumstances. Detailed regulations would have the effect of taking away "from the pharmaceutical chemist, the person who sells the poison, that responsibility which at present is a great safeguard to the public".

The evidence presented to the Select Committee by Professor A.S. Taylor represented the views of the bill's promoters. Taylor was a close friend of John Simon and they held identical views on pharmacy and poisons. Taylor was regarded as the leading authority on poisoning which he had been studying since 1831. He had been engaged in assisting criminal proceedings in all the principal poisoning cases since 1848. He argued that the increasing number of deaths from poisoning, from 270 a year in 1837 to 349 in 1840 and over 530 in 1853 in England and Wales, was a direct consequence of the ease with which poisons could be obtained. Although legislation cannot altogether prevent criminal and suicidal poisoning, it can reduce its incidence. He supplied examples of accidental deaths from poisons supplied in mistake by druggists and argued that such accidents would be significantly reduced by government regulation. Taylor, like Simon, pointed to the strict state regulation of the sale of poisons in France and Prussia as the model to be emulated. In those countries not only were the laws strict, they were also enforced. The machinery of enforcement was just as important as the legislative provision. In detail, Taylor argued that the Arsenic Act should be replaced by one general act restricting the sale of thirteen scheduled poisons. The Privy Council should have the power to add to and amend the list of poisons. After a breathing space of five years, all persons vending drugs should be required to pass an examination before a Board consisting of nine examiners, three from the College of Physicians, three from the Society of Apothecaries, and three from the Pharmaceutical Society. Taylor approved of most of the provisions of the Government's bill: sales by and to adults only, certificates to be supplied, records to be kept, poisons to be coloured, and stored in separate closets, and sold in peculiarly shaped and coloured bottles. Taylor had little sympathy for the public's right of self-medication : the poisonous vegetable alkaloids should be sold only by qualified chemists on the prescription of a qualified medical practitioner.

The views of men like Taylor and Simon ignored the realities of the sale and use of poisons in mid-Victorian Britain. When questioned about the problem of small sales of opium to lower class people, Taylor conceded that the sale of pennyworths of laudanum should be allowed to continue, but added, only to adults and on condition that the drug was drunk in the chemist's shop. In the end he had to admit that severe restriction was not practicable and that opium was a special case, although it accounted for two-fifths of all deaths from poisoning. He was forced to agree with the pharmaceutical chemists, who had pointed out that, if the open sale of opium was suddenly curtailed, "a smuggled sale might go on". Jacob Bell explained that it would be almost impossible to carry the Government's bill into effect in many country districts where pennyworths of laudanum and opium were frequently sold. John Abraham and John Baker Edwards, members of the Pharmaceutical Society and of the Liverpool Chemists' Association, pointed out that restriction would be impossible to enforce and would only produce a growth in illicit sales. Opium would continue to be sold "as it is sold now, by a low class of dealer throughout the villages in the country in defiance of the law". How much better to have its sale in the hands of pharmaceutical chemists exercising their professional judgment and responsibility.

The Select Committee made several important alterations in the bill. It was decided that poisons should be sold only by medical practitioners and licensed vendors; and that the required licence should be granted only to those who passed an examination instituted for the purpose. The examiners were to be six in number, three to be appointed by the Queen, and one each by the College of Physicians, the Society of Apothecaries, and the Pharmaceutical Society. These examiners, or any two of them, were to be authorised to enter and search any shop where poisons were sold to see if the storage regulations were duly obeyed. The revised edition of the bill repeated the exemption of patent medicines from its operation.[49]

The bill was reintroduced in the next session of parliament. "To those who are practically conversant with the subject", wrote Jacob Bell, "it will be obvious . . . that the last state of the bill is worse than the first. The bill, as originally drawn, would have been simply impracticable, and therefore inoperative". The bill, as altered, would nullify all the Pharmaceutical Society's attempts to improve the practice of pharmacy and invest an irresponsible Board with inquisitorial powers. Before the bill could be submitted for discussion, Lord Palmerston's Government was defeated. Lord Derby, the new prime minister, lost little time in producing a bill on the same lines. The new bill proposed to recognise medical practitioners and pharmaceutical chemists as vendors of poisons but would have required all other dealers to submit to a special examination. Persons who could satisfy the examiners that they had been in business for a year as chemists and druggists were to be exempt from examination at the time but would have to come up for a renewed licence in five years. The examiners were to be only three in number: the College of Physicians, the Society of Apothecaries and the Pharmaceutical Society appointing one each.

The Pharmaceutical Society remained adamant in its opposition. In a letter to Lord Derby, written on 7 June 1858, Jacob Bell explained that the Society's principal objection was to

> the proposal to supersede the Pharmaceutical Society by the appointment of a new Board of Examiners, to examine candidates for the distinction of "Licensed Druggist". For about eighteen years the Pharmaceutical Society has been endeavouring to introduce a regular education and examination of all chemists and druggists. During nearly the whole of this time, very little encouragement has been obtained from the Legislature or the Government; the efforts of the society having been met either with indifference or opposition, and the necessity for education and examination having been scarcely admitted to exist. It is now generally acknowledged that some qualification in those who dispense medicines, including poisons, is necessary for the safety of the public, and it is also acknowledged that the Pharmaceutical Society has done service to the public in promoting this object, for which its establishment is expressly designed. Yet in carrying the principle into practice, it is now proposed to appoint another Board of Examiners, the tendency of which would be to divert candidates from the channel of education and examination provided by the society, substituting a qualification which must of necessity be inferior to that of a pharmaceutical chemist, and frustrating the endeavours of the society to raise the standard of education.

The Earl of Derby behaved in an imperious and high handed manner. He replied immediately to Bell's letter denying the validity of the objection. He refused to see the Society's deputation and secured the third reading of the bill in the House of Lords by a procedural sleight of hand. But the prime minister's arrogance backfired. Within two hours from the time at which the third reading had been carried, Elias Bremridge was setting in motion the Society's nationwide protest campaign. Batches of circulars were dispatched, one convening a meeting of members in London, the other informing local secretaries in the provinces how to channel their members' protests in the most effective way. Within twenty four hours petitions came flooding in and members of parliament were inundated by letters from indignant constituents. In the course of two or three days deputations of chemists from various parts of the country clustered in the lobby of the House of Commons to meet their M.P.s and convey their anger to Spencer Walpole, the Home Secretary. Rather bewildered, Walpole invited them to form a delegation to meet him at the Home

Office, but, on the evening before the interview was due to take place, he announced the withdrawal of the bill. In his statement to the House on 19 July 1858 he admitted that the storm of protest aroused by the bill had dissuaded the Government from proceeding with it that session. This was a considerable achievement for the Society and a salutary shock for the Government. In their determination to carry the measure, the Government had seriously underestimated the Pharmaceutical Society's power to mobilise support.

Before the end of the year, however, a calamity occurred which helped to maintain the moral panic about poisons. In a dramatic way, the evils of both food adulteration and carelessness in handling poisons were demonstrated. The Bradford disaster concerned a manufacturer of cheap peppermint lozenges, who habitually substituted plaster of Paris for part of the sugar used in their production. Towards the end of October 1858, the manufacturer, in readiness for market day, sent to a local druggist for twelve pounds of "daff", the name used to disguise the adulterant. The druggist was ill in bed and his assistant, who had been with him only a few weeks on trial with a view to his being apprenticed, was left in charge of the shop. Not knowing what "daff" was, he went to his master's room to inquire. He was told it was a white powder kept in a cask in a corner of the attic, but was not warned that nearby was another cask containing white arsenic and that neither cask had visible labels. The lad finding a cask with white powder (which proved to be arsenic), took the quantity required and supplied it to the manufacturer. It was made into lozenges (with sugar and oil of peppermint) which were sold in the market at less than a penny an ounce. Each lozenge contained about ten grains of arsenic. Twenty persons lost their life and nearly two hundred were made seriously ill. The parties implicated in the affair were put on trial for manslaughter and acquitted, the druggist being merely censured for not having the arsenic cask properly labelled.

The publicity the Bradford catastrophe received almost compelled the Government to again take in hand the regulation of the sale of poisons. A new bill was brought forward early in the session of 1859, this time in the House of Commons and in the charge of Spencer Walpole. In this bill many of the proposals to which the Pharmaceutical Society had objected in earlier bills were modified or abandoned. There was no mention of a purchaser's certificate nor of the examining board. The schedule of poisons was much reduced. The main features of this bill were provisions for labelling vessels or packets containing poisons, in stock and when sold, and for keeping records of sales. Power was given to constables on magistrates' orders to search any shop where poisons were sold. The Pharmaceutical Society urged the Home Secretary to recognise the importance of qualification for vendors of poisons; Spencer Walpole agreed with the reasoning, but refused to add any clauses to his bill. He promised to deal with the matter in a separate measure. The bill passed through the committee stage in the Commons but was then withdrawn in the face of growing opposition. The Government was shortly afterwards defeated on its Parliamentary Reform bill and parliament was dissolved.

There were no more poisons bills until in 1863 Lord Raynham introduced into the House of Commons a short one "for the prevention of accidental poisoning". The bill was summarily rejected when a second reading was sought. Yet, in the same year, a report appeared which showed that the movement for government regulation of the sale of poisons, far from collapsing, was gaining strength. In 1858 Dr. John Simon had been appointed medical officer of health to the Privy Council, a position he held until 1871. In his *Sixth*

Report to the Privy Council, Simon put forward what he considered to be an incontrovertible case for state interference in the practice of pharmacy in Britain. Simon's plan of reform included the examination and licensing of all chemists entitled to dispense poisons, the registration of all sales of poisons and the regulation of the trade in general by the Privy Council (i.e. in effect, by himself). Although Simon's report was regarded at the time, and has been regarded since, as an authoritative, objective inquiry into the keeping, vending and dispensing of poisons and into criminal and accidental poisoning, it should be seen more as a well-timed, forcefully presented piece of propaganda. The report's reputation was founded on the official status of its author and the authority of the Privy Council. Read without such preconceptions, the report can be seen to comprise highly selective evidence, tendentious reasoning, a series of non-sequiturs, and a list of recommendations which seem to have only a peripheral bearing on the problems identified.

Simon begins his report by suggesting that the Registrar General's figures, which indicate that between four to five hundred people die each year from poisoning may seriously underestimate the extent of the problem.

> The list of deaths by poison is at best only the list of the fatal poisonings which are discovered. But here is a cause of death which is peculiarly apt to be undiscovered. For the murderous poisoner of course plans not to be found out. And the accidental poisoner—the careless dispenser, for instance, who supplies a poison instead of an innocent medicine, is at first unaware of his mistake, and may perhaps never be made aware of it.

If the official statistics represent merely the tip of the iceberg, it is important to consider "what security the public enjoys against an indefinite multiplication of such cases". Professor A.S. Taylor was therefore invited by the Privy Council to draw upon his long experience and report on two questions, which had been carefully formulated by Simon:

> (1) to what extent is injury occasioned by the carelessness and incompetence of persons employed in retailing drugs; and (2) to what extent are unnecessary facilities given for the purchase of poison for criminal purposes.

It is not surprising that Taylor's report pointed to a very unsatisfactory state of affairs. First, with reference to the ease with which poison may be obtained for criminal purposes, Dr. Taylor concluded that:

> so long as a person of any age has the command of threepence, he can procure for this sum a sufficient quantity of one of the most deadly poisons to destroy the lives of two adults ... No one wishing to destroy another by poison ... can meet with any difficulty in carrying out his design. If refused at one shop, he can procure the poison at another. If refused by a druggist, he can procure it at a grocer's. If refused at a grocer's, he can procure it at a village general shop ...

In spite of the Arsenic Act, uncoloured arsenic is still used as the instrument of murder.

> Its great cheapness (one penny to twopence an ounce) places it within the reach of the poorest persons. It is sold to any applicant on the most frivolous pretences ... The better class of druggists do not sell arsenic by retail; the grocer, chandler, oilman, and village shopkeeper are the principal vendors of this poison; and it is

> clear from the numerous deaths which take place from white arsenic that they set
> the law at defiance, and sell the poison in an uncoloured state ...

With the sale of other poisons, there is not even nominal statutory interference; and whether they are wanted for murder, suicide, or procuring abortions, "the lower class of drug-dealers, including grocers, oilmen, and the general shopkeepers of villages" have no scruples in supplying the public.

Dr. Taylor then reported on the consequences of allowing "entirely unskilled and heedless persons" to sell powerful drugs and medicines to the public, on demand, without any check or control. He related

> how, for instance, opium and its tincture have often been given in mistake for
> rhubarb and its tincture,—how oxalic acid and other poisons have again and again
> been given for Epsom salts,—how chloride of zinc has on several occasions been
> given for fluid magnesia,—how arsenic has been given instead of calomel and
> instead of magnesia,—and so forth.

The inevitable results of the incompetence and gross ignorance of those who are allowed to retail drugs, "are increased a hundred-fold by reasons of the carelessness displayed in keeping innocent medicines and poisonous compounds resembling each other on shelves or drawers in close proximity". Thus, in ordinary druggists' shops, tincture of opium and tincture of senna and tincture of rhubarb, like one another in colour, may be found standing side by side on a shelf, in bottles of like size and shape, and with labels which, if only half-read, seem identical. Strychnine may be side by side with jalapine, morphia, salicine and quinine. By far the worst instances of this particular danger are found in village general stores where arrowroot, rice and oatmeal may be found alongside arsenic, corrosive sublimate, and oxalic acid, and all under the care of an ignorant boy.

Cases in which the careless custody of poisons has lead to large scale poisonings were cited in the report: cases of orpiment (arsenical yellow) sold instead of turmeric and used to colour buns, of twelve pounds of arsenic sold instead of twelve pounds of plaster of Paris and used in the manufacture of lozenges, and of thirty pounds of sugar of lead (lead acetate) sent, instead of alum, to a miller in Stourbridge for mixing with eighty sacks of flour. In the Stourbridge case some 500 persons were affected (none fatally but some with great severity) by the poisoning of their bread with lead. Taylor also described how, in 1856, 340 children of the Norwood school took, with their morning milk-and-water, about one grain of arsenic each, because a workman had left arsenite of soda in the boiler he was cleaning.

Simon also drew on the reports he had commissioned from Dr. Edward Greenhow and Dr. Henry Julian Hunter on infant mortality in the manufacturing districts and the Fens to point an accusing finger at those who sold opium without restriction by law or conscience. Simon summed up his case vividly:

> The absence of special enactment on the subject seems in most instances to be
> accepted as a ground for concluding that a druggist's carelessness and malpractice,
> however extreme in degree, and however fatal in result, are not in the eye of the
> law criminal carelessness and malpractice. Thus, in nearly all the scandalous cases
> which Dr. Taylor describes, the tradesmen whose ill-conducted business led to loss
> or endangerment of life escaped with absolute impunity ... Even in the Bradford
> case, where, in 1858, 9,200 persons were poisoned, and seventeen of them fatally,

through the sale of arsenic for plaster of Paris, it was ruled that no legal carelessness had been committed ... Evidently this state of things implies more than the legislature can mean to sanction: it implies not merely that the right-doing druggist shall be free from interference, but that the wrong-doing druggist shall be almost secure from punishment.

John Simon wanted the Pharmaceutical Society to become an exclusive, regulatory organisation under the close supervision of the Privy Council. He believed the Society should build upon and reinforce the division between pharmaceutical chemists and the rest of the trade. An Act was needed to divide retail chemists into an upper and lower class. The upper class would initially consist of those who had passed an examination as either pharmaceutical chemists or apothecaries, together with those chemists, who at the time of the enactment, were in practice on their own account, provided their trade was exclusively pharmaceutical. Subsequently, admission to this class, whose members alone would be allowed to sell poisons, would be obtained by passing an examination. The purchase of poisons by the public would be subject to the regulation "which now ineffectually relates to the purchase of arsenic".[50]

* * *

It was not until 11 May 1868 that the Pharmaceutical Society's bill to regulate the sale of poisons and alter and amend the Pharmacy Act, 1852, was introduced in the House of Lords, but it was then brought in under very favourable circumstances. Although the Conservative Government did not, in the end, take charge of it, they did not oppose it. Earl Granville, a leading Liberal politician, who had served as Lord President of the Council between 1858 and 1866, and eleven years earlier had introduced the first comprehensive poisons bill, undertook the task of piloting the bill through the House of Lords. Granville was influenced as much by John Simon as by the Council of the Pharmaceutical Society. Simon kept close tags on the Society's bill and used all his political influence to mould it to his liking. The bill was read a second time on 28 May. There was no discussion on the second reading but when it was considered in committee on 15 June, several issues were raised. Earl Granville explained that the object of the bill was to provide for the safety of the public by compelling all persons keeping shop for the selling of poisons, and all chemists and druggists, to undergo an examination before the Pharmaceutical Society as to their practical knowledge; and no person was to be permitted to keep a shop for the sale of poisonous drugs, or to call himself a "chemist and druggist" unless duly registered. As a further precaution, the bill required that every box or bottle in which any poison was to be sold should be labelled with the name of the article, the word "poison", and the name and address of the seller. Lord Vaux of Harrowden urged that the bill's operation should be extended to Ireland, but the Lord Chancellor and other peers thought it better to draw up a separate bill for Ireland. Lord Redesdale pressed persistently for a clause requiring that poisons be sold only in a peculiarly shaped "poison-bottle"; on the third reading, he took a division on this suggestion and was defeated by 45 votes to 39. The Duke of Marlborough, the Lord President of the Council, obviously instructed by John Simon, made the most significant interventions. He quoted Simon's 1863 report to show the danger to life from the indiscriminate sale of poisons. The Pharmaceutical Society, he continued, was a voluntary body but since it stood alone, having come forward in the public interest to promote examinations, it was not unreasonable that it should have the advantage, which the bill would confer, of conducting throughout the country such examinations of chemists as were necessary for the protection of the public. But as these examinations were to be made compulsory upon all persons undertaking the trade, it was necessary that the Government should have some control over the mode in which the examination was to be conducted. He had therefore proposed an amendment, to which Earl Granville had assented, which would give the Privy Council the authority to see that these examinations were conducted in a proper manner and would also give the Pharmaceutical Society the power to make regulations for the general sale of poisons, subject to the approval of the Privy Council. It was better to look to such regulations as the means of effecting public security than to attempt to embody every minute detail in the strict terms of an Act of Parliament.

The Duke of Marlborough then persuaded the Lords to remove an exemption in respect of poisons bought for photography. In conclusion, he drew attention to the fact that opium and its preparations had been omitted from the schedule of poisons. There was, he said, ample evidence that opium and its preparations were extensively sold in many parts of Britain and was used by men and women and given to infants. The reports on the subject were most distressing and revealed much destruction of life. He would, therefore, be glad to see opium added to the schedule. The Duke of Marlborough knew perfectly well that the Pharmaceutical Society had omitted opium from the poisons schedule under pressure from its own members. An early draft of the bill had provided for the regulation of the sale of opium, but, in June 1867, a deputation of druggists living in Stamford, Sleaford, Lincoln, Peterborough, Norwich and Gainsborough convinced the Pharmaceutical Society's Council that such regulation was undesirable. Elias Bremridge told the Pharmacy Bill Committee of the General Medical Council that:

> the promoters of the bill received such strong representations from chemists residing principally in Cambridgeshire, Lincolnshire and Norfolk against interfering with their business—opium, as they stated, being one of their chief articles of trade— that the promoters felt compelled to strike opium out of Schedule A.[51]

By raising the issue in the Lords, the Lord President of the Council ensured its consideration in the Commons. The bill was read a third time in the Lords on 18 June 1868.

The bill passed through several hands in the Commons. At first it was in the charge of T.E. Headlam, a lawyer and Liberal M.P. for Newcastle, but it was later transferred to Lord Elcho, a Conservative, and in its final stages was taken up by A.S. Ayrton. It was ironic that Ayrton, the radical member for Tower Hamlets, a convinced free trader and opponent of government intervention, should have had a hand in adding to the statute book an act which gave the Pharmaceutical Society and the Privy Council such wide ranging powers over the British drug trade. In the Commons, Robert Lowe, who was a close friend of John Simon and had been carefully primed by him, fought to convert the Pharmaceutical Society's bill into an Act which would incorporate the policies and enhance the powers of the medical officer of the Privy Council. Robert Lowe was already a leading politician. In 1862, while vice-president of the Committee of Council on education, he had been responsible for introducing the policy of "payment by results" in elementary education. In the years 1866-7 he had led the opposition to parliamentary reform. Under Gladstone, he became Chancellor of the Exchequer (1868–73) and Home Secretary (1873–4). Lowe had the distinction of replacing A.S. Ayrton as the most thoroughly disliked member of the House of Commons.

The Sale of Poisons and Pharmacy Act Amendment bill was read for a first time in the Commons on 22 June and a second time, again without debate, on 29 June 1868. On 7 and 10 July Robert Lowe intervened to ensure discussion of the bill. He suspected, with good cause, that Headlam was hoping to see the bill pass through committee in the early hours of the morning without any debate. Lowe maintained that the bill was "a measure of very great importance to the country and particularly to those who vend poisons". The main question was "whether powers of licensing persons to sell dangerous drugs shall be entrusted to persons who are in truth a mere voluntary association. The Government ought to obtain some security from this voluntary association that the provisions of the bill will be properly carried into effect". He hoped, therefore, that "the Government will give some facilities for discussing its principle". When, however, Lowe argued that the bill should not be allowed to pass through parliament that session, Headlam reminded him that the country demanded a poisons bill and Lowe would have to take the responsibility if this bill were rejected.

Once the decision to press on had been made, Lowe proposed amendment after amendment. By his first amendment, registration was made compulsory on all chemists in business. The proposal in the bill was to leave them free to register or not. Headlam explained that the bill had been framed in accordance with the suggestions of the 1865 Select Committee and had been circulated all over the country: chemists would consider there had been a breach of faith if registration were made compulsory. But the Home Secretary argued that "there ought to be a list of all persons who sell poisonous drugs" and Lowe made the obvious point that "unless this registration be insisted upon the Act will not work at all". The Pharmaceutical Society had, since its foundation, favoured compulsory registration. The amendment was carried without a division. Lowe then objected to the proposal in the first clause, giving to the Pharmaceutical Society the initiative in making regulations respecting the keeping and selling of poisons. "The Act ought to be placed under the care of the police and in the hands of a department of the Government", he argued, "and certainly not left in the hands of those who will live by the sale of poisons; if that be so, the restrictions imposed will be of little value". Lord Robert Montagu, the vice-president of the Committee of the Privy Council, not surprisingly, supported Lowe. "The point is", he said, "to restrict the sale of poisons, and probably the Pharmaceutical Society will not publish all the necessary restrictions if the matter be quite left to them. I think the matter should be left with the Privy Council". Henry Austin Bruce, a good friend of both Simon and Lowe, put the case even more strongly:

> more power should, on the part of the public, be given to the Privy Council. There is a medical department of the Council and more power should be given to the chief officer of it, in order that he may say what evils arise from the present practice of selling poisons. It is a department of the State acting for the public interests.

Headlam admitted that "there ought to be some regulations relating to the sale of poisons" but added that "these regulations ought in the first instance to be framed by the Pharmaceutical Society. Then ... they ought to go before the Privy Council for their sanction and approval". Thomas Cave agreed: "I think there will be a great advantage to the public if this matter be left with the Pharmaceutical Society".

Robert Lowe did not press his amendment on this point but the support of several influential M.P.s led him to carry to division his proposal to leave to the Privy Council exclusively the right to make additions to the schedule of poisons. He made use of the fact that opium had been excluded from the schedule to ram home his point. "If there be one poison more used than another, it is opium in various forms, and this will not come under any regulations, not being named in the schedule. The Pharmaceutical Society would leave it out, and it is a most dangerous poison. Perhaps because more profit is got out of the sale of this poison, it is not proposed to deal with it". Headlam's response was equally robust. "What is proposed is to get rid of the Pharmaceutical Society in this matter, and then to enact that another gentleman, the medical officer of the Privy Council, for that will be the effect of it, shall by his own ipse dixit declare what is a poison and what is not. I think that will be most objectionable". Sir R. Collier backed Headlam. "It appears to me that the Pharmaceutical Society will know more about this matter than the Privy Council and that they will attend to it in a much better manner". A.S. Ayrton opposed the whole idea of a poisons schedule. Scientific experts (he had Taylor and Simon in mind) talked "a vast lot of nonsense" on the subject. "Chemists will enlarge their list of poisons just as they like. The Privy Council will give themselves up to any theory ... and this schedule will grow and grow to the manifest injury of trade in this country". On a division, the clause as originally drafted was approved of by 49 votes to 25. The Pharmaceutical Society retained the initiative in adding to the list of poisons.

The registration of chemists and druggists and their assistants was the next issue to arouse Robert Lowe's attention. Both the General Medical Council and John Simon had wanted all chemists and druggists to prove their qualification by examination before being registered, but the bill's promoters, relying on the precedent of the 1815 Apothecaries Act, had arranged for all those in practice, whether as proprietors or assistants, to be registered without being examined. Lowe intervened in two ways. Section 5 of the 1868 Act was drawn up by him and added at his insistence. By providing for registration without fee, it ensured that the initial mass registration of principals did not swell the coffers of the Pharmaceutical Society. Lowe then opposed the clause allowing registration of assistants without examination. Reluctantly he was prepared to swallow the idea that those who owned shops had property interests to protect and should, therefore, be allowed to register without a test of qualification: but assistants were servants and had no vested interest to preserve. In response, Lord Elcho, who had now taken over the responsibility for the bill, thought it would be very hard on those now dispensing medicines to make them pass the same examination as apprentices entering the trade. As a compromise, Lord Elcho suggested the provision of a "modified examination" for assistants, but Lowe was not appeased. The principle of the bill, he said, was to require education on the part of those who sell poisons. The idea of a modified examination was wholly indefensible. It is said that assistants have a vested interest. "A vested interest in what? A vested interest in ignorance—in not knowing enough to pass the examination usually required". Although Lowe won the argument, Elcho won the vote. The House accepted the compromise solution of a "modified examination".

In the bill as drafted, an exemption from its restrictions was provided for "the retailing of arsenic, oxalic acid, cyanide of potassium or corrosive sublimate for use in manufactures or photography". The exemption in respect of photography had been removed, on the suggestion of the Lord President of the Council, in the House of Lords. Robert Lowe now attacked the exemption in respect of manufactures. "We profess to regulate the sale of poisons by this bill", he said, "yet we propose to leave the most subtle poisons to be sold by ignorant and disqualified persons because it is said they are used and required in ordinary manufactures and household duties. I think it is most absurd to attempt such legislation as this". Lord Elcho warned that "in regulating these matters we must not too much interfere with the trade of the country". "We must not be too doctrinaire", he declared. Lowe won the division by 58 votes to 30 and the exemption was removed.

The seventeenth clause, regulating sales of poisons, gave rise to the most extended and convoluted discussion. Robert Lowe, echoing the views of John Simon, sought to apply the provisions of the Arsenic Act to all poisons. Lord Elcho responded by arguing the Pharmaceutical Society's case. The Arsenic Act regulations, he said, "are so stringent as to make the Act a dead letter". Elcho proposed, and the Commons eventually agreed to, a compromise, which involved dividing the schedule of poisons into two parts: poisons in the second part were subject only to labelling restrictions. Lowe rightly pointed out that both sets of poisons were equally dangerous. Elcho urged the House to respect the views of the Pharmaceutical Society.

> They have done great public service since their incorporation. They have a most excellent school of pharmacy; they have excellent and extensive laboratories; lectures of the highest class are delivered at the institution, and it is a body whose opinions are entitled to respect and consideration.

The Pharmaceutical Society's views, representing as they did a half-way house between the free-traders and the medical officer to the Privy Council, were found acceptable to most M.P.s.

Lowe's work was not yet finished. On his suggestion, the words "opium and all preparations of poppies" were added to the poisons list. This was later changed to "opium and all preparations of opium or of poppies" by the Lords. Section 24 of the 1868 Act, applying the Adulteration of Food Act to the adulteration of drugs, was added at Lowe's insistence, but proved, in practice, a dead letter. Lowe even tried to insert into the Act a clause establishing a legal criterion for culpable carelessness in the sale of drugs and poisons, to render such carelessness a punishable offence. This, as we have seen, was one of John Simon's favourite ideas but the Solicitor-General quashed it in three sentences.

> The question of gross negligence is well known to the law and judges have no difficulty in directing a jury upon this point. A man would not be a bit more criminally liable for gross negligence under this clause than he is by the present law. I really think it would be better not to press the clause.

Lord Robert Montagu, as vice-president of the Committee of Council, had also been carefully instructed by John Simon. He secured the addition of two provisions which strengthened the authority of the medical practitioner in his relation to the chemist and druggist. On Montagu's suggestion it was made an offence to compound any medicines of the *British Pharmacopoeia* except according to its formularies. He also secured the insertion of a clause which stated that "registration under this Act shall not entitle any person so registered to practise medicine or surgery, or any branch of medicine or surgery". This latter clause was part of Simon's attempt to use the Poisons and Pharmacy bill to make counter prescribing illegal. Robert Lowe was drawn into this conspiracy. At the report stage of the bill's passage, when it might be assumed that all major issues had already been considered, Lowe tried to slip a short phrase into the seventeenth section of the bill, which would have had the effect of severely restricting self-medication and counter prescribing. Lowe's amendment would have prevented chemists and druggists from selling poisons as medicines except "under the written prescription of a legally qualified medical practitioner". "If you say that chemists and druggists may dispense anything they please themselves", said Lowe, "they will be able to make up compounds of the most deadly poisons and sell them as they like, and this Act will not stop them or give any remedy against them, and consequently all your precautions will go for nothing". Lowe's proposal would have given the medical profession complete control of the supply of powerful drugs to the public. "What my right honourable friend seems anxious to do", pointed out Lord Elcho, "is to prevent any dispensing whatever, except under the signature of some legally qualified medical practitioner". Elcho went on to complain that Lowe had given no warning of this amendment which, if carried, would constitute a breach of contract between the House and the Pharmaceutical Society. Only sixteen M.P.s were left in the chamber: they rejected Lowe's amendment by 14 votes to 2.

The report stage of the bill was successfully used by Lowe's opponents to pull a fast one on him. A.S. Ayrton carried an amendment striking out from clause 2 the words authorising the Pharmaceutical Society and the Privy Council to add new substances to the schedule of poisons, on the grounds that "it is a power which the Privy Council ought not to have under any circumstances whatever", since it "might very materially interfere with the trade of this country". Lowe protested in vain. The amendment, he said, "is equivalent to saying that there shall be no new poison defined without a new Act of Parliament". It was now Lowe's turn to complain of "a breach of faith with the House". He accused the Pharmaceutical Society and Lord Elcho of conspiring to get the amendment carried. If this were in fact the case, their triumph was short-lived. Simon arranged for the words to be restored when the House of Lords considered the Commons' amendments, and, in the end, the Commons acquiesced.

During the passage of the 1868 Act the clause exempting all chemists and druggists from jury service was struck out, without discussion. This decision was the death-knell of the United Society of Chemists and Druggists. The passage of the Poisons and Pharmacy bill through parliament demonstrated how feeble the influence of the United Society was in the corridors of power. The Society's principal demands were unceremoniously rejected by parliament: exemption from jury service, voluntary registration, and admission of assistants to the register of chemists and druggists. Once the bill entered parliament, the Pharmaceutical Society became the one and only representative of the British drug trade and the struggle was between it and the medical officer of the Privy Council. Much of the ground conceded to the United Society in the preliminary discussions was regained by the Pharmaceutical Society as the bill went through parliament. The Council of the Pharmaceutical Society could not be expected to regret the loss of clauses in their bill which had only been included under duress.[52]

NOTES AND REFERENCES TO CHAPTER FIVE

1. William Dickinson, *The Unconstitutional and Illegal Proceedings of the Council of the Pharmaceutical Society* (1853) 35
2. *Annals of Pharmacy and Practical Chemistry; a monthly record of British and Foreign materia medica, pharmacy and chemistry, theoretical and technical* 2 (1853) 209
3. *C. & D.* 22 (1880) 435
4. *Annals of Pharmacy* 3 (1854) 17–9, 83–4
5. *P.J.* 13 (1853–4) 345–8
6. *An address to the Chemists and Druggists of the United Kingdom, issued by the Committee of the British Association of Chemists and Druggists* (1854)
7. *P.J.* 76 (1906) 280
8. *P.J.* 13 (1853–4) 300–2
9. *P.J.* 13 (1853–4) 198–9
10. *C. & D.* (1900) 134
11. *P.J.* 3 [2] (1861–2) 201–2
12. *P.J.* 2 [2] (1860–1) 538
13. *P.J.* 2 [2] (1860–1) 590–601
14. *C. & D.* 2 (1861) 193–5
15. *P.J.* 3 [2] (1861–2) 592; 4 [2] (1862–3) 1
16. *C. & D.* 1 (1859–60) 266–7
17. *C. & D.* 2 (1861) 69–72
18. *C. & D.* 2 (1861) 40
19. *C. & D.* 1 (1859–60) 385
20. *C. & D.* 2 (1861) 40
21. *C. & D.* 3 (1862) 144–5
22. *C. & D.* 3 (1862) 61–2
23. *C. & D.* 3 (1862) 79–80, 121–2
24. *P.J.* 3 [2] (1861–2) 489–90
25. *P.J.* 3 [2] (1861–2) 192
26. *P.J.* 4 [2] (1862–3) 93–102, 285–6
27. *C. & D.* 3 (1862) 335
28. *C. & D.* 3 (1862) 181–2; 4 (1863) 151–9; 5 (1864) 134–6
29. *P.J.* 5 [2] (1863–4) 1–2, 45–6, 93–5, 285
30. *P.J.* 5 [2] (1863–4) 484–5
31. *C. & D.* 5 (1864) 33–6, 39–41, 134–6
32. *C. & D.* 2 (1861) 255
33. *P.J.* 5 [2] (1863–4) 429–31
34. *P.J.* 5 [2] (1863–4) 589–91
35. *P.J.* 5 [2] (1863–4) 444–59
36. 1865 (78) I 107
37. 1865 (84) I 115
38. *P.J.* 6 [2] (1864–5) 298–9
39. *C. & D.* 6 (1865) 33–4
40. *Hansard* CLXXVIII (1865) 470–9
41. *Special Report from the Select Committee on the Chemists and Druggists Bill and Chemists and Druggists (No.2) Bill*, 1865 (381) XII 303
42. *P.J.* 6 [2] (1864–5) 474–6
43. *P.J.* 5 [2] (1863–4) 618–9

44. *P.J.* 6 [2] (1864–5) 476–8
45. *P.J.* 7 [2] (1865–6) 1–2
46. *P.J.* 7 [2] (1865–6) 538–9
47. Royston Lambert, *Sir John Simon 1816–1904 and English Social Administration* (1963)
48. Edward Seaton (ed.), *Public Health Reports by John Simon* (1887) I 150–2, 155–6
49. *Report from the Select Committee of the House of Lords on the Sale of Poisons Bill*, 1857 Session II (294) XII, 551.
50. Edward Seaton (ed.), *Public Health Reports by John Simon* (1887) I, 541–550 and *P.J.* 6 [2] (1864–5) 141–2, 172–88
51. V. Berridge and G. Edwards, *Opium and the People* (1987)
52. *P.J.* 10 [2] (1868–9) 35–41, 57–76

CHAPTER SIX

The 1908 Pharmacy Act

In phiala bene obturata—In a well-stoppered bottle

The 1868 Pharmacy Act—Drug adulteration—The Chemists Defence Association—*The British Pharmacopoeia*—Proprietary medicines—Chloro-dyne—Patent medicines defined—The 1869 Pharmacy Amendment Act—John Simon, the Privy Council and the Pharmaceutical Society—The opposition to regulations for the storage and sale of poisons—The Chemists and Druggists Trade Association—Dentistry—Women in pharmacy—The Pharmacy Acts Amendment Act of 1898—*The Pharmaceutical Society v. The London and Provincial Supply Association*—The multiples, department stores, and co-operative societies—Company trading and professionalism—Unqualified assistants—Carbolic acid and the Privy Council—The Departmental Committee on the Poisons Schedule, 1901–3—*The Pharmaceutical Society v. The Company Chemists*—A maze of pharmacy bills—The Poisons and Pharmacy Act, 1908.

The words of the 1868 Pharmacy Act caused trouble for half-a-century. "It is impossible to disguise the fact that this statute is characterised by great ambiguity, I would almost go to the length of saying confusion of language", observed Lord Watson in 1880. The problem stemmed, in his view,

> from the circumstance that the framers of this Act were dealing with two separate matters: the one, improvements of a society called the Pharmaceutical Society; the other, the regulation of the sale of poisons generally throughout Great Britain.[1]

The Act had a long and stressful gestation. The Pharmaceutical Society, the United Society of Chemists and Druggists and the Government fought one another over its contents. In its passage through Parliament each clause became a tug-of-war between the Pharmaceutical Society and the medical officer of the Privy Council. In its final form the Act was more a patchwork quilt of amendments than a seamless web of legislative thought. After so difficult a birth, the Act remained troublesome throughout its life. Although its words stayed the same, their meaning altered with changing circumstances. Unravelling that meaning proved a lengthy and expensive process.

No summary can do justice to the complexity of the 1868 Act's provisions. The most tangible products of the Act were the registers. Since 1852 the Pharmaceutical Society had had the statutory duty of compiling a register of pharmaceutical chemists. In 1868 it acquired the added obligation of publishing a register of chemists and druggists. Although the new register included the names of pharmaceutical chemists, a separate register of pharmaceutical chemists continued to be published. It contained the names of all members of the Pharmaceutical Society and of all who had passed the Major examination without becoming members. After 1868 passing the Major examination became the sole qualification for admittance to this register, an honour which brought with it exemption from jury service. Although the register of chemists and druggists was a single list of names arranged in alphabetical order of surnames, it comprised several categories of practitioners. The list included the pharmaceutical chemists and all persons who had, at any time prior to the passing of the Act, been proprietors in Great Britain of shops for the compounding of prescriptions of qualified medical men. It also included those assistants who either were associates of the Pharmaceutical Society or had passed the Minor examination. Assistants, who had neither joined the Pharmaceutical Society nor passed its examination, could become registered as chemists and druggists by passing the newly-instituted "modified" examination, provided they had been employed as assistants for a period of not less than three years. In future, however, the sole qualification for admittance to the register of chemists and druggists would be passing the Minor examination.

A chemist and druggist who wanted to register as a person in practice before the Act was required to furnish declarations that he "was in business as a chemist and druggist in the keeping of open shop for the compounding of the prescriptions of duly qualified medical practitioners". The magistrates and doctors who were required to endorse these declarations did so without paying too much attention to the precise wording of the schedule. Elias Bremridge, the registrar, was too busy and too diplomatic to challenge the validity of the declarations he received. Consequently, no one who ran a chemist's shop had any difficulty in getting his name on the register, even though he may never have dispensed a medical prescription in his life. This was a great disappointment for those members of the Pharmaceutical Society who thought the wording of the schedules would effectively exclude from the register all save bona-fide dispensing chemists. John Simon also was dismayed by the open-door policy. There was, however, no alternative. The registrar had neither the inclination nor the authority to question the integrity of magistrates and medical practitioners. Had he done so, he would have aroused the opposition of the general public, many members of parliament and the majority of chemists and druggists. "Let sleeping dogs lie" was the appropriate response to the declarations he received.

For registration purposes, chemists and druggists were defined in the 1868 Act as persons keeping open shop for the compounding of medical prescriptions. The Pharmaceutical Society was wedded to this definition. It had long sought to obtain for its members a monopoly of the dispensing of prescriptions. The bill adopted by its Council in 1865 would have restricted "the dispensing or compounding of all prescriptions of physicians and surgeons" to examined and qualified chemists. The Government, however, was not keen to interfere with the dispensing of medicines: the sale of poisons was its problem. Hence, the 1868 Act created a register of persons qualified "to sell or keep open shop for retailing, dispensing or compounding poisons". Chemists and druggists were licensed to sell poisons, not to dispense medicines. In practice, the distinction was not so clear-cut: the registered chemist alone had the right to dispense "poisonous" prescriptions. The Pharmaceutical Society did not give up its attempt to secure for qualified chemists a monopoly of the dispensing of all prescriptions. Provisions to this effect appeared in the bills to amend the Pharmacy Act promoted by the Society in 1881, 1891 and 1899.

240

The 1868 Act reserved to registered persons the right to assume, use, and exhibit certain titles, namely, "chemist and druggist", "chemist", "druggist", "pharmacist", and "dispensing chemist or druggist". The titles "pharmaceutical chemist" and "pharmaceutist" were already reserved under the 1852 Pharmacy Act to those whose names appeared in the register of pharmaceutical chemists.

The restriction of these titles was a very considerable commercial asset. The unqualified drug seller was forced to take up titles such as "herbalist" or "medical botanist" and to describe his shop as a "drug store" or a "medical hall". The use of the word "pharmacy" to describe a shop where medicines were sold, first gained currency in the hands of unregistered practitioners. The Pharmaceutical Society took the view that the unqualified were debarred from using not only the titles specified in the Act but also any name or title suggesting or implying registration. The law courts tended to agree. In the 1890s the Society obtained two important decisions in Scotland. In *Bremridge v. Hume*, the defendant carried on business as a scientific instrument maker. He had a thorough knowledge of chemistry but was not registered under the Pharmacy Acts. In a printed advertisement and price list he described himself as a "scientific instrument maker and technical chemist". He was held to have contravened the 1868 Act by using the name of "chemist". In *Bremridge v. Turnbull* the defendant was a dealer in photographic requisites and had over his shop a sign designating him as a "photographic chemist". It was held that, as he was not registered, this was an infringement of the 1868 Act. In England the Pharmaceutical Society successfully prosecuted unqualified persons for using such titles as "botanic chemist", "analytical chemist", "shipping druggist", and "photographic chemist". But the decision of the House of Lords in 1880 that the word "person" in the 1868 Act did not include corporate bodies was a severe setback. It meant that companies owned by unqualified persons were free to use the terms that the Act reserved to registered individuals. In the 1868 Act the right to assume protected titles was placed on the same footing as the right to keep open shop for the sale of poisons. In 1880 corporations acquired both: they did not hesitate to use the titles in advertising and in the external description of their premises. The Pharmaceutical Society argued that the object of the Pharmacy Acts of 1852 and 1868 was to create a special right to the titles in persons who had qualified themselves by study and examination. It claimed that the titles were as personal and inalienable as the titles "physician" and "surgeon". It was difficult to sustain this argument. Leading firms of chemists and druggists in London and the provinces retained, purely for trade purposes, names other than those of the persons who carried on the business. John Bell & Co. and Savory and Moore were well known examples of a large class. Within the 1868 Act itself, there was provision for executors to carry on the business of a deceased chemist, in his name and with his titles, provided a qualified assistant was in charge. Jesse Boot argued that, while terms such as "pharmaceutical chemist" and "pharmacist" might properly be reserved to holders of professional qualifications, the words "chemist" and "druggist" traditionally described a type of business, and should be available to anyone engaged in it. In 1868, of course, no one contemplated the possibility of multiple, department and co-operative stores selling drugs and medicines. The premise of the 1868 Act was that the retail trade in pharmacy would be conducted by individual proprietors exercising personal control over their establishment.

The 1868 Act continued the process started by the Arsenic Act of 1851 by prescribing

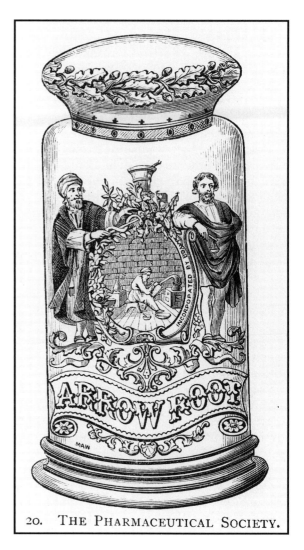

20. THE PHARMACEUTICAL SOCIETY.

42 *Taken from the Book of Illustrations to the* Quarterly Price-Current *of S. Maw Son & Thompson, a catalogue of medical, surgical and pharmaceutical supplies, 1882. The specie jar is decorated with a motif based on the supporters taken from the Society's coat of arms. Adapted in a variety of designs, this became a popular form of decoration on pharmaceutical objects, stationery and advertising in the nineteenth century.*

precautions to be taken in the sale of poisons. Fifteen selected poisons were listed in a two-part schedule. Those in the first part (which included cyanide of potassium, strychnine and corrosive sublimate) could be sold only if the purchaser were known to the seller or had been introduced by someone known to the seller. A detailed entry was to be made in the poisons register of the date of the sale, name and address of purchaser, name and quantity of the article sold, and the purpose for which it was wanted. The container itself had to be clearly labelled "poison", with the name of the article and the name and address of the seller. Only these labelling restrictions applied to poisons in Part 2 of the schedule (which included oxalic acid, belladonna, chloroform and opium). Medicines containing poisons, however, had merely to be labelled with the name and address of the seller; but, in addition, the chemist had to write the prescription and the name of the person to whom the medicine was sold

242

or delivered in a prescription- book. Such regulations could hardly be regarded as onerous. There was, moreover, ample compensation: the inclusion of a substance in the poisons schedule gave chemists and apothecaries a monopoly of its sale. The 1868 Act referred, in sections 1 and 15, to regulations for the keeping and selling of poisons which would have been binding on chemists and druggists alone. But it took the Pharmaceutical Society until January 1899 to issue such regulations.

The obligations under the 1868 Act, like the privileges, were greater in theory than in practice. Section 24 of the Act extended to medicines the provisions of the Adulteration of Food and Drink Act of 1860 and Section 15 made it an offence to compound medicines of the *British Pharmacopoeia* except in accordance with its formularies. However admirable the intentions may have been, the lack of means of enforcement meant that these provisions remained dead letters. It was not until 1872 that comprehensive official control of adulterated drugs was introduced and not until 1875 that any action was taken.[2]

None of the British nineteenth century legislation dealt with the fundamental questions of what constituted drug adulteration and how the existence and degree of adulteration were to be determined. No standards or limits of purity were recognised. The principal elements of the legal definitions of adulteration centred on the intent and knowledge of the manufacturer and vendor. The public analysts appointed under the Sale of Food and Drugs Act of 1875 began by taking a very serious view of their new responsibilities. Their reports gave the impression that not only were drugs frequently adulterated but even the dispensing of prescriptions was rarely performed with adequate care. The chemist who advertised that, in making up prescriptions, "we dispense with accuracy", became a standard joke at this time. The result was decidedly prejudicial to the drug trade.

The majority of early cases brought under the new legislation hinged partly on the problem of an official standard for drugs and partly on questions of trade practice. The resentment of chemists and druggists stemmed largely from the fact that the courts considered it to the prejudice of the purchaser if he asked for any drug, such as mercurial ointment, by a name recognised in the *British Pharmacopoeia*, but instead received one differing at all from its standards. In 1876 several prosecutions were instituted by public analysts against chemists selling milk of sulphur prepared according to the directions of the 1721 *Pharmacopoeia* and consequently containing about sixty per cent of hydrated calcium sulphate. Some of the standards of the *British Pharmacopoeia* were, in fact, inferior to current commercial standards. Some trade practices, made respectable by public acceptance, promoted names that bore no relation to the product itself or else harked back to Pharmacopoeias of former times. The courts, however, did not recognise claims of commercial standards differing from the *British Pharmacopoeia*; but in cases where only the formula or method of preparing a drug, but not its composition, was given in the *Pharmacopoeia*, the courts did not consider this a standard. Such a situation threw a disparaging light on both the drug trade and the administration of the adulteration laws. Analysts tended to concentrate their attention on those products involving "trade questions" and ignored other more flagrant abuses: they also created an unbalanced picture of the real nature and extent of adulteration practices.

The majority of chemists and druggists regarded these proceedings against traditional practices as tyrannical and arbitrary: one of the principal objectives of the Chemists and Druggists' Trade Association was to defend chemists in such cases. It scored a notable early success when the conviction of a Mr. Marshall of Runcorn was quashed by the Knutsford Quarter Sessions. The general reaction of the pharmaceutical and medical press was that it was questionable to treat many of these cases as examples of adulteration and that prosecutions might better concentrate upon products of more immediate concern to public health such as patent medicines. Although the plea of commercial trade standards and time-honoured customs was easily abused, the fact is that the public had been accustomed to expect certain products under names not, or no longer, rationally applicable. The British Pharmaceutical Conference formally condemned non-descriptive trade names. The official view of the Pharmaceutical Society was that fanciful or non-descriptive drug titles was an indefensible trade practice: the correct solution was to call drug preparations by their proper generic names. The Council refused to get involved in the controversies over the sale of effervescent citro-tartrate of soda under the name of "citrate of magnesia"; "milk of sulphur" instead of precipitated sulphur (B.P.); "sweet spirit of nitre" in place of spirit of nitrous ether (B.P.); and "castor oil pills" containing no castor oil. Its refusal, however, contributed to the charges of indifference to trade questions which chemists and druggists repeatedly levelled against the Pharmaceutical Society.

The Society's refusal to defend its members against prosecutions under the adulteration laws led W.S. Glyn-Jones to set up the Chemists' Defence Association in 1899 as an offshoot of his Proprietary Articles Trade Association. The Defence Association was intended to give its members legal advice, to defend them if prosecuted under various trade Acts, to indemnify them against loss for mistakes in dispensing or retailing, to keep them informed about existing laws and on the progress of new legislation, and to watch legislation in the interests of members. The Defence Association was organised as a limited company in which members purchased shares. Glyn-Jones pointed out that his organisation differed materially from previous organisations with similar aims because of the direct benefits accruing to each subscriber. For an annual fee, each member was entitled, if legally prosecuted, to defence up to a value of ten pounds. Besides the services of a well-known lawyer, the Association retained the noted analyst C.G. Moor, author of *Suggested Standards of Purity for Foods and Drugs* (1902). Members were entitled to the free analysis of one sample per year, and might have further analyses made at a stated fee. The Chemists' Defence Association attracted wide attention and a growing membership: the success of its legal proceedings elicited the admiration of non-pharmaceutical organizations.

The Pharmaceutical Society regarded drug adulteration as a professional problem rather than as a trade matter. It sought a solution in professional terms, primarily in the raising of the educational qualifications of pharmaceutical practitioners. It also took the lead in establishing the *British Pharmacopoeia* as a reliable standard for drugs and drug preparations. The increasingly scientific orientation of the *British Pharmacopoeia* in the late nineteenth century was primarily the result of the increased involvement of leading members of the Pharmaceutical Society in its production. When pharmacists first became involved in revising the *Pharmacopoeia*, it was still a recipe book, useful primarily for chemicals and a few "organic" substances, including the vegetable alkaloids, but not for most of the drugs of vegetable and animal origin that formed the bulk of the official materia medica. The *British Pharmacopoeia* appeared under the sponsorship of the General Medical Council, whose members possessed very limited knowledge of pharmacy. It was a wise decision to invite members of the Pharmaceutical Society to participate in the revision of the *Pharmacopoeia* after its disastrous first appearance in 1864. Theophilus Redwood edited the Pharmacopoeias of 1867 and 1885. Leading members of the Pharmaceutical Society realized that, although their work received no official recognition from the General Medical Council, it was their professional duty to help develop higher standards. Following proposals made in 1885, special arrangements were made by the Council of the Pharmaceutical Society for research, related primarily to preparations of the *Pharmacopoeia*, to be carried out in the Society's laboratories. This work was under the direction of John Attfield, the professor of chemistry and director of the laboratories, and H.G. Greenish, the professor of pharmacy and later of pharmaceutics, who reported periodically to a Research Committee of the Society's Council.

The edition of the *British Pharmacopoeia* published in 1898 marked a significant step forward in scientific quality. John Attfield, then president of the British Pharmaceutical Conference, acted as editor. The "assistance of great value . . . rendered" by a special committee of the Pharmaceutical Society was duly acknowledged; and a number of outstanding pharmacists acted as "referees" in special fields, among them the noted botanist and curator of the Society's museum, Edward Morrell Holmes (1843 – 1930) and the former Bell scholar and the expert in essential oils, William A. Tilden (1842–1926). By 1900, however, the work of revising this edition had already begun. The General Medical Council, while still questioning the propriety of recognising the Pharmaceutical Society's role in the preparation of the *Pharmacopoeia*, specifically requested the Society's laboratories to check (1) to what extent the standardization of potent drugs could be carried out with accuracy and success, (2) the percentage of ash in certain drugs, (3) the boiling points of certain substances, and (4) the solubilities of the chemical salts in the *British Pharmacopoeia*. An examination of William Chattaway's *Digest of Researches and Criticisms . . . of the British Pharmacopoeia, 1898* (published in 1903) reveals the extent to which pharmacy contributed to the improvement of the *Pharmacopoeia* and the number of these improvements that first appeared in the *Pharmaceutical Journal*. The work of E.M Holmes, J.C. Umney, J. Barclay and H.G. Greenish deserved more recognition that the General Medical Council was prepared to give.

During the negotiations preceding the enactment of the 1868 Pharmacy Act, the manufacturers of proprietary medicines, with the support of the Commissioners of Inland Revenue, obtained an important concession. Although both the Pharmaceutical Society and the British Medical Association lobbied for restrictions on patent medicines, Section 16 appeared to exempt "the making or dealing in patent medicines" from most of the requirements of the Act. Patent medicines coming within the description of poisons were, however, made subject to the labelling regulations contained in the seventeenth section. Few patent medicines actually deserved the name. Medicinal compounds were rarely patented. Those which were subject to duty were medicines bearing proprietary names protected by trade marks rather than medicines sold under the authority of letters patent.

There was a spectacular upsurge in the sale of proprietary medicines in the 1880s with an increase in working-class purchasing power. From 1855 to 1905 sales increased nearly tenfold while the population just about doubled. The reduction of the medicine licence duty in 1875, however, also led to a marked rise in the number of vendors: over 13,000 licences were taken out in 1874, nearly 20,000 ten years later. The profit to the retail chemist on the sale of proprietary medicines was always small but especially so from the 1870s when

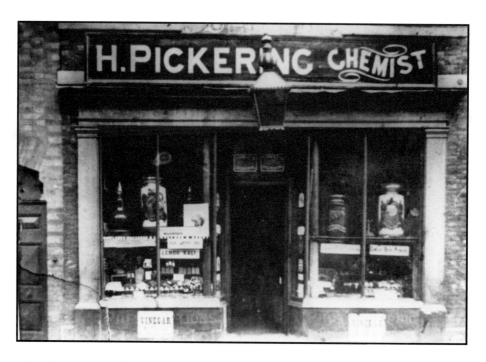

43   *H. Pickering, Chemist, 59½ High Close Street, Leicester, c. 1880. The business was established in 1830. One of the earliest photographs of a shopfront in the Society's museum collection.*

multiple, departmental and co-operative stores joined grocers in selling them at a little above the retailer's wholesale cost. In 1897 the *Chemist and Druggist* lamented that a chemist who sold 2,000 stamped medicines per year would realise a net profit of about £10.

The proprietary medicines offered for sale to the Victorian public ranged from digestive aids and headache powders to cures for syphilis and thinly disguised abortifacients. Many were perfectly harmless, containing little more than soap, sugar, colouring and flavouring. Others contained a moderate amount of active ingredients which did in fact produce their advertised effects upon the taker. A few, however, contained powerful drugs in dangerous concentrations. An analysis of thirteen patent medicines undertaken by the distinguished pharmaceutical chemist, E.F. Harrison, showed that they contained varying amounts of morphine, prussic acid, strychnine and aconite. Only four were labelled "poison" as required by law, and none, of course, actually listed the ingredients on the bottle.

During the 1880s a new campaign was launched to bring proprietary medicines under professional control. Doctors wanted poisonous medicines to be available only on prescription and chemists and druggists wanted to prevent unqualified persons from selling them. Press publicity was given to cases of accidental death caused by taking patent medicines such Holt's Whooping Cough Syrup, Winslow's Soothing Syrup, Martin's Pectoral Balsam and Chlorodyne. Discussions took place between the Home Office, the Privy Council Office, the Institute of Chemistry and the Pharmaceutical Society in 1881 and

1882. No agreement about further legislation could be reached but it was hoped to establish that proprietary medicines did, in fact, already come within the 1868 Act. In January 1882 the Director of Public Prosecutions brought a case at the Hammersmith police-court against a Kensington chemist for selling two bottles of Hunter's Solution of Chloral without labelling them "poison" and without adding the seller's name and address. The medicine was sold with a medicine-stamp attached. The defence argued that the exemption in the sixteenth section of the Pharmacy Act took patent medicines out of the statute but the magistrate decided that the article was a poison and imposed a £2 penalty. The defendant, however, declined to appeal and the situation remained unclear. The Pharmaceutical Society's pharmacy act amendment bill of 1884 would have provided that patent medicines containing poisons should be labelled and sold only by registered chemists; but without government backing the bill was not successful.

The Victorian patent medicine that achieved most notoriety was chlorodyne. The mixture was invented by Dr. John Collis Browne as a cholera remedy while serving with the army in India. Its main ingredients were chloroform and morphia: the name was derived from the words "chloroform" and "anodyne". When Collis Brown left the army in 1856 he went into partnership with John T. Davenport who was then president of the Pharmaceutical Society with premises at 33 Great Russell Street, Bloomsbury. Davenport acquired the sole right to manufacture and market chlorodyne but, despite his many warnings to the public to beware of imitations, he was plagued by competitors. "Towle's Chlorodyne" and "Teasdale's Chlorodyne" were soon on the market. "Freeman's Original Chlorodyne" became the subject of an unsuccessful lawsuit brought by Collis Browne in the early 1860s. Another president of the Pharmaceutical Society, Peter Squire of Oxford Street made his own version and virtually every chemist in Britain followed suit.

Chlorodyne was advertised as a cure for a wide range of common ills: "Coughs, Colds, Colic, Cramp, Spasms, Stomach Ache, Bowel Pains, Diarrhoea, Sleeplessness". Its success was due to the fact that it worked: the formula, which made it such an effective medicine, also made it potentially lethal. While Davenport's sales climbed from £28,000 in 1871 to £31,000 twenty years later, the inquest records filled with the victims: suicides, accidental overdoses, chlorodyne addicts.[3]

The professional scare about chlorodyne was the core of a medical campaign against proprietary medicines conducted in the 1890s and 1900s by Ernest Hart, editor of the *British Medical Journal* and chairman of the B.M.A.'s Parliamentary Bills Committee. It was this committee which instigated the action against chlorodyne and its manufacturer. For general practitioners the widespread consumption of patent medicines meant a loss of income from and control over their patients. In 1892 the Treasury Solicitor prosecuted J.T. Davenport "for having unlawfully sold by retail opium and chloroform contained in a preparation known as Dr. Collis Browne's chlorodyne, without distinctly labelling the wrapper of the bottle . . . with the word 'poison.'" Dr. August Dupre and Dr. B.H. Paul, the editor of the *Pharmaceutical Journal*, proved that their analyses of the article yielded a proportion of two grains of morphia to the ounce and a certain quantity of chloroform. Davenport's defence was that the preparation was a patent one and hence exempt under Section 16 of the 1868 Act. The magistrate, however, took a strict definition of the term: a patent medicine was one "exposed to sale under the authority of any letters patent under the Great Seal", and not one merely paying the medicine duty. The charge was held to be proven and Davenport was fined £5 with five guineas cost.

247

The Association of Owners of Proprietary Medicines and the Grocers' Associations were far from happy with this verdict and decided to contest this new interpretation of the Act. However two cases (1893 – 4) settled the matter. The judge in *Pharmaceutical Society v. Piper & Co.*, stated:

> In my opinion, no satisfactory case has been made in favour of sweeping the very large class of proprietary medicines into the immunity extended to patent medicines, the object of the Act being for the safety of the public to ensure that compounds into which a scheduled poison enters ... shall only be dispensed by persons having a technical knowledge of their properties. Can there be anything more dangerous than to allow a medicine which is called a proprietary medicine, but which may contain poison to any amount, to be sold or compounded by any unskilled person who chooses to compound or sell it? ... That mischief does not exist in the case of patent medicines, for any one can find out the exact ingredients used in them, but the case is altogether different with those which are merely the subject of some proprietary right.

This case was followed and approved by the Court of Appeal in the *Pharmaceutical Society v. Armson*. An action was brought to recover the penalty

> incurred by the defendant in keeping open shop for retailing, dispensing or compounding of poisons, to wit—morphine, or a preparation of opium, contained in and forming part of an article called 'Powell's Balsam of Aniseed', contrary to the provisions of the Pharmacy Act, 1868, sec. 15.

The defendant was a grocer and it was contended, on his behalf, that the article sold by him was a proprietary one which came within the meaning of patent medicines in section 16 and was therefore exempt. The Court of Queen's Bench decided otherwise.

> The reason for the exemption seems to me very clear indeed. Where the medicine is properly speaking a patent medicine,—that is to say, where the exclusive right to make or sell it has been granted to somebody by letters patent under the Great Seal,—the condition of the patent always is, that a specification should be lodged in the Patent Office, describing the whole of the ingredients, and the process of manufacture. Therefore, when people buy a patent medicine, they have the means of ascertaining what ingredients are contained in it ... The term does not extend and is not intended to extend to mere proprietary medicines, or to include a medicine like this, for which the owner or maker has not obtained any patent whatever.

The result of these decisions was that the sale of proprietary medicines containing scheduled poisons was restricted to registered chemists. Various attempts to evade the Pharmacy Act by taking out patents on proprietary remedies were defeated by the prompt action of the Pharmaceutical Society working in conjunction with the Court of Chancery. Such action was expensive but invariably effective. The Society, moreover, vigorously prosecuted unqualified dealers who sold these medicines. Until the enactment of the Dangerous Drugs Act in 1920, which forced manufacturers to lower significantly the morphia content of their remedies, the only safeguard against the abuse of these medicines was the discretion of the professional chemist who might limit the sale to a single bottle per customer. The ineffectiveness of such control was revealed by the comments of a North London chemist in 1906:

I, as a chemist, understand by my qualification that I shall be able to use discretion to whom poisons should be supplied . . . I have had one or two cases myself where I had refused certain articles containing poisons, for internal use, because the parties were becoming habituated to them . . . I recollect a lady was taken to an asylum through taking a certain drug which I personally warned her against.[4]

Unfortunately, the customer whose purchases were regulated by one chemist could always go to others: the professionalism of the North London pharmacist was negated by his customers' ready access to other sources of supply.

Nonetheless, restricting the sale of proprietary medicines containing scheduled poisons to registered chemists had a marked effect on the sale of Collis Browne's chlorodyne. Davenport's sales figures were down by £6,200 in 1899 from the 1891 level: at £25,000 they were £3,000 lower than the total in 1871. This decline probably indicates, not a fall in consumption, but an increase in substitution by local chemists. The large profit margins in the manufacture of proprietary medicines made substitution attractive to both the chemist and his customers.

The campaign against "patent" medicines did not end: any restriction on self-medication was in the interest of the general practitioner. Publications such as Health News' *Exposures of Quackery* (1895–6), a series of articles upon and analyses of various patent medicines, attacked the "widespread system of home-drugging" which had resulted from the easy availability of opiate proprietary medicines. In 1909 and 1912 the British Medical Association published its own investigations into the composition and profitability of patent medicines entitled *Secret Remedies* and *More Secret Remedies*. The work of analysis was carried out by Edward Frank Harrison (1869–1918), a distinguished member of the Pharmaceutical Society. *Secret Remedies*, which was aimed at the educated general public to wean them away from indulgence in proprietaries, sold some 62,000 copies. Although the official policy of the British Medical Association was for legislation against secret remedies, the *British Medical Journal* continued to carry advertisements for proprietary medicines in the inter-war years. The most important development after 1900 was that manufacturers whose remedies once contained opium began to drop it from their formulae. The makers of Owbridge's Lung Tonic and Beecham's Cough Pills found commercial advantage in declaring that opium was not present. Liqufruta Medica, little more than a sugar solution, was guaranteed to be "free of poison, laudanum, copper solution, cocaine, morphia, opium, chloral, calomel, paregoric, narcotics or preservatives". Informed consumer choice reinforced the effects of legislation.

* * *

Within a year of its enactment, the 1868 Pharmacy Act had to be amended. During the passage of the original bill through the House of Commons, Lord Robert Montagu carried, without objection, an amendment substituting the term "apothecary" for "medical practitioner" in the 16th and 17th sections. As the *Lancet* was quick to point out, this meant that medical practitioners, other than licentiates of the Society of Apothecaries, would be denied the right to carry on a pharmaceutical business. However much the College of Physicians might welcome this attempt to restrict doctors' involvement in retail trading, general practitioners were soon up in arms about it. Lord Robert Montagu was prevailed upon to make amends. A short Act was passed in August 1869 making it clear that the exemptions applied to all registered medical practitioners. It went further: by repealing Section 23 of the original Act, it made it possible for registered medical practitioners to register as chemists and druggists as well. The amending Act sorted out two other minor issues. The holders of certificates from the Highland and Agricultural Society of Scotland were given the same right to dispense medicines for animals under their care as members of the Royal College of Veterinary Surgeons. The Pharmaceutical Society stepped in to remedy a grievance created by the insertion, by an unknown scribe, of the word "immediately" in the declaration which assistants were required to make if they wished to avail themselves of the modified examination. By the 1869 Act it was declared sufficient for an assistant to have been employed in dispensing for a period of three years at any time (not necessarily "immediately") prior to 31 July 1868. The time limit for the delivery of certificates was extended until 31 December 1869.

The introduction of a bill to amend the 1868 Pharmacy Act was seen by John Simon as a fine opportunity to steal a march on the Pharmaceutical Society. At the report stage of the original Act, Robert Lowe had attempted to insert a clause preventing chemists from selling poisons as medicines except under the written prescription of a legally qualified medical practitioner. The attempt had been frustrated but John Simon did not abandon his aim of restricting self-medication and counter prescribing. In 1869, therefore, he arranged for Dr. Brewer, M.P. for Colchester, to introduce an amendment identical to that proposed the previous year by Robert Lowe. Dr. Brewer's version of Section 3 of the 1869 Act stated that the word "poison" (with all its legal implications) would not apply to any medicine supplied by a registered medical practitioner or dispensed, under the prescription in writing of any legally qualified medical practitioner, by any person registered as a chemist and druggist. This version was accepted by the House of Commons but, on the representation of the Pharmaceutical Society, the House of Lords omitted the critical phrase "under the prescription in writing of any legally qualified medical practitioner". Thus the 1869 Act placed both medical men and chemists and druggists on the same footing. The medical officer of the Privy Council was once again thwarted.

The 1868 Act established the Pharmaceutical Society as the regulatory authority of chemists and druggists in Great Britain. The Act required the Society to undertake five main functions: maintaining the public registers of pharmaceutical chemists and chemists and druggists, conducting their qualifying examinations, initiating proceedings against unqualified persons, prescribing regulations for the keeping, dispensing and selling of poisons and proposing additions to the schedule of poisons. In carrying out these duties, the Society was subject to the supervision of the Privy Council. The 1868 Act gave the Privy Council the power of approving the Pharmaceutical Society's list of examiners, of inspecting its examinations, and of sanctioning its by-laws, the schedule of poisons, and the regulations concerning their keeping and sale. With John Simon as the medical officer, there was no possibility that the Privy Council's supervision would be purely nominal. Arrogantly regarding himself as the personification of the public interest, he exercised his powers to the full.

The passing of the Pharmacy Act meant that the by-laws of the Pharmaceutical Society had to be altered to carry out the Act's provisions. A special general meeting of members was held on 14 October 1868 to consider and approve the changes. When the new by-laws were submitted to Simon, however, he took exception to several of them and referred them back to the Society. The principal alterations referred to the Board of Examiners. No one over the age of 65 was to be appointed nor was any member of the previous year's Council.

The only Council members who could serve on the Board of Examiners were the president and vice-president, who were ex-officio members. The Society confirmed the amended by-laws on 14 January and they were confirmed by the Privy Council on 6 February 1869. At the end of that year the Privy Council confirmed a resolution of the Council of the Pharmaceutical Society making six important additions to the list of poisons in Schedule A of the Act. At first the relationship between the Society and the Privy Council, although not without friction, was working satisfactorily. The Society's Council welcomed Simon's decision to appoint two of the most eminent doctors of the day, E.H. Greenhow in London and Sir Robert Christison in Edinburgh, to act as the inspectors of the Society's examinations. This ensured that the Privy Council's inspection was not a perfunctory task nominally performed by time-serving mediocrities but an elaborate and meticulous surveillance leading to full public report. The publication of these reports brought nothing but satisfaction and honour to the Pharmaceutical Society.

The first section of the 1868 Pharmacy Act vested in the Pharmaceutical Society the power to prescribe, subject to the consent of the Privy Council, regulations for the keeping, dispensing and selling of poisons. The relevant section had been inserted as an amendment to the Pharmaceutical Society's original bill in the House of Lords by the Duke of Marlborough, acting under instructions from John Simon. Simon intended that during the bill's passage through the Commons the clause would be further amended to give these powers directly to the Privy Council, but Robert Lowe's amendment intended to achieve this was rejected. The result was to prove a major frustration for the medical officer to the Privy Council. Since the Lords' amendment had not been intended to survive the Commons, Simon had not worried unduly about its precise wording. After the Act's enactment, however, it became clear that, while all other powers to be exercised for public purposes by the Pharmaceutical Society were vested in the Society's Council, the language of the first section of the Act vested in the members as a whole the authority to prescribe regulations for the storage and sale of poisons.

In 1869 the Council of the Pharmaceutical Society, under pressure from the Privy Council, prepared a set of regulations, which it published before submitting them to the annual meeting in May 1870. The proposed regulations read:

> 1. In the keeping of poisons, each poison shall be kept in a box, bottle, vessel, or package, distinctly labelled with the name of the article and the word "Poison".
>
> 2. In the keeping of poisons, one or more of the following systems shall be used:-
> (i) The boxes, bottles, vessels, or packages containing poison shall be kept apart from other boxes, bottles, vessels, or packages, and shall be so kept in an apartment, cupboard, compartment, or drawer set apart for dangerous articles.
> (ii) The bottles or vessels used in any shop or dispensary to contain poison shall be distinguishable to the touch as by being angular, fluted, or corrugated, and shall be unlike the bottles or vessels used to contain articles which are *not* poisonous or dangerous in the same shop or dispensary.
> (iii) The bottles or vessels used in any shop or dispensary to contain poison shall be tied over, capped, or secured in a manner distinguishable from the way in which any bottles or vessels not used to contain poisonous or dangerous articles used in the same shop or dispensary may be tied over, capped, or secured.

3. In dispensing and compounding poisons all liniments, embrocations and lotions containing them shall be put into distinctive bottles, or bottles made distinctive, and labels containing some word or words of caution showing that the contents are not intended to be taken, in addition to the name of the compound, or instructions for use, shall be affixed thereto.

As soon as these regulations were published, strenuous opposition emerged to their adoption. At a meeting of the North British Branch held in December 1869 member after member voiced his opposition. The correspondence columns of the *Pharmaceutical Journal* filled with letters of protest. The local associations became involved and several sent petitions to the Council objecting to the proposals. Although the regulations would not have proved burdensome to well-established chemists, the majority of whom already observed similar precautions, any enforced additional expenditure was dreaded by the smaller, less secure proprietors. Moreover, all chemists and druggists, prosperous or struggling, resented the fact that medical practitioners, with or without retail shops, would be exempt from these regulations. The idea that the protection of the public required chemists and druggists to have regulations imposed on them from above while medical practitioners could be safely left to their own devices was wrong in principle and in fact.

The annual meeting held on 18 May 1870 was distinguished by the large attendance of members, especially from the provinces; by the importance of the subjects under discussion; by the acrimonious character of several of the speeches; and by an episode which led to the withdrawal from the Society of that stormy petrel, William Dickinson. There was good reason to anticipate a lively meeting. The country members were determined to make their weight felt in the election of Council and in voicing their opposition to the proposed poisons regulations. Most members believed that these were neither necessary nor desirable and, after heated discussion, the matter was conveniently deferred for another year. George F. Schacht from Bristol made a plea for the development of pharmaceutical education in the provinces and urged the desirability of distributing the Society's resources more generally over the country rather than concentrating them on the London school of pharmacy. For the first time the subject of trading as chemists and druggists by the recently-formed Civil Service Co-operative Society was raised. William Dickinson argued that anybody found encouraging such trading should be thrown out of the Society and Edwin Vizer raised the meeting's temperature by asking whether it were true that the firm which the president, H. Sugden Evans, represented was the medium for supplying the Civil Service stores with drugs. Despite an emphatic denial by the president, the meeting became increasingly rowdy. The real scandal occurred later, during the scrutiny of the votes cast in the Council election. William Dickinson was forced to admit that he had tampered with the returns and misled his fellow scrutineers: he removed over a hundred votes cast for Sugden Evans and added them to those cast for other candidates. His resignation relieved the Council from the unpleasant task of expelling him from the Society. Dickinson, a regular fly in the ointment, never attempted to establish himself as a leader of opposition. His attacks were motivated by spite and jealousy rather than attachment to causes or general grievances.

The failure of the annual meeting to approve the poisons regulations convinced John Simon that the Society was a monopolising trade association that could not be trusted to carry out public duties. In his twelfth annual report (1870), he drew the Privy Council's attention to the fact that the Society's inaction left the public "still without the protection which such regulations might give and which notoriously is much needed against the danger of having poisons dispensed or used in mistake for harmless preparations". This public rebuke concentrated the minds of the Pharmaceutical Society's Council members, who decided, on 5 October 1870, to appoint a committee to examine the whole issue. In its report, two important alterations in the poisons regulations were suggested with a view to securing the approval of the membership. In the first regulation it was proposed to use some distinctive mark rather than the actual word "poison", which it was thought might unduly alarm customers: the third regulation, which referred to the dispensing, compounding and selling of poisons, was to be omitted altogether.

Before the revised version of the regulations could be placed before the members, the Society's Council received a letter from John Simon, dated 23 December 1870. My Lords of Her Majesty's Council, wrote Simon,

> think it right to inquire whether the Pharmaceutical Society intends, within any time you can specify, to propose such regulations to their Lordships. They direct me, therefore, to request that you will have the goodness to give me, at your earliest convenience, the information required . . .

In response, the Council forwarded a copy of the revised proposals. Simon was not amused. The president of the Society, G.W. Sandford and the secretary, Elias Bremridge, were summoned to the Privy Council Office. Simon explained that a complete body of regulations for the keeping, dispensing and selling of poisons was absolutely necessary for the public safety. The regulations were remodelled and a copy of them, together with a statement of the reasons which induced the Council to suggest them, was sent to every member of the Society and to each associate in business. The result was a spontaneous outburst of indignation and protest. In Birmingham, Glasgow, Halifax, Hull, Leeds, Liverpool, Manchester, Nottingham and Sheffield meetings of chemists and druggists passed resolutions condemning the compulsory nature of the proposals. In London chemists gathered at the Freemasons' Tavern and unanimously pledged themselves to resist any attempt to impose compulsory regulations upon them. The Metropolitan Chemists' Defence Association was formed to co-operate with similar associations in the provinces. Memorials and petitions began to pour into Bloomsbury Square. At the Council meeting held on 5 April 1871 the following resolution was carried:

> That, considering the numerous and strongly expressed objections, by members of the Society and others who will be affected by them, to the compulsory character of the suggested regulations for the keeping and dispensing of poisons, and in order to obtain the more cordial adoption of these regulations by chemists throughout the country; it is resolved to present them to the annual meeting with such alterations as will divest them of a compulsory character, but accompanied by the earnest recommendation of this Council that all "pharmaceutical chemists" and "chemists and druggists" in business in Great Britain do make use of these recommended regulations . . .

On a division, out of eighteen members of Council present, two did not vote, fifteen voted for the motion, and one, the president, voted against. G.W. Sandford then explained that he had held office during the last few months simply that his successor should not commence his term with such a troublesome question as the poisons regulations on his hands. The Council had now, in effect, withdrawn them and, as he felt that the president should at the annual meeting represent the views of Council, he considered it his duty to resign immediately. G. Webb Sandford had been president continuously from 1863 to 1869: he played a major role in bringing about the reconciliation between the leaders of the United Society of Chemists and Druggists and the Council of the Pharmaceutical Society which paved the way for the 1868 Act. He was the helmsman who steered the Society through the difficult negotiations with the Government which enabled the Pharmacy bill to pass through parliament. It was G.W. Sandford who listened to John Simon's expostulations in the Privy Council Office. Political realism was the minority of one.

The Council's decision inevitably brought down the wrath of the Privy Council. In his annual report Simon deplored the Society's failure to exercise its powers and added:

> It is perhaps not surprising that a large body of tradesmen should be slow to take the initiative in imposing even the most reasonable penal restrictions on themselves: but I have to submit to your Lordships, as a fact which you may deem deserving the consideration of Parliament, that this non-fulfilment of the Society's duty, to make rules against dangerous slovenliness in the keeping, dispensing, and selling of poisons, is a breach of the implied contract under which the Legislature in 1868 gave powers and privileges to the Society.

Simon wrote a threatening letter to the Society's Council informing them that the Privy Council would propose new legislation if the Society failed to submit poisons regulations for approval after the next annual meeting. This letter was read to the annual meeting on 17 May 1871, but a motion was carried, by a majority of nineteen, rejecting compulsory regulations. On 1 June Simon wrote again to the president asking what steps the Society had taken with regard to poisons regulations. Without waiting for a reply, the Lord President of the Council introduced a bill transferring the power of action in the making of poisons regulations from the Society to the Society's Council and giving power to the Privy Council to act under certain conditions. The bill was read a third time and passed in the House of Lords on 15 June 1871. On 22 June a deputation representing the Pharmaceutical Society and all registered chemists met W. E. Forster, the vice-president of the Privy Council (and now remembered in association with the 1870 Education Act), at his official residence in Downing Street. John Simon was also present. G.F. Schacht presented the chemists' case. Compulsory regulations, he said, were unwise, unjust and unnecessary: unwise because they upset the work of thirty years, unjust because medical men were not included, unnecessary in view of the great progress in pharmaceutical education. Neither Forster nor Simon were willing to argue. In their view the 1868 Act required the Pharmaceutical Society to lay down regulations. It had failed to do so. Doubtless the fact that, out of 12,000 chemists, only 3,000 chose to join the Society weakened its authority. In that case it became the duty of the Privy Council to protect the public: hence the new bill. The only encouragement the deputation received came from Forster's acceptance of the argument that medical men should be subject to the same regulations as chemists. If an amendment to that effect were moved, he promised to give it careful consideration.

The Privy Council bill divided the Council of the Pharmaceutical Society into two factions. The older members such as George Edwards, A.F. Heselden, Thomas Hyde Hills,

George Sandford and John Williams were not totally opposed to the bill. They welcomed the proposal to transfer power from the Society's members to its Council. The function of Council in their view was to lead and even control the membership. The other faction, which included Alexander Bottle, Thomas Greenish, Richard Reynolds and Messrs Atherton and Betty, represented the new democratic wing of the Society. Its members were the heirs of the United Society in which several had played prominent roles. They believed the Council should respond positively to the views of the majority of members. The Society's strength derived from the rank and file not from co-operation with the Government. This group favoured the unfettered reporting of Council meetings by both the *Pharmaceutical Journal* and the *Chemist and Druggist*.

The general body of chemists and druggists, organised by local defence associations, demonstrated their opposition to the Privy Council's bill. Meetings in Birmingham, Bolton, Bradford, Glasgow, Halifax, Leeds, Liverpool, Manchester, Newcastle, Nottingham, and Sheffield were solid in condemning it. Petitions against it were presented in the House of Commons from over two hundred towns. The second reading was to have taken place on 26 June but was postponed first until 6 July and then until 17 July. Mr. W.E. Gladstone, the prime minister, then announced that the bill would clearly require considerable discussion and would in the meanwhile be withdrawn. It was never re-introduced.

By 1872 the question of poisons regulations had reached an impasse. The members of the Pharmaceutical Society had not only blocked their Council's attempt to introduce regulations for the storage and dispensing of poisons but had also secured the election of Council members specifically committed to resisting the introduction of such regulations. At the same time the limits of the power of the Privy Council Office had been exposed. The collapse of the 1871 bill revealed the capacity of the rank and file chemists and druggists to obstruct legislation emanating from that office. John Simon's threat to use parliament to impose his will on the nation's chemists had been exposed as mere bluff. Members of parliament were not easily persuaded to support bills which seemed neither popular nor particularly important. Between 1869 and 1908 both the Privy Council and the Pharmaceutical Society's Council wanted to amend the Pharmacy Act and both made repeated attempts to do so. Each attempt failed because neither Council could get its bills accepted without the support of the other. They could obstruct one another but independently they could not initiate change.

* * *

For most chemists and druggists the 1870s were a depressing decade. The monopoly of the sale of poisons promised by the passing of the 1868 Act was breached by the activities of medical practitioners, the unqualified and the vendors of patent medicines. New threats began to emerge. The analysts appointed under the drug adulteration acts of 1872 and 1875 took their responsibilities very seriously and started a campaign to rid the drug trade of nefarious practices. A more serious form of oppression was perpetrated by the Medical Defence Association in its endeavour to put down counter prescribing. Many general practitioners feared that the registration and official recognition of the qualifications of chemists and druggists would lead to an upsurge in counter practice. A gullible public would be encouraged to believe that those who were now legally authorised to sell dangerous drugs were also qualified to practise medicine. The public's credulity was strengthened by the fact that those who were licensed to practise medicine were also permitted to keep open shop for the sale of poisons. The Medical Defence Association, formed to protect the commercial interests of general practitioners, adopted a decidedly aggressive stance in the 1870s. At the same time, co-operative and company trading began to affect retail pharmacy. On top of harassment by public analysts and disgruntled doctors, chemists and druggists had to face a new and rampant form of competition.

The reluctance of the Pharmaceutical Society to make the protection of trade interests a priority encouraged a small group of wholesalers and prominent retailers to believe that the time had come for the creation of a new trade association. In July 1876, a trade conference of chemists and druggists, organised by Southall Brothers and Thomas Barclay and Sons, was held in Birmingham. Richard Reynolds, one of the founders of the British Pharmaceutical Conference, presided and, thanks to his skilful control, a wide-ranging discussion on various trade topics took place. At the close of the meeting a Chemists and Druggists' Trade Association was formed. The new association made the by-now customary pledge of loyalty to the Pharmaceutical Society and declared its intention to supplement rather than supplant the older institution. In a bid to recruit the whole trade, the annual subscription was fixed at five shillings. Within two years the Association claimed a membership of 4,000.[5]

Among those taking a leading part in the formation of the new association was Robert Hampson (1833–1905). Hampson was secretary of the Manchester based Chemists' Defence Association which had been formed primarily to oppose the adoption of the poisons regulations. After passing the Major examination in July 1864, Hampson practised in the Manchester area and became prominently involved in the activities of the United Society of Chemists and Druggists. When Cyrus Buott's ambition to become the new registrar under the 1868 Act was thwarted, Hampson organised a relief fund to compensate the United Society's energetic secretary for his loss of earnings. In 1872, after a vigorous campaign designed to inject new blood in the system, Hampson, together with Scott Brown and James Woolley, who all came from Manchester, were elected to the Council of the Pharmaceutical Society. At the first meeting he attended, Hampson seconded an unavailing motion to admit a reporter from the *Chemist and Druggist* to Council meetings. Sometime in 1875 Hampson moved to London and established a pharmaceutical business in Islington. His wife, Caroline Winifred, had studied midwifery in Manchester and in 1876 they started a home in North London "for the rescue of young women who had fallen into evil courses". This was such a success that it became, in due course, Winifred House, Tollington Park, with a new building costing £2,300. Hampson remained a Council member for twenty-six years and held the post of treasurer for nine of them (1890–8). He was active in promoting controversial causes (the admission of women to the laboratories, the closure of the School of Pharmacy, opening up the membership to all registered chemists) but never shirked the more mundane work of committees.

During the 1870s the operation of the Society's democratic constitution and the efficiency of the railways produced a Council more nearly representative of the rank and file than had previously been the case. The Council came under increasing pressure to take steps, in the words of the Charter, "for the protection of those who carry on the business of chemists and druggists". In 1876 Robert Hampson urged the Council to test the legality of co-operative traders keeping open shop for the dispensing of poisons. The problem, however, was not as straightforward as Hampson and his fellow radicals thought. The Law and Parliamentary Committee had already considered the question many times without reaching agreement on appropriate action. When a deputation from the Chemist and Druggists' Trade Association was received, the Committee explained that its failure to act was due not to lack of will but of a suitable occasion. In the same year the Council discussed the advisability of defending the case of any registered chemist who might be proceeded against for alleged infringement of the Apothecaries Act. After a long discussion it was decided, by nine votes to eight, that, if circumstances warranted, the Society would undertake the defence.

The enactment of the 1858 Medical Act, with the consequent publication of the Medical Register and the establishment of the General Medical Council, was an important landmark in the process by which general practitioners became accepted as members of a profession. Although the 1858 Act did not make unqualified practice illegal, it created a monopoly of practice for registered practitioners in all public institutions. Moreover, by bestowing the prestige of the state on licensed practitioners, the 1858 Act gave them a competitive advantage in the open market. It did not, however, provide the general practitioner with any sense of financial security, nor did it lessen his involvement in business and commercial activities. Doctors who did their own dispensing (and this included the great majority) were sellers of drugs just as much as those who kept open shop (and many continued to do this). The temptation to adopt a prescribing strategy to maximise earnings struggled with the doctor's professional conscience. The impression, which is often created, that the competition between medical practitioners and chemists and druggists was a contest between, on the one hand, members of a learned profession, and, on the other, profit-seeking tradesmen is grossly misleading. General practitioners who sought a share in the status of the physician, were determined to cling on to the profits of the druggist. During the 1870s the battle between the Medical Defence Association and the Chemists and Druggists' Trade Association was a struggle, neither pure nor simple, between two groups of businessmen with equal claims to professional status.

In January 1876 the Medical Defence Association scored a notable triumph. Proceedings were taken by the Society of Apothecaries, at the instigation of the Defence Association, to recover a penalty of £20 for an infringement of the 1815 Apothecaries Act by a chemist and druggist named Nottingham. Nottingham was a registered chemist living in Shadwell in the East End of London. He was in partnership with a duly qualified medical man but this gentleman was not always on the spot. When applied to for advice and medicine, Nottingham responded as most chemists would have done. There was, however, no evidence that he ever went from his shop to attend patients, and it was proved, that in cases of serious illness, he always referred the patient to the doctor with whom he was in partnership. Nottingham admitted he had, on various occasions, prescribed medicines in trivial cases. In a summing up which ignored both history and the chemists' exemption clause, Baron Bramwell remarked:

> I feel some difficulty in putting the case to you, for on the defendant's own admission he says he prescribed, and that, if a person brought a child to him suffering from, say diarrhoea, and asked what was good for it, he gave the medicine: if, however, the case was serious, he sent the doctor. Surely this is acting and practising as an apothecary within the meaning of the Act.

Armed with this opinion, the Medical Defence Association became remarkably agitated and dealt out threatening notices to chemists right, left and centre. The Apothecaries

Company was encouraged to institute a series of prosecutions of counter prescribing druggists in various parts of the country, from Bermondsey to Birmingham, from Redruth to Bradford. The Chemists and Druggists' Trade Association, already heavily involved in defending chemists prosecuted under the Food and Drugs Act, was stung into action: it decided to take up the case of George Shepperley who had fallen victim to the jealousy of the medical profession in Nottingham. Shepperley was an established market-square chemist whose success riled the local G.P.'s. They employed a man with the well-chosen name of Jolly Death to visit Shepperley's shop to secure evidence for a conviction under the 1815 Act. Shepperley was fined £20 for looking in the jaws of Death and prescribing a gargle. The verdict produced a storm of protest in the local press and some cool replies from "Medicus" who had obviously been briefed by the local medical profession to be as economical as possible with the truth. Leave was given to appeal and the case was taken to the High Court of Justice, Exchequer Division, and came on for hearing on 20 November 1877 before the Lord Chief Baron Kelly and Baron Cleasby. A new trial was ordered in that court and this took place a year later before Baron Pollock and a special jury. After a trial lasting two days, the jury found for the defendant. The successful outcome owed much to the consummate skill, particularly in cross-examination, of Sir Henry James, the defence counsel selected by the Chemists and Druggists' Trade Association. However, the legality or otherwise of counter prescribing was in no way settled by the verdict. The jury merely decided that, in this particular instance, Mr. Shepperley had not infringed the Apothecaries Act.[6]

In August 1877, on a motion proposed by Robert Hampson, the Council of the Pharmaceutical Society decided, by twelve votes to four, to authorise its solicitor, Mr. Flux, at his discretion and at the expense of the Society, to defend George Shepperley. Since the Trade Association had already taken on the case, Flux decided not to involve the Society. An even wiser decision was made not to take on the Wiggins case, which badly burnt the fingers of the Trade Association.

The Society of Apothecaries v. Wiggins was an action against a registered chemist for practising as an apothecary which the Trade Association defended in the hope of securing exemption from the 1815 Act for all chemists and druggists. Evidence was given by three venerable chemists to show that counter prescribing by chemists was the norm before 1815: their testimony merely demonstrated the weakness of oral history. They succeeded in conveying the impression that, prior to the Apothecaries Act, chemists and druggists confined themselves to the treatment of simple cases. The cases Wiggins had been taking on were serious: the jury found him guilty. At the close of the case, Mr. Justice Field expressed his unease about the wisdom of the Apothecaries Company taking such action against chemists:

> I think it might be considered by chemists and druggists whether they should not communicate with the Apothecaries Company and see whether something might be done. I cannot help thinking there might be some modification.

The Council of the Pharmaceutical Society had, in point of fact, already adopted this approach. In October 1878 George Schacht had suggested that an effort should be made to arrive at some understanding with the Society of Apothecaries about the type of cases which should be open to prosecution under the 1815 Act. No one seconded his motion at the time but two months later the Council instructed its solicitor to get in touch with the solicitor of the Apothecaries Company to seek a practicable settlement along the lines indicated by Mr. Schacht. The Society of Apothecaries claimed that it had no desire to institute vexatious proceedings against chemists in the ordinary exercise of their business which it admitted necessarily involved giving their customers a certain amount of advice. In response, the Pharmaceutical Society declared that, although it regarded counter practice as protected by law and as a necessity for both the trade and the public, it would do nothing to encourage it. Without making any concessions, the Council of the Pharmaceutical Society sought and obtained the basis of an agreement with the Society of Apothecaries which left the majority of chemists and druggists undisturbed. Behind the surface expression of conciliatory attitudes, there existed the realisation of common interests. In both societies, wise heads saw the danger of allowing the situation to get out of hand: in both societies, the tail was beginning to wag the dog. The Medical Defence Association was taking decisions which committed the Society of Apothecaries to initiate prosecutions: the Chemist and Druggists' Trade Association was seeking to determine the policy of the Pharmaceutical Society. In each society, the Councils acted to regain the reins of power. By shaking hands, authority was restored.

Going to law has always been an expensive pursuit. The Chemists and Druggists' Trade Association soon discovered its funds depleted by its wide ranging legal activities. In July 1878 Mr. Fairlie, a member of the Trade Association and of the Pharmaceutical Society's Council, attempted to persuade the Council to allocate £100 to help the Association fight the Shepperley case. Although the motion received little support, the matter was raised again in December, this time by Robert Hampson. He claimed that the defence of Shepperley came within the objects of the Society as defined by the Charter. According to his version of history, the Society had been formed in 1841 out of similar opposition to medical oppression and the 1814–15 Defence Fund had then been transferred to the Society specifically for such purposes. The Council was not impressed by the logic of history: Hampson's motion was defeated by nine votes to six. Nonetheless, a requisition was then presented, signed by some fifty members, requesting a special meeting of the Society to consider the advisability of rendering substantial pecuniary aid to the Trade Association. The meeting was held on 9 January 1879. About a hundred members and associates-in-business turned up. The president, John Williams, arrived, armed with counsels' opinion on the limits within which the discussion would need to be confined. According to the lawyers, the resolution, if passed, would have no legal force. The management of the Society's funds was not subject to the control of members but was vested in the Council. Indeed the Council itself could not legally vote a sum of money to be administered by another body, unaccountable to the Society. Any money applied to the protection of the trade must remain under the direct control of the Council.

The majority of members present had no intention of allowing lawyers to hijack their meeting. Robert Hampson and Thomas Barclay presented the argument in favour of the resolution with great skill and judgment. G.W. Sandford and George Schacht spoke against. The meeting was noisy and boisterous: speeches were punctuated by frequent interruptions and heckling. The resolution was carried by a large majority. And that was the end of the affair. The Shepperley case ended without an appeal: the occasion to act on the resolution never occurred. The members, having expressed their anger and indignation, turned their attention to more serious matters.

The struggle to protect the chemists' right to advise over the counter was fought not only in the law courts but also in parliament. Three bills to amend the 1858 Medical Act, introduced during 1877 and 1878, contained clauses which would have severely restricted the prescribing activities of chemists. The opposition of the Pharmaceutical Society contributed to their demise. The diplomacy of the Society did more to protect the rank and file chemist and druggist than the battles fought by the Trade Association. No decisions on particular legal cases would define the perimeters of counter prescribing. Support for the Trade Association withered away. Its annual report in June 1886 revealed a desperate plight. "Failing the most liberal donations from the wholesale houses, in many instances repeated again and again, the Association must inevitably have long since collapsed for want of funds". During the early part of 1887 special efforts were made to place the Association on a sound financial footing, but these were unavailing. On 27 June 1887 a sparsely attended gathering decided to wind the Association up. The experience of the past eleven years had been disheartening in the extreme. The final verdict was that the Trade Association had provided evidence yet again "of a thorough want of public spirit and capacity for combined action among a large part of the chemists and druggists of this country".[7]

One of the most profitable portions of thousands of chemists' businesses in late Victorian Britain was the extraction and adaptation of teeth and the supply of artificial ones. Until the Dentists Act of 1921 many registered chemists and druggists maintained a substantial dental practice. Attempts to create a separate profession of dentistry followed very closely the pattern set by the Pharmaceutical Society. When John Tomes set up the Odontological Society in 1855 he drew heavily on the advice and experience of his friend, Jacob Bell. Tomes and his associates were led to the conclusion that two things were required: an Act of Parliament to create a register of qualified men, who alone would be empowered to practise and the formation of a voluntary association of those registered. The first Dentists Act, introduced as a private measure by Sir John Lubbock, was passed in 1878 and the British Dental Association was founded in 1880. The Dentists Act of 1878 was modelled on the Pharmacy Acts, and on the 1858 Medical Act. To ensure the subjection of the dental profession to the medical profession, the administration of the Act was placed in the hands of the General Medical Council. A register of dentists was set up to be compiled and kept by the G.M.C., upon which the duties of supervising examinations in dentistry and of erasing names from the register were laid. The Act did not prohibit practice by the unregistered but gave the registered certain privileges.

> A person shall not be entitled to take or use the name or title of "dentist" (either alone or in combination with any other word or words) or of "a dental practitioner" or any name, title, addition or description implying that he is registered under this Act or that he is a person specially qualified to practise dentistry unless he is registered under this Act.

An unregistered person was not to be entitled to recover any fee or charge "for the performance of any dental operation or for any dental attendance or advice".

When the Dental Practitioners Bill was first introduced, it contained a clause which might easily have been construed to exclude from the register those who practised dentistry in conjunction with pharmacy. John Williams, the president of the Pharmaceutical Society, wrote to Sir John Lubbock calling his attention to this possible construction of the clause and suggesting a modification. Lubbock replied that he had no intention of excluding chemists and druggists. The clause was rewritten so as to admit to the dental register all licentiates in dental surgery or dentistry and "any person who is at the passing of this Act bona fide engaged in the practice of dentistry or dental surgery, either separately or in conjunction with the practice of medicine, surgery, or pharmacy". It was in this form when the bill became law on 22 July 1878. When the first edition of the register appeared in 1879 it contained the names of 5,289 persons of whom 2,049, or well over one-third, were registered as combining the practice of dentistry with that of pharmacy. The 1878 Act, however, failed: its statutory defences proved to be shams, the privileges it gave the registered turned out to be useless. The growth of a large class of unqualified practitioners continued unabated until 1921.

*   *   *

When the Pharmaceutical Society was founded, it was taken for granted that its members would be men. This was not because there were no women in business as chemists and druggists. On the contrary, the 1869 register records the names of 215 women practising pharmacy, i.e., nearly two per cent of the total number of 11,638 registered chemists and druggists. It was simply that the Society's founding fathers shared the conventional Victorian view about the role and status of women. When Jacob Bell made his tours of

Census, England and Wales 1841–1891
Chemists and Druggists

Men and women over the age of 20

	Men	*Women*
1841	7,526	148
1851	11,701	298
1861	12,638	365
1871	15,540	441
1881	14,819	481
1891	16,581	871

The census returns make no distinction between qualified and unqualified, master and servant, dispenser and general assistant. In 1871 there was a difference of nearly 4,000 between the number of persons over the age of twenty returning themselves as chemists and druggists in the census and the number of persons on the statutory register. Unqualified persons could set up in business to sell drugs and medicines provided they did not sell scheduled poisons. A licence from the Commissioners of Inland Revenue was required for the sale of patent medicines. The number of licensed vendors rose from 10,922 in 1865, to 12,619 in 1871, to 18,754 in 1881, and to 27,295 in 1891. Many of these were qualified chemists. Unqualified dispensers (working for medical men, or for qualified chemists, or for company chemists, and in institutions such as hospitals, infirmaries, workhouses, asylums, prisons, barracks, etc.) would be classified in the census as chemists and druggists, as would the holders of the Society of Apothecaries' Assistants' certificate. General assistants working in chemists' shops might return themselves as chemists and druggists.

Between 1868 and 1900 the number of women on the statutory register fell while the number of women returning themselves as chemists and druggists in the census rose. Women constituted a growing proportion of the pharmaceutical labour force between 1841 and 1891. In 1841 two per cent of those calling themselves chemists and druggists were women: by 1891 the proportion had risen to five per cent.

Britain, drumming up support for the new Society, he regarded the presence of women chemists in an area as a symptom of the backward state of pharmacy there. But this was sheer prejudice on his part. Most of these women were carrying on the business started by a dead father or husband and some employed male assistants to help them: but the majority were running the shop themselves and successfully performing all the duties of a chemist and druggist. The 1868 Pharmacy Act, more by default than design, accorded women the same right as men to sit the qualifying examinations and to be registered. The first woman to qualify by passing an examination was Fanny Elizabeth Potter of Kibworth, near Leicester, who was registered on 5 February 1869 and remained on the register until 1930. Before the passing of the 1868 Act she worked as an assistant to her father and qualified by passing the Modified examination. She was followed six months later by Catherine Hodgson Fisher of Botcherby, near Carlisle. The first woman to qualify by passing the Minor examination was Alice Vickery of Camberwell in Surrey, who registered on 18 June 1873. Two years later, on 15 December 1875, Isabella Skinner Clarke became the first woman to pass the Major examination and register as a pharmaceutical chemist. While the right of women to practise pharmacy was firmly established in law, many members wanted the Pharmaceutical Society to remain a male preserve.

The first mention of women infiltrating the student body at Bloomsbury Square occurs in the minutes of the Library, Museum and Laboratory committee for 9 October 1861. "The Committee, having heard a lady has had a ticket of admission to the lectures without sanction", decided that ladies "must be regarded as attending upon sufferance". Next year a proposal to admit women to the lectures was firmly rejected by Council. The lady in question was Elizabeth Garrett, making use of the lectures in the School of Pharmacy to prepare herself for the examinations of the Society of Apothecaries, whose licence to practise medicine she acquired in 1865. After the passing of the 1868 Pharmacy Act, the Society was eager to welcome as members the newly registered chemists and druggists—provided they were men. In 1869 a woman, registered in December 1868, applied for membership and was rejected three times. Elizabeth Leech was an experienced chemist. She spent seven years learning the trade in her father's shop. When he died, she ran the shop for six years with her brother and then, for a further nine years, on her own. When the Lancashire cotton famine forced her out of business, she went to join her sister who was a lady superintendent of a lunatic asylum in Fulham. For the past five years she had worked as the dispenser at Munster House Asylum, compounding and dispensing the prescriptions of medical practitioners. She produced testimonials from two of them in support of her application. Miss Leech was not looking for trouble. She merely wanted to get back into business and thought it might help if she were a member of the Pharmaceutical Society. "I have no wish upon any occasion to interfere with the Council or its meetings. All I want is the Membership", she explained. Six members of Council supported her, but it was not enough.

Nonetheless, the influx, during the 1870s, of new radical members of Council, drawn from the provinces, ensured that the "eternal feminine question" would be placed prominently on the Council's agenda. In the Council meeting of 2 October 1872 Robert Hampson moved a resolution to admit women to both the lectures and the laboratory. Since women were already admitted to the Society's examinations, he argued, it made little sense to deny them the means of instruction. As a matter of expediency, in view of the limited accommodation in the laboratory, the word "laboratory" was withdrawn, and it was then unanimously resolved to admit women as students to the lecture classes. The next move was to obtain admission for women as members. At the Council meeting held on 6 November 1872, Robert Hampson put forward the name of a woman in business on her own account for election to membership of the Society. After some discussion, he withdrew her name to allow further consideration. At the next Council meeting, in December, Hampson returned to the subject by another route. He proposed that women students should be eligible to compete for all the prizes, certificates and scholarships awarded in the School of Pharmacy. This sparked off a general discussion of the advisability of encouraging women to become students, which carried over to the first council meeting of the new year, when the motion was lost by one vote.

In the meanwhile, two women students sat for the preliminary examination, and the name of one of them, Rose Coombes Minshull appeared at the top of the list of the 166 who passed; the other, Louisa Stammwitz, was about half-way down the list. At the Council meeting in February 1873 these two names, together with that of Alice Marion Hart, whose certificate from the Society of Apothecaries was received in lieu of the preliminary, were brought forward for admission as "registered students" of the Society. G.W. Sandford moved an amendment rejecting their names, and, when this failed, another amendment, deferring the decision until after the next Council elections, was put. Nine voted for, and nine against. The chairman, A. F. Heselden gave his casting vote in favour of the amendment, and the women's admission was blocked.

The subject of women pharmacists had by now aroused the interest of the general body of members and letters in prose and verse began to fill the pages of the *Pharmaceutical Journal*. Few members felt constrained to restrict themselves to the point in question, which was the admission of women to the Pharmaceutical Society. Instead they roamed over the whole question of the role of women in society, often with the flippancy characteristic of those whose intellect has succumbed to the weight of their prejudices. The editors of both the *Pharmaceutical Journal* and the *Chemist and Druggist* came out strongly in favour of admitting women to the Society, as did several members of Council. G.F. Schacht could find no "reason for alarm if ladies were elected to membership. It did not at all follow that they would be elected to the Council table or to the presidential chair; though if the majority of the members desired to confer that honour upon them, he saw no reason why they should not be elected". Another Councillor found good practical reasons for admitting women. It would enable a man to train his daughter to take a part in his business and later to set up on her own account. "He had known two instances in which a business which had not prospered very well under the care of the husband had thriven much better when conducted by the widow". In a letter to the *Pharmaceutical Journal*, Rose Minshull, Louisa Stammwitz and Alice Hart put forward their demands modestly but firmly:

> All that we ask is to be allowed the same opportunities for study, the same field for competition and the same honours, if justly won.

The leader of the opposition was George W. Sandford, who was rapidly acquiring the reputation of a dyed-in-the-wool reactionary. "The tendency of the present day", he wrote, "is too much towards upsetting that natural and scriptural arrangement of the sexes which has worked tolerably well for four thousand years". He saw clearly that the admission of women as members would act as an encouragement to their taking up the business of pharmacy: for him, that was a most undesirable development. He opposed the admission of women "both on behalf of the Society and of the women themselves". The Pharmaceutical Society was intended to be society of men: major disadvantages would arise from its becoming a mixed society of men and women. A large inflow of women would endanger progress towards professionalism in pharmacy. "There were many other means of earning a living open to women and he was opposed to encouraging them to enter a business where they would have, day by day, to deal in things which he should be very sorry for any near, female friends of his own to have any knowledge of". "There may be more fitting occupations for them than listening to the description of bodily ailments over our shop counters". The main objection to women chemists, as another writer explained, was "the common occurrence of prescriptions and remedies dealing with maladies of the most revolting nature which have the power to appal and disgust the sternest member of the sterner sex". The innocence of the fair sex was part of the Victorian romantic myth.

A very full debate took place on the admission of women at the annual meeting in May 1873. Robert Hampson's advocacy of their cause was lucid and closely argued. The Pharmaceutical Society, he said, was not a private club, but a public body carrying out national duties. The admission of women "is a question of simple justice and common fairness". "You cannot prevent them being chemists, and why should you prevent them entering the Society as men do?" He told the members that "we shall do no dishonour to ourselves by admitting women but shall be simply acting fairly at least to a few women who wish to join us". The supporters of Hampson's motion dominated the debate, won all the arguments, and were heavily defeated at the end of the day.[8]

For five years the question was shelved. By the time it was reintroduced, at the annual meeting in May 1878, events outside the world of pharmacy made resistance to women's demands more difficult. The London School of Medicine for Women opened its doors in 1874 and, two years later, Russell Gurney's "Act to remove the restriction on the granting of qualifications on the ground of sex" gave qualified women the right to be placed on the Medical Register. The University of London was brought to recognise, in 1877, that since it had been founded to admit persons "of every kind, without distinction", and "all classes and denominations", it could not very well refuse to admit women. "If sex is to be no hindrance to the pursuit of the medical profession", said the *Lancet* in 1875, "it can be to no other. In other words, the legislation which would admit women to medicine will mark a new era in social and political history, the effect of which may be more felt in other professions than in ours".[9] Since women had never been barred from practising as chemists and druggists, their exclusion from membership of the Pharmaceutical Society was becoming increasingly anomalous. The annual meeting in May 1878 resurrected the issue but left it in confusion. At the end of the debate, a vote of 59 to 57 was recorded, but no one knew which side had won. At the next Council meeting in June, members divided equally, eight on each side, on a motion to admit women, but the president, John Williams, cast his vote to maintain the status quo. Inevitably, the motion was repeated at the next annual meeting: again the voting was close, 81 to 79, but the motion was lost. With the members equally divided, Messrs. Hampson and Woolley brought the matter up once more in Council. On 1 October 1879 the motion that Isabella Skinner Clarke and Rose Coombes Minshull, both of London, be elected members of the Society was carried with only the president, G.W. Sandford, dissenting. At last the sex of otherwise eligible persons was no longer a bar to their admission as members of the Pharmaceutical Society.[10] But if the question of the admission of women was finally settled, the struggle for equal opportunities had only just begun.

It required a high level of ability and determination for a woman to enlist as a student in the School of Pharmacy. At the beginning women were cold-shouldered and forced to keep very much to themselves: they were not even allowed through the same entrance as the men students. Despite, or perhaps because of, the obstacles placed in their path, women, once admitted, did exceptionally well. By 1925 there had been five Pereira medallists, seven Redwood scholars, five Jacob Bell scholars and fifteen Burroughs scholars among them. In 1908, after Gertrude Holland Wren became the first woman to be awarded the Pereira medal, a columnist of the *Chemist and Druggist* observed:

> the Male Intellect is evidently not equal to the contest with feminine rivals in the class rooms and in examinations. Miss Wren annexes three out of four silver medals which the Pharmaceutical Society contributes annually ... and at the same time establishes her claim to the Pereira medal. Miss Neve supplements this demonstration of the superiority of the sex by scooping in exactly the same proportion of the bronze medals awarded in the Minor course. This appropriation of the Society's bullion by two very young ladies ... leaves but a scanty "distribution" of honours ... among the masculine majority of competitors. Moreover the ominousness of the event is that it is not merely occasional or accidental. It is just the climax of a consistent progress which has been noted again and again ... Undoubtedly the average of the academic work of the ladies at schools of pharmacy (and not in this country alone) has been much higher than that of the male students ...

It was, however, reassuring that men remained firmly in control.

> ... But there remains the consoling fact that though women have been demonstrating their capabilities in pharmacy for thirty years or more, it is still men who teach them, men who examine them, and men who hand them out their medals.[11]

The newly-qualified women encountered many difficulties when it came to getting a job. Prejudice and discrimination ensured that they were employed in the worst paid and least demanding areas of pharmacy. By 1908 the number of registered women pharmacists had fallen to 160, constituting about one per cent of all qualified chemists. Of the 160 only two-thirds were actually practising pharmacy, the rest having married, gone abroad, or left pharmacy for medicine or for some special application of chemistry. Of those still practising, more than sixty per cent. were working in hospitals and institutions; eighteen to twenty per cent. were in retail pharmacy, either running their own businesses or more often employed as assistants; twelve per cent. were dispensers to medical men in private practice; a few were employed by wholesale firms; and still fewer were engaged in analytical work, in teaching or in research. Fathers seemed unwilling to invest capital to launch their daughters in business but were not averse to using them as managers and assistants. One or two wholesale houses employed women for the supervision of packed goods, tablet-making and other mechanical tasks, scarcely deserving consideration as work for pharmacists. At least

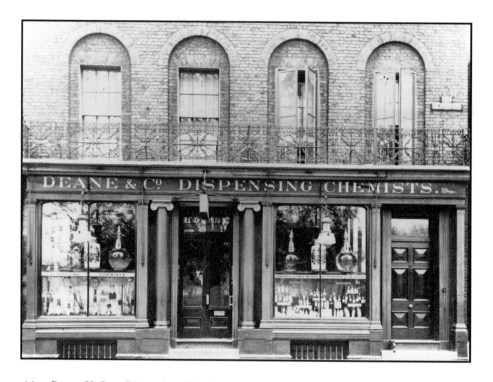

44   *Deane & Co., Dispensing Chemists, 17 The Pavement, Clapham, early twentieth century. Established by Henry Deane in 1837, from 1914 this pharmacy was staffed and run entirely by women. One of a series of exterior views of pharmacies in the museum collection.*

eighty-five per cent. of women pharmacists were employed in positions in which they were not only poorly paid but also directly subordinate to men. The average salaries for full-time posts (54 hours a week) in institutions were £118 per annum (or £70, if resident). This was less than an elementary school teacher, a bank clerk or a clerical grade civil servant would earn. Female managers or assistants in retail pharmacy received between £50 and £80 a year, with board and lodging. Qualified pharmacists working in hospitals and institutions and for medical practitioners were competing with dispensers who held the Assistants' Certificate of the Society of Apothecaries, who invariably accepted low wages. The jobs consisted mainly of routine dispensing with little scope to demonstrate powers of intellect and initiative or even to make use of the skills acquired in training. Nonetheless, more than one hospital management committee had cause to recognize the value of "the rigid economy of a woman's administration and dispensing". With reference to hospital and infirmary dispensing, Margaret Buchanan, in 1908, observed that:

> In such a position the orderliness and attention to detail, the tact and desire to please, which are supposed to be natural to most women, are a most necessary part of their stock-in-trade, and there have been not a few instances where women's

business capacity and an up-to-date knowledge of drugs and economical methods have led to practical appreciation on the part of committees.[12]

Until the foundation of the Association of Women Pharmacists on 15 June 1905, women pharmacists stood isolated and unorganized. Although many of them were members of the Pharmaceutical Society, their needs and aspirations were almost completely ignored. The Association was founded as a rallying point and as a centre for social intercourse. Its objects were severely practical. They were : (1) to discuss the employment of women in pharmacy from an ethical and practical standpoint, (2) to keep a register of all qualified women and their appointments, (3) to keep a register of members requiring assistants or locum-tenens and to put them in touch with members desiring employment. The Association's employment bureau compiled a black list of badly paid posts and put pressure on hospitals and other institutions to improve salaries and terms of employment. The Association was not hostile to the Pharmaceutical Society. Members of the Association were encouraged to join the Society and those who did, paid an annual subscription to the Association of only five shillings, while non-members paid half-a-guinea. Membership of the Association was confined to women who had passed either the Major or Minor examination. The first committee consisted of five women of awesome intellect and steely determination. The president was Isabella Skinner Clarke (by then, Mrs Clarke Kerr, Ph.C.), with Margaret Buchanan Ph.C., as vice-president, Hilda B. Caws, Ph.C., treasurer, and G.E. Barltrop and Elsie S. Hooper, B.Sc.(London), Ph.C., as secretaries. About fifty pharmacists joined immediately and the Association grew steadily as invariably the sixteen or so women who qualified each year became members. Co-operation and education were the keystones of the Association. Women were encouraged to co-operate in a variety of ways; by using the Association's employment bureau and its special insurance and annuity scheme; by participating in a training programme which involved the interchange of apprentices between retail and hospital pharmacy; and in setting up in business. To overcome the difficulties faced by single women, the Association suggested that "two or three qualified women of congenial tastes, each with a knowledge of some special branch of work" should join together and launch their own enterprises. Co-operation was also needed "in mutual defence against unjust statements and misrepresentations in the Press". The Association was deeply committed to the value of education. "Education not merely of ourselves, but of the public, of the medical men and women with whom we come into contact, and of those who are entering our craft". Medical practitioners must be educated

> as to the value of the education and status of the examination we have undergone . . . Every qualified chemist may help towards the recognition of the qualification by being able and willing to give needed information on chemical, pharmaceutical, and botanical questions such as are constantly cropping up when dealing with medical men and the public . . . Then, too, we must educate the public as to the position of pharmacists who . . . are . . . not mere tradesmen but should possess that professional skill and morality which can alone guarantee the safety and protection of the public. If there be a calling where competent skill and professional honour must be combined, pharmacy is surely that one".

Although the Association of Women Pharmacists believed in the need to "stand shoulder to shoulder with our brother-pharmacists in the field of pharmaceutical education, politics and defence", it contained within its ranks a lively group of militant feminists. On Saturday 17 June 1911 they joined more than 40,000 other women in marching from the Victoria Embankment to the Royal Albert Hall to express their solidarity with the Suffragette movement. Their banner proudly bore the slogan, "Women Pharmacists Demand the Vote". Among their number that day were Elsie Hooper, Mrs. A. Freke, who became a member of the Council of the Pharmaceutical Society in 1926, and Miss A. Gilliatt, who became the first woman mayor of Fulham in 1935.[13]

Shortage of manpower during the First World War (1914–18) enabled women to increase significantly their representation within the profession: by 1920 seven per cent. of the names on the register were women's. By 1922, with growing fears of widespread unemployment, the inevitable male backlash occurred. Acrimonious correspondence on the subject of women in pharmacy became a regular feature of the correspondence columns of the *Pharmaceutical Journal* between 1922 and 1929. "The mass influx of women" rose to the top of every sensible man's list of the forces destroying pharmacy as a worthwhile occupation. During this period qualified women received much help and encouragement through their membership of the Association of Women Pharmacists (now the National Association of Women Pharmacists). The Association enabled women to stand firm and convert the beach-head that they had gained during the war into a permanent foothold in the profession. In 1918 Margaret Buchanan was elected the first woman member of the Council of the Pharmaceutical Society and in 1923 Miss A. Borrowman was appointed to the Society's board of examiners. The Association's employment bureau helped newly qualified women to find scarce jobs and many of the more experienced women owed their promotion to positions of greater responsibility to the Association's influence. By 1937 there were 2,227 women on the register, ten per cent. of the total of 22,195. In that year Mrs. Jean Irvine, whose flair for administration was evident in her work as superintendent of the South-eastern Pricing Bureau for National Health Insurance prescriptions, was elected to the Society's Council. In 1947 she became the first woman President.

The Association of Women Pharmacists encouraged its members to take an active part in the public life of pharmacy especially at the local branch level. All the women who were elected to the Society's Council were prominent members of the Association and became well known for their work within it: their candidature was strongly supported by the Association. During the 1939–45 war women pharmacists made further advance. The Association's employment bureau worked in close collaboration with the Central Pharmaceutical War Committee and was able to give valuable help in ensuring the efficient use of women power in pharmacy. By 1941 the number of women on the register had risen to 3,562, fifteen and a half per cent. of the total. A further indicator of women's progress in pharmacy was the fact that 166 women held the post of superintendent in registered companies. By 1945 nearly forty per cent. of newly qualified chemists were women. Since the coming of the National Health Service the proportion of women in the profession has grown steadily from eighteen per cent. in 1953 to twenty-six per cent. in 1964 to thirty-six per cent. in 1984. Women students comprised two-thirds of the intake at schools of pharmacy in 1982.[14]

* * *

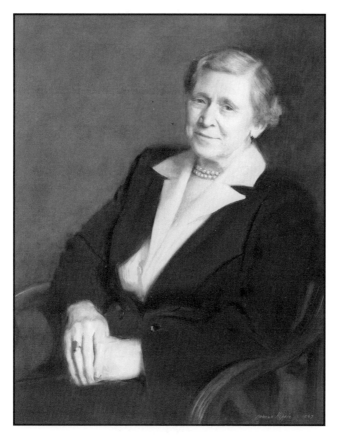

45 *Mrs Jean Kennedy Irvine MBE who qualified in 1900, lived to 85 years and died in 1962. The first woman President of the Pharmaceutical Society, 1947–8. Oil portrait by Norman Hepple ARA.*

From the Pharmacy Act of 1852 to the Pharmacy and Poisons Act of 1933 the distinction between registration under the Pharmacy Acts and membership of the Pharmaceutical Society was retained and persisted. The first statutory register, the Register of Pharmaceutical Chemists, was set up by the Pharmacy Act of 1852, which also made the use by a non-member of a description implying membership of the Society a statutory offence. But the distinction between members of the Pharmaceutical Society and pharmaceutical chemists was carefully preserved, and each person who passed the Major examination remained free to decide whether or not to become associated with the Society. The new "chemist and druggist", who was legally brought into existence by the 1868 Act, was carefully distinguished from the pharmaceutical chemist, who continued to be registered separately. The 1868 Act provided the same legal status, that of "chemist and druggist", to a wide range of pharmaceutical practitioners: those in business prior to the Act's passing, associates of the Pharmaceutical Society, assistants who passed the new

The Statutory Registers, Pharmacy Acts 1852 and 1868

[A] *The Register of Pharmaceutical Chemists*

   (1) All members of the Pharmaceutical Society before 1868, examined and unexamined.

   (2) All who have passed the Major examination.
   Pharmaceutical Chemists are exempt from jury service.

[B] *The Register of Chemists and Druggists*

   (1) All pharmaceutical chemists

   (2) Unexamined, but in business on their own account prior to 1868.

   (3) Associates of the Pharmaceutical Society before 1868, examined and unexamined.

   (4) Assistants of three years standing prior to 1868, who have passed the Modified examination.

   (5) All who have passed the Minor examination.

Although the Pharmaceutical Society compiled the statutory registers and conducted the qualifying examinations, the distinction between registration under the Pharmacy Acts and membership of the Pharmaceutical Society was maintained until the passing of the Pharmacy and Poisons Act in 1933.

"modified" examination, and everyone who passed the Society's Minor examination. The statutory registers made no distinction between employers and employed: the intention was to make, in the long run, the difference between the pharmaceutical chemist and the chemist and druggist simply a matter of educational attainment.

   Although educational qualification was to become the criterion for admission to the professional registers, the basic requirement for membership of the Pharmaceutical Society remained, until 1872, ownership of property. Chemists who did not own their own shops, whether they were registered as pharmaceutical chemists or chemists and druggists, continued to be treated as second-class citizens within the Pharmaceutical Society. To this general rule there was one minor exception. "Confidential superintendents", the managers of the retail outlets of the major wholesale firms, could be specially elected to membership by the Council: their number was kept very low. The lack of congruence between educational attainment and employment status created the anomaly which was rectified in 1872. Before that date employers who had never passed an examination in their life could become president of the Pharmaceutical Society, while their employees, who might have achieved the highest honours in passing the Major examination, were denied the right to attend meetings and vote. In 1872 the Council decided to abolish the grade of "major associate". All pharmaceutical chemists who wished to be associated with the Society were

Composition of Pharmaceutial Society 1868–1872
Association voluntary. Men only

[A]   *Those in business on their own account* (i.e. proprietor-chemists)

(1) *Members who are Pharmaceutical Chemists*
   (a) Unexamined members before 1868, i.e. those who joined the Society in 1841, 1843, or 1852.

   (b) Those who passed the Major examination.

(2) *Members who are Chemists and Druggists*

   Those in business prior to 1868 who joined in 1868 or later (unexamined or passed Minor examination before 1868).

All members eligible for election to Council but Council not to contain more than seven members (from a total of twenty-one) who are not pharmaceutical chemists.

(3) *Associates-in-business*

   Those who qualified as chemists and druggists by passing the Minor or Modified examination after 1868.
   Associates-in-business "shall have the privilege of attending all meetings of the said Society and of voting thereat, and otherwise taking part in the proceedings of such meetings, in the same manner as members of the said Society: provided always that such associates contribute to the funds of the said Society the same fees or subscriptions as members contribute".
   Associates-in-business were not eligible for election to Council.

[B]   *Those NOT in business on their own account*
(e.g. employed managers and assistants)

(4) *Associates*

   Those not in business on their own account who are either pharmaceutical chemists (having passed the Major examination) or chemists and druggists (having passed either the Minor or the Modified examination.)

(5) *Associates admitted before 1 July 1842*

   Unexamined assistants who joined the Society at its foundation.

(6) *Registered Apprentices and Students*

   Those who have passed the Preliminary examination, and registered with the Society. It was not necessary to pass the preliminary examination, register with the Society, or serve an apprenticeship to sit the statutory examinations.

Associates, apprentices and students paid half the annual subscription for which they received the *Pharmaceutical Journal*. They were not allowed to attend meetings or vote.

now required to become full members, whether they were in business on their own account or employed as assistants. By this decision the property qualification for membership was abolished. Registration as a pharmaceutical chemist, not ownership of a shop, became the *sine qua non* of membership. A society of proprietor chemists became an association of professional pharmacists.

The decision taken by the Council in 1872 was an attempt to preserve the distinctive quality of the Major examination. Before 1868 the Major examination had been regarded as the qualification for starting up in business. The Minor examination was a more rudimentary test designed for assistants. The Pharmacy Act of 1868 turned the Minor examination into the legal license to practise pharmacy and made the Major examination an unnecessary appendage. In 1872 the Council tried to rescue the Major examination by underlining the fact that it was still the qualification required of members of the Society. Those who had only the Minor qualification were classified as "associates". They could register as chemists and druggists and set up open shop to practise pharmacy but they could not become members of the Society. In 1872 one hundred and forty nine pharmaceutical chemists were transformed from associates to members at the stroke of a pen. Even though they were only employees, they acquired the right to attend and speak at meetings, to vote, and to be elected to Council. Not all of them were grateful. Several expressed outrage at the doubling of their subscription: more than a third left the Society altogether.[15]

The rationalization of 1872 did not eliminate all the anomalies in the constitution of the Pharmaceutical Society. The disjunction between the Society's constitution and the structure of the statutory registers was aggravated by the provisions of the 1868 Pharmacy Act. Not only was there no necessity for the chemist and druggist to join the Pharmaceutical Society, his association with it was hedged about with numerous restrictions. Men employed as assistants who qualified by passing the Minor examination were admitted only as associates, although unexamined chemists who owned shops before 1868 were welcomed as members. But their membership carried with it restricted access to seats on Council. This may account for the fact that, although the number of unexamined chemists who secured registration under the 1868 Act was large, the number who took advantage of the Pharmaceutical Society's offer of membership was noticeably small. The new generation of proprietors who qualified by passing the Minor examination was even more reluctant to become associated with the Society. This is hardly surprising in view of the fact that they were debarred from membership and offered instead the inferior status of "associates-in-business". They were expected to pay the same fees and subscriptions as members but were denied the right of being elected to Council. Such curmudgeonly treatment was not calculated to gain their allegiance to the Society.

It was the perennial need to recruit new members that led to the Pharmacy Acts Amendment Act of 1898. The original bill, drafted in February 1890, merely proposed extending membership to associates-in-business. But the 1890 bill was received with so little enthusiasm from the body of chemists generally that it was rapidly withdrawn. During the years 1890 and 1891 Michael Carteighe, the president of the Society, went on a tub-thumping, fact-finding tour of Britain, with meetings in Aberdeen, Birmingham, Brighton, Cardiff, Carlisle, Dundee, Edinburgh, Exeter, Glasgow, Hull, Leeds, Liverpool, Manchester, Plymouth and Sheffield. He argued that constitutional reform of the Pharmaceutical Society was a prerequisite for more fundamental pharmaceutical legislation.

His visits kindled some interest in reform and convinced the president that all registered chemists and druggists should be made eligible for membership of the Society. The idea was taken on board by the Council and incorporated into the Society's pharmacy bills of 1891, 1894, and 1895. The only one of this series of bills to prove successful was drafted in 1897. It was introduced into the House of Commons on 3 March 1898 and received the Royal Assent on 25 July that year.

The Pharmacy Acts Amendment Act of 1898 gave all registered chemists and druggists, whether employers, self-employed or employed, the right to become full members of the Pharmaceutical Society and to be elected to its Council. The discrimination between "members who are pharmaceutical chemists", "members who are chemists and druggists", "associates-in-business", and "associates" was swept away. The only division to survive was between "members" and "student-associates". Although the distinction between pharmaceutical chemists and chemists and druggists was maintained by the statutory registers, it lost its relevance in the Society's constitution. The reservation of two-thirds of the Council seats for pharmaceutical chemists was abolished. In future the seven Council members who had been longest in office without re-election would retire each year. Every member, including the retiring Councillors, would be eligible to fill the vacancies. Previously, two-thirds of the Council had retired each year.

The origins of the 1898 Act are to be sought, not in the Council chamber in Bloomsbury Square, but in the provincial cities that Michael Carteighe visited in 1890 and 1891. One of the most striking developments of the last quarter of the nineteenth century was the growth of local associations of chemists and druggists. Even before the formation of the Pharmaceutical Society, the druggists of Aberdeen, Leicester and Colchester had small trade associations. After 1841 local branches of the Society were started, on the recommendation of Jacob Bell, for the reading of papers and the promotion of social intercourse among members. As education was such a strong feature of the Society's work, the establishment of branch schools of the Pharmaceutical Society became the primary responsibility of these local associations. In Bath, Bristol, Manchester and Norwich branch schools were set up and aided by grants from the Society's funds. These branches consisted entirely of members of the Pharmaceutical Society and the member's fee to the Society included membership of the branch. But the Pharmaceutical Society did not, in the beginning, make great strides in the provinces and some of the branches came to an untimely end. These branches of the Society have to be carefully distinguished from the local associations which developed in the 1870s. In these, membership was thrown open to all registered chemists and druggists. They met to discuss current pharmaceutical politics, to arrange hours of business and fix local prices, and, above all, to promote good fellowship. In 1874 there were, throughout Britain, more than twenty-five flourishing local associations some of which had been established for several years. By 1896 their number had risen and by 1906 there were about seventy in full working order. It was the manifest success of these local associations that convinced Michael Carteighe and his fellow Councillors that the constitution of the Pharmaceutical Society needed drastic revision.

* * *

The forty years between the Pharmacy Act of 1868 and the Poisons and Pharmacy Act of 1908 saw radical changes in the trade of chemist and druggist. The position and methods of the independent proprietors were challenged by the emergence of new types of retailing ushered in by multiples, co-operatives and department stores. In the 1870s a number of limited liability companies, including the Civil Service Co-operative Society and leading department stores such as Harrods, began selling drugs and medicines. To attract customers they used the term "chemist" for the part of the shop that dealt in drugs and, if a qualified person was in charge, they also sold poisons. The Pharmaceutical Society, having campaigned for over twenty years to secure the 1868 Act, was determined to defend the privileged status that Act accorded the proprietor chemist. The Society held that the professional practice of pharmacy required the qualified chemist to retain the ownership and control of the practice. Professional service depends on individual qualities and individual judgment, supported by individual responsibility. Professionalism is destroyed when unqualified laymen, driven solely by the profit motive, acquire the ownership and control of the professional enterprise. The demands of the owners may be expected to clash with the conscience of the professional. If, by forming limited companies, unqualified persons acquired the right to use professional titles and employ registered persons to carry on professional practice under their control, the independent professions would be destroyed. This was true, not only for pharmacy, but for medicine and the law as well. Laymen could form joint-stock companies, call themselves physicians and surgeons and employ registered medical practitioners to treat patients. The laymen would control the quality and the cost of the services and pocket the profits. The Pharmaceutical Society maintained that since a corporate body could not sit its examinations and be registered, it had no legal right to operate a chemist's business. The 1868 Act had been passed to prevent those who could not fulfil these conditions from keeping open shop for the sale of poisons. Most members of the Society, however, were probably more interested in maintaining their own profit margins against the threat of a new type of retailing than they were in upholding the purity of a professional ideal.

The Pharmaceutical Society v. The London and Provincial Supply Association was the most important case decided under the 1868 Pharmacy Act. It was contested, with varying fortunes, up to the highest court of the realm. The London and Provincial Supply Association carried on a general retail trade at 113 Tottenham Court Road. The business included a drug department which was managed by H.E. Longmore, a qualified chemist and druggist, who had two qualified men under him. The sole proprietor was an unregistered man, William Mackness. In January 1878 the Pharmaceutical Society's solicitor wrote to Mackness indicating that the Society intended to take legal proceedings against him in respect of a sale of oxalic acid (a scheduled poison); as an unregistered person, he was liable to a penalty of £5 under the 15th section of the 1868 Act. Mackness, admitting he was in the wrong, paid the money to the Society without going to Court and intimated that he was taking steps to end any further violation of the law. This he did by simply converting the business into a limited liability company. Not that this involved any material change in the method of conducting the business or in the matter of proprietorship. The new company, with a nominal capital of £6,000, consisted of ten persons, of whom Mackness held £5,640 worth of shares, paid up, while nine other persons held between them £360 worth, £82–10s. of which was paid. W.E. Longmore continued as a salaried servant in charge of the drug department, but also became a shareholder with £50 worth of shares, £12–10s of which was paid up. The London and Provincial Supply Association had been registered under the Companies Acts with the deliberate intention of thus allowing an unqualified person to keep open shop for the sale of poisons.

The Pharmaceutical Society decided that this was an appropriate opportunity to determine the legal position. In May 1878 the Society applied for a penalty under the 15th section of the Pharmacy Act against the Association for unlawfully keeping open shop for the sale of poisons. Judge Russell, in the Bloomsbury County Court, gave judgment for the defendants. He said:

> If Mr. Longmore had sold these things for himself alone, he would not have committed any offence whatever. It is said, however, that it was committing an offence because the business was so conducted that money is acquired and the profit so made goes into the pockets of other people. That obviously is not within the mischief intended to be remedied by the Act.
>
> It does not become unlawful when done on behalf of the company, so long as the business is conducted by a duly qualified chemist and druggist who, if carrying it on for his own benefit, would not be within the penalties of the Act.

The Pharmaceutical Society appealed against the County Court decision and the case came before the Court of Queen's Bench on 15 March 1879. The Attorney-General, Sir John Holker, appeared for the Society and Mr. Wills, Q.C. for the defending company. At the outset, Mr. Wills intimated that his case rested on the argument that companies, not being persons, were not affected by the 15th section of the Act. He could not see his way to support the view taken by the judge in the County Court that it made any difference for the purpose of this action, whether the company did or did not employ qualified assistants. He maintained that when the Act was framed corporate bodies were not thought of; that this was, in fact, a *casus omissus*. It was not for the Courts to impose penalties which the legislature had not envisaged, however desirable it might be in order to complete the round of legislation. He argued that there was a well-known distinction in law between a corporation and the individuals of a corporation. The Pharmacy Act applied only to persons: a number of persons forming a company could not be held guilty of an offence within an Act of Parliament relating to individual persons. He quoted various sections of the Act, such as those relating to examinations, which it was evident a corporation could not fulfil, to show that all consideration of them had been overlooked. The Attorney-General, in reply, maintained that if the corporations could not fulfil the requirements so much the worse for the corporations. The Act was passed to prevent anyone who could not fulfil these conditions from carrying on such a business.

The point whether, in law, the word "person" included a company was argued at great length. The Attorney-General, with the intention of showing that "corporation" was within the term "person", drew attention to certain cases in which actions were brought against corporations. The Court was much influenced by this argument and, on 23 April 1879, gave judgment in favour of the Pharmaceutical Society. Both judges agreed that the 1868 Act was intended to prevent the mischief of the sale of poisons by unqualified persons; that qualified persons only should be allowed to keep open shop for the sale of such articles; and that therefore artificial as well as natural persons could not trade as chemists and druggists if they were not or could not be qualified.

The case came next before the Court of Appeal in the form of an appeal by the defendants. The arguments were heard on 23 and 25 February 1880 by Lords Justices Bramwell, Baggallay and Thesiger. Mr. Wills contended that, although the term "person" was capable in law of including "corporation", in modern Acts of Parliament that was not so, but where "person" was intended to include "corporation" there was an interpretation clause saying so. He cited several Acts to support this view. In addition to the strictly legal part of his speech, Mr. Wills argued that the Pharmaceutical Society had used the poisons scare of the mid-sixties to obtain this Act of Parliament, which did a good deal for them, but that now their real object was to shut down the co-operative stores, which were hitting them so hard. This was all very clever and well calculated to prejudice the Society's case. In 1880 co-operative stores were synonymous in the public mind with "self help" and "social amelioration"; while the idea of protection for any social group was anathema.

In presenting the case for the respondents, the Attorney-General pointed out that the important point to determine was, what did the legislature intend when the 1868 Act was passed? He argued that it was not enacted in the interests of chemists but of the public. In proof of this he instanced the wording of the preamble, "whereas it is expedient for the safety of the public ..."

Judgment was given on 16 March reversing that of the Court below. Lord Justice Bramwell found that in all modern Acts of Parliament "corporations" were expressly named if they were intended to be included. In this Act they were clearly not included. Nor did their exclusion affect the public safety. If the servant of a corporation, not being a qualified chemist, sold poison, he was the offender. It might then be asked, how could the offence of "keeping open shop" be reached? The servants do not keep it open. No, but directors or managers do; they are the offenders in that case. He could not see how they could deny that they keep open shop: they do, they do it in fact.

> If the statute—it can have no object except this—means to impose the penalty on him who commands the prohibited act to be done, unless he is qualified, this opinion will not affect his liability and if the penalty attaches to several, unless all are qualified, they will be liable, notwithstanding this opinion.

Lord Justice Thesiger took a similar view.

> I feel bound to add that I am by no means satisfied that, although a corporation as a separate entity be not liable to the penalty, ... the individual members of the corporation, whether directors of the company or otherwise, may not be liable, and thus the mischief be remedied.

Lord Justice Baggallay came to similar conclusions, and added:

> The object of the Act is to prevent the selling, dispensing or compounding of poisons by unqualified persons. A corporation cannot of itself sell, dispense or compound; it can only do so by the aid of a servant or assistant, and if that servant or assistant is duly qualified in the manner required by the Act ... the object of the Act is attained.

This confident assertion overlooked the fact that, even with the precautions mentioned, an unqualified individual proprietor was subject to the penalties in the Act. A major consideration influencing the Court of Appeal's judgment is indicated by Lord Justice Bramwell's comment that the verdict had the advantage of not needlessly restraining trade.

> There is this advantage, as I have said, in this construction, that it does not exclude a corporation from the benefit of carrying on this business, nor the public from dealing with them ... The statute never meant to infringe the rules of free trade, nor to grant protection to chemists, but only to the public ...

The Pharmaceutical Society appealed from this decision to the House of Lords and the case was opened on 20 July 1880 before the Lord Chancellor (Selborne), Lord Blackburn and Lord Watson. On this occasion more than at any previous hearing, the argument was very sharp, counsel and judges being all well acquainted with the points in dispute. In general, the rival counsels followed the same lines of contention as previously. The judgments were unanimously, and, in the main, confidently, against the Pharmaceutical Society. The Lord Chancellor thought that the word "person" might—in his view did—*prima facie* include in a public statute a person in law as well as a natural person; yet, in a popular sense and in ordinary usage, it did not extend so far. In reading this Act, however, it seemed to him that the legislature had only natural persons in mind. He showed this by several citations. There was no general prohibition of the trade but merely a declaration that it shall be unlawful for a person to carry on the business unless he complies with certain conditions. It was sound to hold that only such persons were contemplated as might, by taking appropriate action, comply with the conditions. The argument that the object of the Act would be defeated unless a corporation were included could not be successfully maintained because the act of selling, the act of compounding, or any act mentioned in the sections by which penalties are imposed, is struck at, whether done by the principal or by the person whom he employs. The liberty of the subject should not be more restrained than the words of a statute require. He thought, therefore, it would be wrong to impose on the word "person" such a construction as would render illegal the carrying on of business by corporations, when, from the beginning of the Act to the end, there was not a single reference to them.

Lord Blackburn was of the same opinion. He would have found no legal difficulty in applying the word "person" to corporations, if it were necessary. But the object of including corporations was certainly not avowed on the face of the Act. Whether the promoters of the Act had any such idea in their minds, he could not tell, but they had not brought it forward; and he thought that if they had boldly said bodies corporate and joint-stock companies shall not deal in poisonous drugs "unless they pay blackmail to us", it was exceedingly unlikely that the legislature would have consented. No mischief was done by corporations keeping open shop if sales were conducted by qualified persons. There could be no sale, whether a corporation were the ultimate vendor or not, unless a natural person managed the sale, and that natural person, if unqualified, would be liable under the Act. He was, moreover, inclined to think that if a corporation, or anyone else, caused an unqualified person to make such sales, they might themselves be liable to penalties; but he was not certain about that.

Lord Watson said that the statute was characterised by great ambiguity, almost confusion, of language. If the legislature had intended to impose penalties on corporations for keeping open shop for the sale of poisons, it would have been very simple to have said so. If that had been the intention, the draftsman had entirely failed to use language adequate for the purpose.

The House of Lords decided that a corporate body was not liable to a penalty if it kept an open shop for the sale of poisons, but it did not say that individual members of a company, who were not registered chemists and druggists, were not liable to penalties. Indeed, in the Court of Appeal, two judges had hinted at the possibility of action against individual company directors. Encouraged by such remarks, the Council of the Pharmaceutical Society took an early opportunity to test their validity by instituting proceedings against unregistered individual directors and shareholders. In June 1887 the Society commenced a suit against the seven partners in a limited company trading as chemists and druggists in Edinburgh. The action was brought in the Summary Court. After hearing the evidence and arguments, Sheriff Rutherford concluded that the shareholders had infringed the Act and gave judgment against them individually for certain fines. But the defendants appealed to the High Court of Justice, where three judges, guided by the House of Lords' decision of 1880, agreed in reversing the Sheriff's decision. Since there could be no appeal from this ruling, the Pharmaceutical Society abandoned the attempt to demonstrate that directors of companies were personally liable for keeping open shop.

The House of Lords' decision opened the door to the carrying on of the business of a chemist and druggist by limited liability companies even though none of the shares of the company was owned by a chemist and the business was not managed by a chemist. The decision was construed as permitting the use by companies of titles restricted to chemists and druggists by the 1868 Act, provided only that a qualified person was employed to conduct the sale of poisons. The decision made possible the development of large-scale pharmaceutical businesses based on the branch system and of the development of the practice of pharmacy by co-operative stores. Firms with an interest in the drug trade were not slow to take advantage of this special dispensation. During the next fifteen years (1880–95) more than two hundred limited liability companies were registered for retail trade in drugs and dispensing, numbers of them by grocers, provision merchants and other retail tradesmen with multiple interests. The first multiple-shop firm specialising in drugs was that of the unqualified druggist, Jesse Boot of Nottingham who, taking advantage of the House of Lords' decision, called himself a "Cash Chemist" in 1880 and had formed a limited company with some 10 branches by 1883.[16] By 1890 there were three other firms in the trade with over ten branches each; Taylors Drug Company Ltd. of Leeds and Yorkshire, W.T. Warhurst of Liverpool, and Timothy White of Portsmouth. The 1890s saw a big increase in the number of multiple chemists' companies. Day's Southern Drug Company of Southampton, which dated back to 1874, expanded rapidly in the 'nineties, and Lewis & Burrows Drug Stores Ltd. was founded in 1895 by the incorporation of eleven cut-price private chemists in London's West End. Other firms which emerged in these years were Magor Ltd. (Birmingham), Needhams Ltd. (Yorkshire), Sussex Drug Co. (Brighton), Hodders (Bristol), Wands (Leicester) and H.B. Pare (Manchester). The Chemists' Co-operative Society was set up to buy forty going concerns, fifteen in London and its suburbs, and twenty-five in leading provincial cities.

From the start both the multiples and the department stores adopted a strategy of selling drugs and proprietary medicines at reduced prices. When, in 1898, Lewis & Burrows Ltd., opened branches in the Pimlico area of London, circulars were distributed announcing that the firm, "the popular store chemists, have declared war against the extortionate prices charged by chemists in the district". Boots, in the same year, used an advertisement in Guernsey, headed, "Great Robbery in the Drug-Trade at Guernsey—Thousands of Pounds". William Day employed boys to walk the streets with placards announcing in bold red and black type:

> Who brought down the chemists' extraordinary prices?—Undoubtedly the Southern Drug Co. Ltd., the original Cash Price List Chemists!

The aggressive selling methods and blatant commercialism of the company chemists inflicted incalculable damage on the burgeoning profession of pharmacy. The Pharmaceutical Society found itself powerless to prevent the growth of either the root cause or the gaudy blossom. It would, however, be quite wrong to believe that the growth of the company chemists had only negative consequences for the development of pharmaceutical professionalism. Once the multiple shop firms became established, they added dispensing and the sale of poisons to the retailing of proprietary and other medicines, and this created new employment opportunities for qualified pharmacists. By 1906 Boots Cash Chemists had 329 branches and employed 434 qualified pharmacists. The multiple stores gave qualified chemists, who lacked the capital to set up in business on their own, the opportunity to become managers and superintendents of branch shops. The company chemists injected a much needed element of competition in the pharmaceutical labour market and did much to transform the conditions of work for the growing number of pharmacists who had no prospect of owning a shop but would remain employed all their working life. The salary and status of the assistant chemist was transformed.

The qualified chemists who went to work as managers in the new multiple stores were roundly abused as "traitors to the craft". In 1898 the president of the Pharmaceutical Society referred to "the disastrous and suicidal conduct of men in our own ranks", and others spoke of "registered chemists who, by their Judas-like treachery in selling their services to unqualified persons . . . have degraded pharmacy, as carried on in joint-stock drug stores, to the lowest depths of mere commercialism".[17] In later years, Jesse Boot acknowledged, "it took some courage for a qualified man to join us". A branch manager was likely to be ostracised by his fellow chemists in the town. Consequently, the companies had to pay salaries and provide benefits that were significantly better than those offered by proprietor chemists. In a letter to the *Chemist and Druggist* in 1893, Jesse Boot explained:

> We have several qualified men with us, who have come to us from the service of firms where they worked fourteen hours daily, fifteen on Saturdays, and had to be on call on Sundays. With us the daily hours are much shorter; there is a complete half-holiday weekly (excepting at one town, where, however, we are arranging this); there is no Sunday duty; and we make arrangements to send qualified relief every year to enable assistants to have a holiday. Under these conditions our managers are, we contend, much better off than the average assistant in middle-class trade. We are not, of course, making the comparison with the cream of West-End pharmacy.
>
> Taking one consideration with another, the shorter hours, the yearly holiday, the fact that in cases of illness qualified relief is at once supplied, whereas numbers of men in a small business are never able to leave their place all the year round—no half-holidays, no annual holidays, and in cases of illness must drag on as best they can—we consider it is far preferable for a man to be engaged in business as a manager with us than in a small way on his own account . . . We have managers with us who have considered it an immense relief to be free from the grind and anxieties of a small business.

Among the replies to Boot's letter was one from a chemist who complained that in his experience West-End pharmacies were no better than any others as employers, and another correspondent observed that "in some of the best-known West-End businesses the accommodation provided for the assistants is disgusting". The advantage of not having to "live-in" was much appreciated by qualified men who went to work for the multiple stores. Assistants described the "poor and ill-cooked food", the "dirty and slovenly surroundings" and the humiliations heaped on them by arrogant and bullying employers owning "legitimate premises".[18]

In contrast, the "business-like courtesy and treatment" received by qualified men at the hands of Boots Ltd., and the majority of stores was frequently remarked upon. The company chemists realised that the future of their business depended on their ability to recruit and retain qualified pharmacists to manage their retail branches. Jesse Boot paid his chemist-managers a commission on branch sales and launched a non-contributory pension scheme for them in 1897. As his retail outlets grew in number and size, a career structure was developed by promoting managers from smaller to larger branches.

Although the qualified men who went to work for the co-operative, department, and multiple stores were branded as quislings to the profession by proprietor chemists, they were, in an important sense, more professional than their detractors. The proprietor chemist embodied the entrepreneurial ideal. In theory, at least, he was a self-made man who gained modest wealth and a secure livelihood by investing his capital in and actively managing his own business. His position and success was dependent upon the ownership of capital. In contrast, the employed chemist-manager embodied the professional ideal. His livelihood, too, depended upon the possession of a scarce resource, but, in his case, it was human, intellectual capital rather than property. His position and success depended upon trained and certified expertise and selection by merit. Although the 1898 Pharmacy Acts Amendment Act made all qualified chemists, whether employers or employed, eligible to be elected not only members but also councillors and officers of the Pharmaceutical Society, the Society maintained a hostile attitude towards the qualified chemist-managers who worked for the co-operative societies, department stores and multiple shop companies. Local branches usually ostracized them, and Michael Carteighe, for fourteen years president, devised a disreputable scheme to have their names erased from the statutory register for infamous conduct in a professional sense.

* * *

The 1868 Pharmacy Act was intended to ensure that the dispensing of dangerous drugs and the sale of poisons was in the hands of qualified chemists and druggists. When it was passed it was assumed that the unqualified assistants employed by chemists and druggists would be under the close supervision of the registered proprietor and that he would himself be responsible for the acts of his assistants. The safety of the public would be protected because the qualified proprietor would be responsible for the overall running of the business. Unqualified persons, such as apprentices, might be employed to assist in the general running of the shop and might even be involved in the dispensing and sale of poisons, provided the owner exercised close personal supervision. The development of multiple stores and branch shops, whether owned by limited companies or by registered chemists, raised a host of new problems. In the case of *The Pharmaceutical Society v. The London and Provincial Supply Association* several of the judges expressed the view that, although limited companies could not be prevented from carrying on business as chemists and druggists, the act of compounding, the act of dispensing and the act of selling must be performed by qualified persons. Before 1880 only the well-established chemists and druggists in London and the provinces employed qualified assistants but, for many years after the House of

Lords' judgment, the Pharmaceutical Society took no action against unqualified assistants selling poisons. Then, in September 1889, at an inquest held by Mr. Braxton Hicks, the energetic coroner for mid-Surrey, it emerged that a servant-girl had purchased a packet of Battle's Vermin Killer, a preparation containing strychnine, at a chemist's shop one Sunday evening and that the actual seller of the poison was an unregistered assistant named Wheeldon, who for the time was in sole charge of the shop. Braxton Hicks reported the case to the Pharmaceutical Society, who sued Wheeldon in the Wandsworth County Court. Judge Holroyd declared: "the Act says that any unqualified person who sells poison is liable to a penalty of £15. The person who sells is liable, whether he be master or servant or apprentice".

After the judge expressed the hope that the case would go to a higher court, a fund was raised and an appeal lodged. The case was argued in the Queen's Bench Division in February and the judgment delivered in April 1890. The Court held that the County Court judge was right and dismissed the appeal. The judgment had important implications for the general conduct of chemists' shops.

> It had been contended . . . that it was not unlawful . . . for an unqualified assistant to a duly-qualified chemist to sell poisons in his master's shop; . . . that the sale being a sale by him as a servant, the master was in law and in fact the seller, and that as the master was qualified the sale was lawful. It was further suggested that great inconvenience and hardship would result to small chemists who could not afford to employ properly qualified assistants . . . We do not agree with the view thus presented, nor are we at all impressed by the suggestion of inconvenience or hardship . . . Nothing, to our minds, can be clearer than that the object of the Act was, beyond all other considerations, to provide for the safety of the public, and to guard, as far as possible, all members of the community from the disastrous consequences so frequently arising from the sale of poisons by persons unacquainted with their baneful properties; and the whole object of the Act would be frittered away, and the Act itself become a dead letter, were we to declare, by our judgment, that an unqualified assistant can lawfully and with impunity sell any of the poisons to which the Act applies, unless upon each occasion of such sale he acts under the personal supervision of a qualified employer, or a qualified assistant to such employer. By personal supervision we mean not mere presence in the shop or room where the sale takes place, but actual personal supervision, so that every individual sale shall be so guarded round by those precautions prescribed by the Act that the safety of every member of the public may be provided for, as far as the law can accomplish that object.

Mr. Justice Hawkins, in delivering the judgment, went on to dismiss the argument that the legislature intended to leave the selection of assistants to the discretion of the employer, without regard to any qualification.

> In our opinion the object of the legislature was to insist upon one uniform qualification for every person who should sell, whether on his own account or for any other person, such poisonous commodities—namely, registration under the section, based upon a certificate of fair skill and knowledge, granted after examinations by examiners carefully selected and specially appointed for that purpose. With such a certificate the holder of it may fairly be deemed to possess knowledge, not only of the general effect and operations of the various poisons with

which he may be called upon to deal, but—what is quite as important, if not more so, for the public safety—the quantities in which such poisons may be harmlessly or beneficially taken, and the quantities which, if taken, would inevitably result in death.

After this declaration of how the need for uniform professional qualification established a legal equality of master and assistant by making them both professional colleagues, the learned judge dealt with the responsibilities of the smaller chemists.

> Those who cannot afford to keep qualified assistant, if they desire for a longer or shorter period to absent themselves from their shops, must take precautions, either by locking up their poisons or by other means, to prevent the sale of any poisons in their absence ... We need hardly say that if mischief arose by reason of the master's negligently leaving an unqualified person in charge of his poisons, no punishment of the assistant would exonerate the master from liability to civil proceedings; nor, if death ensued from such negligence, and the jury found it to be of a criminal and culpable character, would he be exonerated from the charge of manslaughter.

Since 1880 the Pharmaceutical Society had sought powers to ensure that only qualified assistants were employed in chemists' shops and that branch establishments were run by qualified persons. Provision to secure these objectives were included in the abortive pharmacy bills of 1881 and 1883. The further growth of company chemists, multiple stores and branch shops forced the Society to elaborate its policy. The unsuccessful Pharmacy bill of 1901 gives a clear indication of how the Pharmaceutical Society was trying to bring the mounting crisis under control. The 1901 bill was designed to check the growing practice of registered chemists opening several shops without employing qualified persons to run them; to require that companies carrying on the business of chemist and druggist should be managed by registered chemists as directors; and to authorise the Society to compile a register of shops where poisons may be sold and of the duly qualified chemists in charge of them.

Parliament was reluctant to grant these powers but, in the interim, the Society used its existing powers to try to prevent unregistered persons selling poisons. All manner of unqualified sellers were prosecuted: drug store proprietors, grocers, herbalists, seedsmen, florists, oilmen, drysalters and ironmongers as well as assistants employed by companies and registered chemists. Table A below reveals that the unqualified assistant working for a registered chemist could expect no favours: he was at least as likely to be prosecuted as assistants in other establishments. The difficulty the Society found with prosecuting assistants was that, although convictions might be secured, the penalties, in many cases, could not always be enforced, owing to the systematic removal of the defendants from one branch to another by their employers, who were not themselves liable for the penalties incurred by their assistants. The Society was not in the least interested in prosecuting the hapless assistants: its aim was to embarass the employer and to establish the principle that he was responsible for contraventions of the 1868 Act. As part of this policy, the Society brought actions under section 17 of the Act against certain companies for selling poisons without observing the statutory regulations. In 1907 A. W. Gamage (Ltd) was convicted for selling mercuric sulpho-cyanide in the form of "serpent's eggs" without a poison label and later in the same year, Boots Cash Chemists (Southern) Ltd., was convicted for selling strychnine, contained in Easton's Syrup tabloids, across the counter without obtaining the required signatures. These cases established that companies were themselves liable if they expressly or impliedly authorised illegal practices. Jesse Boot, no doubt anxious to demonstrate to the Pharmaceutical Society that its point had been well taken, immediately instituted proceedings against Richard A. Robinson, three times president of the Pharmaceutical Society, who traded as W. Walter Malden and as Malden and Co., for

---

PROSECUTIONS UNDER THE 1868 ACT

[A]   Prosecutions under Section 15, Pharmacy Act 1868, undertaken by the Pharmaceutical Society from 1896 to 1901.

	Three year periods	
	1896–8	1899–1901
Unqualified proprietors of drug stores and their unqualified assistants	139	132
Unqualified assistants of members of the Pharmaceutical Society and of other registered chemists and druggists	115	109
Unqualified assistants to limited companies carrying on business of chemist and druggist	35	36
Unqualified assistants in doctors' open shops	23	22
Unqualified assistants to Executors	3	5
Grocers	40	23
Herbalists	5	9
Drysalters and oilmen	6	7
Seedsmen and Florists	4	6
Other traders	25	5
TOTAL	395	354

[B]   Proceedings under Section 17, Pharmacy Act 1868, instituted by the Pharmaceutical Society from 1896 to 1901

	Three year periods	
	1896–8	1899–1901
Limited Companies	1	6
Members of the Pharmaceutical Society	1	4
Doctors of medicine	0	2
	2	12

In the period 1899–1901 one limited company was prosecuted under Section 12 of the 1852 Pharmacy Act.

Source: Report of Departmental Committee to consider Schedule A to the Pharmacy Act 1868, 1903 (1442,1443) xxxiii Appendix VII.

selling these same tabloids—Easton's Syrup tabloids—without complying with the provisions of the 1868 Act. Robinson was convicted.

In spite of all the efforts of the Pharmaceutical Society to ensure that only qualified persons should dispense and sell poisons, one glaring anomaly persisted. The law required no qualification of any kind for the thousands of persons engaged in dispensing poisons in doctors' surgeries and dispensaries unless these were kept as "open shops". More than four fifths of the medicines prescribed in Britain were dispensed in doctors' surgeries without any legal restriction as to the qualification of the dispenser or regulation as to the mode of dispensing. Advertisements in which doctors stipulated that they required unqualified men to dispense for them appeared regularly in the *Lancet* and the *British Medical Journal*. In 1864 the *Chemist and Druggist* high-lighted the dangers "from errors and ignorance in surgeries when the medicines are dispensed by doctors' wives, errand boys and other useful servants". In October 1898 the Chemists' Assistants' Union drew the attention of the Pharmaceutical Society to the evil of the dispensing of poisons by utterly incompetent persons in doctors' surgeries. An inquest at Heaton Norris in January 1899 revealed that the dispensing error which killed Patience Broderick was as much attributable to the ignorance as to the carelessness of the unqualified dispenser employed by Dr. Greenhalgh. An isolated case does not prove that such occurrences were common but the facilities possessed by doctors to prevent inquests by giving a certificate of death may have covered up many such incidents.

Every success in the Pharmaceutical Society's struggle to reserve to qualified chemists the right to dispense poisons enhanced their employment opportunities and furthered the development of the profession of pharmacy. However, since the 1868 Act dealt only with the sale of poisons, it left completely untouched the whole field of public institutions. Hospitals, infirmaries, asylums, sanatoria, dispensaries and poor law institutions, whether supported out of public funds and by public authorities or by charities and voluntary subscriptions, were exempt from the legal requirement to employ qualified dispensers and to adhere to the regulations relating to the storage and supply of poisons to their patients. There was a long way to go before the employment of registered pharmacists in public institutions was recognised as a necessity.

* * *

By the 1868 Pharmacy Act certain substances were from time to time declared by law to be poisons. Schedule A of the Act was the authentic statutory list of poisons. No additions could be made to the list except on the proposal of the Council of the Pharmaceutical Society, subject to the approval of the Privy Council. The poisons schedule was based on the standard Victorian technique for promoting public safety: legal restriction upon access to the sources of danger. The professed object of poisons legislation was to reduce the danger to human life, first, by preventing the indiscriminate sale of the more dangerous poisons by unqualified persons, and, secondly, by enabling persons who purchased them for criminal purposes to be more easily traced. The Pharmaceutical Society contended that the way to limit the misuse of poisons, to prevent accidents, murder and suicide, was to prohibit their sale except by registered medical practitioners and chemists and druggists. The public health lobby believed that accidents could be prevented by full and clear labelling; potential murderers deterred by the systematic recording of sales details; persons bent on suicide deflected by delays in purchase and by sentinel professionals. With the benefit of hindsight, it is now clear that the most beneficial effect of the regulation of the sale of poisons was the gradual transformation of their public perception. Scheduling a substance initiated a long term process of health education. By making the purchase of poisons more difficult, linking it with the chemist's shop and surrounding it with special procedures (the register, the prescription book, labels, peculiarly shaped and coloured bottles) their dangerous character was etched in the public mind. The ritual of buying poisons set the act apart from ordinary shopping and impressed upon the layman the need for special care in their handling and use.

Nineteenth century suicide statistics suggested that the availability of poison determined the method if not the act of suicide.[20] Of the suicides committed by chemists, photographers, and doctors, and their assistants, 86%, 85% and 60% respectively were by poisoning. By 1900 the growing popularity of photographic developing at home made swallowing cynanide of potassium a common method of suicide for middle class men. Working class women preferred oxalic acid which was very cheap and in continual household use for cleaning brass. Vermin killer, an essential part of routine domestic equipment, was frequently used by women for suicide in the period between 1869 and 1882. The most popular suicide poison for women, and the second most popular for men, in the years 1863–82, was opium. Victorian families kept opiates in the home as most families keep aspirin today. Before the First World War laudanum was regarded as the best all-round remedy for the domestic medicine chest. The first edition of *Black's Medical Dictionary* (1906) described it as "perhaps the most valuable remedy in the whole range of medicine".

The daily habits of life and work, "the trivial round, the common task", determined the use of poisons for suicide. What was potentially fatal was for a person in a suicidal mood to have lying around, at the critical moment, on a shelf or in a cupboard, some substance familiar in daily life, known to be easy to use to bring about death. Restricting the availability of such substances by statute seemed to many people to be a worthwhile contribution towards reducing the death rate.

Ironically, the ready accessibility of one of the most popular suicide poisons of the 1880s and 1890s was intended to promote health not destroy life. From the 1870s every respectable urban household kept a supply of carbolic acid at hand for use as a disinfectant. The corollary was that, by 1899, one in eight of the women who took their own lives did so by drinking carbolic acid. Accidental deaths were also frequent. A former editor of the *Chemist and Druggist* once described how:

> This deadly poison is still sold to all comers without question by oilmen and other uneducated persons in common gallipots and similar receptacles bearing no label to indicate the nature of the contents. The stuff is not in appearance, upon a slight scrutiny, unlike porter, and many men and women, presumably in a more or less inebriated condition, have lost their lives through drinking it in mistake for that beverage.

The Council of the Pharmaceutical Society first recommended that carbolic acid be added to the poisons schedule in February 1882, at a time when sales to householders were increasing but well before its use for suicide was noted. Under the second section of the 1868 Act the resolutions of the Pharmaceutical Society's Council remained ineffective until confirmed by the Privy Council. In 1882 it took the Lords in Council six months before deciding not to sanction this proposal. The Pharmaceutical Society, undaunted, repeated its resolution in 1886, 1888 and again in 1893. On each occasion, the Privy Council refused to sanction the proposal. In the meanwhile, the case for restricting the availability of carbolic acid grew in strength. It took until August 1900 before the Privy Council relented and authorised the addition of certain preparations of carbolic acid to the second part of the poisons schedule.[21]

Between 1886 and 1900 carbolic acid was first in the list of poisons selected by both men and women who took their own lives. In 1895 347 men and 233 women deliberately poisoned themselves: one third of the men and one half of the women did so by swallowing carbolic acid. In that year only 68 persons killed themselves by taking opium; 224 did so by taking carbolic acid, a much less pleasant method of dying. The scheduling of carbolic acid in 1900 had an immediate effect on its use as a poison for suicide. In 1899 carbolic acid accounted for 13% of all female suicides; by 1907 for less than 6%. Dr. W. Wynn Westcott, the coroner for North East London, noted in his carefully researched book, *On Suicide* (1905), that "in my district the number of deaths from carbolic acid was at once halved", as a direct consequence of its scheduling.

Although the Pharmaceutical Society was the first and most persistent advocate of restrictions on the sale of carbolic acid, many others supported the cause. Judges, coroners and juries made repeated representations to the Privy Council to try to get carbolic acid added to the poisons schedule. Dr. W. Wynn Westcott, author of *Suicide: Its History, Literature, Jurisprudence, Causation and Prevention* (1885) and co-author, with William Martindale, of *The Extra Pharmacopoeia*, asserted that scheduling a poison significantly reduced the number of its victims. People bent on suicide, he argued, gave up an intended purchase of poison when they found they had to go from shop to shop, answer questions, and sign a register to get a dose. In May 1897 the *Medical Chronicle* published "Notes on the Statistics of Carbolic Acid Poisoning" by Professor Dixon Mann, M.D., F.R.C.P., the professor of forensic medicine and toxicology at Owen's College, Manchester. Mann demonstrated that the number of suicidal deaths from carbolic acid poisoning was increasing rapidly from 43 in 1890, to 117 in 1893, to 224 in 1895. He argued that the statistics "very forcibly demonstrate the urgent need for restrictive legislation as regards the sale of carbolic acid". Although restriction would not save every life taken by carbolic acid, it would undoubtedly save a very large proportion. "Facility of access to a poison", he concluded, "is a direct incentive to the suicidal act".

The Pharmaceutical Society's efforts to get carbolic acid defined as a poison were supported by both the Coroners' Society and the British Medical Association. The Coroners' Society had over 200 members who came from almost every part of England and Wales: their observations on the control of poisons were the product of personal experience. In June 1896 they explained to the Privy Council why they felt that carbolic acid should be added to the poisons schedule.

> Although it is such a deadly poison, no restrictions are placed upon its sale—the result is that in many cases it is looked upon as being entirely innocuous. Some manufacturers at present take the trouble to label it "poison", and place it in distinctive bottles, but the cheap and crude carbolic, which is mostly purchased by the poorer classes, is sold by oilmen and similar shopkeepers without restriction or any precautionary measures being adopted. It is generally placed in such vessels as the purchasers may take with them, such as beer bottles, old tin cans, and other receptacles in daily use amongst them for containing household and harmless

liquids. The result is that no precautions being taken by the vendors of carbolic acid, none are exercised by the purchasers themselves to keep it in a safe place, or to specially identify it, and adults and children frequently take it in mistake for beer, etc.

The Coroners' Society further urgently desire that the sale should be under some reasonable restriction. If it is not considered advisable to include carbolic acid in the first or second part of the schedule, so as to restrict its sale to chemists and druggists, at least it should only be sold in some distinctive vessel, which should be plainly labelled "Poison" in large letters. It is clear that no precautions could prevent the article being used in all cases; but if a warning were given as to its nature, with directions to place it in safety, many accidents, and possibly suicides, would be prevented. It is to be further noted that during an epidemic and at other times, Parochial Authorities not infrequently gratuitously distribute carbolic acid for disinfecting purposes in a way equalled by the careless methods in vogue at oil and other shops.

Such indiscriminate distribution of carbolic acid without providing any action or advice as to its poisonous nature, did more harm than good.

The views of the Coroners' Society made little impact on the Privy Council Office. A brief note was sent to its secretary informing him that the matter was "under consideration", as, indeed, it had been for the past fifteen years. Eighteen months later, the British Medical Association took up the attack on the Privy Council's policy. In a powerfully argued editorial in the *British Medical Journal*, the insouciance of the Privy Council was made to look like criminal negligence.[22] For a long time past, it was pointed out, coroners, magistrates, juries, medical men and others have expressed their belief that the existing provisions for restricting the supply of poisons are insufficient security against accident or misuse. But the persistency with which this opinion has been expressed by persons in official and representative positions has been insufficient to overcome the inertia of the authorities. A comprehensive inquiry is needed to confirm or refute the idea that more stringent restrictions are needed. For years past, carbolic acid

has been pre-eminent as a cause of death by accident and misuse, but from a legal point of view it is not a poison. More deaths are caused by carbolic acid than by any single article in the schedule . . . and fifteen years ago that fact had become so obvious that the Council of the Pharmaceutical Society, in the performance of its public duty, submitted to the Privy Council a recommendation that carbolic acid should be added to the schedule of legal poisons. That recommendation of the body entrusted by Act of Parliament with the duty of providing for public safety in the matter of poisons, has not yet been acted upon, although it has been repeatedly endorsed by various authorities, and the fatal consequences of its practical disregard have been manifest from the constant reports of cases in which death by accident or suicide has been due to carbolic acid. Nor has there been any attempt to furnish a satisfactory explanation of reasons—if such there can be—for not adopting the recommendation to add carbolic acid to the poison schedule . . . the long-continued hesitation of the Privy Council to confirm the recommendation made by the Council of the Pharmaceutical Society remains quite inexplicable.

So common are deaths from carbolic acid, the editorial continued, that the press frequently infers that no regulations about the sale of poisons exist. The provisions of the Pharmacy Act may be relied upon as sufficient to protect the public from danger and were they carried out in regards to carbolic acid, as recommended by the Council of the Pharmaceutical Society, there is every reason for believing that there would be a large reduction in the number of deaths, both by suicide and accident, which now occur as a result of neglecting to carry out those provisions.

The British Medical Association received a reply from the Privy Council, which, though worded differently from that sent to the Coroners' Society, meant the same. The B.M.A. were told that a bill dealing with the subject of carbolic acid was under the consideration of the government, and pending its introduction, the Privy Council was not prepared to include that substance in the schedule to the Pharmacy Act. The Privy Council trotted out the same evasive answers whenever the carbolic acid issue was raised in the House of Commons. In December 1888 Mr. Picton was the first M.P. to draw attention to the need to control the sale of carbolic acid: further questions on the matter were asked in November 1893 by Mr. Macdona, in March 1898 by Mr. Woods, and in March 1899 by Dr. Farquharson. Each time the House of Commons was told that the matter was "under consideration". An article in the *Chemist and Druggist* in 1896 made an appropriate riost:

> We are surprised that even a Government official should not be ashamed to repeat this threadbare reply. The "Lords of the Council" have had this pressing subject "under consideration" for at least twenty years and hundreds of victims of their indecision have been sacrificed meanwhile. This country has gone into dozens of great wars with a fraction of the "consideration" which, if we are to believe official statements, has been devoted to this question. What is there to consider? ... Has not carbolic acid yet established its claim to be considered a poison? And who are these "Lords of the Council" who take it upon themselves to defeat the obvious intention of an Act of Parliament in this way?

The history of the addition of carbolic acid to the poisons schedule shows how wrong it would be to think of the Privy Council as continually striving to establish, in the public interest, an efficient system of poisons control but being thwarted by the Pharmaceutical Society. It is difficult to find in this episode any evidence that the officials of the Privy Council Office had any conception of the public interest other than an unthinking commitment to an economic doctrine which had long since outlived its usefulness. After the departure of John Simon, whose credentials as a proponent of state intervention in the field of public health are indisputable, the Privy Council became obsessed with the need to foster competition and remove restraints on trade and industry. Although the primary intent of poisons legislation was to restrict availability in the interest of public safety, the Pharmaceutical Society's attempts to add to the schedule were frustrated by the Privy Council. Between 1870 and 1900 only chloral hydrate (in 1877) and nux vomica (in 1882) were added to the list of poisons. The Privy Council, at various times, rejected proposals to include in the schedule, sulphuric, hydrochloric, and nitric acids, butter of antimony, hellebore, vermin killers containing phosphorus, digitalin, savin, nitrobenzol, lobelia, indian hemp, soluble oxalates and nitroglycerine.

The Privy Council Office had no need to justify its decisions in public and made no effort to do so. Some indication of official thinking, however, can be gained from the memoranda which circulated at the time within the Privy Council Office. The civil servants who ran the office deeply resented the Pharmaceutical Society's failure to promulgate regulations for the storage and sale of poisons. This failure was for them proof that the Society was simply a trades union whose only interest in poisons was to make their sale "a monopoly in the hands of chemists and druggists". The Society's 1881 bill to amend the Pharmacy Act was dismissed as "trades unionism pure and simple". "The Pharmaceutical Society", said Lord St. Aldwyn, "have been endeavouring throughout to secure by legislation a trade monopoly in order that they may raise, to their own benefit and to the public injury, the prices of their goods".[23] Adding a substance to the poisons list restricted its sale to chemists and increased its price to the public. Such reasoning underlay the Privy Council's refusal to sanction the Pharmaceutical Society's resolutions. Yet not a shred of evidence was produced to substantiate the charge and no attempt was ever made to ascertain the facts. The price of substances did not rise when they were deemed poisons: opiates did not become more expensive after 1868, nor did the price of carbolic acid go up after 1900. So fierce was the competition within the ranks of chemists and druggists that prices were not affected by scheduling. The rise of chain stores, like Boots, and of co-operatives forced the prices of all drugs down.

The conversion of the Privy Council to the idea that its duty lay in ensuring the unrestricted availability of poisons to the public at low prices coincided with the growing influence on its policies of the large-scale commercial manufacturers of poisons. The refusal of the Privy Council to sanction the inclusion in the poisons schedule of carbolic acid was not due to a conviction that its utility as a disinfectant precluded any limitation of its sale. The Privy Council's reluctance reflected the influence of F.C. Calvert & Co., the principal manufacturers of carbolic acid. Mr. R. Le Neve Foster, the managing director of Calverts, a Manchester firm, was a good friend of A.J. Balfour, M.P. for East Manchester from 1885 to 1906, who led the Conservative party in the House of Commons before becoming prime minister in 1902. It was Calverts, with a near monopoly of the manufacture of carbolic acid, who determined its price and not the retail chemist. If the price of carbolic acid to the general public and local health authorities was maintained at an artificially high level, the reason was the lack of competition between Calverts and Blagden Waugh & Co. of London, who together controlled its manufacture and distribution.

Calverts were, nonetheless, anxious to prevent any restriction on their retail outlets. A letter from the firm appeared in the *Times* on 24 January 1882 opposing controls on the sale of poisons. "It is absolutely impossible to stop the abuse of poisons", it asserted: "an analysis of 80 poisoning cases occurring within a seven months period shows that 52 were by scheduled poisons: further restrictions, instead of saving life, would merely interfere with the manufacture of chemicals, used largely for commercial purposes". The statistics which Calvert & Co. managed to conjure up made a deep impression on the civil servants in the Privy Council Office. On 5 December 1893 Calverts had a letter opposing the scheduling of carbolic acid published in the *Chemist and Druggist*. The statistics of deaths from carbolic acid poisoning contained in this letter were used by Sir Charles Peel, K.C.B. of the Privy Council Office, in an interview with Michael Carteighe, president of the Pharmaceutical Society, to justify the Privy Council's refusal to schedule carbolic acid. Carteighe ventured to suggest that the figures used by Peel would not bear the weight of his argument. The following day Carteighe sent Peel a discreet letter presenting the correct figures:

14 December 1893

With reference to my interview with you yesterday, I find that the deaths from Carbolic Acid poisoning in 1887 were 52, but in 1891 had risen to 94;

showing a serious increase which will certainly continue unless some restrictions are placed upon the sale of the article.

By way of correction to the published statement of Messrs. Calvert & Co., I submit the following record of deaths by Carbolic Acid during the five years 1887–1891:

1887   52
1888   91
1889   68
1890   69
1891   94

Total 374 deaths: statistics for England and Wales only.

I find also that my statement that Carbolic Acid was responsible for a larger number of deaths in 1891 than any other poison is correct.

A junior official at the Privy Council Office did his own research and eagerly informed his superior that the Registrar General's return for 1891 showed that only 41 persons had

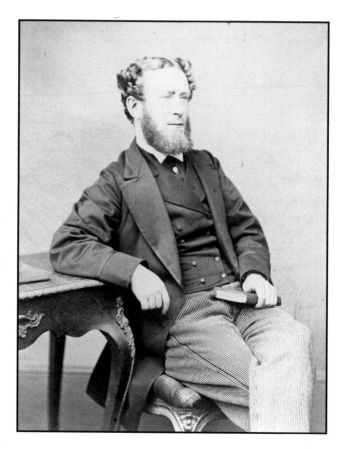

46   *Michael Carteighe (1841–1910). An examiner and a member of Council. He was one of the longest-serving Presidents of the Society, from 1882 to 1896.*

died from carbolic acid poisoning that year. Peel, in triumph, wrote to Carteighe, demanding an explanation for the discrepancy in the figures. Carteighe, politely and without even a trace of sarcasm, replied that his figure of 94 was for the whole year rather than for the six-month period to which Sir Charles' data referred. Sir Charles Peel was not the sort of person to allow facts to cloud his prejudices. It needed much more than rational argument supported by empirical data to change the Privy Council's mind.

No action relating to carbolic acid was contemplated by the Privy Council Office without first consulting Mr. R. le Neve Foster. It is not surprising that his views were somewhat slanted: but it would not be unreasonable to expect advice from so-called experts to be more objective and of a higher quality. During this period, the Privy Council Office referred matters relating to the regulation of the sale of poisons to three eminent authorities; Sir George Buchanan and Sir Richard Thorne Thorne, both, in turn, medical officers to the Local Government Board, and Lord Playfair, who had served as Vice-President of the Committee of Education. The reports they submitted lead the reader to suspect that the authors were more interested in reaching conclusions acceptable to the Privy Council Office than in demonstrating the virtues of scientific objectivity. Dr. Buchanan, in 1883, expressed his reservations about legislation, "which confers certain monopolies upon pharmacists", and added:

> I would leave the function of adding to the Schedule with the Privy Council who would do as it pleased, either on its proper motion, or at the instance of those whose counsel it saw fit to accept.[24]

Since the Privy Council resisted adding carbolic acid to the schedule for twenty years, Buchanan's advice was a recipe for inaction. Buchanan's memoranda are, nonetheless, of a much higher calibre than those of Sir Richard Thorne Thorne. Thorne was content to repeat Buchanan's opinions and add a few prejudices of his own. In 1894 he wrote a report opposing the scheduling of carbolic acid, but advocating its being clearly labelled when sold. Thorne, who was trained as a doctor but clearly fancied himself as an economist, began by stating that the Pharmaceutical Society was not really interested in regulating the sale of poisons in the public interest. "If the Privy Council were to sanction the resolution which the Pharmaceutical Society have submitted to them, it would mean the chemists would have a complete monopoly of the sale of carbolic acid", that in hamlets it would be unobtainable as a disinfectant, "and that judging by precedent the monopoly would mean an advance in the price of the article to which the monopoly applies". In contrast, Calvert & Co., argued Thorne, showed commendable public spirit. Each bottle of carbolic acid sold by them "is of a peculiar shape and ribbed on two sides: each has a patent poison stopper and each bottle is distinctly labelled 'Poison'". Thorne did not seem to appreciate the purely commercial advantages gained by selling in such distinctive bottles nor the fact that Calverts had a large trade in carbolic acid powders which were sold without any form of cautionary label. In any case, Thorne's enthusiasm for labelling is difficult to reconcile with his comment on suicide in the same memorandum:

> Carbolic acid is an article which is largely used in households for public health purposes, and to encourage in numberless houses, where the word "Poison" is rarely seen, the presence of a bottle often standing ready to hand, and having on its face the suggestive word in question, might easily extend, instead of diminishing its use for suicidal purposes.

Lord Playfair held the same view. Putting the word "poison" on bottles for domestic use might increase the number of suicides and murders "by constant obtrusion of the word on diseased minds". Like Thorne, Playfair was very ready to derive firm conclusions from the minimum of evidence. Noting that in one year 21 men and 42 women used carbolic acid to commit suicide, he pontificated "that women from ignorance select poisons which produce trouble and agony and that men generally avoid such poison". The Privy Council Office got the advice it asked for: Calverts got the privileges they sought.

After 1880 the Privy Council Office sought ways of reconciling its belief in the virtues of the free market with the demands of the public health lobby for restrictions on the sale of poisons. In 1883 certain "important Government officials" came up with a scheme calculated to undermine the chemists' monopoly which the 1868 Act had set up.[25] The proposal was to create a third schedule of "poisonous articles" which could be sold, if properly labelled, by anyone. The establishment of a third part of the schedule, however, required an amending Act of Parliament: and that required the co-operation of the Pharmaceutical Society. The House of Commons had not time to spend on contested poisons bills: it had more pressing problems to tackle. The idea of a "third schedule" was highly objectionable to the Pharmaceutical Society: it seriously eroded the principle embodied in the 1868 Act that dangerous substances should only be sold by educated and qualified persons.

From 1885 all the Privy Council's attempts to legislate on poisons featured two main objectives: a tripartite schedule and transfer of responsibility for poisons regulations and the schedule from the Pharmaceutical Society to the Privy Council. In June 1898 the Duke of Devonshire, Lord President of the Council, introduced a "poisonous substances" bill restricted to these two objectives. The bill, which had been drafted as early as November 1896, had been prepared in compliance with a pledge that the government would provide some additional restrictions on the sale of carbolic acid and other dangerous substances which the Privy Council were determined not to include in the existing schedule to the 1868 Act. The bill was also designed to enable the Privy Council to enforce on chemists regulations for the storage and sale of poisons which the Pharmaceutical Society had refused to issue. The bill aroused opposition from all sides: the public health lobby wanted more restrictions, the manufacturers none at all. The collapse of yet another poisons bill convinced Almeric FitzRoy, the clerk to the Privy Council, that the best way of dealing with the demand to restrict the sale of carbolic acid might, after all, be to schedule it under the existing Act. The Privy Council had already been embarrassed by the decision in June 1898 of the Lord Lieutenant of Ireland to add carbolic acid to the list of poisons in Ireland. On 23 March 1899 FitzRoy wrote to a colleague in the Board of Agriculture:

> As however the only substance upon the use of which we are pressed to do something is carbolic acid, I am not sure that the best plan would not be to insert it in some qualified form in the schedule of the Pharmacy Act and leave legislation alone.[26]

The Privy Council's change of policy was closely linked to events within the Pharmaceutical Society. At the beginning of 1899 the Council of the Pharmaceutical Society had been successful in persuading the members to accept regulations under section one of the 1868 Act for the keeping and dispensing of poisons. An important source of friction between the Society and the Privy Council was removed. On 23 June 1899 Sir M.White Ridley of the Home Office responded to Sir John Leng's question in the House of Commons about the refusal of the Privy Council to schedule carbolic acid, by stating that "the objections to scheduling this poison in England have now been lessened by the fact that regulations for the keeping, dispensing and selling of poisons ... have now been prescribed".

On 5 July the Council of the Pharmaceutical Society resolved that "carbolic acid in crystals, commercial carbolic acid and other liquids containing more than 3% of phenols" be deemed poisons. "This is going considerably further than we can approve", commented Almeric Fitzroy; and both Calverts and the Board of Agriculture raised objections to the scope of the resolution. "I observe that Mr. Le Neve Foster writing on behalf of Calverts shows much suspicion of the proposals of the Pharmaceutical Society and I think he is justified in doing so considering the trade union character of that society", wrote one civil servant, anxious to see the public interest protected. The same conscientious official had no difficulty in equating the general good with the interests of F.C. Calvert & Co. Le Neve Foster suggested that any restriction should apply only to liquid preparations of carbolic acid. This would have little effect on Calverts' business: liquid disinfectants containing carbolic acid were being largely superseded by other more effective preparations. Calverts' trade was now mainly in carbolic acid powders: in 1897 they sold a quarter of a million packages (or over a hundred tons) of 15% Carbolic Disinfecting powder. Such powders, they said, should be exempt from regulation.

The Board of Agriculture became involved. It was keen to promote the interests of the manufacturers of carbolic acid sheep dips, of whom William Cowper & Nephews of Berkhampstead was the largest. Negotiations involving the Pharmaceutical Society, the Privy Council, the Board of Agriculture, the Parliamentary Counsel (Sir C.P. Ilbert), Calvert & Co., Blagden Waugh & Co., and the Association of Coal Tar Distillers went on from November 1899 to June 1900. The Privy Council Office used its muscle and charm to persuade the Council of the Pharmaceutical Society to revise the wording of its resolution. On 2 July 1900 Almeric FitzRoy sent a letter to the Pharmaceutical Society instructing its Council to pass the necessary resolution using the wording that had been agreed. On 4 July the Society's Council passed the following resolution:

> That liquid preparations of Carbolic Acid and its homologues containing more than three per cent. of these substances, except any preparation prepared for use as sheep wash or for any other purpose in connection with agriculture or horticulture and contained in a closed vessel, distinctly labelled with the words "Poisonous", the name and address of the seller, and a notice of the agricultural or horticultural purpose for which the preparation has been prepared, ought to be deemed poisons within the meaning of the "Pharmacy Act, 1868", and ought to be deemed poisons in the second part of the schedule A of the said "Pharmacy Act, 1868".

The resolution was approved by order of council on 26 July and the official announcement appeared in the *London Gazette* on 31 July 1900.

The story of the struggle to bring the retail sale of carbolic acid under professional control provides a reminder to treat with scepticism the claim that government departments act in an impartial way to secure the public interest. If the public interest exists, it is not easy to discover where it lies. It is, of necessity, intertwined with private, sectional interests. On any particular issue, the interests of the majority may be fostered as much by a voluntary association, like the Pharmaceutical Society, as by a public department of government, like the Privy Council. The most obvious feature of the carbolic acid story is the attempt by the Privy Council Office to increase its own powers, to wrest control of the regulation of the sale of poisons from the Pharmaceutical Society. In 1904 a Home Office official provided an apt quotation to end the story:

> Personally I don't think the Privy Council are a very good authority to deal with this question, and I am not anxious to see them have too many powers.[27]

The Council of the Pharmaceutical Society could be forgiven for having similar thoughts.

The scheduling of carbolic acid did not lessen the Privy Council's determination to revise the Pharmacy Act of 1868. Its principal objectives remained the introduction of a third schedule designed to undermine the chemists' monopoly and the augmentation of its own power to regulate the sale of poisons at the expense of the Pharmaceutical Society. At the same time the government was coming under increasing pressure from the manufacturers of poisons used in manufacture and agriculture to free the retail trade in them from all restriction. In June 1901 the Lord President of the Privy Council set up a departmental committee to consider what alterations were necessary in the poisons schedule and whether a third part should be added. The members of the committee and its terms of reference were carefully chosen to ensure that its recommendations would pave the way for legislation on the lines advocated by the Privy Council Office.[28]

The committee reported in January 1903.[29] The majority report took as its starting point the great increase in the use of poisons in agriculture and horticulture since the passing of the 1868 Pharmacy Act. Sheep dips containing strong poisons had become indispensable to the modern sheep-farmer. Poisons were now widely used for killing weeds, parasitical insects and fungoid growths on growing plants: they had become the regular auxiliaries of agriculture and horticulture. Restricting the sale of these poisons to chemists and druggists had enhanced their price and inconvenienced farmers and gardeners. The prosecution of unregistered sellers of poison was characterised by uncertainty and irregularity. The Pharmaceutical Society had no staff of inspectors nor other regular machinery for detecting the sale of poisons by unregistered persons. Its powers can only be exercised on voluntary information and extemporised means which renders the working of the restrictive provisions inadequate and uneven. In the West Midlands the sale by unregistered persons of poisons used in agriculture and horticulture has been completely stopped; in part of Kent it has been stopped temporarily; whereas in Scotland and the North of England it is carried on by such persons with impunity. Thus the effect of the 749 prosecutions undertaken by the Pharmaceutical Society during the six years from 1896 to 1901, and of the numerous cases in which penalties were exacted without prosecution, has been very unequally felt. For while the law has been enforced in some areas, it has been wholly inoperative in others. The obligation laid upon the Pharmaceutical Society by the 15th Section of the 1868 Act is unduly onerous. Even the limited extent to which they have taken action under it, has involved them in a net loss of £700 a year, beyond the sum received as penalties, which the Society has been allowed to retain.

In districts where there is no qualified chemist and druggist within easy reach, farmers and gardeners have experienced great inconvenience, which would have amounted to a very serious interference with legitimate industry had the 15th Section been universally put into effect. In the Highlands and Islands of Scotland, where sheep-farming is the principal occupation, farmers are sometimes more than fifty miles away from the nearest registered chemist. Here the law is disregarded and the sale of sheep dips is regularly carried on by ironmongers and other traders. H. Cannell, a nurseryman and florist of Swanley in Kent, alleged that extreme inconvenience had been given to cultivators, when the sale of weed-killers and insecticides was discontinued by nurserymen, following the successful prosecution of a firm of seedsmen. He maintained that there were numerous small cultivators and amateurs who would use poisons, if they could get them, to the advantage of their greenhouses and gardens; but chemists do not know what to recommend, whereas nurserymen do, and ought, therefore, to be in a position to supply them.

The committee thought that the lax way in which arsenic was handled in transit to and from wholesale dealers constituted a source of danger to the public. It recommended that the traffic in arsenic should be regulated either by an amendment of the 1851 Arsenic Act or by more stringent enforcement of the 17th Section of the 1868 Pharmacy Act. The committee also recommended certain additions to Parts 1 and 2 of the poisons schedule and tried to eliminate the inconsistencies between the two parts. Its most important recommendation was that preparations for use in connection with agriculture, horticulture or sanitation should be placed in a third part of the schedule, to be sold only by licensed persons and subject to regulations to be made by the Privy Council.

One of the members of the committee was Alexander Cross (1847-1914), the Liberal M.P. for the Camlachie division of Glasgow from 1892 to 1910, and the senior partner of Alexander Cross and Sons, a long established firm of seed merchants and chemical manufacturers. It was Cross who spearheaded the manufacturers' agitation against the restrictions embodied in the 1868 Pharmacy Act. From the early 1890s Cross had been encouraging farmers' organizations, such as the Scottish Chamber of Agriculture, to petition the Privy Council to change the law relating to poisons. At the same time he helped to persuade the Board of Agriculture to take up the manufacturers' case. In June 1898 J.H. Elliott, the Board's secretary, wrote to J.H. Harrison of the Privy Council Office, that

> it appears to the Board that agriculturists are entitled to ask that the sale of such articles as fertilisers, sheep-dips, insecticides and other chemical preparations used for agricultural or horticultural purposes should not be restricted to pharmacists.

The Board of Agriculture's complete disregard for public safety provoked the usually compliant Dr. Richard Thorne Thorne to point out that, if poisonous substances used by farmers

> can be purchased, they can be used as poisons; whereas the object hitherto aimed at has been to control the sale of poisonous preparations . . . . It is not so much the purpose to which a poisonous preparation is commonly put, as the uncontrolled power of purchasing the poison that is in question. . . .[30]

The Privy Council Office had a habit of ignoring advice it did not wish to receive. The advice of Alexander Cross, however, was published as a supplement to the main report. While fully concurring with that report and with the committee's recommendations, Cross wanted, in addition, greater latitude in the sale of poisons employed in manufacture. The use of these substances for trade and technical purposes, he said, was developing continually but industry was being hampered by the restrictions. He advocated

> the removal of all such matters from the control of the Pharmaceutical Society which is a private association existing for purposes quite apart from the public interest. In my opinion such control as the sale of such substances demands should be elastic, automatically adapting itself to the conditions of manufacture and trade as such arise. And as the Privy Council are in possession of the best information and have the necessary well-qualified staff and have been long associated with this subject ... full powers of regulating and controlling sales of such poisonous substances as may be required in trades and manufactures ... should be placed in their hands.

To demonstrate how far he considered de-regulation could go without harming the public, Cross added that country medical practitioners and their assistants, even though keeping open shop for the sale of poisons, should be exempt from the 1868 Act. Local authorities should be given power to grant licences to suitable persons to assist medical men in dispensing. Country doctors cannot be expected to keep a qualified man on the premises.

The relationship between the evidence collected by the committee and the report it issued is tenuous. A mass of data pointed to the need to improve the machinery for enforcing the 1868 Act. The case for increasing the powers and resources of the Pharmaceutical Society was unimpeachable. The Society had strained its finances to carry out the public duties imposed upon it. The administration of both the 15th and 17th sections of the Act needed tightening. Yet the committee recommended increasing the powers of the Privy Council, whose reluctance to protect the public with respect to sales of carbolic acid had drawn widespread condemnation. At no point did the committee address the public health issue. There was no attempt to discover whether the 1868 Act had been effective in fulfilling its principal objective. The views of the Coroners' Society that the poisons restrictions should be increased rather than diminished were ignored. The legitimacy of the demand for the relaxation of statutory restrictions, which came from the manufacturers and distributors of poisonous substances, was taken for granted. No reliable evidence was presented that the administration of the 1868 Act by the Pharmaceutical Society had interfered with the legitimate use of poisons for technical or manufacturing purposes or that any practical inconvenience had been experienced in obtaining poisonous compounds for use in agriculture or horticulture. Only two witnesses were users of poisons: neither had any difficulty in procuring what was necessary for his own requirements.

Not a shred of evidence was offered to support the oft-repeated charge that chemists' prices were excessive. The committee swallowed the allegation and regurgitated it as gospel in their report. Yet the prices of poisonous substances in the West Midlands, where chemists were supposed to have a monopoly, were no higher than those in the North of England or in the Highlands of Scotland, where open competition supposedly ruled. This fact could easily have been obtained by the committee: but it only looked for evidence to buttress its predetermined conclusions.

The real objection to confining the sale of poisonous compounds to chemists and druggists was not the inconvenience it caused to farmers and market gardeners nor the enhanced prices predicted by economic theory, but the fact that chemists and druggists did not push the sale of weedkillers and insecticides in the way seedsmen, nurserymen and ironmongers did. The manufacturers wanted to pour onto the market a constant stream of "poisonous novelties". Yet the basic premise of the 1868 Act was that professional chemists should act as a restraint upon the irresponsible supply of poisons to the public. Michael Carteighe emphasized this point in his evidence to the committee:

> The restrictions of this Act do not apply in restraint of any form of trade, agricultural or otherwise. The Act was passed to prevent the distribution to the public in an open shop of small quantities of poison. We have never sought to interfere with the use of a poison . . . for the purpose of manufacture; but when a poison is put into a popular form and put into an open shop and the public are invited to buy it, we conceive (and I think rightly), whatever the demands of agriculture may be, that it is a danger to the public.

The committee's recommendations used the language of control to conceal a policy of de-regulation. The report referred to a schedule, licensed persons and Privy Council regulations: but it meant that any poison on the Privy Council's list would be available from ordinary shopkeepers without restriction.

In 1904 the main recommendations of the departmental committee were embodied in a bill drafted by the Unionist government led by A.J. Balfour: its progress was halted by the opposition organised by the Pharmaceutical Society. While the Privy Council was attempting to relax the provisions of the 1868 Pharmacy Act, the Pharmaceutical Society was endeavouring to tighten up the law. During the fourteen years, 1882–1896, that Michael Carteighe occupied the presidential chair, persistent efforts were made to promote legislation to reverse the House of Lords' decision in the notorious case, *The Pharmaceutical Society v The London and Provincial Supply Association (Limited)*. The Society's Council had no doubt that its primary obligation to the profession was to keep retail pharmacy in the hands of the independent proprietor. Since 1880, therefore, its priority was to prevent limited liability companies from trading as chemists and druggists. An amendment of the 1868 Act defining persons to include corporations was the most effective way of achieving this. Another solution, ingenious but somewhat disreputable, was mooted by Carteighe. His idea was to apply to parliament for powers to erase from the register of qualified chemists the names of those found guilty of infamous conduct in a professional sense. Once this power was obtained, he proposed to introduce a by-law making it infamous conduct for a qualified person to act as cover for an unqualified person or corporation, thereby eliminating both the co-operative societies and the multiple shop companies as competitors in the sale of poisons.[31]

Simmering discontent among the members of the Society and the continued growth of company pharmacy induced Michael Carteighe in 1895 to collect evidence to submit to the Departmental Committee on the Companies Acts, 1862–1890.[32] Since the House of Lord's decision of 1880, Carteighe argued, the Pharmacy Act was no longer capable of providing adequate safeguards to the public. It was now open to any person, without training or knowledge, to associate with six others, equally ignorant and unfitted, to obtain sanction under the Companies' Acts to sell, dispense and compound any potent poison or dangerous drug. He had gathered particulars of more than two hundred companies registered by unqualified persons to trade in drugs and gave details of eight of them, including Day's Southampton Drug Company and J.H. Inman and Co., of Newcastle-upon-Tyne. Rather surprisingly, the unqualified Jesse Boot was not included in his list. He pointed out that, in 1882, William Day, a grocer of Southampton, had been convicted of selling poison and was fined £5. In April 1886 he formed the Southampton Drug Company, consisting of six persons, who held 6,000 shares between them, of which Day held 5,995 himself. Persons who had repeatedly failed the qualifying examination were able to circumvent the law by setting up as a limited company. John Oakley failed the Minor examination eighteen times but traded as Price and Co., William Herbert Warhurst (Warhursts Ltd.) failed eight times, Edgar H. Wand (Wands Ltd.) and John Sarsfield (Sarsfield and Co.) had each failed six times.

In 1898 the Pharmaceutical Society sought to insert a clause in the Companies Acts Amendment bill stipulating that "it shall be unlawful for any number of persons to form a company or corporation under the Limited Liability Acts to engage in any business or profession which as individuals it would be unlawful for them to engage in". This provoked Jesse Boot to circulate an open letter in which he accused the Society of concealing the fact that, under the existing Acts, no company could keep open a chemist's shop which was not under the supervision of a registered pharmacist. At first the Society's proposal was welcomed by the Lords, but Jesse Boot's timely intervention led the Lord Chancellor to revise the amendment to read:

> A company may carry on the business of a pharmaceutical chemist or chemist and druggist if and so long only as the business is bona fide directed by a manager or assistant being a duly registered pharmaceutical chemist or chemist and druggist.

The Pharmaceutical Society, faced with the prospect of company pharmacy receiving fresh legitimation, persuaded the Lord Chancellor to withdraw his amendment. Later that year, during the passage through the House of Lords of the Pharmacy Acts Amendment bill, the Lord Chancellor and Lord Herschell announced that a clause to prevent grocers and similar retailers trading as company chemists was required. Although the editor of the *Chemist and Druggist* saw in this the salvation of the independent chemist, the Pharmaceutical Society's Council was less enthusiastic.[33] It smelt a rat. A clause designed to halt company pharmacy would stick out like a sore thumb on such a purely domestic bill. It could be guaranteed to arouse enough opposition in the House of Commons to ruin the whole bill. The Council's defensive instincts were right. The Lord Chancellor and Lord Herschell were really trying to bring back the clause affirming the legality of company pharmacy when conducted by qualified managers. In 1899 the Lord Chancellor made another attempt to gain the object of the clause by promoting a bill which would have given companies the right to carry on business and use the titles "pharmaceutical chemist" and "chemist and druggist", subject to the employment of qualified persons. The bill was defeated by the active opposition of the Pharmaceutical Society. A further attempt to enact its provisions, in a slightly altered form, was made in the Companies bill of the same year. Delaying tactics by the opposition led to the bill's reintroduction in the following session, but the clause affecting pharmacy was withdrawn when the Society decided to oppose it.

A bill drafted in 1899 by the Pharmaceutical Society would have driven company chemists out of the trade altogether. It provided that the word "person" in the Pharmacy Acts should include a limited company or a partnership and that it should be unlawful for any person other than a pharmaceutical chemist or a chemist and druggist to sell, dispense or compound medicines. Thus limited companies would have been debarred from keeping open shop not only for the sale of poisons but for the sale of any medicines whatsoever. The Pharmaceutical Society had always regarded the chemist and druggist as the supplier of drugs and medicines to the nation. His proper role was the dispensing of prescriptions, whether these came from the medical practitioner or directly from the patient. It was the unfortunate legacy of the United Society of Chemists and Druggists that the 1868 Pharmacy Act had identified the qualified pharmacist with the sale of poisons. The Pharmaceutical Society, for both professional and trade considerations, continued to seek for the chemist the exclusive right to compound and dispense prescriptions. The granting of such a monopoly would be the most effective protection against the competition of grocers, general shops and drug stores.

Meanwhile the fear of legislative interference led Jesse Boot and William Day to form the Drug Companies' Association to protect the interests of the company chemists in Parliament and the courts. The other founder members were Hodders, Inmans, Taylors, Parkes, and Lewis and Burroughs. Boot was elected chairman at the inaugural meeting and was able to report that the immediate danger was passed. Boot was already engaged in a fierce war against the Proprietary Articles Trade Association (P.A.T.A.), which William Glyn-Jones had created in January 1896, and now tried to make use of the Drug Companies' Association to further his campaign. Glyn-Jones, however, out-manoeuvred him. He announced in *The Anti-Cutting Record* that some of the company chemists were actually members of the P.A.T.A. and added:

> We should like the D.C.A. to know that the P.A.T.A. occupies a perfectly neutral position with regard to these companies and the parliamentary strivings respecting them...[34]

Within a year, Glyn-Jones, at the age of thirty, was elected to the Council of the Pharmaceutical Society. With characteristic energy he set about trying to get the Society's leaders to adopt a more realistic policy towards the drug companies. At his very first meeting, he startled the "reverend, grave and patient seigniors" of the Council by interpellating them as to their policy on the company pharmacy question. Glyn-Jones realised it was far too late to try to stop companies from trading as chemists. They had built up a considerable vested interest and had the resources to make friends and influence people in high places. Their operations satisfied public demand and were in tune with current economic opinion. The Pharmaceutical Society, however, could and should use its influence to try to regulate company pharmacy in the interests of the profession as a whole. The independent proprietor could not hope to compete successfully with bulk-buying companies that cut prices: but if companies could be persuaded to maintain prices instead of cutting them, the small private chemist could find a niche in the market-place. The P.A.T.A. had been created for that purpose. Similarly, if companies were obliged to employ only qualified persons to run their branches, their labour costs, compared to those of the self-employed chemist, would enable the latter to survive. At the same time new careers would be created for pharmacists unable to set up their own businesses. It was the Pharmaceutical Society's task to force companies to recruit qualified chemists. The basic grievance of the profession was, in Glyn-Jones' view, that a company could have a hundred shops, "and employ not a single qualified man". In an exchange of letters to the press in 1902, Boot replied that the problem was the same for private chemists, "for there are many cases where a private chemist runs several shops with an unqualified manager in each . . ." The use of unqualified assistants was widespread. Taylor's Drug Stores, a Leeds-based chain founded by a qualified chemist, W.B. Mason, were probably the worst culprits but were certainly not the only firm in which qualified men were thin on the ground. However, when the Pharmaceutical Society, in 1903, prepared a bill to compel companies keeping open shops for the sale of poisons to appoint only qualified chemists as directors, Boot replied with a sequence of whole-page advertisements in the London and provincial newspapers headed— "Company Chemists versus the Pharmaceutical Society". It listed the names of 364 qualified men employed at his 278 branches.

The Pharmaceutical Society's bill was drafted in 1901. Its principal aims were:

(1) to provide that companies carrying on the business of a chemist and druggist should be managed by qualified chemists as directors and their shops bona fide conducted by registered persons.

(2) to render it unlawful for any company, even if employing qualified chemists, to use the description "chemist" or "druggist", or "chemist and druggist", or any title implying registration under the Pharmacy Acts.

(3) to check the growing practice of duly qualified persons carrying on several shops for the sale of poisons without providing that each shop is under the bona fide personal conduct and supervision of a duly qualified person.

(4) to prohibit unqualified persons keeping open shop for the dispensing of prescriptions.

(5) to put an end to the abuses attending the hawking of poisons and to better regulate the sale of them by providing that no poison shall be sold except in a shop which shall first be duly registered.

(6) to provide for a register of shops where poisons may be sold and a register of the duly qualified chemists running each shop.

(7) to acquire power to accept for registration persons with colonial qualifications.

(8) to acquire power to divide the qualifying examination into two parts, the practical and the scientific, and to impose compulsory courses of study and practical training as a condition of entry.

On 2 March 1901 the draft bill was sent to Almeric FitzRoy, the Clerk to the Privy Council, with a request that a deputation from the Pharmaceutical Society's Council be received by the Lord President of the Council. Almeric FitzRoy decided to send copies of the bill to the Lord Chancellor and to the Board of Trade for their comments. His advice to the Lord President revealed a certain lack of enthusiasm.

> The main objects of this Bill are to effect the alteration in the law which the Lord Chancellor proposed to do by clause 2 of the Companies Bill 1899 and to make it necessary that every branch shop shall be conducted by a qualified person . . . but there are other provisions of doubtful utility and obscure import about which we shall have to make enquiries in various directions before any useful purpose would be served by a deputation. Eventually it may be expedient to incorporate the useful part of the Bill in any measure that the Government propose for the amendment of the Pharmacy Acts and by this means neutralize the opposition of the Pharmaceutical Society to any unpalatable changes.

At the beginning of April the Board of Trade returned their comments. They thought that the clause which would make it unlawful for a company to retail poisons or compound and dispense medical prescriptions, unless the business was managed by one or more directors registered as chemists and druggists, "would seem unduly to fetter the employment of capital and go beyond what is really necessary for the protection of the public". It is sufficient that the actual keeping of shops and the retailing and dispensing of drugs should be carried on only by such registered and qualified persons. By the end of the month, Almeric FitzRoy had made up his mind.

> It would be a waste of time to receive a deputation in support of such a Bill which will probably never be introduced and, of course, has not the slightest chance of passing. Hereafter certain portions of it, in which the Society are specially interested, might be made the subject of negotiation with them, if any amendment of the Pharmacy Act is attempted by the Government.

In October the Pharmaceutical Society wrote again, appealing to the Privy Council to support its bill: "without the support of a Public Department to legislative proposals of this kind the attempt to pass them into law will be futile". By this time the Privy Council had appointed the departmental committee for recasting the poisons schedule. Almeric FitzRoy reminded the Lord President of this and added:

> . . . in the result of their deliberations some amendment of the law will probably become necessary and it will then be time to consider which of the provisions in the Society's draft Bill can be accepted and in what shape. I would therefore have nothing to do with the Draft Bill as it stands and let the Society know we are contemplating legislation as a sequel to the Committee's deliberations.[35]

He hastened to add that "we must not commit ourselves to bringing in a Bill".

Despite the advice of the Privy council, the Pharmaceutical Society decided to go ahead with its bill: it was introduced on three separate occasions in the House of Commons—in 1903, 1904 and 1905—by Thomas Lough, M.P. for Islington and an entrepreneur in the tea trade. The Drug Companies' Association actively opposed it by lobbying M.P.s, printing a series of leaflets and publishing articles in the advertisement columns of *The Times*. Jesse Boot was particularly incensed by the proposal to prevent companies using the description "chemist and druggist".

> This has all the appearance of an unworthy device, the object of which is to discredit, and draw trade away from, the companies and stores carrying on the business of chemists. Moreover, it is so worded that it would apply to existing companies, unjustly throwing upon them the expense of altering all their labels, memorandum and account forms, and everything else, such as plate glass windows, facias, etc., bearing the word "chemists".

He had recently spent £15,000 advertising "Boots the Chemists" and the title was invaluable to him as a trade name. The clause, he argued, would have deplorable consequences:

> A large shop, owned by a company, managed by a licensed chemist, stocked in the most complete manner with medicinal drugs and chemists' goods, is not to be called a "chemist's." No sign of any kind may be displayed bearing the designation of "chemists and druggists" to attract the notice of passers-by. This would inevitably have the effect of causing the companies' shops to be overlooked by thousands by

prospective customers; many more would be deterred by suspicion, by ignorance of the real reason why the companies' shops could not use the title of "chemists and druggists". The benefit of the trade thus diverted would accrue to the nearest chemist's shop owned by a member of the Pharmaceutical Society, who is not more a chemist than his fellows in the companies' shops, but may use the title and description on his premises in as bold and noticeable a form as he may desire.[36]

There was little chance that prospective customers would fail to notice Boot's shops: they were usually decorated with huge signs covering a large part of the upper storeys. A typical one in Sheffield proclaimed, "Boots the Largest Chemists in the World".

Each time the Pharmaceutical Society's bill was brought in, the friends of the Drug Companies' Association in parliament blocked it. Upon its third appearance in 1905, an important modification was made. It was no longer required that all directors of a company involved in retailing poisons should be registered chemists but merely that the pharmaceutical side of the business should be managed by a director who was qualified. This modification was continued in the bills introduced after 1906.

The Pharmaceutical Society's campaign took a new turn after the Liberal landslide in the general election of 1906. 330 of the elected candidates had promised support for legislation on the basis of the Society's bill. One of the newly elected M.P.s was Richard Winfrey, a newspaper owner of Stamford in Lincolnshire, who had spent the early part of his career in retail pharmacy. He had served a four year apprenticeship and worked as a qualified assistant for five years. Winfrey was still a member of the Pharmaceutical Society, although he had left pharmacy twenty years before. Winfrey was responsible for introducing the Society's pharmacy bill in 1906, 1907 and 1908. The main objects of the bill were declared to be to check:

> (a) The evils arising from unqualified management of shops in which medicines are dispensed and poisons retailed; and (b) the assumption of the statutory title of "chemist" by unregistered persons.

The Drug Companies' Association, however, believed that the bill was directed against its members and was designed to curtail their activities.

In March 1906 the Government published its own bill, "an act to regulate the sale of certain poisonous substances and to amend the Pharmacy Acts". Lord Crewe, Lord President of the Council, was sponsor. The main provisions were:

(1) to alter and extend the schedule of poisons

(2) to authorise persons who are not registered chemists, if licensed for the purpose by local authorities, to sell sheep-dips, weed-killers and other poisonous substances for use in agriculture and horticulture

(3) to place restrictions on the sale of certain poisonous mineral acids and other dangerous substances used in manufacture without limiting their sale to registered chemists.

(4) to require branch shops in which a chemist's business is carried on to be conducted by duly-qualified managers

(5) to empower the Pharmaceutical Society to impose courses of study in connection with the qualifying examination.

(6) to bring companies within the provisions of the 1868 Pharmacy Act.

For three years there followed a see-saw struggle between the promoters of the two bills.

302

In 1906 the Pharmaceutical Society and the Drug Companies' Association managed to block the Government's bill. In 1907 the society's bill was re-introduced and the following month the Government retaliated by bringing back their bill, without the clause regulating companies. Neither bill was successful. In 1908 the Government bill was re-introduced in the same form as in 1907, but accompanied by a statement of the Government's intention to refer the measure to a Joint Committee of both Houses to obtain an independent decision on the terms upon which the companies' question should be settled. The Pharmaceutical Society then re-introduced its bill for the purpose of informing the Joint Committee of its proposals, but the provision requiring companies to have a qualified director was omitted.

After considering Lord Crewe's bill and examining numerous witnesses, the Joint Select Committee reported the bill with several amendments.[37] On the vexed question of the use of titles by limited companies, the Committee proposed an amendment which the Pharmaceutical Society found quite unacceptable. The Committee recommended that companies should be allowed to describe themselves as chemists provided each branch were run by a qualified assistant whose name and certificate of qualification were conspicuously exhibited in the shop. This proposal meant that companies, under the control and management of unqualified persons, would be allowed to use titles implying professional qualification. As long as one junior registered assistant was employed in each shop, the company could legally describe itself as "chemists and druggists", without any member of the profession being involved in policy making or management. The qualified assistant would be working under the direction and supervision of laymen.

When the Pharmaceutical Society's renewed opposition to Lord Crewe's bill threatened to wreck it, a last minute compromise was arranged by William Glyn-Jones and Jesse Boot. Boot as chairman of the Drug Companies' Association had been a leading opponent of the Society's bill. According to Richard Winfrey's reminiscences,

> before the Bill got to Committee we discovered that Mr. (now Sir) Jesse Boot was very active in lobbying against the Bill. Being an invalid, he was wheeled in his chair every afternoon into the strangers' smoke room on the terrace. Then one of his friends, a Member of Parliament [Sir James Duckworth] ... used to bring M.P.s downstairs to hear Sir Jesse's story of how this Pharmacy Bill would adversely affect his multiple business. This went on for ... several weeks; and it became evident that if the Bill was to become law some compromise would have to be made ...[38]

As Winfrey anticipated, some kind of compromise had to be found, and it was Jesse Boot and William Glyn-Jones, now the Pharmaceutical Society's parliamentary secretary, who found it. On 26 October 1908 a deputation waited on Herbert Samuel at the Home Office. The members of the deputation included J. Rymer Young, the Society's president, T.H.W. Idris, M.P., the mineral water manufacturer and a member of the Pharmaceutical Society, William Glyn-Jones and Jesse Boot. Glyn-Jones did practically all the talking and outlined what he and Boot had concocted.[39] Their solution was that corporate bodies should be allowed to carry on the business of a chemist and druggist provided that the part of the business connected with poisons was under the control of a qualified superintendent. At each shop the business must be conducted by a registered chemist under the direction of the superintendent. Only if the superintendent was a member of the board of directors would the company be allowed to use the description "chemist and druggist". Subject to these provisions, the Pharmacy Acts were to apply to companies in the same way as they applied to individuals. Herbert Samuel, the Home Secretary, was surprised and baffled by the sudden outburst of friendship between the Pharmaceutical Society and the Drug Companies' Association, but the Government happily incorporated the agreed solution in its bill, which received the royal assent on 21 December 1908. The compromise had been carefully worked out. The Pharmaceutical Society, as the professional association of pharmacists, gained a much greater measure of control over company pharmacy than the Joint Select Committee had proposed. Jesse Boot, who, on the surface, conceded most, gained more. Not only did Boots get the right to call themselves "chemists", they were also given a headstart over rival companies. The new arrangements involved no alteration in the Boots organisation but implied considerable restructuring for others.

The Pharmaceutical Society had for some years sought the power to allow pharmacists, who had qualified within other countries of the British Empire, to practise in the mother country. Provision for this had been included in the Society's draft bill of 1901. But only with reluctance did the Society succumb to pressure from the Government to accept the qualifications of army and navy dispensers as being equivalent to the Minor examination. At the same time an association representing the holders of the assistants' dispensing certificate of the Society of Apothecaries saw in these development an opportunity for angling in troubled water with some hope of success. They arranged for certain amendments to the pharmacy bills to be placed on the Order Paper which would have secured the admission of their members to the Pharmaceutical Register. At a late stage, the Government informed all the parties interested in Earl Crewe's bill, that if it was to be passed, it must be an agreed measure and, as we have seen, various attempts were at once made by those concerned to negotiate agreements. Among the compromises then reached was the insertion of an agreed amendment giving power to the Pharmaceutical Society to make by-laws admitting to the Register, without examination, "certified assistants to apothecaries, who produce evidence satisfactory to the council of the society that they are persons of sufficient skill and knowledge to be so registered". In Committee the Government spokesman expressed the opinion that legally the exercise of this power was not obligatory. Later, however, the Privy Council Office took a very different view.

An Act to regulate the sale of certain Poisonous Substances and to amend the Pharmacy Acts, or the Poisons and Pharmacy Act, 1908, as it is usually called, came into operation on 1 April 1909.[40]

Section 1 replaced the schedule of poisons in the 1868 Pharmacy Act by a revised and rationalised schedule. The Pharmaceutical Society retained its power to deem a substance a poison, subject to approval by the Privy Council, and acquired new powers to ask for the removal of any substance from the schedule or its transfer from one part of the schedule to the other.

Section 2 provided for the granting by local authorities, subject to certain conditions, of licenses to sell agricultural and horticultural poisons to dealers other than registered chemists. The Privy Council was given the power to make relevant regulations and to amend the list of such poisons. Local authorities were directed to grant such licences only in cases where, in their opinion, the needs of the neighbourhood were not adequately met by the existing facilities.

Section 3 legalised the position of limited companies carrying on the business of chemist and druggist. These were permitted to carry on such business provided that the poisons department was under the control and management of a legally qualified superintendent whose name was registered with the Pharmaceutical Society and who did not act at the same time in a similar capacity for any other body. If the business was not personally carried on by the superintendent it had to be conducted, under his direction, by a qualified manager whose certificate of qualification was required to be conspicuously exhibited in the shop. If these conditions were observed and if, in addition, the superintendent was a member of the board of directors, the company could use the description of "chemist and druggist", or "chemist", or "druggist", or "dispensing chemist" or "dispensing druggist". But companies were, in effect, forbidden to use the titles "pharmaceutical chemist", "pharmaceutist" and "pharmacist". By the 1852 Pharmacy Act the titles "pharmaceutical chemist" and "pharmaceutist" were restricted to persons registered as Pharmaceutical chemists. By the 1908 Act the title "pharmacist" was restricted to persons registered as chemists and druggists (which included pharmaceutical chemists). This right was purely personal and in no case was a limited company entitled to use any of these titles.

Section 4 extended the powers of the Pharmaceutical Society to make by-laws relating to the courses of study and the examinations to be undertaken by candidates for registration as pharmaceutical chemists and chemists and druggists. By this section the Pharmaceutical Society was no longer required to come to parliament for fresh powers to regulate the education and examination of prospective pharmacists. Since the 1880s the Council of the Society had been seeking powers to modify the Minor examination by dividing it into two parts, the practical and the scientific, and by requiring candidates to produce evidence of attendance at systematic courses of instruction. Between 1887 and 1891 five bills were drawn up to achieve these objectives but failed to attract enough support in the House of Commons. This section also gave the Pharmaceutical Society power to make by-laws providing for the registration, without examination, of persons with colonial diplomas, military dispensers, and certified assistants to apothecaries.

Section 5 set up, in effect, the third part of the poisons schedule which the Privy Council had sought to establish since the early 1880s. By this section, sulphuric, nitric, and hydrochloric acid and soluble salts of oxalic acid could, if suitably labelled, be sold by anyone. The Privy Council was given the power to add to the list of substances.

As soon as the 1908 Act became law, a great storm of protest from the trade burst on the steps of 17 Bloomsbury Square. Those officers of the Pharmaceutical Society who were held responsible for the passing the Act, J. Rymer Young, the president, Richard Bremridge, the secretary, and William Glyn-Jones, the parliamentary secretary, were accused of having sold the pharmacist's birthright by agreeing to allow companies to call themselves "chemists" and unqualified persons to sell poisons. The grass-roots reaction was predictable but wrongheaded. The 1908 Act was a government measure and the government were adamant on the issue of agricultural poisons. Moreover, a large section of opinion in both Houses of Parliament were in favour of giving companies the right to use all the titles reserved to qualified chemists by the Pharmacy Acts. It was no mean achievement for the Pharmaceutical Society to retain its control of the poisons schedule, to bring companies within the orbit of professional regulation and make them subject to the legislation on poisons, and to reserve for qualified chemists titles which distinguished them from companies of unqualified persons. After the passing of the 1908 Act both the Pharmaceutical Society and the individual pharmacist were in a stronger position than they had been at any time since the decision of the House of Lords in 1880.

NOTES AND REFERENCES TO CHAPTER SIX

1. On pharmacy law in this period see: [Alfred Charles Wootton] *The Pharmacy and Poison Laws of the United Kingdom* (The *Chemist and Druggist*, 1892); Hugh H. L. Bellot, *The Pharmacy Acts, 1851–1908* (1909); and W. S. Glyn-Jones, *The Law Relating to Poisons and Pharmacy* (1909).
2. Ernst W. Stieb, *Drug Adulteration* (1966)
3. Terry M. Parssinen, *Secret Passions, Secret Remedies* (1983)
4. *C. & D.* 68 (1906) 618
5. *P.J.* 7 [3] (1876–7) 932
6. *P.J.* 9 [3] (1878–9) 368–402
7. *P.J.* 18 [3] (1887–8) 6–12
8. *P.J.* 3 [3] (1872–3) 268,366–7,480,698–9,936–41
9. *Lancet* 1875 (2) 213
10. *P.J.* 10 [3] (1879–80) 263, 265–7
11. *C. & D.* 73 (1908) 15 and 103 (1925) 515
12. *P.J.* 80 (1908) 675–8
13. *P.J.* 74 (1905) 893–4: *C. & D.* 73 (1908) 592 and 78 (1911) 904
14. *P.J.* 146 (1941) 163: Dorothy M. Jones, "Progress of Women in Pharmacy", *C. & D.* 172 (1959) Centenary Issue 185–7: J.G.L. Burnby, "Women in Pharmacy", *Pharm.Hist.* 20 (June 1990) 6–8
15. *P.J.* 3 [3] (1872–3) 612–3, 618
16. Stanley Chapman, *Jesse Boot of Boots the Chemists* (1974)
17. *P.J.* 61 (1898) 638–45, 647
18. *C. & D.* 68 (1906) 618–9
19. *P.R.O.* PC8/531
20. Olive Anderson, *Suicide in Victorian and Edwardian England* (1987)
21. *P.R.O.* PC8/484
22. *B.M.J.* 1897 (2) 1441
23. *P.R.O.* HO45/10284/107339
24. *P.R.O.* PC8/281
25. *P.J.* 63 (1899) 473
26. *P.R.O.* PC8/531
27. *P.R.O.* HO45/10284/107339
28. *P.R.O.* HO45/10059/B892
29. 1903 (1442,1443) xxxiii, 1, 17
30. *P.R.O.* PC8/531
31. *The Indian and Eastern Druggist* (March 1921) 61
32. 1895 (7779) lxxxviii, 151
33. *C. & D.* 53 (1898) 88–9, 188–9
34. *Anti-Cutting Record* (1898) 205
35. *P.R.O.* PC8/549
36. *The Proposed Pharmacy Acts Amendment Bill* (The Drug Companies' Association Limited, 1905) 11–13
37. 1908 (150,359) IX, 521, 611
38. *C. & D.* 102 (1925) 21–2, 57–9, 93–4, 127–9
39. *P.R.O.* HO45/10284/107339
40. 8 Edw. VII c.55

CHAPTER SEVEN

From National Health Insurance to National Health Service

Tunicatae prius, denique in folio argenti volvendae—First varnished and then rolled in silver leaf

1. THE PROPRIETARY ARTICLES TRADE ASSOCIATION AND RESALE PRICE MAINTENANCE 1896–1976

A retailing revolution?—William Samuel Glyn-Jones—The Chemists Federation—The Resale Prices Act 1964—Exemption for medicines 1970.

The last quarter of the nineteenth century was a period of growing price competition in many branches of retailing. New types of retailing establishments were rapidly gaining ground. The middle class co-operative stores (the Civil Service Supply Association, the Civil Service Co-operative Society, and the Army and Navy Co-operative Society), the new department stores (William Whiteley's Universal Provider, Spiers & Pond's, and Harrods), and the multiples (Express Dairy, Home and Colonial, Lipton's, Hepworth's, Foster Brothers, Freeman Hardy & Willis, W.H. Smith, Maynard's, and Salmon & Gluckstein) offered the public extensive price reductions. The working class co-operative societies, whose main attraction was the quarterly dividends paid to customer-members, were steadily expanding and extending their operations geographically. Membership of co-operative societies passed the 100,000 mark in 1863 and by 1881 there were 971 societies, still mainly in the North of England, with over 547,000 members. By 1914 there were 1,385 societies, some of them by now very large, with over three million members. Annual turnover rose from £15.4 million in 1881, to £61 million in 1905, to £87.9 million in 1914. Co-ops and multiples concentrated initially on a narrow range of standardised products for which there were steady demand and ready sources of supply. To reduce costs they negotiated discounts with suppliers for bulk purchases or diversified vertically into production. Some manufacturers dispensed with middlemen to sell directly to the public. Sewing machines, bicycles and footwear were sold by the maker direct to the user. By the beginning of the present century the novel variety stores like Marks and Spencer and Woolworths made their appearance.

In the early phase of multiple shop trading low prices combined with high turnover and low margins ("small profits, quick returns"), plus uninhibited advertising and salesmanship were the most important factors in its rapid advance. Most multiple shop organisations in this period were handling what were virtually entirely new types of products, that is, mass-manufactured goods for which the producer, not the retailer, took the responsibility and the credit. Soaps, teas, coffees, and a host of other articles were made up by the makers in packages suitable for retail. By 1900, for example, there were over 300 different types of biscuit on the market baked by nationally known firms like Carr, Huntley & Palmer, Peek Frean, Macfarlane Laing and McVitie. The merits of the respective proprietary brands were kept prominently before the public by newspaper advertisements, pictorial appeals on the hoardings, distribution of free samples and other promotional devices. In this way a demand for the particular article was created, the retailer was obliged to stock it and was placed under a constant temptation to cut the price of branded goods and use them as "leading lines" to attract trade to his shop.[1]

For the chemist and druggist there was little that was new in all this. The chemist and druggist owed his origin to the policy of under-cutting the apothecary. Since the mid-eighteenth century chemists and druggists had promoted the practices of cash trading, of working on low margins, of "ticketing" (that is of marking definite prices uniform to all customers), and of disregarding the traditional divisions between the various branches of retailing. In its early years the Pharmaceutical Society was regularly urged to take action against chemists who could not be distinguished from grocers and against "cutting chemists" who "ticketed" their drugs. An article on "Company Chemists" in 1897 pointed out that "the cutter was with us before the company chemist appeared on the scene but except in his own immediate locality he was loftily ignored".[2] Proprietary medicines had flourished since the beginning of the eighteenth century: in 1748 the author of an article in the *Gentleman's Magazine* had listed over two hundred, all readily available.

Even before the foundation of the Pharmaceutical Society, the established chemists and druggists sought to preserve profit margins by local agreements on retail prices. Local associations of chemists in various towns attempted to introduce minimum price lists and to secure adherence to them. Although some of these associations achieved short term success, local price-fixing agreements without effective sanctions against non-members or newcomers were bound to fail. Members themselves found it difficult to honour their undertakings when outsiders were cutting below the agreed prices, whose one-sided maintenance made new entry and price-cutting profitable. The numerous reports of the failure of price-fixing agreements constantly refer to the "troublesome minority" and to the fact that "one cutter makes many".

The half-century after 1860 saw a marked upturn in the sales of patent medicines in Britain. Sales rose from £600,000 in 1860 to £3 million in 1891 and to £5 million by 1914. The population of England and Wales increased from 17.9 million in 1851 to 32.5 million by 1901. It was an increasingly urban and affluent population. The proportion of the population living in towns increased from one-half to two thirds. Certain sections of the manual working class, the skilled unionised "aristocracy of labour", experienced a substantial rise in real income from the mid-1870s, despite occasional trade slumps and cyclical unemployment. A broad-based white collar professional, managerial, commercial and clerical middle class emerged during this period. Proprietary medicines, which had been a small item of popular consumption up to this time, took a significant share of this growing consumer power. A small group of entrepreneurs, with a taste for showmanship,

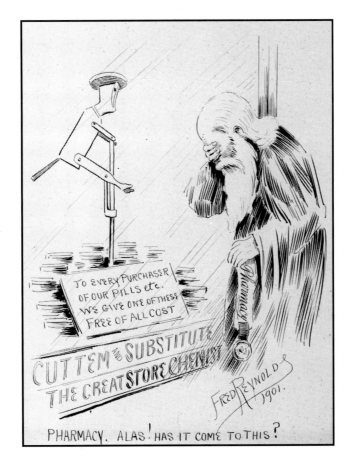

TO EVERY PURCHASER
OF OUR PILLS etc.
WE GIVE ONE OF THESE
FREE OF ALL COST

CUTTEM & SUBSTITUTE
THE GREAT STORE CHEMIST

PHARMACY. ALAS! HAS IT COME TO THIS?

47 Pharmacy; Alas! has it come to this? *Pen and ink drawing by R.F. Reynolds, 1901. Published in the* Chemist and Druggist, *1901* **58** *920 under the title "Window-dressing".*

men like Thomas Holloway (1800–83) and Thomas Beecham (1820–1907), built up a vast market for their products by uncontrolled advertising. Holloway's advertising expenditure rose steadily from £5,000 in 1842 to £50,000 at the time of his death; Beecham's went up from £22,000 in 1880 to over £120,000 in 1891. The fortunes they accumulated were later dissipated on the promotion of classical music and women's education.

The coming of the mass market for advertised proprietary medicines did not bring the chemist and druggist the prosperity that might have been anticipated. His share of the sale of patent medicines was eroded by increased sales by grocers and general stores and, more damagingly, by the emergence of the multiple drug store. The rise of Jesse Boot in the Midlands, Lewis & Burrough's and Parke's in London, Day's and Timothy White's in the South and Taylor's and Inman's in the North created a new and very threatening form of competition.

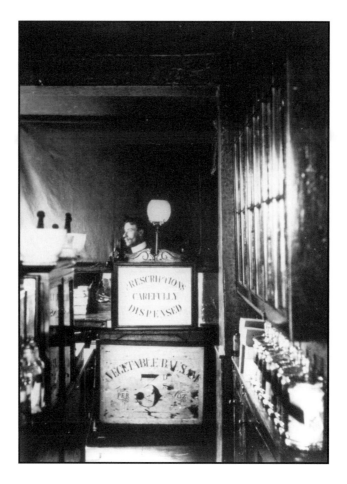

48   *Interior of Wallis Pharmaceutical Chemist, Patent Medicine and Drug Stores, 78 Essex Road, Islington, 1902. "End of the Shop with Mr Keasley": from an album assembled by T.E. Wallis, a unique collection of personal photographs recording both his family business and his long connection with the Society's School of Pharmacy and Museum.*

The advantages of the company chemists' chains can be seen in the price lists issued by Holloway's and Beecham's. A new Holloway's price list of June 1896 offered profit margins of 14.5 per cent. for orders of £5 or over but only of 5 per cent. for the normal orders of the small retailer. Beecham's in September 1898 provided profit margins of 35 per cent. for small orders but 42 per cent for orders of £5 and over. The largest chains, in fact, negotiated even more favourable terms for bulk purchases. The practice of granting substantial quantity discounts encouraged price competition at retail and manufacturers were often censured for supporting the cutters and making cutting possible. A letter to the *Chemist and Druggist* in 1896 pointed out that "it was the owners of 'proprietaries' who made the cutting movement possible to the stores" because suppliers granted such generous discounts to the company chemists that it "permitted them to cut the goods down to, and sometimes below, the prices which the retailer had to pay the selfsame supplier".[3]

The rapid growth of Boot's in the early 1890s soon made its owner the principal target for the chemist and druggist's resentment of the new-style competition.[4] An editorial in the *Chemist and Druggist* in November 1893 drew attention to Boot's twenty-nine shops as "by far the most extensive experiment in company pharmacy we have yet heard of". This development, it was maintained, "threatens the annihilation of pharmacy proper in this country" for within a few years, it forecast, "a few companies will supply all the pharmaceutical requirements of the country". The editorial produced a flood of letters from angry chemists whose livelihoods were being put at risk by the company chemists. One independent proprietor from Hanley, where a new branch of Boot's had just opened, detailed some of Boot's cut-price offers and commented: "To a chemist in a small way, and with limited capital, the above prices are the cost of purchase".[5]

The Pharmaceutical Society sought a political solution to the problems created by the company chemists. At first it attempted, by legal and political means, to eliminate the company chemists. When this proved impossible, it settled for the regulation of their activities through the operation of the 1908 Pharmacy Act. There was, however, another way of protecting the small independent chemist against the unmitigated competition of the multiple stores. If the resale prices of proprietary medicines could be fixed and enforced upon all types of retailer, price competition between the small retailer and the large company would be eliminated. In 1895 a twenty-six year old chemist in a small shop in London's East End took up the formidable challenge of leading the country's independent chemists in a crusade against price-cutting.

William Samuel Glyn-Jones, the son of George Griffith Jones, who became registrar of marriages for Aberdare, was born in Worcester in 1869, but received his early education in South Wales.[6] After attending Merthyr Grammar School, he served a three year apprenticeship at a dispensary in Aberdare run by a Mr. J. Richards, a strict disciplinarian. He then moved to London where, on the fifteen shillings a week he earned as a dispenser to a Bermondsey medical practitioner, he kept himself and paid the fees for evening classes in a private school of pharmacy in Chancery Lane. After qualifying in 1891, he did the dispensing for Dr. Hildreth Kay of Commercial Road in the East End. During this time, Glyn-Jones made the acquaintance of John Evans, a young Welshman who had opened a draper's shop in the same locality, and met his future wife, who was a sister of Evans. In 1894, with the help of a £500 loan from his brother-in-law, he started in business on his own account, under the trading name of Glyn & Co., in the East India Dock Road. The business was in a poor neighbourhood and he found that the sale of proprietary medicines represented more than half the turnover. His profit margins were so slender (his gross profit was around seven and a half per cent), that he realised there was no future in the trade in such a location. Instead of applying for posts with the wholesalers, however, he resolved to tackle the root cause of the problem, which he identified as price-cutting. No one wanted to cut, he observed, but everyone did so. "It was positive madness for intelligent people, all of whom said it was a suicidal game we were playing, to go on playing it".[7] Glyn-Jones decided it was time to stop. With great courage, he launched a modest, monthly, circular called the *Anti-Cutting Record* with the object of organising retail chemists to press manufacturers for fair profit margins. 5,000 copies were distributed throughout Britain.

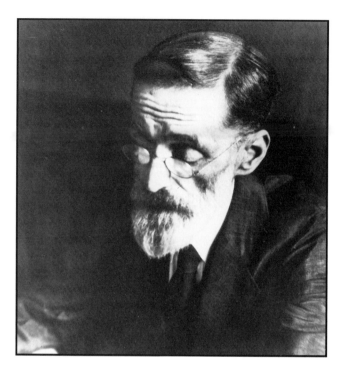

49   *Sir William S. Glyn-Jones (1869–1927).*

"Chemists are the chief sufferers; from them must come the initiative", he wrote in the first issue in November 1895. "The time has arrived when something must be done if the rank-and-file of the retail drug trade are not to be completely wiped out". He suggested twenty-five per cent minimum profit on articles containing poisons (which only qualified men could sell) and fifteen to twenty per cent. on others. In the next issue Glyn-Jones was able to announce that he had received six hundred favourable replies and that his initiative had the support of the *Chemist and Druggist* (though not of the *Pharmaceutical Journal*). This was enough for him to announce in January 1896 the formation of the Proprietary Articles Trade Association (the P.A.T.A.) to promote the policy of protected prices. At the first meeting he was appointed secretary and immediately embarked on a tour of the southern counties to address meetings of the local chemists' associations to gather support. Glyn-Jones had developed his ability as a platform speaker while serving as a lay preacher in the Presbyterian Church. During the spring he spoke at Birmingham, Bradford, Bristol, Brixton, Edinburgh, Exeter, Leeds, Nottingham, Plymouth, Sheffield, South Kensington, and other centres. His reception was one of sympathy tinged with scepticism.

At the same time, he started negotiations with the manufacturers. Although some firms, such as Allen & Hanbury and Burroughs Wellcome had already tried their own schemes to maintain retail prices, the initial response was scarcely encouraging. After six months' work he was able to announce that the owners of twelve proprietaries had subscribed to his list, and the only popular item was "Dr. Scott's Little Liver Pills". The *Chemist and Druggist* commented that this was not very impressive and in October Glyn-Jones complained that "five chemists out of six have done nothing towards assisting us". Undaunted the founder of the P.A.T.A. persisted with his campaign, visiting a new round of towns, including Glasgow and Manchester, in the autumn. Glyn-Jones realised that protected prices or resale price maintenance (to use the modern term) was the most promising device for maintaining or raising the retailer's gross margins and for depriving the company chemists of their most important method of attracting customers and enlarging their trade. He was aware that

> the public did not expect chemists to work for nothing, but they would certainly go where they could get things cheapest. That was the only reason of their forsaking the chemist for the stores. But if the prices were all fixed, there would be no inducement to go to the stores or such places.[8]

To him resale price maintenance

> . . .was not only a question of ensuring a better profit on proprietary articles, but, what was more important to them, to rob the cutter and stores of the advantage which followed their sale of these goods to the public.[9]

Jesse Boot had built his business on price-cutting and Glyn-Jones' campaign deeply antagonised him. He was afraid that the mainstay of his trade would contract and that the independent chemists would be the chief beneficiaries.

> I am sure from my very large and long experience of the patent medicine trade that any rise in prices after the public have for a long series of years been accustomed to a reduced price, will have a most detrimental effect on sales.[10]

He believed the bulk of the patent medicine trade was moving into the hands of the grocers and the company chemists.

> The small retail chemists who persist in doing business on old-fashioned lines are practically shut out, and this movement [the P.A.T.A.] is simply organised by them in order to regain the trade out of the hands of the grocers and the progressive firms and bring it back to themselves at full prices.

Boot was determined to smash the P.A.T.A. In 1896 he paid for large advertisements protesting against the price ring of the P.A.T.A. which he described as "a nice little plot hatched for the benefit of the retailer and the wholesale middleman". He advised the public to refuse to buy any article on the list of the chemists' ring. In a sequence of letters to the *Chemist and Druggist* in August and October 1896, Jesse Boot made his intentions clear:

> Rather than be defeated we are prepared, if need be, to buy all proprietary articles at full retail prices, and label every one of them to inform the public of the point at issue between ourselves and the ring . . .
>
> In order to clear out our stocks, we may be driven, as a last resource, to get up a special sale to dispose of them at very cut rates indeed . . .[11]

Boot and William Day (of Day's Drug Stores) came together to plan a mammoth sale of protected goods to demoralise the chemists who backed the P.A.T.A. Day rented a disused chapel in south London and in 1897 and 1898 began to build up a large stock of P.A.T.A. goods by buying through grocers and other retail chemists. Then, as Glyn-Jones expressed it, "the fire of the Lord fell" and the chapel and all its contents were destroyed. The fact that the company chemists took the P.A.T.A. so seriously made the ever-cautious chemists and druggists see "more in this Association than they had thought".[12] Membership jumped from 1,600 in February 1897 to more than 3,000 in July 1898.

The growing support of retailers was a necessary condition for the ultimate success of the P.A.T.A. but, as Glyn-Jones was aware, the "first axiom is that the key to the situation lies in the manufacturer's hands; he it is who can control supplies and without this control . . . it would be impossible to arrange matters by mutual consent of the traders". Proprietary medicines offered prospects of securely enforced minimum retail prices because each manufacturer was in a position to control the supply of his brands to particular retailers and so to discipline price-cutters by withholding supplies. Glyn-Jones had the difficult task of persuading manufacturers that a system of protected prices was in their interests as well as in the interests of the independent retailer.[13]

The manufacturer faced a complex problem of assessment in considering whether or not to yield to Glyn-Jones' demands. He had to judge the relative strengths of the two broad groups of supporters and opponents of protected prices, as well as the relative severity of the damage each group was likely to inflict on him if dissatisfied with his decision. The manufacturers were told that they had to choose between "the legitimate trader or retailer of proprietary articles and the stores, and that they could not obtain the friendship and goodwill of both".[14] "The case of the retail druggist must be considered by manufacturers and wholesale dealers, in spite of the fact that Mr. Boot and similar pushing men are valuable customers".[15]

For the patent medicine proprietor the greatest risk involved in resale price maintenance was that the public would find cheaper substitutes. Jesse Boot was not averse to conjuring up the spectre of independent chemists increasing the substitution of new remedies for advertised proprietaries.

> The worst substitutors in the trade are the smallest men, who having any amount of time on their hands and very little capital, are too glad . . . to sell two pennyworth or three pennyworth of their nostrums in the place of a proprietary article . . .[16]

Manufacturers could not in any way be certain that those retailers who were agitating for price maintenance would refrain from substitution once resale prices were protected. Retail members of the P.A.T.A. were not required to bind themselves not to substitute for protected articles. The chairman at a P.A.T.A. meeting announced that

> there was an impression abroad that the members of the Association must agree not to substitute. Nothing of the kind would be asked, and it would be left to the discretion of the members.[17]

Glyn-Jones provided considerable encouragement for chemists to substitute their own preparations for proprietaries. In 1903 he gained a famous victory through the decision of the High Courts in *Farmer v. Glyn-Jones* which restored to chemists the dormant statutory right to sell "known, admitted and approved remedies" unstamped. Since the medicine stamp duty amounted to about twelve per cent. of the retail price, the chemist's own preparations were given a considerable comparative advantage. This was reinforced in 1904 when the Pharmaceutical Society published the *Pharmaceutical Journal Formulary*, which included the formulae of several hundred proprietary medicines regularly sold by pharmacists. The Board of Inland Revenue accepted all the formulae published therein as "known, admitted and approved" remedies and therefore not requiring a patent medicine stamp. In this way, widely advertised proprietary remedies could be reproduced by the independent chemist, at greater profit to himself and lower cost to his customer.

The question of substitution raised two issues. Would the independent chemist be more or less likely to substitute if his profit margins on proprietaries were adequate? Did the patent medicine manufacturer have more to fear from the substitution practised by small retailers or by the multiples? Glyn-Jones contended that, in the long run, the support of the numerous "legitimate" retailers was more valuable to manufacturers than that of the large stores, the multiples, and the co-operative societies. He argued that the price-cutters used proprietary articles to build up a reputation for low prices; but that, having eliminated the small retailer, they would progressively dispense with the proprietary medicines and substitute their own products for them. The opponents of resale price maintenance were large firms, well able to advertise widely and to finance production. Boot already manufactured his own range of proprietaries and was in a strong position to produce cheaper alternatives to popular brands; moreover, he gave his counter staff a good commission for selling Boots' own lines.

The manufacturers, however, feared that the introduction of resale price maintenance would actually provoke the multiples to commence or extend their own production. In 1906, after the P.A.T.A. had decided that the payment of dividends to customers was a breach of minimum price stipulations, the Co-operative Wholesale Society notified the retail societies that P.A.T.A. articles would no longer be available.

> Wherever practicable, we propose to manufacture or pack articles to replace those withdrawn, which, together with preparations manufactured by firms unconnected with the P.A.T.A., will enable you to supply your members with little, if any, inconvenience.

A later circular from the Co-operative Wholesale Society listed its own preparations and the brands for which they were replacements. The list included substitutes for eight brands which were not on the protected list.

There were other ways in which price maintenance could defeat its own ends. The Civil Service Supply Association produced its own proprietary medicines, the sales of which were no doubt stimulated by the appearance of the following notice in its catalogue of 1906:

> Pressure from traders combined in an association for the purpose of keeping up the retail prices of proprietary articles has caused certain manufacturers to fix minimum prices below which their articles must not be sold. Whilst the Civil Service Supply Association, for the convenience of its members, continues in some cases to supply those goods at the prices fixed by the makers—prices frequently much higher than the committee of management would desire to charge—the extra profits derived from the sale of those articles are utilised in reducing the prices of the great variety of other goods in which there is and can be no limitation of price.

The independent chemists, particularly if well organised, were also in a position to take direct action against the interests of manufacturers of branded goods. Dispensing chemists had the facilities and skill to devise and prepare substitutes for many proprietary lines: they could refuse to co-operate in manufacturers' sales—promotion efforts and, more generally, could keep lines with low profit margins in the back of the shop or under the counter. To reassure the manufacturers, the P.A.T.A. developed an anti-substitution policy.

> The retailer has a right to persuade the customer to take something else, and each man must settle his business policy in this respect for himself. But a different consideration arises where the proprietor has added his article to the P.A.T.A. By so doing he recognises the retailer's right to a profit, and he takes upon himself the burden of securing that profit for the retailer. Common fairness dictates that the least he has a right to expect is that when his article is asked for it will be handed over the counter without any attempt to sell anything in its place.

After persuasion came the threat. "Cases of substitution in relation to P.A.T.A. goods", announced the report for 1905–6, "have been investigated, and the Council will in future deal with such cases as they do with those of cutting".[18]

Many manufacturers were unwilling to have their brands placed on the P.A.T.A. list unless their competitors did likewise: they were anxious not to give their rivals any competitive advantage. The representative of Oppenheimer, Sons & Co., Ltd., a manufacturer of chemists' goods and a member of the P.A.T.A., stated that "they were not without competitors, but if the proprietors of kindred articles agreed to add their articles to the list, his firm would be most happy to do so".[19]

The reluctance of maufacturers to commit themselves to the P.A.T.A. was due to the difficulty of weighing the conflicting considerations and the uncertainty of the outcome of the adoption of price protection. Manufacturers had had many years of a highly competitive retail market in which the severity of price-cutting was a good index of the popularity of a brand. Without compelling reasons, they would not readily interfere with the supply of their goods to the most successful retail competitors. As late as 1904 a manufacturer of a popular proprietary medicine in turning down an invitation to join the P.A.T.A. observed that the Association had "considerably under 2,000 retail members and that 2,000 could not be placed in the balance for sales of proprietaries against the various big firms". Those supporters of resale price maintenance "who expected an immediate capitulation of the great proprietors expected a very foolish thing" warned the editor of the *Chemist and Druggist*. Glyn-Jones in 1899 recorded that

> the negotiations are exceedingly tedious, but we find there is no help for it. The issues for the large firms are very grave, and they are naturally cautious.[20]

He realised that his arguments would not impress manufacturers unless he was accepted as the spokesman for a large number of retailers. Both his offers of support and his threats of trade opposition would lack substance. What was insignificant when practised by isolated small retailers became serious when individuals were organised and could act with a high degree of solidarity. "The retailers held a powerful weapon", Glyn-Jones pointed out, "for it was evident that manufacturers must join [the P.A.T.A.] if retailers combined to boycott their goods". The success of the P.A.T.A. was assured "if chemists joined the Association in sufficient numbers" for the manufacturers "could not withstand the organized opposition of a combined trade".[21]

The speed at which the manufacturers' reluctance to join the P.A.T.A. was overcome depended largely upon the strength of the retailers' organization. Glyn-Jones rightly "emphasized the fact that the size, length and importance of the protected list would be almost in direct proportion to the support given to the movement by retailers".[22] The more conspicuous the support of the "legitimate" retail trade, the easier it was to convert wavering manufacturers. The testimony of firms who discovered that the policy of protected prices was rewarding was given wide publicity. The proprietors of Hall's coca wine, one of the first items on the P.A.T.A. list, announced that

> we are more than satisfied that it pays us to support the ordinary shopkeeper in a fair minimum profit. In maintaining this position we have lost the goodwill of some of the large co-operative societies, but our loss in this direction has been more than made up by the increased sales of the retail trade.[23]

The proprietors of Scott's pills were

> glad to say that the increased sales of their pills proved that they were right in their belief . . . Formerly they had the greatest difficulty in getting [chemists] . . . to exhibit showcards or distribute handbills, or in any way assist the sale of their pills. Now, however, they were having application for handbills, etc., from hundreds of retailers in all parts of the country.[24]

The Proprietary Articles Trade Association was formed in January 1896 to unite the interests of manufacturers, wholesalers and retailers. It was governed by a council of thirty members, ten from each group. Manufacturers and wholesalers paid an annual subscription of five guineas, retailers five shillings. In the first year the income of the Association was £677 and the expenditure £626. By 1923 the income was £6,800 and the expenditure £5,000. At first its functions were confined to resale price maintenance. A protected list of proprietary articles was drawn up, the owners of which agreed to supply them only on condition that they were retailed at specified prices. The P.A.T.A. council insisted on retail profit margins of between 20 and 25 per cent. for goods when purchased from wholesalers in ordinary quantities. The P.A.T.A. undertook all the protection work. The list of articles was sent in the *Anti-Cutting Record* to all chemists in business in Britain and to a large number of grocers and others holding patent medicines licences. The P.A.T.A. appointed officials and private inquiry agents in every town: information about hostile cutters and those who supplied them was systematically collected. Every wholesale house signed an undertaking to withhold supplies of P.A.T.A. goods from cutters on the "stop list"; and any cutter refusing to conform with P.A.T.A. prices was liable to be placed on the "stop list". The P.A.T.A. Year Book for 1905–6 reported:

> With the very large accession to the protected list of articles of extensive sale, there has naturally been an increase in the work entailed by reported cases of cutting. The council are glad to report that whilst the reported cases of cutting have been numerous, the cases where the association has been defied are rare. The council have now no fear of their ability to ultimately bring any offender into line . . . Every credit should be given to the members of the wholesale trade who so loyally support the council in their efforts to prevent supplies of articles on its list reaching cutters.

The Association started with a list of 16 articles: by the end of 1897 it comprised 142 and by the beginning of 1924 over 2,000. After ten years activity, 214 manufacturers and 3,647 retailers paid subscriptions (compared with 81 manufacturers and 1,989 retailers in 1902.)

By 1924 there were 430 manufacturers, 61 wholesalers and 8,000 retailers. The official journal, the *Anti-Cutting Record*, had a circulation, by 1908, of 10,500.

The success of the P.A.T.A. was dependent upon the groundwork carried out over half a century by the Pharmaceutical Society. Chemists and druggists were by far the most strongly organised of the retail trades. Their organisation derived from the fact that entrance to the "legitimate", higher status branches of the trade was guarded by the traditional mechanism of apprenticeship and the statutory requirement of the Pharmaceutical Society's examinations. "The qualification", acknowledged Glyn-Jones, "is the foundation upon which all else is built". If the qualification were to go, everything else that the P.A.T.A. and the Chemists' Defence Association stood for, would be lost. "The qualification, so far as the public is concerned, is regarded as the hallmark of skill and qualification to carry on the whole business".[25] The local associations of chemists and druggists were the substructure on which the P.A.T.A. was constructed. Without this pre-existing base of solidarity, the trade could never have been organised to defeat the cutters. In 1902 the P.A.T.A. convened a conference attended by delegates from forty-four local chemists' associations. A strong resolution in favour of the P.A.T.A. method of securing retail profit margins was carried. "The result has been that since the conference about fifty proprietors have joined the association, some of them representing articles of the largest sale".

The manufacturers of proprietary medicines could not afford to alienate the "legitimate" trade. Through legal action, the Pharmaceutical Society had established by 1894 that only qualified chemists could sell proprietary medicines containing poisons. The manufacturers knew how much the sales of their products depended upon public confidence in their efficacy. That confidence was in danger of being undermined by the B.M.A.'s campaign against secret remedies. Ernest Hart, the editor of the *British Medical Journal* and chairman of the B.M.A.'s parliamentary bills committee, intensified that campaign during the 1890s. In 1909 the B.M.A.'s booklet, *Secret Remedies; what they cost and what they contain*, revealed that nearly all the widely-advertised patent medicines contained only well-known and inexpensive drugs. More than ever, the manufacturers needed the support of the qualified chemist: their products gained respectability by being recommended and sold in the traditional shops of the proprietor-pharmacist. The manufacturers could not afford to become exclusively associated with the less respectable price-cutting retailers: they feared this would damage the public image of their brands. There is strong evidence that before 1914 patients were reluctant to take prescriptions to company shops that sold cut-rate drugs. Glyn-Jones observed that some patients would tear off the bottom part of a doctor's prescription form, on which some proprietary article had been prescribed. The part of the prescription requiring something to be dispensed would be presented to a reputable proprietor-chemist and the proprietary article would be obtained from a cut-price company store.[26] It was the fact that the traditional, qualified chemist stocked the same proprietary medicine as the multiple stores that gave the customer the confidence to buy it at the cheaper rate. Consumer demand for proprietary medicines was partly dependent on their being sold by qualified chemists. It was one of Glyn-Jones' tasks to convince manufacturers that price protection was required to enable the small retailers, who provided the demand-creating services, to capture the benefit of the sales which resulted from their investment in education and training.

Several years before Glyn-Jones founded the Proprietary Articles Trade Association, a number of manufacturers attempted to protect the retail prices of their products. Ellimans Ltd., Allen & Hanbury, and Burroughs Wellcome were among the first manufacturers to realise how damaging the price-cutting activities of companies like Boots and Taylors could be. These manufacturers wanted to maintain the reputation of their products by preserving the traditional professional retail outlets for their brands. The more scientifically based manufacturers had difficulty in launching new and relatively expensive products except through the "legitimate" trade. There was a great gulf between the products of firms like Holloway's and Beecham's and those of new manufacturers like Burroughs Wellcome. Burroughs Wellcome insisted upon strict laboratory control of raw materials and finished products and concentrated upon the manufacture of accurate dosaged medicaments. In 1894 Henry Wellcome set up the first physiological research laboratory in Britain and two years later established chemical research laboratories in London. Firms like Burroughs Wellcome and Allen & Hanbury had every reason to want to protect the qualified proprietor-chemist from the onslaught of the price-cutting stores. Thus in the trade papers of 1894 we find manufacturers' advertisements of which the following is a typical example:

> If you buy two dozen 1s. size . . ., and sign our agreement not to sell to any person whatever below the present cutting price of 10 1/2d. per bottle, we will charge you 9s.6d. per dozen, and will allow you as a bonus for non-further cutting 2s. on every dozen. This will leave you a profit of 3d. per bottle at the cutting price of 10 1/2d., or 40 per cent. on your outlay . . . If any one, after having signed our agreement, infringes the same, we will proceed, against him according to the terms of the agreement for the recovery of the bonus given to him, as well as for damages, costs, etc., and an injunction will be applied for to restrain him from repeating his breach of contract. Besides this, we shall refuse to supply him with goods, except at the full price of 9s.6d. net, without bonus, so that he could not make any reasonable profit by selling under 10 1/2d. per bottle.

The initiative to introduce resale price maintenance did not come from Glyn-Jones, nor from the independent retail chemists, but from certain manufacturers who saw that intense price competition was prejudicial to their interests. But the wholesale houses could not conduct their business on the basis of a multitude of individual agreements; nor could these separate agreements be adequately policed and enforced. It was the genius of William Glyn-Jones to create the Proprietary Articles Trade Association and bring together the interests of manufacturers, wholesalers and the independent chemists. It remained, nonetheless, a herculean task for Glyn-Jones to persuade manufacturers and retailers that it was in their own interests to join the Association.

The acceptance of resale price maintenance by the company chemists after 1900 was a further triumph for the diplomacy of Glyn-Jones and a major factor in the ultimate success of the P.A.T.A. In the political struggle between the Pharmaceutical Society and the Drug Companies' Association, Glyn-Jones maintained the P.A.T.A. on a strictly neutral course. Within the counsels of the Pharmaceutical Society, he adopted a conciliatory position, believing in the need to regulate but not to suppress the activities of company chemists. Glyn-Jones and Jesse Boot eventually built up a good working relationship: they knew when and how to compromise. When the Chemists' Defence Association was formed to defend pharmacists in prosecutions under the Food and Drugs Act, Jesse Boot sent Glyn-Jones a donation of £100. In 1899 Boot and William Day quietly abandoned their campaign against the P.A.T.A. In the following ten years three multiple shop organisations joined the Association while others, like Boots, although not formally taking out membership, agreed to adhere to its fixed prices. By 1914 resale price maintenance was becoming the rule in the trade both in regard to chemists' goods proper and to the widening range of toilet preparations and requisites being sold. The company chemists were by now taking the initiative in pressing patent medicine manufacturers offering low profit margins to go on the P.A.T.A. list. Over a fifteen year period Jesse Boot's policy towards the P.A.T.A. moved from bitter opposition to tacit acceptance: he discovered that the advent of resale price maintenance did not ruin his trade. Fixed retail prices did not imply uniform wholesale prices; bulk purchasers like Boots continued to buy at much more favourable terms than the independent chemist.

The introduction of price protection brought its benefits to both the independent chemist and the customer. It gave the small retailer a breathing space to enable him to adjust to a rapidly changing world. With reasonable profit margins assured, the private chemist was given the incentive to maintain extensive stocks of proprietary medicines and to provide professional advice on their use. Despite higher retail prices, the public received an improved standard of service with an increased emphasis on health education and drug information and a wider geographical dispersion of chemists' shops. The chronically ill, the disabled, the elderly and the poor were the principal beneficiaries of the survival of the small local chemist's shop.

The structure and methods of the P.A.T.A. were widely copied. By 1938 it was estimated that between 27 per cent. and 35 per cent. of all consumer goods sold to the private domestic consumer were sold at prices fixed by the producers.[27] After the First World War the expansion of resale price maintenance attracted official scrutiny. A sub-committee of the Standing Committee on Trusts was appointed

> to report the extent to which the principle of fixing a minimum retail price by manufacturers or associations prevails; what are its results, and whether the system is, in the interests of the public, desirable or otherwise.

The Committee could find no fault with the fixing of retail prices.

> ... where, as at the present time, the demand is in excess of the supply, the method of fixing retail prices has undoubtedly restrained or tended to restrain any undue inflation of prices ... In times of plenty it tends to ensure to all classes, including labour employed in manufacture and distribution, a fair rate of remuneration ...[28]

The next general inquiry took place in 1930–1. A committee was set up jointly by the Lord Chancellor and the President of the Board of Trade to consider resale price maintenance as well as other trade practices involving withholding supplies from particular retailers. The Committee concluded that:

> no significant case has been made out for interfering with the right of the manufacturer to sell his goods upon conditions which permit him to name the terms on which such goods shall be re-sold.

The Committee was

> quite unable to say that the interests of the public would be better served by an
> alteration in the law which would prevent the fixing of prices of branded goods . . .
> We have been impressed by the volume and force of the testimony as to the harmful
> effects of price cutting upon the manufacturers and distributors of advertised
> branded goods and ultimately, as was contended, upon the public.[29]

After the Second World War, however, official policy changed. The Monopolies
Commission was set up in 1948 and the Restrictive Practices Court in 1956. In the course
of major inquiries into particular industries, resale price maintenance was one of the
practices subject to investigation: but it was also singled out for special scrutiny and,
eventually, in 1956, 1964 and 1976, for special legislation. In 1947 the President of the
Board of Trade set up a general inquiry into resale price maintenance. The Lloyd Jacob
Committee's report, which appeared in 1949, indicates the change in direction of official
thinking. The Committee concluded:

> We are satisfied that the elimination of price competition over the greater part of
> the distributive trades is not consistent with the need for the maximum efficiency
> and economy in production and distribution . . .

Moreover, the collective withholding of supplies involving "the use of extra-legal sanction
which may deprive a trader of his livelihood" could not be justified.

Although the Lloyd Jacob Committee was critical of resale price maintenance, it
nonetheless saw much good in it. The Committee accepted the argument

> advanced by some manufacturers that the uncertainty brought about by prolonged
> price-cutting may make it difficult and sometimes impossible for them to maintain
> the quality and continuity of production of their branded goods . . . Past experience
> appears to have shown manufacturers that if a nationally advertised brand is sold
> at varying prices in neighbouring shops the demand for it—as reflected in the
> distributors' orders to the manufacturer—substantially decreases . . . Price
> reductions . . . may not reflect any actual or expected saving in operating expenses
> but may be used as an aggressive weapon of competition . . . The disruption of
> trade in popular lines which is brought about by these activities appears to bear
> particularly heavily upon the retailer who, by carrying in addition a wide range of
> relatively slow selling lines and in some trades by offering skilled technical advice
> to his customers, provides a service whose value may not be recognised until it has
> disappeared.

The Committee was forced to acknowledge that retail price competition could be damaging
to manufacturers, retailers and "to the wider interests of the public".[30] In *A Statement on
Resale Price Maintenance* in 1951, the Government promised that, in drafting legislation, it
"will take account of any cases where it may be established that exceptional conditions
would render the operation of the proposed provisions unworkable or undesirable in the
public interest".[31]

The Restrictive Trade Practices Act of 1956 made illegal the collective enforcement of
resale price agreements, the method devised sixty years previously by William Glyn-Jones
to give the P.A.T.A. teeth. The Act also set up the Restrictive Practices Court which, in
1958, ruled that the restrictions imposed by the Chemists Federation (the so-called

Chemists' Friends Scheme) were contrary to the public interest and therefore void. The Chemists Federation was a by-product of the work of the P.A.T.A. For pharmacists one of the undesired consequences of the P.A.T.A.'s success was the encouragement it gave to grocers and drug stores to sell proprietary medicines. Provided its resale conditions were observed, the P.A.T.A. did not concern itself with the kinds of channel through which proprietary medicines might be distributed. While the P.A.T.A. clearly benefited pharmacists by maintaining the price of the articles they sold, it also had the effect of making the sale of proprietary medicines very profitable for other retailers. To meet this situation, the Chemists' Friends Scheme was developed by the National Pharmaceutical Union. Under this scheme, which was started in 1935, manufacturers of proprietary medicines were asked to restrict to pharmacists the retail distribution of their products and those that agreed to do so were placed on the Chemists' Friends list and their products were given special prominence by those retail pharmacists who supported the scheme. By 1958 there were about 4,000 articles (out of a total of some 9,000) on the C.F. list, the products of 122 manufacturers (out of a total of 356). C.F. products accounted for one third of the value of all proprietary medicines sold in this country. Had the C.F. list been restricted to medicines that required the advice and guidance of the pharmacist to accompany their sale to the public, the Chemists Federation would probably have survived the scrutiny of the Restrictive Practices Court. After the Court's decision, the Chemists Federation wound itself up.[32]

Resale price maintenance leapt into prominence again early in 1964 when John Stonehouse, a highly regarded Labour M.P., introduced a private member's bill to abolish it, except in those instances in which the Restrictive Practices Court found the practice compatible with the public interest. The bill did not survive its second reading but may have helped to precipitate the Conservative Government's decision to legislate. The Resale Prices bill was introduced on 10 March by Edward Heath who was then the Secretary of State for Industry, Trade and Regional Development and President of the Board of Trade. He proposed to

> facilitate the introduction of new and improved methods of distribution by ending resale price maintenance, except when it can be shown that it helps the consumer and is not contrary to the public interest.[33]

His bill, which helped to destroy the small shopkeeper's instinctive faith in the Tory Party, had a stormy passage through parliament. Those who were most alert to the damage the bill would cause—chemists, newsagents, garage owners, tobacconists, wine merchants and scores of other independent retailers—co-ordinated their protest in the Resale Price Maintenance Co-ordinating Committee in Wimpole Street. Pamphlets were published, M.P.s were lobbied. The *Daily Express* added momentum to the protest. A Tory back-bench rebellion, led by Sir Hugh Linstead, secretary of the Pharmaceutical Society since 1926 and Conservative M.P. for Putney since 1942, harassed Mr. Heath from January till April. The rebellion reached its climax on 11 March 1964 when 21 Conservatives voted against the Government and at least 17 others abstained. On a later division, when Mr. Heath refused to exempt medicines from the provisions of the Act, the Government's majority fell to one. Edward Heath emerged from the struggle with the reputation of a determined politician, capable of carrying through unpopular measures in the face of deep-rooted opposition from within his own party. In the General Election held later that year, the Labour Party was returned to power after thirteen years of Conservative government. Sir Hugh Linstead was one of many Tory casualties: he was narrowly defeated at Putney and never returned to the House of Commons.

The Resale Prices Act 1976 consolidated a number of different enactments, of which the Resale Prices Act of 1964 was the most important. Like its 1964 predecessor, the 1976 Act makes it unlawful to establish or seek to establish minimum prices for the resale of goods in the United Kingdom. However, there is a provision in Section 14 of the 1976 Act (which corresponds to Section 5 of the 1964 Act) whereby the Restrictive Practices Court may, upon application to it, make an order exempting goods of a specific class from the Act's provisions. An application may be made by the Director General of Fair Trading, a trade association, or any supplier of the goods in question. Under Section 14, the Court may grant an exemption order where it appears that, without resale price maintenance, the consumers or users of the goods would suffer detriment greater than the detriment resulting from the maintenance of minimum resale prices. The 1976 Act, like its predecessor of 1964, requires the Court to have regard exclusively to the interests of consumers. In piloting the 1964 Act, Mr. Heath stubbornly resisted attempts to introduce additional grounds for exemption, such as the protection of the interests of retailers and their employees, the promotion of exports, or the maintenance of employment. Section 5 of the 1964 Act (now Section 14 of the 1976 Act) specifies the particular kinds of benefit to consumers which alone are to be considered by the Court. An exemption order may be granted where the absence of resale price maintenance would result in any of the following undesirable consequences:

(1) The quality or variety of the goods available for sale would be substantially reduced to the detriment of the public.

(2) The number of establishments in which the goods are sold by retail would be substantially reduced to the detriment of the public.

(3) Retail prices of the goods would in general and in the long run be increased to the detriment of the public.

(4) The goods would be sold under conditions likely to cause danger to health in consequence of their misuse by the consumer.

(5) Any necessary services provided with or after the sale of the goods would be substantially reduced to the detriment of the public.

The Restrictive Practices Court has made only two exemption orders: the first, in 1968, for books; the second, in 1970, for medicines. In the case of medicines, the application was made by, amongst others, the P.A.T.A.; the exemption order was granted on 5 June after a 28 day hearing. The order was made because the Court was convinced that medicines are fundamentally different from other goods on sale to the public: they have the power to do harm even when the consumer believes they are doing good. The Court decided that, because medicines can damage health when used to excess or for the wrong condition, the public should not be encouraged by cut-price and special offers to buy more than they need. Moreover, the Court was satisfied that if minimum resale prices were not maintained, small pharmacies might go out of business in the face of competition from larger firms with the resources to undercut their prices. If this were to happen, the consequences would be particularly serious for people living in remote areas who rely upon their small local pharmacies and would suffer considerable hardship if these were forced out of business. Ease

323

of access is specially important to those members of the public who make most use of pharmacies, such as the old, the chronically ill, the disabled, and mothers of young children. The Court considered that a plentiful and well distributed supply of pharmacies was very much in the public interest and felt that the removal of price maintenance on medicines could cause disastrous changes in their viability. The Court also decided that it was important for the proper functioning of the National Health Service that there should be an adequate and efficient supply of household remedies available to the public, especially through pharmacies. The purchase of household medicines, particularly if accompanied by the advice and guidance of the pharmacist, is an essential supplement to other forms of medical care. In short, it was recognised that retail pharmacy is of a unique character because of the wide variety of medicines stocked, the slow rate of turnover, the importance of the service provided and the professional skill required.[34]

2. NATIONAL HEALTH INSURANCE TO NATIONAL HEALTH SERVICE 1911–1948

> The Poor Law, Friendly Societies, and Industrial Insurance Companies—David Lloyd George and National Health Insurance—The insurance industry, doctors and pharmacists *versus* The Friendly Societies—The separation of prescribing and dispensing—Pharmacists and National Health Insurance—Pharmacists in the National Health Service—Hospital pharmacists.

During the reign of Queen Victoria state provision for the destitute was based on the Poor Law of 1834. Its aim was not to relieve poverty but to force the working man onto the labour market. The fundamental premise was that an able bodied person's application for parish relief constituted an interference with the operation of the free market economy. Relief, therefore, ought to be offered only on the most humiliating and degrading terms and its acceptance should be made to carry the stigma of the semi-criminal. Any relief given to the individual that lessened his desperation for work harmed both the individual and the economy. At the beginning of the twentieth century, J.S. Davy, permanent head of the Poor Law Division of the Local Government Board, argued that the poor must be deterred from applying for relief by the threat of

> firstly ... the loss of personal reputation (what is understood by the stigma of pauperism); secondly, the loss of personal freedom, which is secured by detention in a workhouse; and thirdly, the loss of political freedom by suffering disfranchisement.

The Victorian Poor Law was highly successful. At the time Davy made this statement, thirty per cent. of the population lived in poverty, but less than three per cent. were in receipt of poor relief. Fear of pauperism was burnt into the very heart of the British working class.

A system of public relief which was deliberately made hideous for its recipients forced those who could do so to make more humane provision for themselves by relying on mutual help. The Friendly Societies in particular had become, by mid-Victorian times, major institutions for social security. Friendly Societies were the product of the increasing social interaction created by the growth of towns in eighteenth century England. They were originally created for conviviality as well as mutual help. People drawn together by sectarian belief, occupation or residence would help one another in time of misfortune, not by passing round a hat, but by creating a common fund designed to provide security against impoverishment by illness or the expenses of a funeral. By 1815 it was reckoned that eight and a half per cent. of the population belonged to a Friendly Society of some kind. During the period 1825–75 the movement grew rapidly, both in number of societies and in membership, so that by 1900 the Registrar of Friendly Societies reported the existence of nearly 24,000 registered societies and branches, with nearly four and a half million members, or very roughly half the adult male population of Great Britain. Every middle-sized town had scores of national societies represented among its population as well as innumerable local societies. In 1901 Seebohm Rowntree estimated that 636 societies had 10,662 members among the 75,812 inhabitants of York. For the better-paid Victorian artisan, membership of a Friendly Society was taken for granted. It was the symbol of his independence and respectability. Within the social and moral fraternity of the lodge, opportunities for leadership and increased status were provided. Membership also guaranteed a measure of financial independence. In return for a contribution of between 4d. and 8d. a week (about one to two per cent. of the weekly wage) the society gave sick pay, ordinarily around ten shillings a week, medical care, usually provided by a doctor under contract to the society, and a death benefit of £10 to £15, enough for a respectable funeral. Small local societies, such as had been normal at the beginning of the nineteenth century, still existed at the end of it, but they now shared the field with the great affiliated societies, which were nation-wide bodies. The two largest of these, the Manchester Unity of Odd Fellows and the Ancient Order of Foresters each had well over 700,000 members. Of the large societies, Hearts of Oak, with some 400,000 members, was distinctive in having its main offices in London and in not being organised into lodges.

Overlapping with the world of Friendly Societies, but much more exclusive, were the trade unions. Most of them offered sickness and death benefits, and in many cases the added security of unemployment pay. The numbers benefiting from such arrangements were, however, very limited. In 1900 for every four Friendly Society members in Britain there was only one trade unionist.

This still left about half the adult male population outside the reach of both the Friendly Societies and the trade unions. Part of this is explained by the fact that neither appealed to those above the lower middle class. At the other end of the social scale, more than a third of the working class were too badly paid or too intermittently employed to be able to make such provision for themselves. Yet men who could not afford to pay for sickness benefits tried at least to insure themselves and their families against the humiliation of a pauper's funeral. They paid their weekly pence to the Industrial Assurance Societies whose agents called regularly at the door. A funeral grant of £10, although no security against the misfortunes of life, was a protection against social degradation at death. Charles Booth in 1899 found that in East London even the poorest households saved a weekly average of three and a half pence for so-called life assurance. Playing upon the fear of burial by the parish, commercial insurance companies built up a gigantic and immensely profitable business. By 1913 they employed about 100,000 men of whom 70,000 were full-time door-to-door agents, selling nearly ten million new policies each year, worth together over £101 million, a sum slightly larger than half the total national budget. For each ten new policies sold in a year, there were nine that lapsed.

In the years immediately before the First World War there were about 75 industrial insurance organisations. Of these 50 were organised as collecting friendly societies but most of these were small local "Burial Societies". Ninety per cent. or more of the business of collecting insurance, the "industrial insurance industry", was in the hands of twelve companies. Of these nine were limited liability corporations and three were "collecting" Friendly Societies. By far the largest of the twelve companies was the Prudential which had an industrial insurance reserve fund nearly nine times as large as its nearest competitor, the Pearl. The Prudential was the largest private owner of freehold properties in the United Kingdom. It was the largest shareholder of Bank of England stocks, and of Indian and colonial government bonds and stocks. Each month its investment committee had to find a profitable situation for about half a million more pounds. Its premium income was about one third of the £20 million per year received by the twelve largest companies together.

Only two of the collecting Friendly Societies ranked in size with the private companies. These were the Royal Liver, based in Liverpool, and the Liverpool Victoria, based in London. By 1911 the Liverpool Victoria was the largest collecting Friendly Society. In 1908 it enjoyed an income of £1,199,574 and during the year spent £390,355 in benefits and £489,606 on management. The rest went to swell its three and a half million pound reserve. Between 1909 and 1913 it spent 45 per cent. of its premium income on salesmen's commissions and managerial expenses.[1]

For most people before the Second World War, social reform meant Part 1 of the National Insurance Act of 1911. In health insurance David Lloyd George provided 14 million British men and women with medical care from general practitioners and pharmacists and payments for the support of the family while the breadwinner was ill. Health insurance was by far the most expensive and most controversial of the welfare reforms of the 1905–14 Liberal government. Through the wage-earner, it touched five-sixths of the families of the United Kingdom, bringing them in contact with the State in an unprecedented way. The national scheme of insurance against sickness and disability applied to all wage-earners over the age of sixteen with an annual income below £160, this being then the limit for exemption from income tax. In return for a 4d. contribution from working men or a 3d. contribution from women, with 3d. from the employer, the scheme provided unlimited primary medical care for the insured person and income support during illness. The sickness benefit was intended as a contribution towards the maintenance of the breadwinner and his family while illness prevented his earning. When the Act was introduced it amounted to 10s. per week for men and 7s. 6d. per week for women contributors during the first thirteen weeks of illness and 5s. per week for both for the next thirteen weeks. When sickness benefit ran out, a disability benefit of 5s. per week was payable, which could continue indefinitely. In addition, the plan offered a 30s. lump-sum payment at child-birth for the wife of an insured man, although medical or midwife attendance was not provided. If both husband and wife were contributors the payment was doubled. Finally, there was entitlement to treatment in a TB sanatorium for both the insured and members of his family.

Two entirely dissociated pieces of machinery were created to administer the two types of benefit guaranteed to the insured. The medical services (general practitioner and pharmaceutical services) were provided by local Insurance Committees, composed of local doctors, pharmacists, and representatives of the local authorities and of the insured. All cash benefits, on the other hand, were provided by so-called Approved Societies, either the

Friendly Societies or the national insurance sections of the industrial insurance companies and collecting Friendly Societies.

The scheme of national health insurance that became law in mid-December 1911 bore practically no resemblance to the plan originally conceived by Lloyd George. The reconstruction of his plan was brought about under the powerful and conflicting political pressures exerted by the major social institutions most affected by compulsory health insurance, that is, the Friendly Societies, the industrial insurance companies, and the medical and pharmaceutical professions.

David Lloyd George's original conception of national health insurance grew out of his experience with non-contributory old age pensions which he had piloted through parliament in 1908 soon after he became Chancellor of the Exchequer. Like many other social reformers, he was looking for a way of superseding the Poor Law by a far-reaching programme of unconditional State payments. Such a comprehensive plan could not be supported by taxation alone: to a large extent, it would have to be paid for by the beneficiaries themselves. With this in mind, he travelled, in August 1908, to Germany to look into the widows', orphans', and invalidity pensions established there in 1889 as part of Bismarck's general scheme of compulsory social insurance. He came back full of enthusiasm for the German system and in the autumn of 1908 began the planning of a contributory scheme to provided benefits for workers' sickness and disability and for widows and orphans.[2]

Lloyd George realised, however, that any such scheme would come into competition with the Friendly Society movement, which already offered these benefits. From the start, therefore, he proposed to bring the Friendly Societies into his programme by offering some sort of government subsidy which would extend mutual aid to those sections of the working class which had hitherto been unable to insure for themselves. In the House of Commons on 29 April 1909 he said:

> At the present moment there is a network of powerful organisations in this country, most of them managed with infinite skill and capacity, which have succeeded in inducing millions of workmen in this country to make something like systematic provision for the troubles of life. But in spite of all the ability which has been expended upon them, in spite of the confidence they generally and deservedly inspire, unfortunately there is a margin of people in this country amounting in the aggregate to several millions who either cannot be persuaded or perhaps cannot afford to bear the expense of the systematic contributions which alone make membership effective in these great societies. And the experience of this and of every other country is that no plan or variety of plans short of a universal compulsory system can ever hope to succeed adequately in coping with the problem.

This proposed extension of the power of the State was by no means welcomed by the Friendly Society movement. They regarded self-help as morally and socially preferable to compulsory State provision and believed that State Welfare reforms were devised to enable employers to evade the just demands of the working class for higher wages and regular employment. Welfare reforms were a shoddy substitute for increasing wages, since, with a regressive tax system, the working class paid the cost of such welfare provision through indirect taxes on such items as tea, cocoa, tobacco and alcohol.[3]

Nonetheless, between the autumn of 1908 and the autumn of 1910, Lloyd George negotiated with the National Conference of Friendly Societies a plan involving Friendly Society membership for all the working men the Societies cared to accept and a slightly less advantageous State scheme for their rejects. The two programmes—one State-subsidised, the other entirely State-operated—would be democratically controlled like the Friendly Societies and much of the administration would be handled by the members themselves.

Then, in the middle of these negotiations, probably early in August 1910, the Chancellor of the Exchequer learned that his plans concerned not only the Friendly Societies but the industrial insurance industry as well. Since a widows' and orphans' pension would reduce a wife's financial desperation at the time of her husband's death, it would interfere with the sale of funeral insurance. The industrial assurance companies and the collecting Friendly Societies were organised into a powerful trade association called the "Combine", which forced a major revision of Lloyd George's plans. Widows' and orphans' pensions were dropped and, in compensation, the worker's sickness benefit was raised from 5s. to 10s. a week. Industrial insurance companies and collecting societies were given the right to become, along with the Friendly Societies and the trade unions, approved societies in the administration of the scheme. What had originally been intended as a boost to the Friendly Societies worked in practice overwhelmingly to the advantage of the commercially run insurance companies. Although they were not permitted to make a profit from administering the national insurance scheme itself, their status as approved societies gave them ample opportunity to expand the profitable side of their business. Their collecting agents now had access, in their health insurance capacity, to homes not previously open to them and under conditions which minimized resistance to the private policies they had to sell. Their agents had a dual role as quasi-civil servants administering State-controlled funds and as full-blooded salesmen in a highly profitable and more than dubious business. The vast growth of the life insurance industry in the years between the two world wars owed much to their success in obtaining approved status under the 1911 Act.

In the original version of Lloyd George's national insurance scheme, the Friendly Societies were accorded a privileged position. It was intended that they should become the principal administrators of both the cash benefits and the medical and pharmaceutical services. The industrial insurance industry had no desire to administer any form of medical treatment: nor did it want local management committees clogging up its collecting system. Such local committees were useful only if the doctors and pharmacists did work for the approved societies. In its fight against the Friendly Societies, the Combine found ready allies in the British Medical Association and the Pharmaceutical Society. Neither the doctors nor the pharmacists wanted to work for the Friendly Societies: they did not want the approved societies to administer the medical and pharmaceutical services. It was not difficult, then, to form a temporary alliance between the Combine, the British Medical Association and the Pharmaceutical Society to extract concessions from the government at the expense of the Friendly Societies.

The medical profession had long resented the dominance of the medical consumer. From the late eighteenth century doctors had sought to gain control over the demanding and independently-minded patient by curtailing the practice of self-medication and the prescribing of chemists and druggists. In the late nineteenth century the doctors' quest for medical autonomy found new opposition with the rise of the Friendly Societies. Friendly

328

Society practice was contract practice: the doctor was an employee of the Society and under its control. He had to treat any patient the Society chose to send him; he felt that he was poorly paid and under-resourced. The British Medical Association particularly resented the fact that "medical gentlemen" could be hired, fired and disciplined by committees of labouring men. To attract members, the Friendly Societies offered medical treatment at bargain prices. The B.M.A. believed that a large proportion of those members were well able to afford private medical fees. But it was a good deal more difficult to recruit Friendly Society members than it was to replace an unsatisfactory or unsympathetic doctor. An overstocked profession was in no position to impose its terms on the Friendly Societies. The famous "Battle of the Clubs", fought during the years 1903 to 1905, was an attempt by the B.M.A. to gain control of Friendly Society medical practice. Although it failed in this aim, it did much to solidify doctors' opinions against the Societies and helped to determine their attitude towards Lloyd George's scheme of health insurance.

Lloyd George gave details of his proposals to the House of Commons on 4 May 1911. Not only were the Friendly Societies to administer the medical services without any form of medical representation, but despite their reputation for "sweating" their doctors, they were to work out their own system of remuneration and dictate other conditions of service to medical practitioners. The medical reaction was immediate and hostile. The doctors' hatred of the Friendly Societies was not concealed. The B.M.A. insisted that the administration of medical benefits should be undertaken, not by the approved societies, but by the governmental local health committees. The B.M.A. was rightly far more suspicious of working class than of government control. The Friendly Societies were far less likely to permit medical control over their affairs than a public authority and far more likely to administer medical services with an eye to economy rather than professional standards.[4]

Only two weeks after the first printed text of the National Insurance bill became available, the British Medical Association held a special representative meeting which passed unanimously the "Six Cardinal Points" which were the minimum conditions under which doctors would agree to serve under the scheme. The six points were:

(1) Medical and maternity benefits to be administered by the local health (later "insurance") committees, not the Friendly Societies.

(2) The method of payment in the area of each insurance committee to be decided by the local medical profession, and all question of medical discipline to be settled by medical committees composed entirely of doctors.

(3) Payment should be "adequate". This was later defined as a capitation fee of 8s. 6d. per patient, per year, excluding the cost of medicines. (The government calculations had assumed the doctor would be paid 4s. per year for each insured person).

(4) An income limit of £2 a week for the insured. No one earning more should be permitted to receive medical benefit without extra payment to the doctor.

(5) Free choice of doctor by the patient, subject to the doctor consenting to act.

(6) The medical profession to have adequate representation upon the various administrative bodies of national health insurance.

Simultaneously with the action of the British Medical Association, the Pharmaceutical Society took steps to promote the interests of chemists and druggists. To some extent the interests of medicine and pharmacy were parallel and to that extent joint action was taken. But in certain areas the interests of general practitioners and pharmacists diverged and the

329

Pharmaceutical Society needed to remain alert to stop the British Medical Association obtaining concessions from the government at the chemists' expense.

The Friendly Societies were quickly identified as a common enemy: neither the doctors nor the pharmacists wanted to see the medical and pharmaceutical services under Friendly Society control. When Lloyd George introduced his bill in May 1911 he announced that the Friendly Societies were to arrange with chemists for the supply of medicines and appliances under the scheme. He added that he had no doubt they would make as advantageous terms with the chemists as they had in the past made with the medical profession. Immediately afterwards a spokesman for the Friendly Societies indicated that they would not necessarily use the chemists but would instead establish their own dispensaries in all the large towns. The Manchester Unity of Odd Fellows proposed the setting up of a central drug store and branch dispensaries to be controlled and administered by themselves. Soon the Friendly Societies began to canvass the possibility of setting up a factory for the preparation of galenicals, drugs, chemicals and sick-room requisites, which would then be distributed to depots throughout the country.

The Pharmaceutical Society was quick to point out that these new projects would come under the jurisdiction of neither the Pharmacy Acts nor the Food and Drugs Act. They would, moreover, deprive qualified chemists of some fourteen million customers a year. "The effect on pharmacists would be disastrous", declared the *Pharmaceutical Journal*, and argued that, instead of creating new establishments, the existing network of chemists' shops should be used. Yet even if the Friendly Societies did not adopt these radical solutions, any participation of the pharmacist in the national insurance scheme would be subject to negotiation with them. This was not an inviting prospect. "Chemists and druggists do not want to bargain with friendly societies", said the *Pharmaceutical Journal*, "if there is any bargaining to be done, it should be done with the Government". "Do we desire to be under the thumb of the friendly societies?" asked G.T.W. Newsholme, a past president of the Pharmaceutical Society. "See what the friendly societies have done for the medical profession", was his answer.[5]

As soon as Lloyd George's bill was published the Council of the Pharmaceutical Society set up a committee to consider its likely effect on the activities of chemists and druggists. W.S. Glyn-Jones was the key member. He had been appointed parliamentary secretary to the Society in 1908 and had played a crucial part in securing the Poisons and Pharmacy Act of that year. In the general election of December 1910, after a campaign which was a masterpiece of strategy and organisation, he won the Stepney seat for the Liberal Party after years of Conservative domination. He soon made his mark in the House of Commons which always listened to him with respect. The thorough mastery he showed of all the details of the National Insurance bill gained for him the ear of the House and the respect of the Chancellor of the Exchequer. By 1911 Glyn-Jones had built up such a formidable array of connexions and such a store of first-hand knowledge of all aspects of the trade that his leadership of the world of pharmacy during the crisis of 1911 was both authoritative and unchallenged. By establishing the Proprietary Articles Trade Association he had achieved success in a task which at the outset had seemed doomed to early collapse. By sheer perseverance he gained the support and admiration of manufacturers, wholesalers, independent and company chemists. He followed this by creating the highly effective Chemists' Defence Association and won the gratitude of all retailers. In 1904, after eating the required number of dinners at the Middle Temple, he was called to the Bar and five years later published the standard text on the law relating to poisons and pharmacy. He had served on the Council of the Pharmaceutical Society and had won the respect of Jesse Boot, the strong-willed founder of the Drug Companies' (later the Company Chemists') Association. By 1911 William Samuel Glyn-Jones embodied the unity of the British pharmaceutical trade.

On 1 June 1911 a strong deputation of pharmacists organised by the Council of the Pharmaceutical Society was received by the Chancellor of the Exchequer in his rooms at the House of Commons. The deputation, introduced by William Glyn-Jones, was representative of the whole of the drug trade. It included J.F. Harrington, the president of the Pharmaceutical Society and the immediate past president, J. Rymer Young; two members of Council, C.B. Allen and Edmund White; Richard Bremridge, the secretary, and A.J. Chater and J.R. Hill, assistant secretaries; two representatives of the Pharmaceutical Society of Ireland; a representative of the Drug Companies' Association and one from the Chemists' Defence Association; and the editors of the *Chemist and Druggist*, the *British and Colonial Druggist*, and the *Pharmaceutical Journal*. The most impressive feature of the delegation was the unprecedented unity of all sections of the legitimate trade. This unity, of course, did not just emerge: it was realised by the diplomacy and tireless energy of William Glyn-Jones.

J. Rymer Young began by outlining to the Chancellor the views which had been expressed by chemists and druggists up and down the land. Then Glyn-Jones took over and detailed the seven principles which pharmacists wanted incorporated in the National Insurance bill. They were:

(1) that no agreement for the supply of medicines for insured persons should be made except with a person, firm or corporate body entitled to carry on the statutory business of a pharmaceutical chemist or chemist and druggist in conformity with the 1908 Act.

(2) that the dispensing under the Act should be done under the direct supervision of a pharmacist.

(3) that the control of medical and pharmaceutical services to insured persons should be in the hands of the County Health (later "Insurance") Committees and not under the control of Friendly Societies.

(4) that a panel of all qualified pharmacists in a particular district willing to supply medicines under the scheme should be set up, so that insured persons could choose their own suppliers.

(5) that remuneration for pharmacists should be on a scale system and not on a per capita basis.

(6) that pharmacy should be represented on the County Health Committees, the Advisory Committees, and the Insurance Commission.

(7) that medical benefit should not be extended to persons earning more than £160 per annum.

In response, Lloyd George said that in his opinion his bill would greatly improve the position of pharmacists, but he promised to consider carefully the representations made to him. He strongly approved of the mission to Europe undertaken by Professor Henry Greenish and Glyn-Jones to obtain first-hand information about the supply of medicines to State-insured persons in Germany, Austria and Italy. Finally, referring to Glyn-Jones, he "expressed the conviction—derived from personal experience of his pertinacity—that with such a parliamentary representative, the pharmacists of the country might feel assured that their interests would be quite efficiently safeguarded".[6]

The seven principles listed by Glyn-Jones were the Pharmaceutical Society's basic desiderata with regard to compulsory health insurance. The Society believed that insured persons should be supplied with medicines in exactly the same way as the rest of the public by using the facilities already provided by private enterprise. In this way the sick would be able to obtain their medicine promptly and with the minimum of inconvenience.

> The overwhelming majority of the insured will find a pharmacy, managed by a qualified chemist, at their door, and under the scheme, it should be and can be made possible for the insured sick to get the prescriptions given them by the doctor dispensed there.

Since medical treatment under the scheme was to be given only by duly qualified medical practitioners, so medicines supplied to the insured should be dispensed only by legally qualified chemists. Moreover, since doctors were insisting on the establishment of a panel system with free choice of practitioner by the insured, so pharmacists wanted the same system and for the same reasons. Neither profession wanted laymen, whether from Friendly Societies or on Insurance Committees, to appoint and dismiss medical officers and pharmacists. Nor did they want to see a system in which a few selected practitioners reaped all the rewards from the insurance scheme: such an arrangement would be both invidious and divisive for the professions. G.T.W. Newsholme made the point well:

> We want recognition for ourselves as pharmacists. We do not want to be limited by the Government or the friendly societies to a certain number of chemists; we want every chemist to be recognised as a dispenser of medicines and we must try and see that under the Bill every chemist in the country will have the privilege of dispensing whatever medicine is required and be paid for so doing by the State. There must be no limitation of numbers and no selection of certain chemists.

The pharmacists' demands closely paralleled those of the doctors. Both professions wanted to be involved in policy making at all levels of the service. They put forward the view that their advice and co-operation would be needed to ensure that the system worked fairly, efficiently, and smoothly: that the suppliers of services should be represented on all administrative and decision taking bodies.

One of the medical profession's principal demands was that there should be a solid and very low income limit above which contributors could not claim medical benefit. The British Medical Association wanted a limit of only £104 a year: the Pharmaceutical Society was quite happy to go along with Lloyd George's suggestion of £160, the starting point for income tax. The medical profession was keen to gain by compulsion patients who had previously been unable or unwilling to pay its fees but was anxious to preserve the full extent of private medical practice. This was much less of a problem for the retail chemist. The poor had always gone to the chemist's shop and would continue to do so, unless forcibly diverted by the Friendly Societies or the doctors. "My experience is that a good many of them did go to chemists' shops in times past", said Glyn-Jones in 1913, "but they will go into chemists' shops in future in a different capacity. They will go as the bearers of prescriptions. They used to go before for the old-fashioned remedies of general drugs, sometimes with and sometimes without the advice of the chemist".[7] For the qualified chemist, the main effect of the national insurance scheme would be to attract customers to his shop from the drug stores run by the unqualified.

Both the medical and pharmaceutical professions were opposed to a full-time State salaried service but they differed on the way they wanted to be paid. The doctors wanted to be paid an annual sum for each registered patient: the pharmacists wanted an item-of-service system of payment. The medical profession argued that a per capita system of remuneration would encourage the doctor to practise preventive medicine by making use of early diagnosis and treatment. The chemists, on the other hand, pointed out that no one could say in advance what medicines and appliances would be required and a per capita system of payment would lead either to imposing upon the chemist or to depriving the insured of what was necessary for their effective treatment. Henry Greenish and Glyn-Jones discovered that in all European countries payment for medicines supplied to State-insured persons was on a tariff or scale basis. Moreover, a per capita system of payment for the chemist would have entailed a system of patient registration. The insured person would have lost his freedom to take the doctor's prescription on each occasion to whichever chemist suited him. In arguing for an item-of-service system of payment, the Pharmaceutical Society made the assumption that the insurance fund would be adequate to meet the total cost of medicines and appliances prescribed. But a cash limit of 2s. per insured person was imposed on the cost of pharmaceutical services; and the retail chemist was left with the burden of picking up the bill after the doctor had freely prescribed.

On 1 August 1911 the House of Commons sitting in Committee of the Whole House voted 387 to 15 to deprive the approved societies of supervision of insurance medical and pharmaceutical practice and to vest it in the local health committees. The pharmacists, as Glyn-Jones pointed out in the debate, "were at one with the doctors in asking that the control of the medical benefits should be transferred to the local Health Committee".[8] But although pharmacists were glad to have the threat of Friendly Society control removed, they were not yet out of the wood. There was still the danger that the British Medical Association would persuade Lloyd George to reverse his initial decision to separate prescribing and dispensing.

"The first thing which I think should be done", Lloyd George said in May 1911, "is to separate the drugs from the doctors". He had "provided in the Bill that, in future, all the drugs should be dispensed by somebody else rather than by the doctor".

> It should be for the chemist to dispense . . . there should be a compulsory separation of the two . . . [in remote areas] the doctor would have to do both the doctoring and the supplying of the drugs he prescribes . . . if there is no chemist available, the doctor should be allowed to go on as at the present moment, but
> · wherever there is a chemist available, there should be a separation.

He had, he explained, special reasons for that. "There ought to be no inducement for underpaid doctors to take it out in drugs". The Government "wanted to be quite sure when the doctor prescribed a certain medicine that that medicine would be provided for the patient, so they were going to separate the doctors and the drugs".[9]

The experience of both the Poor Law and the Friendly Societies was that whenever doctors received an inclusive fee for attendance and medicines, the temptation to use cheap drugs was not easily resisted. Glyn-Jones told the House of Commons that he had spent twelve years dispensing in a doctor's service. He knew from practical experience how dreadful the club-practice system was and how disgraceful the treatment of the poor was in dispensaries in all the large towns. The conditions were such that effective treatment was impossible. The *Pharmaceutical Journal* reported that "a vast number of doctors do use the cheapest drugs it is possible to buy . . . their selection of drugs is woefully insufficient . . . and . . . sometimes the manner of mixing them is an abomination".[10]

In public Lloyd George emphasized the benefits to the patient of separating dispensing from prescribing and spoke as if cost was not a consideration. He told the House of Commons:

> You are separating the drugs from the medical attendance and that in itself will increase the charge . . . In many cases drugs of the most expensive character were not supplied when they might have been. In future they will be. There will be no inducement to any man not to prescribe them. That will increase the cost very considerably, and the experience of Germany is that it will do so very rapidly.[11]

Yet the cost to the taxpayer was uppermost in the Chancellor's mind when he decided to separate prescribing and dispensing. Paying doctors to supply the medicines they recommended would encourage excessive prescribing: anyone who had received an apothecary's bill knew that. When the national insurance scheme was established, doctors were given a financial incentive to prescribe economically. In October 1912 it was decided that the total sum for medical benefits should be 9s. per insured person, of which only 1s. 6d. was to be allotted for the payment of drugs and a further 6d. (later known as "the floating sixpence") should be available for paying chemists if the drug bill exceeded 1s. 6d. per insured person. If, however, such allocation was unnecessary that sum would be credited to the doctors' accounts. This extraordinary arrangement meant that doctors could increase their incomes by denying their patients expensive drugs, while chemists would be denied full payment if doctors prescribed excessively.

The Pharmaceutical Society welcomed the statutory establishment of the principle of separating the prescribing from the dispensing of medicines. This was also supported by a joint committee of the British Pharmaceutical Conference and the British Medical Association, and by the General Medical Council. The Society of Apothecaries, however, had a very different opinion. In whatever shape or form the national insurance bill is finally passed, they declared, it must profoundly and, it is feared, prejudicially affect the future of the medical profession in this country. The right of dispensing his own medicines has always been "the inalienable right of the holder of the Medical Diploma granted by the Society". "It is a great injustice that these and other medical practitioners who have been in the habit of making up their own medicines should be deprived of this privilege".[12]

On this occasion, the Society of Apothecaries spoke for the rank and file of the medical profession. Most general practitioners provided attendance and medicine for an inclusive fee. They argued that they had gained the confidence of their patients not only in their skill in diagnosis but also in the rightness of the medicines they supplied. It was an unnecessary inconvenience for patients to be sent to a chemist for medicine which they would rather obtain direct from the doctor.

With pressure from the grass roots, the British Medical Association soon adopted the same stance. It argued that the patient should be free to make special arrangements with his doctor to supply him with medicines where the doctor had, before the passing of the Act, been in the habit of so doing; and that under such circumstances the doctor had the right to claim remuneration for the cost of the medicines and for dispensing them. In August 1911 Dr. Christopher Addison M.P. proposed an amendment to the National Insurance bill, on behalf of the B.M.A., to give effect to this policy, but the move was not successful. In March 1912 the B.M.A. revived the same proposal in negotiations with the Insurance Commissioners. The *British Medical Journal* claimed that:

> The profession had no desire to interfere with any established right of pharmacists but it will strongly resent any attempt by pharmacists to usurp what is the undoubted right of medical men to dispense their own medicines, when they think proper, for their own patients.[13]

This was one of the few battles that the British Medical Association lost. Although local insurance committees were permitted to make special arrangements for doctors to dispense in rural areas where no chemist was available for some miles, a clause was inserted in the Act stating that:

> no arrangement shall be made by the Insurance Committee with a medical practitioner under which he is bound or agrees to supply drugs or medicine to any insured person.

Although prescribing and dispensing were to be separated, it was still necessary for the Pharmaceutical Society to ensure that only qualified chemists were given the right to dispense medicines under the Act. There was still a residual fear that local health committees might establish "a species of communal trading in drugs and medicines subsidised by public money" on the lines originally proposed by the Friendly Societies. A slightly more serious threat was posed by the Incorporated Society of Pharmacy and Drug-Store Proprietors of Great Britain, the organisation of the unqualified drug sellers. When the Pharmaceutical Society prepared a pamphlet, "The Case for Pharmacists", and circulated it to all M.P.s, the Incorporated Society responded by issuing M.P.s with a broadsheet entitled, "The Case against the Pharmacists or Registered Chemists". The unqualified chemists argued that the supply of registered pharmacists was inadequate to meet public demand; that registered practitioners lacked practical training and were a danger to the public; that it would be unjust to crush out of existence established but unregistered men who were already serving the public well; and that establishing a further monopoly was contrary to British traditions. Whatever the strength of the Drug-Store proprietors' arguments, their proposals were unrealistic. They suggested that insured persons should be required to pay for the dispensing of their prescriptions and the supply of medical and surgical requisites but that they should be free to purchase such services from whomsoever they wished. Competition, it was believed, would keep prices down.[14]

The Pharmaceutical Society and the Company Chemists' Association came together to ward off the threat from the Incorporated Society. Jesse Boot and William Glyn-Jones together devised an amendment to Section 14 of the National Insurance bill designed to give the independent proprietor pharmacist and the company chemist an equal right to contract with the health committees to supply pharmaceutical services under the Act. "If the present crisis had arisen prior to the 1908 Poisons and Pharmacy Act", Glyn-Jones observed, "he

335

did not know where pharmacists would have been, because they would never have got the agreement they now had". The settlement of the companies issue, which Glyn-Jones had helped to secure in the 1908 Act, made possible the joint action of the Pharmaceutical Society and the Company Chemists' Association.

When the Incorporated Society of Pharmacy and Drug-Store Proprietors presented their case to M.P.s, Jesse Boot, in his capacity as chairman of the Company Chemists' Association, published a statement in support of Glyn-Jones' amendment:

> Section 14 makes "provision for the supply of proper and sufficient drugs and medicines to insured persons."
>
> An amendment supplementary to this is proposed by Mr. Glyn-Jones, M.P. (Stepney), to the effect that this provision shall be made with "persons, firms, or corporate bodies lawfully entitled to carry on the business of a Pharmaceutical Chemist or Chemist and Druggist."
>
> The interests of such corporate bodies or companies entitled to carry on the business of a chemist and druggist are represented by this Association, which is fully in accord with the amendments to the Bill proposed by Mr. Glyn-Jones, on behalf of the Pharmaceutical Society and the aforesaid companies jointly.
>
> This amendment will ensure that only persons qualified to do so shall dispense medicines to insured persons under the Act, and will also ensure that all who are lawfully entitled to carry on the business of chemists shall be allowed an equal opportunity of doing so.
>
> There is no monopoly in this, as now, and in the future all qualified persons and all corporate bodies employing qualified persons will without limit be able and entitled to commence at any time to dispense medicines to insured persons under the conditions laid down in the Act.[15]

Glyn-Jones was successful in securing his amendment but was, nonetheless, forced to yield a little. Attempts were made to get Army dispensers, apothecary's assistants, and dispensers to medical practitioners and public institutions recognised as qualified to dispense national insurance medicines. Glyn-Jones rightly objected to his opponents' tactic of using the National Insurance bill as a way of creating new pharmaceutical qualifications, but conceded that dispensers with at least three years experience should be recognised. He was also forced to give an assurance that the Pharmaceutical Society would, in due course, promote, in consultation with the General Medical Council, the Society of Apothecaries, and the War Office, a bill dealing with the qualifications of dispensers.[16] In its final form, the fourteenth section of the National Insurance Act read as follows:

> ... the regulations shall prohibit arrangements for the dispensing of medicines being made with persons other than persons, firms, or bodies corporate, entitled to carry on the business of a chemist and druggist under the provisions of the Pharmacy Act, 1868, as amended by the Poisons and Pharmacy Act, 1908, who undertake that all medicines supplied by them to insured persons shall be dispensed either by, or under the direct supervision of, a registered pharmacist, or by a person who, for three years immediately prior to the passing of this Act, has acted as a dispenser to a duly qualified medical practitioner or a public institution.

It is sometimes argued that the Pharmaceutical Society was misguided in agreeing to allow corporate bodies to contract with insurance committees to supply professional services. The

Society, it is held, should have insisted that a clear distinction be drawn between the ownership of a pharmacy and participation in the national insurance contract by an employed pharmacist. The contract, it is said, should have been with the pharmacist and not with the employer. This criticism of the Society is historically ill-founded. In 1911 the Society needed all the support it could muster. The Glyn-Jones amendment got the muscle of the Company Chemists' Association on its side. The only issue of principle at the time was whether the Pharmaceutical Society should have encouraged unqualified employers (such as Jesse Boot and other company chemists) to make contracts with the State to have medicines dispensed by qualified chemists in their employ. No one at the time imagined that the contract should be made only with the person who would actually perform the professional services. It was not at all unusual for panel doctors to leave their insured patients to be treated by their assistants while they looked after the private patients. Similarly the independent pharmacist proprietor might employ managers and assistants in the running of his business. In any event, the national insurance contract was not simply a contract for the supply of professional services but also one for the provision of commercial resources. The contractor had to meet the capital cost and recurrent expenses of the premises (surgery or pharmacy), means of transport, and of necessary equipment and stock. Since the 1908 Poisons and Pharmacy Act had already established that companies of unqualified persons employing registered superintendents and qualified assistants could legally carry on the business of a chemist and druggist; it would have been absurd and self-defeating for the Pharmaceutical Society to attempt to deny them the right to make contracts with the insurance committees to supply medicines to the insured.

It would be wrong to give the impression that William Glyn-Jones was alone responsible for securing such a favourable outcome for the pharmacist in the struggle over the National Insurance Act of 1911. It was essential from the outset that the active support of every chemist and druggist in the land should be mobilised behind the policies of the Pharmaceutical Society. At this time the Statutory register contained the names of nearly 16,500 pharmacists but less than half were members of the Society. Nonetheless, the Council gave a firm lead to everyone on the register and tried to enlist their support for the "seven principles". The Fifeshire Pharmaceutical Association was one of the first to realise the importance of the situation and to institute an active campaign in support of the Council's policies. Since the passing of the Pharmacy Act Amendment Act of 1898 there had been an increasing interchange of ideas and co-operation between the Council and the local associations of chemists throughout the country. These bonds were strengthened during the passage of the 1908 Act, but the National Insurance bill led to many new associations being formed and to the appointment of W.J. Uglow Woolcock, later Secretary of the Society, as Local Associations Officer. In addition there was in each parliamentary constituency, a divisional secretary of the Society who had the duty of communicating with his M.P. on matters affecting pharmacy. During the summer of 1911 the local associations sprang into activity: well attended meetings were addressed by members of Council and resolutions in support of Council policy were adopted. Local M.P.s were canvassed for their support of the amendments to the bill proposed by Glyn-Jones.

On 6 July 1911 the Pharmaceutical Society organised a mass meeting of pharmacists in the King's Hall of the Holborn Restaurant. Long before the meeting was due to start the 600 seats in the Hall were taken: over 1,000 pharmacists from all parts of Britain eventually crowded in. Contingents arrived from Birmingham, Dewsbury, Leeds, Liverpool, Manchester, Nottingham and Sheffield in England and from Aberdeen, Edinburgh and Glasgow in Scotland. London and the Home Counties were well represented. The *Pharmaceutical Journal* reported that it was the largest gathering of chemists ever held. The new president, Charles Allen was in the chair; representatives of all the leading pharmaceutical organisations in Britain attended; on the platform sat three pharmacists with recent parliamentary experience, T.H.W. Idris, the former Liberal M.P. for Flint, Richard Winfrey, Liberal M.P. for South-West Norfolk, and William Glyn-Jones. Support was given to this meeting in every way; those who were unable to be present expressed their solidarity by sending post-cards and greetings to the meeting. In their speeches both Glyn-Jones and Winfrey urged pharmacists to write to their M.P.s in support of the "seven principles". The government, pointed out Glyn-Jones, had already stated that doctors were to leave the dispensing (except in rural areas) to chemists: if, in addition, the seven principles were secured, "it would enormously enhance their position in the country". Richard Winfrey also saw the bill as "a great step forward". "He was convinced the chemists of the country were going to gain materially by the Bill".[17]

The National Insurance bill held the attention of parliament from the beginning of May until the middle of December 1911.[18] At first, Lloyd George seems to have hoped that the bill would be passed in a few weeks. When, at the beginning of June, he realised that a detailed discussion of the clauses was unavoidable he clung to the hope that the bill might pass through all its stages before the end of August. But on 18 August, out of the 87 clauses of which the bill consisted in its original form, only 17 had been carried and those not without serious amendment. An extraordinary session in the autumn became necessary. In the meanwhile the Chancellor undertook laborious negotiations with all the vested interests involved. On 21 October parliament reassembled. The Government announced that 19 sittings would be sufficient to finish the dicussion of the bill. In the end two additional sittings were needed, 21 in all. The bill was divided into a fixed number of "compartments" and when the time allotted to the discussion of a particular compartment had been used up, all the clauses which the Commons had not had time to debate, would be passed automatically. The closure prevented the inclusion of many of the amendments which Glyn-Jones wanted to move: he used every opportunity, however, for urging the inclusion of pharmacists on the various representative bodies set up by the bill. In its final form the bill comprised 115 clauses with additional schedules. When it was before the House of Lords further amendments were moved by Lord Weardale on behalf of the Pharmaceutical Society urging the inclusion of pharmacists on the Advisory and Insurance committees. The National Insurance bill passed its third reading in the Commons on 6 December and received the Royal Assent on 16 December 1911.

The Act set up a small body of Insurance Commissioners furnished with administrative, judicial, and legislative powers. The new service of health insurance became an independent branch of administration. The names of the first Commissioners were announced in the Commons on 28 November. Sir Robert Morant, an energetic and politically astute civil servant, was moved from the Board of Education to head the new body. The Commission was made responsible for the administration of health insurance and empowered to issue regulations and to judge, in most cases without right of appeal, infractions of the law. The Act set up, subject to the Commissioners, Insurance committees, on which pharmacists were represented, in every county and county borough to administer the medical and pharmaceutical service. The first National Advisory Committee on Insurance was also established and of the 159 members, two were pharmacists, W.J. Uglow Woolcock and J.P. Gilmour, later editor of the *Pharmaceutical Journal*. Another pharmacist, P.F. Rowsell, was appointed chairman of the National Pharmaceutical Committee, which undertook the difficult task of preparing the first Drug Tariff showing the rates at which chemists would undertake dispensing.

The National Insurance Act became law on 15 July 1912 but the provisions relating to medical benefit were postponed a further six months and the first prescriptions did not reach the chemists' shops until 15 January 1913. The bill had left many details unsettled including the question of doctors' remuneration. Negotiations between the Government and the B.M.A. on this question proceeded during 1912. The Government had originally offered 4s. 6d. per annum as a basic capitation fee: by December 1912 the offer had been increased to 7s. 6d. per head. The extent of this concession is all the more remarkable in the light of the report made by Sir William Plender during the negotiations. With the agreement of the B.M.A., he examined the books of medical men in five representative towns, and found that the average annual cost of visits, consultations, and drugs for all classes of the population amounted to only 4s. 2d.[19] Nevertheless, the Representative Body of the B.M.A. decided on 21 December to hold out for 8s. 6d. and to call upon the 26,000 doctors, who had signed an undertaking not to accept service under the Act except under conditions approved by the B.M.A., to boycott the system. But the Government refused to budge and by 10 January 1913 over 15,000 doctors had intimated their willingness to serve on the Government's terms. Faced with this large-scale desertion of its members to the panels, the B.M.A. was forced to release from their commitment those doctors who were still in favour of the boycott.

It was afterwards said that "the trouble with the B.M.A. is that it doesn't know when it has won".[20] The majority of its members, however, could recognise a good bargain when they saw it. Throughout the Government's negotiations with the B.M.A. leaders, Lloyd George realised that their public pronouncements did not represent the consensus of the profession. Privately, he professed a low opinion of medical deputations:

> . . . it is difficult to ascertain the true feelings of doctors as a whole on any proposal affecting them, since a Deputation of Doctors is always a Deputation of swell Doctors: it is impossible to get a Deputation of poor Doctors or of slum Doctors.

In the winter of 1912, the poor doctors of Britain realised that a capitation fee of 7s. 6d. was an offer they could not refuse. The increased cost of the medical service meant that the worker's weekly contribution to the insurance fund had to be raised to 7d. for men and 6d. for women. The 1911 Act entailed a considerable transfer of income from manual workers to the medical profession by means of a regressive poll-tax, the flat-rate national insurance contribution. Although the financial arrangements for chemists were by no means as advantageous as those offered to medical practitioners, British pharmacists did not hesitate to serve under the Act. Chemists were much more accustomed to standing on their own feet than medical men and much less dependent on financial support from the State and philanthropy. It was felt that the national insurance scheme might help the chemist in working class areas by providing him with a useful supplement to his income and an opportunity to practise his dispensing skills: but no pharmacist was going to make a fortune from a drug fund with a cash limit of 2s. per head.

On 15 January 1913 dispensing began: the *Pharmaceutical Journal* recorded that the first insurance prescription was dispensed at 8.40 a.m. on the first day.[21] The influx of prescriptions varied according to the social class composition of the area. In West London one business obtained only £25 11s. 1d. and another £190 16s. 1d. for the first years's work, representing 0.98 and 7.83 per cent., respectively, of total turnover. In Rotherhithe and Canning Town, however, two businesses showed £616 9s. 8d. and £511 14s. 1d., amounting to 58.11 and 44 per cent. of total turnover. Pharmacies which had previously dispensed only one or two prescriptions were receiving several hundred a week in the densely populated working class areas.

The pharmacist who began dispensing prescriptions in January 1913 faced many problems spared his modern counterpart. He had to price his own prescriptions. Contractors had to be on the panel of each area for which they dispensed prescriptions so that pharmacies in central London were on the lists of numerous insurance committees. Copies of many prescriptions had to be entered in the prescription book to satisfy the poisons legislation. Dispensing was truly extemporaneous as there were no formularies. The Middlesex County Chemists' Association advocated the use of the formulae in the *British Pharmaceutical Codex* and in Yorkshire, the "Doncaster Pharmacopoeia", consisting of 21 mixtures, became the forerunner of many local formularies. The direct profit arising from insurance dispensing was at the start negligible because the basis of remuneration was unsound. The Tariff had been fixed for the country as a whole but there was no substantive basis for the agreed maximum of 2s. per head per year. The authorities had worked on the experience of the Friendly Societies in supplying medicines. The charge for dispensing was the cost price of the drugs contained in the prescription plus 50 per cent. plus a fixed scale of dispensing fees. The dispensing fee for 8 fluid ounce mixtures was 2d. and those formed more than 50 per cent. of the average dispensing. The highest fee was 6d. for an extemporaneously dispensed plaster. There was no dispensing fee for many simple drugs, solids, pills, capsules, powders, tablets, ointments and plasters included in the Tariff. The initial contract was for three months and payments were not made until the end of that period. For that first quarter the number of insured persons was not known and local committees did not receive enough money for distribution and hardship was caused to many contractors. W. J. Uglow Woolcock had warned Lloyd George that the sum of 2s. per head would be "possibly inadequate", and the prospect of discounting was foreseen: even before they agreed to be on the lists, chemists realised the danger that they might not be paid in full. Pharmacists would have been satisfied with the Tariff if they had been able to get their money, but when the accounts came to be paid it was found that the total cash available was insufficient. A system of discounting the whole of the accounts was therefore adopted which inevitably generated widespread dissatisfaction.

The participation of pharmacists in the National Health Insurance scheme led to intense activity within the Pharmaceutical Society and considerable reorganisation. More meetings of local associations were held than at any earlier period. The zenith of this activity was reached on 7 May 1913 when a conference comprising two representatives from each local assocation was held in London: this was the precursor of the modern Branch Representatives' meeting. In an attempt to help the chemist contractors in their negotiations with the Insurance Commissioners, the Pharmaceutical Society encouraged under its auspices a Local Associations Executive, which in 1915 secured the appointment of a Departmental Committee to examine the question of chemists' remuneration.[22] The result was a new tariff of dispensing fees and charges, introduced in 1916.

The National Health Insurance scheme was important to retail pharmacy in two ways: first, in the recognition it gave to the principle that dispensing should be limited to pharmacists, and, second, in the volume of business which it brought to pharmacy. In the first thirteen years of the service, medical benefit was provided for 15 million persons each year at a cost of nine and a quarter million pounds. Of this more than seven and a quarter million pounds went to the doctors and the rest was allocated to medicines, appliances and dispensing fees. Some 50 million prescriptions were issued each year by 15,000 doctors and dispensed by over 10,000 chemist contractors. In 1937 the P.E.P. report on *The British Health Services* estimated that, under the National Health Insurance scheme, eleven million pounds went on doctors' fees and three million on pharmacuetical services. By that date the number of shops where the proprietor was under contract with insurance committees to supply medicines was about 13,000 in England and Wales and about 1,800 in Scotland. Practically all chemists' shops were in the scheme. The average number of prescriptions per shop in 1937 was about 5,000 in England and Wales and 1,800 in Scotland. The total average payment per shop was £175 for England and Wales and £98 for Scotland.

By the 1930s insurance committees in England and Wales were grouped into 15 areas each with a pricing bureau for prescriptions. The "floating sixpence" was abandoned in January 1920 and the practice of discounting the amount payable to chemists, according to the state of the insurance fund, was discontinued after 1926. By 1937 chemist contractors were paid on the basis of the cost of the ingredients calculated according to a standard price list and a dispensing fee regulated according to the nature of the article dispensed: the average figures for 1937 being 3.96d. for ingredients and 4.35d. for the fee. In Scotland the chemist was paid in addition a profit on the cost of materials, the average figures for 1937 being 5.67d. for ingredients, 2.83d. for profit, and 5.23d. for the fee.

The statutory restriction to pharmacists of dispensing under the N.H.I. scheme did not bring to an end dispensing by doctors. The bulk of private dispensing in England and Wales continued to be carried out by doctors or by their assistants who were rarely pharmacists. "It is part of the law that insured persons shall have their medicines prescribed by doctors and dispensed by registered pharmacists", Lord Dawson of Penn reminded the House of Lords in 1931. "That is a very proper provision", he continued, "but, by some curious anomaly, if you are a non-insured person no such protection is given". Neither medical men nor the majority of their assistants could claim to have enough knowledge and training to undertake dispensing. Many doctors employed assistants holding the dispensers' certificate of the Society of Apothecaries. In 1926 the Royal Commission on National Health Insurance refused to recognise the holders of this qualification as fit to dispense medicines to panel patients. "The evidence given before us", stated the Report, "has left no doubt in our minds that the qualification of the holders of the Apothecaries' Assistants' Certificates is inferior to that of a registered pharmacist".[23] Even the doctor's training in pharmacy and dispensing was very rudimentary. These subjects were not treated seriously in the medical curriculum and their testing was neither rigorous nor practical. Moreover, the overcrowding of the medical curriculum meant that the doctor's education in materia medica and prescribing was seriously deficient. While the range and complexity of drugs and medicines were increasing, the knowledge obtained of these matters in medical school was declining. Thus the supply of medicines to private patients in England and Wales was carried out in a less professional manner than that to insured persons. When a doctor dispenses there is no independent check on his prescribing as a safeguard against error. In the interests of efficient prescribing, to say nothing of the safety of the patient, every prescription ought to pass through the hands of a pharmacist so that the doctor can be advised should the prescription appear to be unsatisfactory.

Although general practitioners in England and Wales secured a more than generous settlement in the setting up of the N.H.I. system, they continued to cling tenaciously to their right to act as apothecaries and dispense medicines to their private patients. Indeed the only way in which the principle of separating prescribing and dispensing could be established in this country was by the extension of public provision for medical care. It is not surprising, therefore, to find the Pharmaceutical Society an enthusiastic supporter of proposals to extend the N.H.I. scheme to the dependants of insured persons and to persons with higher incomes than those covered by the original scheme. National Insurance was, in fact, never extended to cover dependants but the income limit was progressively raised, partly because of inflation, from £160 to £250 in 1920 and to £420 in 1942. By 1938 over twenty million workers (43 per cent of the population) were covered by the system: by 1946 the number had risen to twenty-four million, roughly half the British population. In 1946 the average pharmacy in England dispensed a total of 9,652 prescriptions, of which 7,433 or 77 per cent were N.H.I. prescriptions. Only about 20 per cent of doctors in England and Wales sent their prescriptions for private patients to pharmacies. In Scotland, however, the average pharmacy in 1946 dispensed a total of 10,102 prescriptions of which 6,553 or 65 per cent were private prescriptions and only 3,549 were N.H.I. About 90 per cent of doctors in Scotland wrote prescriptions for their private patients to take to the chemist's shop.[24]

The establishment of the National Health Service in 1948 effectively separated prescribing and dispensing in Britain, although in certain so-called rural areas doctors continued to practise as apothecaries. After 1948, 94 per cent of the population obtained their medicines from registered pharmacies. By enlarging their dispensaries, chemists were able to meet the increased volume of business without difficulty. Little delay was experienced by patients in getting their prescriptions dispensed, and there was an almost total absence of public complaints. The dispensing of private medicines dwindled to less than ten per cent. of the total number of prescriptions. The public could now get the medicines they needed, when they needed them and regardless of price. The role of the pharmacist took on an entirely new dimension. Relations with the medical profession improved so much that Hugh Linstead, the secretary of the Pharmaceutical Society, went so far as to describe them as "cordial".[25]

In the early stages of planning, the pharmacists' major concern was the extent to which the proposed new health centres would employ salaried pharmacists and thereby compete with private contractor chemists. Early planning documents referred ominously to patients choosing to obtain "their supplies on the prescription of their doctor either from shops or other premises of a pharmacist or from any health centre where dispensing services are provided". Fears were kindled similar to those invoked by the Friendly Societies' dispensing plans in 1911. However, the Pharmaceutical Society and the National Pharmaceutical

Union were assured that health centres would be limited to a few carefully controlled experiments and that the question of including pharmaceutical services would only arise on new housing estates. Since the supply of chemists' shops was more than adequate to meet the needs of the population, pharmacy services did not figure prominently in early health centre planning.[26] Despite the unambiguous commitment to health centres in the 1946 N.H.S. White Paper, the Labour Government's policy on health centres faltered and failed. By 1963 there were only eighteen purpose-built health centres in England and Wales.

For the chemist contractor, the new National Health Service was, in most respects, simply the old National Health Insurance scheme writ large. Insurance Committees, which had served as administrative agencies, were replaced by Executive Councils, but the same personnel were retained to do the work. The staff, of course, had to be enlarged, since the pharmaceutical service, like the rest of the health service, was now available to the entire population. Pharmacists, like other professions in the N.H.S., played an important part in policy-making and administration. On the national level, the Standing Pharmaceutical Advisory Committee gave technical advice to the Minister of Health. The Central Health Services Council comprised 41 members of whom two were pharmacists. In each Executive Council area, local chemists elected a pharmaceutical committee of ten or more members who looked after the interests of the chemist contractors and co-operated with the Executive Council in various matters. The local pharmaceutical committee chose two members of the Executive Council and also selected one half of the pharmaceutical service committee which investigated complaints and generally assisted the Executive Council in securing compliance with the terms of service.

The chemist contractor, who might be an individual, a firm or a company, displayed a "form notice" in his shop window and his name and the address of his shop appeared in a list available at post offices and at the Executive Council offices. In addition to regular shop hours, he was expected to enter a rota so that one or more pharmacies within a given area would be open for a short period in the evening, on Sundays and on public holidays. Most pharmacists who lived in or near their shops dispensed urgent prescriptions at any time.

The Ministry of Health, in co-operation with the National Pharmaceutical Union, devised a plan to make sure that the drugs and appliances supplied by chemists reached accepted standards. Each Executive Council put into operation a scheme to test samples. A chemist normally received a test prescription once every two years. The clerk of the Executive Council, guided by the chairman of the pharmaceutical service committee, would select the pharmacies to be visited and the medicines or appliances to be examined. A prescription in duplicate would be obtained from a medical practitioner without disclosing to him the name of the chemist to whom it would be given. An agent, after getting the prescription dispensed, notified the pharmacist that it was a test prescription. If a drug or an appliance were found to be deficient in quantity or quality the matter was referred to the pharmaceutical service committee for investigation. During 1952 only 8.6 per cent of samples required further investigation and in 1959 only 5.1 per cent. More than 7,000 samples were tested in 1959 and less than 375 warranted formal investigation. 207 chemists (out of a total of 18,000) were warned in that year but only 96 had money deducted from their remuneration as a disciplinary measure. The drug-testing programme provided ample proof of the high standards of dispensing in the N.H.S.[27]

343

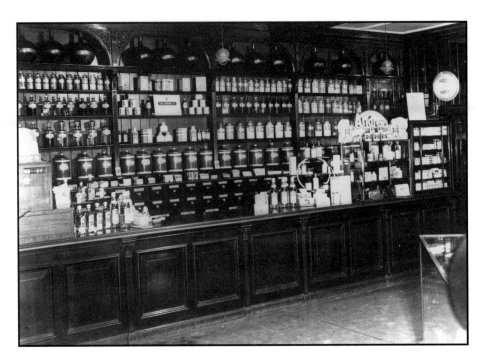

50   *Interior of Rankin & Borland, Kilmarnock, 1921.*

Negotiations concerning the terms of remuneration for chemist contractors in England and Wales were completed on 18 June 1948 and in Scotland on 1 July. The agreement was essentially an update of the N.H.I. scale. The chemist was paid for each prescription dispensed. Payment was made in accordance with the Drug Tariff, which specified the quality of the materials and their prices or the methods of computing them. The Ministry of Health prepared the Tariff and revised it frequently. Under the N.H.S. the chemist contractor received (1) the wholesale cost of the appliance or ingredients, as provided by the Drug Tariff, (2) an on-cost allowance of 33-1/3 per cent. to cover all overhead expenses and to provide a modest profit margin, (3) an average dispensing fee of 1s., with separate rates for certain special services, and (4) a container allowance of 2 1/2d. per prescription. Of these payments the first two repeated the N.H.I. pattern, the third increased the N.H.I. rate of 6d. to 1s., and the fourth was a new payment compensating the chemist for supplying a container for medicine. Under National Health Insurance, the working-class patient brought his own bottle or paid a deposit. A more civilised arrangement was thought appropriate for the new comprehensive, classless system. Assuming a constant cost of ingredients and the on-cost, the N.H.S. rate per prescription to chemists amounted to 30 1/2d. compared with the N.H.I. rate of 22d. The report of a working party headed by William Penman, which was completed in April 1948, demonstrated the peculiarities of the Scottish system of dispensing and justified the continuance of the differential paid under the N.H.I. scheme. In Scotland, therefore, chemists retained their higher dispensing fee, which was fixed at 1s. 3d. instead of 1s. Dispensing doctors were treated very generously: they could choose either to be paid on the same basis as chemists or to receive a capitation fee and receive additional payments for certain expensive drugs and appliances.

In 1948 some 16,800 chemists in Britain contracted to supply medicines under the National Health Service (14,000 in England and Wales; 2,800 in Scotland). The difficulties they experienced in the early years of the new service were not dissimilar to those encountered by chemists in 1913. Their first and most persistent grievance related to the change introduced in pricing the prescriptions submitted to the pricing bureaux. The bureaux were understaffed and unable to cope with the enormous upsurge in the amount of work: the annual number of prescriptions increased immediately from 70 million to 241 million. The full pricing policy which had been followed in the later years of the N.H.I. was abandoned and in its place payment to contractors was made on the basis of a 25 per cent. sample for all prescriptions under 2s. 6d., with full costing for more expensive items. Despite the change, the work of the pricing bureaux rapidly fell into arrears. It took until 1952 in Scotland and the end of 1954 in England before the arrears were cleared, and even then both pricing systems continued to be based on averages. By 1958 about 70 per cent. of all prescriptions were fully priced. Full pricing was the rule for chemists who dispensed less than 500 prescriptions per month. Every prescription with an ingredient cost of 5s. or more was priced. All regions in turn received full pricing three months in every year. Otherwise, only 20 per cent. of the prescriptions, selected at random, were priced and the others were averaged on the basis of the sample. The pharmaceutical profession continued to argue for a policy of full pricing and received support from the Hinchliffe Committee's *Report on the Cost of Prescribing*. After consultation with the Joint Pricing Committee and the Central N.H.S. (Chemist Contractors) Committee, the Ministry of Health decided to introduce full pricing in three stages, beginning in spring 1959. One year later the final stage was reached, and all prescriptions were then fully priced.

From 1 May 1950 the dispensing fee in England was increased to 1s. 1d., while in Scotland the fee was raised from 1s. 3d. to 1s. 6d. and backdated to 5 July 1948. But these gains were nullified by the reduction of the on-cost allowance from 33 1/3 per cent. to 25 per cent. and of the container allowance from 2 1/2d. to 1 1/4d. Such elements as the dispensing fee and the container and on-cost allowances were determined by negotiation between the Ministry of Health and the Central N.H.S. (Chemist Contractors) Committee and carried on within the framework of the Pharmaceutical Whitley Council. The Hinchliffe Committee in 1959 found that what the Government paid to chemists for the medicines dispensed was less than the price would have been if the medicine had been sold privately over the counter.[28]

* * *

Under the National Health Service Act of 1946 almost all hospitals, public or voluntary, were taken over by the Ministry of Health. The state-owned, exchequer-funded hospital service was the jewel in the N.H.S. crown: for the first time comprehensive hospital care was made available to all and without imposition of direct charges. With the advent of a national hospital service, hospital pharmacists had high hopes of at last achieving the status and remuneration appropriate to their important work. No longer would the legacy of the Poor Law drag down the status of those who worked in the municipal hospitals nor would the perpetually poverty-stricken voluntary hospitals impede progress in salary negotiations.

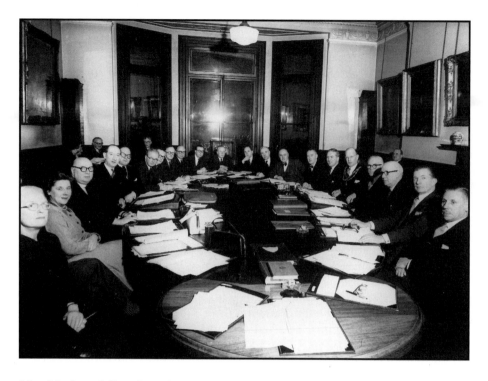

51   *Members of Council meeting 5 January 1955. This was only one of the several rooms to be occupied as the Council Chamber at Bloomsbury Square.*

There was a general expectation that, with the establishment of salary-negotiating machinery in the form of the Pharmaceutical Whitley Council (the first of the N.H.S. Whitley councils to be convened), a new and just salary structure would be devised to reflect properly the professional status of the hospital pharmacist. But this elation was short-lived. It was apparent after the first meeting of the Whitley Council that, however sympathetic to the pharmacists' demands the Hospital Management Committees and Boards of Governors might be, the power rested in the hands of the Treasury representatives. A salary structure was devised based on a points scheme related to the numbers of occupied beds and out-patient attendances in different types of hospital: but this structure could not be agreed by negotiation within the Whitley Council. In the summer of 1949, therefore, the two sides argued their case before an Industrial Court, which, although finding in favour of the pharmacists, made recommendations, influenced by the state of the British economy, that fell way below their expectations.[29]

The representatives of the hospital pharmacists on the Whitley Council came primarily from the Guild of Public Pharmacists, which in 1948 had a membership of nearly 1,000. The Guild had been formed in 1923 by the amalgamation of the Public Pharmacists Association and the pharmacy section of the Hospital Officers Association. Its creation was an attempt to ensure that the status division between the public service and the voluntary hospitals would not be reproduced in the organisation of pharmacists. The Public Pharmacists Association traced its origins back to the formation of the Poor Law Dispensers Association in 1897: the pharmacy section of the Hospital Officers Association was not set up until 1919. The Guild of Public Pharmacists was closely associated with the Pharmaceutical Society but not a part of it. Nonetheless, only persons whose names appeared on the register of chemists and druggists could be elected members. The Guild set out to improve the training, remuneration, and the quality of work of the public pharmacist.[30]

Before the establishment of the National Health Service, the pharmacists who worked in the voluntary hospitals and the public sector were very much the poor relations of the pharmaceutical family, an underprivileged minority usually hidden behind the dispensing screen. The institutions that employed them were chronically under-financed and originally intended only for the poor. The hospital, the asylum, the workhouse, and the prison were closely associated in nineteenth century thought. Hospitals for wealthy people were called "nursing homes".

By the end of the Second World War, the local authority hospital service was impressive in size and depressing in quality. About half the public hospital system consisted of public assistance institutions: the rest were former Poor Law infirmaries incorporated into the local authority service under the Local Government Act of 1929. Despite its size, the public hospital system never challenged the medical importance of the voluntary hospitals. A large proportion of the 130,000 beds in public hospitals in 1945 were occupied by the aged and the chronically and mentally ill. Voluntary hospitals did almost all the complex medical work and monopolised the training of doctors and nurses. Although established for the poor, the voluntary hospitals were rapidly losing their exclusively charitable character. The more affluent sections of society could not be denied access to the more advanced technology and the best facilities. There is a direct relationship between the increasing effectiveness of hospital treatment and the shift in voluntary hospital finance from philanthropy to patient charges. Once hospitals began to cure patients, pay beds were introduced. Gradually the voluntary hospitals acquired a dual character: a service for the wealthy grew alongside the old charitable work. But although income derived from patients or private insurance schemes grew steadily from the 1920s, the voluntary hospitals continued to depend heavily on voluntary donations.

The London Teaching Hospitals, which led the way in the development of medical science, were the first to employ qualified pharmaceutical chemists to run their dispensaries. Until the 1850s it was customary to employ apothecaries to act as resident medical officer and chief dispenser. The need to employ properly trained pharmacists was not recognised until the 1860s. The London and Westminster hospitals led the way, followed, in 1868 by University College Hospital, where the authorities had the sense to appoint the young William Martindale, not only to run the pharmaceutical services but also to lecture to the medical students. In the 1870s, A.W. Gerrard, who later became the recognised authority on plasters and a regular contributor to the British Pharmaceutical Conference, took charge of the dispensary at Guy's Hospital. By the end of the nineteenth century St. Bartholomew's and St. Mary's had appointed pharmaceutical chemists and the leading provincial hospitals had begun to follow London's example.[31]

The appointment of a handful of pharmaceutical chemists to run the dispensaries in major voluntary hospitals must not be allowed to disguise the fact that the great bulk of dispensing in public institutions was carried out by poorly-paid and often inadequately-trained staff. It is perhaps not surprising that chronically under-resourced institutions should practise the false economy of employing under-qualified persons (former army dispensers and holders of the Apothecaries Society Assistant's certificate) to prepare drugs and supply medicines and appliances. Even if fully qualified pharmacists were appointed, the tendency was to appoint women whose weakness in the labour market was exploited by those who managed the institutions. In its early days, the Association of Women Pharmacists was necessarily drawn into the struggle to improve the status and salaries of publicly employed pharmacists.

On the eve of the Second World War, the Pharmaceutical Society carried out a pioneering but rather sketchy survey of hospital pharmacy. It revealed that, although the supply of medicines in many hospitals was still undertaken by medical men, nurses or under-qualified dispensers, considerable progress had been achieved in recent years, particularly in the larger hospitals. In 1938 283 of the 397 hospitals containing a hundred beds or more employed a full-time pharmacist and a further 13 hospitals made use of the services of a pharmacist from the local community. Of the 543 hospitals with less than a hundred beds only 83 employed their own pharmacist but a further 247 called on a pharmacist from outside to supervise the dispensing. The report, with prescience, pointed out that as hospitals came to serve the whole community, so the pharmaceutical service would grow in stature.

> The steady improvement in the conditions under which medicines are supplied in hospitals is probably due in the main to the greater attention that has been paid in recent years to the value of hospital treatment for the whole and not only for the poorest section of the community and consequently to the need for the proper equipment and staffing of hospitals. Hospitals are no longer regarded as places for providing the indigent population with the minimum of medical and surgical treatment but as a vital part of the health service of the nation with an increasingly important role to play as that service becomes more and more organised on a rational and systematic basis. It can be said with confidence that in the future the institutional as opposed to the domiciliary treatment of disease will in one form or another be the principal form of treatment and therefore the hospital service offers a field for the employment of pharmacists which will expand rather than contract and which may ultimately become the main if not the sole field of pharmaceutical practice.

The range and significance of the work of the hospital pharmacist was accurately portrayed in the report.

> Hospital pharmacy provides the pharmacist with a greater opportunity of applying his professional knowledge and ability than is afforded by any other branch of pharmacy. In addition to being responsible for the purchase, custody and dispensing of drugs, medicines and dressings, the pharmacist can ... carry on the manufacture of galenical preparations, assist the medical staff in the selection of the most suitable medicines, conduct research work with a view to the improvement of old and the preparation of new remedies, undertake analyses of hospital supplies ... and act generally as chemical adviser to the hospital. The increasing use of

proprietary articles makes the pharmacist's knowledge of particular importance and value in enabling the medical staff to discriminate between such articles and to evaluate the claims made for them . . . The economic administration of his department is an important part of the hospital pharmacist's work . . . In the larger hospitals the pharmacist may be responsible for the purchase of supplies involving an outlay of many thousands of pounds annually.

The report suggested that "the role of the pharmacist as a hospital supplies officer needs greater stress". It was especially important in connection with municipal health services, which, in addition to general and special hospital services, included ante-natal care, infant welfare, public assistance and the school medical services. A central supply service, with a pharmacist in charge, should be established in every local authority as the most efficient way of obtaining and distributing the large quantities of medical and semi-medical supplies these services require.

Pharmacists in teaching hospitals were seen to have special responsibilities.

The head pharmacists in these hospitals are responsible for the training of medical students in such knowledge of pharmacy as they are required to have. They are also brought into contact with newly-qualified practitioners who remain at the hospitals as house-surgeons. They are therefore those who can do most to influence the attitude which the medical practitioner adopts towards pharmacy . . . The impression of pharmacy which the medical practitioner gains during his student and immediate post-graduate days is of vital importance for pharmacists . . .

The report emphasized the need to encourage "the best-qualified and the most enterprising pharmacists to take up hospital posts". It suggested that only persons with "the Pharmaceutical Chemist qualification, preferably obtained through the medium of a Bachelor of Pharmacy degree" should be appointed to hospital posts. "An honours degree in chemistry to supplement the Ph.C. qualification is also advisable, while in hospitals where manufacturing is undertaken a knowledge of chemical engineering is an advantage". "The role of the pharmacist as a supplies officer makes it advisable for him to acquire a knowledge of economic administration . . ."

The report underlined the contradiction between the responsibilities of the hospital pharmacist and the rewards. The Pharmaceutical Society was under no doubt that the hospital pharmacist had an essential and strategic part to play in the development of pharmacy practice. But how could the most highly educated and the most dynamic members of the profession be recruited to posts which offered lower incomes than those of either the independent proprietor or the manager of a company shop? To this question, the Pharmaceutical Society had no answer.

Prior to 1945 there was no national salary scale for hospital pharmacists. Each local authority determined the salaries it paid to its hospital employees and the staffs of the voluntary hospitals negotiated their own salaries with their boards of management. The first national salary scales were agreed in 1945 and for the first time the Guild of Public Pharmacists became active in the field of salary negotiations. The later experience of the Pharmaceutical Whitley Council led to demands from some members that the Guild seek the services of a professional negotiator or turn itself into a trade union. Despondency about salaries and recruitment in the hospital pharmaceutical service grew during the 1950s and 1960s, although the rationalisation which the N.H.S. brought to the hospital service strengthened the hands of pharmacists in their early struggles with hospital supplies officers. In the 1950s the Guild managed to convince the Ministry of Health that the acquisition of pharmaceutical supplies should be the responsibility of pharmacists.

In spite of the unsatisfactory conditions in which hospital pharmacists continued to work, the professional aspects of pharmacy were carefully nurtured in the hospital sector. The Guild, in 1959, organised a weekend school at Nottingham University with lectures on drug addiction, work study in hospitals and modern sterilising techniques. Hospitals provide an excellent location for pharmaceutical education but understaffing and rapid staff turnover severely limit the opportunities for utilising this valuable resource.

In the early 1960s the Guild of Public Pharmacists, with the support of the Pharmaceutical Society, began to press the Ministry of Health for a thorough examination of the organisation and managerial structure of pharmacy in the hospital service, and, in the early part of 1968, an ad-hoc working party, under the chairmanship of Sir Noel Hall, was set up by the Labour Government. Its terms of reference were:

> To advise on the efficient and economical organization of the hospital pharmaceutical service with particular reference to: (1) the most suitable unit(s) of organization for the whole or parts of the service; (2) the best use of pharmacists, including the need and facilities for their post-graduate training; (3) the best use of supporting staff (including their recruitment and training); (4) a suitable career structure for pharmacists and supporting staff.

The Noel Hall Report, which was published in 1970, followed a period of growing concern at the shortage of pharmacists in the hospital service. Evidence presented to the working party revealed the high turnover and wastage in the basic and senior pharmacist grades, the unacceptably high number of part-time pharmaceutical staff, and shortages in both pharmacist and technician classes. A number of themes were developed in the report which embodied principles applicable not just to pharmaceutical services but to a wide range of professional activities in the health service. These themes emerged in earlier reports on other aspects of the hospital service such as the Salmon report on senior nursing staff structure (1966) and the Zuckerman report on hospital scientific and technical services (1968).[32] These themes were: the need for larger units of organisation to make the most effective use of available staff; the delegation of tasks that do not require the skills of a trained pharmacist to less highly qualified staff; the provision of a career structure offering improved promotion possibilities; and the training of pharmacists to meet their increased managerial responsibilities. The report also included recommendations on training at varying levels for both pharmacists and supporting staff.

Although evidence was presented in the report of the serious shortage of pharmacists in the hospital service (43 per cent of established posts in the basic grade in England and Wales were vacant in 1966), the working party argued that the difficulties of hospitals were aggravated by failures to put available staff to the best use and to delegate suitable tasks to technicians and other support staff. The problems of attracting and retaining younger pharmacists were seen in terms of inadequacies in organisation, salary and career structure. Although pay was not included in the working party's terms of reference (since this was a matter for the Whitley Council), it was obviously intended that the improved career structure would provide opportunities for higher earnings.

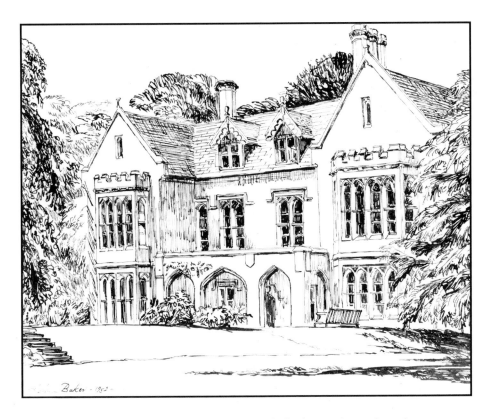

52 *Pen and ink sketch of Birdsgrove House, the Society's convalescent home in Derbyshire. John Baker, 1952.*

There was a mixed reaction in the working party to the suggestion of the Zuckerman Committee that pharmacists and pharmaceutical technicians "might be appropriate for inclusion" in the proposed hospital scientific service. Those who opposed the idea pointed out that "the pharmacist is closely connected with the treatment of the patient, and he has professional responsibilities in this respect which would have to be safeguarded". The development of clinical pharmacy in hospitals since 1970 has underlined the wisdom of those who objected to the proposed classification of pharmacists as laboratory scientists. Hospital pharmacists have played a leading part in the promotion of clinical pharmacy: they have emphasized the need for pharmacists to act as drug information specialists and to work directly with patients on the wards. The day, if it ever existed, when hospital pharmacists could perform their role satisfactorily while remaining hidden in the dispensary, has certainly gone.

The implementation of the recommendations of the Noel Hall report were delayed by the reorganisation of the National Health Service in 1974. Although considerable improvements were made in the career structure, hospital pharmacists continued to be paid less than other scientists in the hospital service, such as physicists and biochemists, and less than community pharmacists. Thus, even after the Noel Hall report, the hospital pharmaceutical service still experienced difficulty in recruiting to the basic grade and labour turnover remained high. Yet the recruitment problem is partially masked by the fact that young pharmacists are attracted to hospital work by the greater opportunities it offers for the exercise of their professional skills. Hospital pharmacy continues to be a predominantly female occupation. In 1984 61.4 per cent of hospital pharmacists, but only 35.7 per cent of all pharmacists, were women.

On 2 December 1972 a special general meeting of the Guild of Hospital Pharmacists (the name was changed in 1971) agreed that its Council should begin negotiations with the Association of Scientific, Technical and Managerial Staffs to seek affiliation with that trade union and at the same time should pursue the possibility of the formation of a hospital pharmacists group within the Pharmaceutical Society. Following negotiations, both objectives were acheived. When the details of the terms of the merger with A.S.T.M.S. were circulated, the Guild members, in a postal vote, voted by 894 to 147 in favour of becoming a separate membership group and this decision became effective on 16 April 1974. In 1975 a Hospital Pharmacists Group was established within the Pharmaceutical Society. Membership is open to pharmacists employed, either on a permanent basis or as a locum-tenens, in a hospital, or by a Health Authority in hospital administration or in a health centre. Among the aims of the Group is the promotion of the application of pharmaceutical knowledge within the hospital service: among its duties is the provision of advice to the Council of the Pharmaceutical Society on all aspects of hospital pharmaceutical practice.

At the end of 1952 there were just over 1,300 full time pharmacists in the hospital service, together with 140 part-timers and 80 students or trainees. Hospital pharmacists represented no more than 7 per cent of all pharmacists. By 1985 there were just over 4,000 pharmacists working, either full-time or part-time, in hospitals: almost all of them were employed by the National Health Service. They constituted about 16 per cent of all working pharmacists.

3. *THE JENKIN CASE, 1933 ACT, DANGEROUS DRUGS AND EDUCATION*

> The Pharmaceutical Society and the First World War—The Apothecaries' Assistants' affair, 1919—Setting up a Whitley Council—The Jenkin case—The Retail Pharmacists Union—The Supplemental Charter 1953—The Dickson Case—Sir William Glyn-Jones—The British Pharmaceutical Conference—Glyn-Jones on the Pharmacy Acts—The Departmental Committee on the Poisons and Pharmacy Acts, 1926–30—The Pharmacy and Poisons Act of 1933—The Dangerous Drugs Acts—Towards the 1968 Medicines Act—The history of pharmcaceutical education—The Pharmacy Act of 1954

Britain declared war on Germany in August 1914 almost totally unprepared both mentally and institutionally for the great upheaval that was to follow.[1] There was an almost total lack of comprehension on the part of both the Government and the people of the effect that the struggle would have on the nation. The expectation that the war would be short gave way to the feeling that it would never end. The excitement of 1914 developed into the confusion and exasperation of 1915 and then to despair and anger in 1916. Military defeats, production failures, shortages of essential supplies, manpower mismanagement, food queues and watered beer led after the first two years of war to the discarding of the old style of constitutional government and its replacement by a more dynamic and authoritarian system geared to the task of winning the war. The new style of government first began to emerge with the setting up of the Ministry of Munitions under David Lloyd George in 1915. The next seventeen months saw a series of running battles within government, parliament and the wider society over such issues as military conscription, direction of civilian manpower, regulation of wages, prices and profits, and the scope and content of government emergency powers. At the end of 1916 these conflicts led to the ousting from the premiership of Asquith, the cautious traditionalist, by Lloyd George, the dynamic innovator. By 1917 food rationing, price controls, the compulsory purchase and requisitioning of raw materials, bulk importation of essential supplies, control of rents and housebuilding, registration and direction of labour involved a degree of centralisation and regulation unthinkable in the pre-war era. In the later years of the war, the establishment of the Ministry of Reconstruction seemed to indicate that the planning which had served the country so well during war was to be carried over into peacetime. "There is no doubt at all", Lloyd George declared in March 1917, "that the present war . . . presents an opportunity for reconstruction of industrial and economic conditions of this country".

When Lloyd George became prime minister, he was succeeded at the Ministry of Munitions by Dr. Christopher Addison, who, a year later, was made the first Minister of Reconstruction. Addison, who was Liberal M.P. for Shoreditch, had trained as a doctor at St. Bartholomew's and was a prominent member of the B.M.A. It was as if professional etiquette determined that his parliamentary secretary at both Munitions and Reconstruction should be the pharmacist William Glyn-Jones. In addition to his work for Addison, Glyn-Jones continued as the parliamentary secretary for the Pharmaceutical Society. There was scarcely a single bill of the many affecting pharmacy the original proposals of which were not materially improved by his direct intervention, whether in debate or privately. He was concerned not merely to represent the interests of pharmacists but also to assist the Government by drawing on the knowledge and the organisational network of the Pharmaceutical Society. During the war a relationship of mutual benefit developed between the Society and government departments. Glyn-Jones has left us his own recollections of the war years:

> The outbreak of the Great War came as a shock for which pharmacy and pharmacists—like every other section of the community—were unprepared. Such a contingency had not been contemplated and no plans made to meet it. The economic structure upon which our work, our habits, our customs as a people were based was shattered, and a new order had to be rapidly improvised. Pharmacy and pharmacists were involved in the upheaval. Parliament was forced by abnormal circumstances to legislate for, and regulate, almost every detail of the work of the pharmacist. Government Departments—many specially created for the purpose— with improvised, well meaning, but ill-equipped staffs administered both the provisions of hurried Acts of Parliament and the more numerous regulations which Parliament, in too great a hurry to make themselves, empowered the Departments to make. We lived from day to day in fear of fresh Parliamentary and Departmental decisions which followed each other in rapid succession, ill thought out and conflicting, for want either of time or knowledge.[2]

The Pharmaceutical Society's activities during the war centred on two problems: the supply of pharmaceutical materials and the allocation of pharmacists and their assistants for military service, while retaining a due proportion to maintain essential pharmaceutical services for both the Forces and the civilian population. The general lines upon which pharmacists were selected under the Scheme of National Service were laid down in consultation with the Society. Pharmacy was declared a reserved occupation and a national register was compiled. The fact that the Local Associations Executive, which had been set up to promote the interests of pharmacists involved in the National Health Insurance scheme, was a part of the Society's organisation was of great service in helping to avoid the haphazard depletion of the ranks of pharmacy and the severe dislocation of business. The Society issued a War Emergency Formulary and War Emergency Notes as an aid to the conservation of essential drugs and other scarce items such as glycerin and sugar. The Society's laboratories and staff were placed at the disposal of the War Office for the examination of drugs required by the Royal Army Medical Corps and for the preparation of special charcoal for anti-gas purposes. The researches of Lieutenant-Colonel E.F. Harrison, a distinguished analytical chemist and pharmacist, who became Director of Chemical Warfare in 1918, led to the saving of many thousands of servicemen's lives.

Despite the links between the Society and the War Office, the question of the employment of pharmacists in the Army, raised from time to time by Glyn-Jones, made no progress. The Society sought in vain to persuade the Government to form an Army Pharmaceutical Corps with commissioned ranks. During the war Glyn-Jones made a tour of inspection of military hospitals and dispensaries in France and produced a comprehensive report detailing the wasteful manner in which military medical supplies were distributed and used and the unprofessional way in which dispensing was done. In 1924 a committee consisting of a military chairman, three representatives of the War Office and three of the Pharmaceutical Society, issued a report recommending reforms. But the Army authorities persisted in their view that the needs of the Army were adequately met by the employment of men trained as dispensers at the Army School of Dispensing.

In August 1918 the Council of the Pharmaceutical Society issued an appeal for subscriptions to a War Auxiliary Benevolent Fund for helping pharmacists who might need financial assistance as a result of the war then nearing its end. The response greatly exceeded expectations: £23,112 was collected within a year. The Fund was administered by the Benevolent Fund Committee and used to deal with cases of hardship among ex-servicemen. By 1924 over 1,500 cases had been dealt with and a total of over £11,000 expended in relief—mostly in supplementing the Government Training Grant or in providing training facilities for those too late to obtain grants. In 1924 the Charity Commissioners approved an extension of the objects of the Fund to include the education of the sons, daughters or dependants of those who served in the Forces and the giving of assistance to ex-servicemen and their dependants even though their need did not arise directly from the war.

After the signing of the Armistice in November 1918 the Pharmaceutical Society was responsible for expediting the demobilisation of thousands of pharmacists and their assistants. It then became involved in the administration of two schemes for demobilised men. First there was a scheme for assisting those who, through disablement, were unable to take up again their own occupation but who would be capable of earning a living by some new trade, business or profession. The Government undertook to train them and the

Pharmaceutical Society agreed to assist. The National Trade Advisory Committee was formed: but there were few disabled men fit and willing to take up pharmacy. The much bigger problem was that of the hundreds of thousands of young men who, when war broke out, were either on the threshold of training for a vocation, or had been forced to abandon the training they had already started. The Government introduced a scheme intended to reduce as far as possible the handicap caused by this break in their careers. The young men were divided into two classes, those whose apprenticeships had been interrupted and those who had been studying at University or for professional qualifications. The provision made for the latter class was much more elaborate and expensive than that for the former. To the dismay of the Pharmaceutical Society, the Government started to treat aspirants for pharmaceutical qualifications as budding shopkeepers under the Interrupted Apprenticeship Scheme. Immediately, Glyn-Jones went into action, pulling every string at his command to get this decision changed. He managed to persuade Dr. Addison to intervene and secure for pharmaceutical apprentices the status and treatment of those training for a profession or studying in higher education. The result was that some 4,000 pharmacy students who had served in the armed forces received the Government Training Grant, covering college fees, examination fees, and maintenance costs for the full nine months' course, at a total cost to the taxpayer of about £400,000. The Pharmaceutical Society organised the selection process and allocated the successful candidates to suitable courses.

The Government's decision to pay the students' fees enabled the Society's Council to put into operation the powers given in the Poisons and Pharmacy Act of 1908 to require attendance at a course of instruction as a condition of entry for the Qualifying Examination. With 4,000 students suddenly returned to civilian life and with the government grant at their disposal, it became a matter of urgency for the Society to find institutions in which they could be trained. E.S. Peck was given the job of visiting universities and technical colleges to arrange the facilities. After three months hard travelling and interviewing, he was able to report to the Council that he had arranged for a complete course of instruction (Parts I and II) to be given in twenty-five universities and technical colleges and for an even larger number of institutions to teach Part I (Chemistry, Physics and Botany) only. After receiving Peck's report, the Council decided, as a general policy, that the number of schools recognised for both Part I and Part II should be strictly limited, but no restriction should be placed on the number recognised for Part I only. This was done so that instruction in these subjects could be provided as near to the home of each student as possible.

In June 1918 the post of secretary and registrar of the Pharmaceutical Society became vacant. William James Uglow Woolcock, who had held the position since 1913, resigned on being appointed general manager of the Association of British Chemical Manufacturers. For a short period the vice-president, E.T. Neathercoat, did the work. Eventually William Glyn-Jones was persuaded to leave parliament to take on the job. He decided not to contest the next election although as a Lloyd George Coalition Liberal his chances of success were good. Curiously, when the "Coupon" election came in December 1918, Uglow Woolcock was returned as Coalition Liberal M.P. for Central Hackney. Glyn-Jones and Woolcock swopped places.

The most discussed event of 1919 in pharmaceutical circles was the admission of apothecaries' assistants to the register of chemists and druggists, without examination, a new departure provided for in Section 4(b) of the Poisons and Pharmacy Act of 1908.[3] When that Act was passed, there was a clear understanding among all parties concerned, that the provision was permissive, not mandatory. Later, however, the Privy Council Office took the view that, whatever the legal status of the provision, its insertion had secured the withdrawal of hostile amendments and that, therefore, there was a moral obligation on the Pharmaceutical Society to exercise the power. This the Society steadfastly refused to do in spite of growing insistence by the Privy Council. The position was finally reached where it became clear that continued defiance of the Privy Council's wishes would involve the Society in damaging controversy over such matters as the scheduling of poisons and the approval of by-laws.

A way out was sought by a series of private conferences between the Society's Council and the Association of Certificated Dispensers held at the Privy Council Office under the chairmanship of Sir William Job Collins. The outcome of these meetings was that the Society's Council agreed to formulate a by-law permitting the registration of Apothecaries' Assistants, who had been continuously employed for seven years as wholetime dispensers in a responsible position in an institution approved by the Society, provided that application to be registered was made before 1 January 1921. As an additional safeguard, it was provided that registration could be refused if the Society's Council considered that the applicant did not possess the necessary skill, qualifications and fitness.

Indications of trouble ahead appeared when the by-law was read a first time at a meeting of the Society's Council on 6 May 1919: three Council members dissented. The case for the opposition was that the Society was under no obligation to make the by-law; that the Privy Council was violating the right of the Society to originate its own by-laws; that the by-law amounted to a dilution of the register and a lowering of the value of the qualification; that the admission of an unspecified number of less well trained persons would create a precedent for further concessions and act as an encouragement to others on the flanks of pharmacy to advance similar claims; and that the real remedy was the creation of a statutory register of assistants. It was clear that the majority of those likely to apply for registration would be dispensers in such institutions as voluntary hospitals, Poor Law infirmaries, asylums and prisons, and that, by passing this by-law, the Society would be helping to undermine the work of the Public Pharmacists Association and the Association of Women Pharmacists. A strong objection on these grounds was recorded by Herbert Skinner, a future president of the Society, in a letter to the *Pharmaceutical Journal* of 28 June in which he maintained that the effect of the by-law would be "to reduce the public service to a farce".

The opposition steadily gained momentum and by the time of the Special General Meeting required for the final adoption of the by-law it became clear that a large and vociferous section of the membership was strongly hostile. The General Meeting was arranged to begin at 3.30 p.m. on 2 July at the Memorial Hall, Farringdon Street. In the circumstances Glyn-Jones thought it wise to call a preliminary private meeting of members at 2.30 p.m. to rehearse the arguments for and against. The afternoon was hot and some 700 to 800 members were packed in the hall. From the outset the meeting was unruly. Representatives of the Council speaking from the platform found it difficult to obtain a hearing: the proceedings were frequently interrupted. It soon became obvious that the by-law would not be adopted by this gathering. At the hour appointed for the start of the

General Meeting, Glyn-Jones announced that thirty-one members had signed a statement that they were unable to gain admission to the hall. The Society's solicitor, who was present on the platform, advised the president, William Currie, that the meeting could not be duly constituted and should be postponed so that it might be held in a hall large enough to hold all members wishing to attend. This announcement was not well received and the discussion continued in a more heated fashion. The opponents of the by-law came forward with the idea that the opinion of the whole membership should be obtained by a referendum. The president expressed doubt of the legality of such a procedure, but undertook to obtain counsel's opinion. By this time tempers on both sides were becoming frayed. A speaker from the platform described the opponents as "idiots", an explanation by the secretary was greeted with cries of "rot", and there were moments of utter chaos. When the members insisted on taking a vote, the president ruled that the General Meeting was not constituted. In desperation he left the chair and was followed from the hall by the secretary and most of the members of Council. The ordinary members who remained elected a new chairman and passed by acclamation a resolution declaring the by-law "unfair, unjust and unnecessary".

Alexander Macmorran, K.C., was invited to advise on the legal status of a referendum. His opinion was that a General Meeting was essential for the approval of by-laws, but that a referendum would have value in ascertaining for general information what the opinion of members unable to attend was. The Council decided that a referendum should be taken before the Special General Meeting, which was arranged for 6 August at the Central Hall, Westminster. In the meantime a conference of Local Association Officers was called for 25 July. At this conference Edmund White, a past president of the Society, explained the circumstances which had led the Council to the conclusion that the by-law should be passed. Then the president, William Currie, made it unmistakably clear what the underlying issue now was. The question members now had to decide, he said, was: who was to control the policy of the Society? Was it to be the majority of the elected members of Council or a small minority of Council members supported by an organised opposition outside the Council? He finished by reading a letter signed by sixteen members of Council indicating their intention to resign if the by-law were not passed: he added that, in such circumstances, Glyn-Jones would also resign. The conference strongly recommended every member to vote for the by-law.

The meeting at the Westminster Central Hall was no less rowdy than its predecessor. Uproar broke out when it was confirmed that the seventeen councillors supporting the by-law had, at their own expense, sent telegrams to known supporters urging them to attend. The Council's failure to publish the promised list of institutions to be approved also provoked angry criticism. The result of the referendum, however, destroyed the popular basis of the opposition's case: 4,294 members had voted in favour and only 1,667 against the by-law. Nonetheless, it was the vote in the Central Hall that was crucial. There was general disorder when it was taken with shouting and unanswered questions ringing out. The result was declared, recorded the *Pharmaceutical Journal*, "in an atmosphere surcharged with electricity". The by-law was adopted by 682 votes to 434. The electricity was discharged by the enthusiastic singing of the National Anthem.

The direct consequence of the new by-law was minimal. After all the talk of diluting the register and cheapening the qualification, only fifty-two holders of the certificate of the

Apothecaries Society were actually registered as chemists and druggists before the dispensation lapsed on 1 January 1921. Yet the by-law controversy had important repercussions. The divisions within the Council widened. Wounds which had been inflicted festered in an atmosphere of hostility and ill-will. The results of the Council election of 1920 suggest that the most active and committed members of the Society continued to find the Council's policies unacceptable. Alexander Keith, the chairman of the committee opposing the by-law, was elected to the Council at the top of a poll in which over two-thirds of the members voted.

The affair of the apothecaries' assistants raised fundamental issues about the nature and constitution of the Pharmaceutical Society. Even in the days of Jacob Bell, the idea of all the members turning up at Bloomsbury Square in person to attend annual general meetings and to approve the by-laws was nothing more than a convenient fiction, made plausible by the fact that the Society was essentially a metropolitan association, with at most two or three thousand members. But, by 1919, the Society had over 9,000 members, scattered throughout Britain. In the interests of either democratic participation or tighter executive control, a new constitution was required. "The cumbrous provision" requiring the by-laws to be confirmed and approved by a special general meeting of members was repealed by the Pharmacy and Poisons Act of 1933. That Act dealt also with the more fundamental issue of the relationship between the Privy Council, the Society's Council, and the members. The by-law controversy of 1919 was an important stage in the process of adjusting the balance between the three parts of that relationship.

When Glyn-Jones agreed to abandon his promising political career to take on the post of secretary and registrar of the Pharmaceutical Society, he did not doubt that his experience as a politician and his standing among pharmacists would enable him to take up the reins of power within the Society. That status was further enhanced by the knighthood he received in 1919. When Glyn-Jones became secretary, he became, in effect, the chief executive of the Society. In the past Elias Bremridge and later his son Richard had acquired a degree of power simply by staying in office for so long. Inevitably, by a process of slow accretion, they acquired a unique knowledge of the ways and means of pharmaceutical decision-making. But the Bremridges were not innovators; they preferred the quiet life of clerical routines. They were preoccupied with the task of keeping the ship afloat on an even keel, without paying too much attention to the direction in which it was sailing. Glyn-Jones was as far removed from this tradition as it is possible to conceive. He was a man of enormous energy and enterprise. He believed in setting himself clearly defined goals and pursuing them relentlessly. "The bigger the mountain", Michael Carteighe once said of him, "the more keen he was to scale it". When Glyn-Jones became secretary, he set himself the task of transforming the Pharmaceutical Society into an organisation as powerful as the British Medical Association. To do that he would need to bring together every section of the trade, business and profession of pharmacy: to unite in one organisation, manufacturers and wholesalers and the pharmacists they employed in the laboratory, office, warehouse, and on the road; independent proprietor chemists and their qualified assistants; the pharmacists employed by Boots and the other company chemists and by the co-operative societies and the department stores; the pharmacists working in voluntary hospitals, Poor Law institutions, prisons and other branches of the public service; and the pharmacists who worked as administrators and teachers.

The British Medical Association was for Glyn-Jones the model professional organisation. It united within its ranks all sections of the profession, from the highest consultant to the lowliest G.P. Its branch organisation and its branch representatives meeting seemed an ideal constitution for a large, nationwide, democratic association. Its annual meetings, moving from town to town, like some medieval king's court, strengthened its members' allegiance and symbolised its leaders' dependence. The mixture of science and politics at these yearly jamborees was a public affirmation that the material interests of its members were but the necessary foundation for the advance of medical knowledge. The unceasing vigilance of the B.M.A. in defence of each and every one of its members made its accumulated power felt wherever medicine was practised.

The most important consequence of the by-law controversy of 1919 was the effect it had on Sir William Glyn-Jones. His political skills were used to engineer the adoption of the by-law but he must have found the experience depressing. "The intense interest taken in this strenuous controversy", observed the Society's Annual Report for 1919, "gave striking evidence of the latent powers possessed by pharmacists for defending their legitimate interests against attacks from outside". Glyn-Jones had devoted his life to mobilising "the latent powers possessed by pharmacists for defending their legitimate interests". Single-handedly he had created the P.A.T.A. and the Chemists' Defence Association: his contributions to the construction of the 1908 Poisons and Pharmacy Act and the 1911 National Insurance Act had been crucial for pharmacy. Yet on this occasion he found himself on the wrong side. The by-law was justifiably unpopular: its adoption was clearly against the best interests of pharmacists. It was being foisted upon the Society by the Privy Council; but the Society's Council and its chief officer were being made to do the dirty work. They were in a cleft stick. The Privy Council had the power, at the very least, to deprive the Society of all means of initiating change. Yet, at the same time, the Society's officials were exposed to rancid comment. In June 1919, the *Drug Union News* carried an article accusing them of placing "care for their own personal advancement" above the interests of members. It went on to argue that their policy was to conciliate the Privy Council in order that sources of revenue other than members' fees might be substantially increased and the members' control over the Society correspondingly reduced. Although there was not a grain of truth in these specific accusations, Glyn-Jones knew that, if the Society was to remain dependent on the voluntary subscriptions of its members, it could not grow and flourish, unless it were free to pursue with vigour their legitimate interests.

When Glyn-Jones was parliamentary secretary at the Ministry of Reconstruction during 1917 and 1918, the Committee on the Relations between Employers and Employed (the Whitley Committee) issued its famous five reports. The decade immediately preceding the outbreak of the First World War had been a period of growing industrial conflict with increasingly militant trade unions and aggressive hard-line employers. The Liberal government, following a policy of social harmony, sought to restrain the more extreme tendencies on the part of both employers and workers by discreet intervention. The Labour Department of the Board of Trade attempted to use the Conciliation Act of 1896 to mediate in industrial disputes but effective conciliation depended upon achieving the consent and co-operation of both sides and in those years of rising costs of living and relatively full employment this was not readily forthcoming. During the war labour shortages and inflationary pressures coupled with government control of such key industries as shipping and the railways led to compulsory arbitration for disputes affecting munitions work and the regulation of wages on a national basis. The Whitley Committee was established in October 1916 to prepare the way for the statutory containment of industrial relations after the war.[4] Its terms of reference were:

> (1) To make and consider suggestions for securing a permanent improvement in the relations between employers and workmen.
> (2) To recommend means for securing that industrial conditions affecting the relations between employers and workmen shall be systematically reviewed by those concerned, with a view to improving conditions in the future.

The Committee argued that it was vital that there should be a permanent improvement in the relations between employers and employed in the main industries of the country and that any arrangements proposed should offer workpeople better conditions of employment and invoke their active co-operation. It recommended the formation in well-organised industries of Joint Industrial Councils comprised of representatives of associations of employers and employed. In badly organised trades, Trade Boards should be set up to provide regular machinery for negotiation dealing with wages, hours, and conditions of work. The Committee emphasised the "advisability of a continuance, as far as possible, of the present system whereby industries make their own arrangements and settle their differences themselves" and gave their "considered opinion that an essential condition of securing a permanent improvement in the relations between employers and employed is that there should be adequate organisation on the part of both".

At the beginning of 1919, Lloyd George was promoting, through the Ministry of Labour, three schemes for reorganising industrial relations in Britain, one by means of Joint Industrial Councils (Whitley Councils), another by Joint Negotiating Committees, and the third through Trade Boards. Between January 1918 and December 1921, 73 Joint Industrial Councils and 33 Joint Negotiating Committees (or Interim Industrial Reconstruction Committees) were formed. On 20 March 1919 representatives of the Pharmaceutical Society attended a meeting called by the Ministry of Labour to discuss the setting up of a Trade Board for the distributive trades. The Society's Council was strongly opposed to the inclusion of pharmacy in such an arrangement: it feared that Ministry of Labour officials, with the minimum of consultation, would impose minimum wage rates and other employment conditions within the drug trade. On Glyn-Jones' advice, the Council decided instead to set up a Whitley Council for the whole pharmaceutical industry. "The whole country was engrossed in the question of the relationship between employers and employed", recalled Glyn-Jones in 1924. "All branches of industry were engaged in setting up machinery, Whitley Councils, Joint Negotiating Committees, and Trade Boards, for dealing with these questions. Rightly or wrongly, the Society tried to meet this demand on the part of pharmacists and their assistants". Since the Society included among its members both employers and employees, it seemed the ideal institution to preside over negotiations between them.

On 4 April 1919 the Council of the Pharmaceutical Society called a meeting at 17 Bloomsbury Square of representatives of all sections of the drug trade, or business of pharmacy (wholesale and retail, employers and employees). The plan was to set up a Joint Industrial Council with the following objectives: the regulation of wages, hours and working conditions, the regulation of production and employment, the settlement of disputes within the trade, the adoption of measures for securing the inclusion of all employers and employees in their respective organisations, the collection of statistics and information, the improvement of health conditions and the provision of special treatment for workers. Immediately after the meeting, the Society put into motion the formation of a chemists' assistants' association to represent employee pharmacists. It was assumed that proprietor chemists were already adequately represented by the Society. Unfortunately things soon began to fall apart.

Jesse Boot's antagonism towards anything smacking of trade unionism led him to oppose the Society's attempt to set up the chemists' assistants' association. He rapidly established instead his own Managers' Representative Council to represent the pharmacist-managers of his retail branches. Moreover, the proprietor chemists, who formed the great majority of members of the Pharmaceutical Society, did not exactly take to the idea of the Society devoting resources to helping their employees form a union to fight for higher wages, shorter hours and better working conditions. Their confidence in the leadership of the Society was already being weakened by the controversy over the proposed new by-law. Worse was to follow. The chemists of Scotland displayed their independence by cocking a snoot at the Pharmaceutical Society. They had already set up a body independent of the Society, the Pharmaceutical Standing Committee, to conduct negotiations for Scottish chemist contractors under the National Health Insurance scheme. They now proceeded to ignore the Society's decision to establish a Joint Industrial Council and instead set about making their own arrangements. At a meeting in Edinburgh on 30 April 1919 they formed the Scottish Pharmaceutical Federation to take charge of the trade interests of employer pharmacists in Scotland. One of its first acts, illustrative of its defiant mood, was to obtain counsel's opinion on the powers of the Pharmaceutical Society conferred by its Charter. The opinion of the Scottish lawyers was that the 1843 Charter gave the Society no authority to assume duties connected with the regulation of wages or other conditions of employment. Indeed, in June 1919, the secretary of the Scottish Pharmaceutical Federation, Alexander Murray, categorically stated that the Pharmaceutical Society could legally do none of the things that Glyn-Jones was proposing.

Glyn-Jones decided to reply in kind. He arranged for the Society's Council to obtain counsel's opinion on a parallel though not identical set of questions. Not surprisingly, the London lawyers came up with the view that the "protection" indicated in the Royal Charter was wide enough to cover all the interests of the trade. Glyn-Jones decided to continue with the establishment of the Whitley Council. He believed in the general principle of regulating industrial relations and in the particular need to keep the regulation of the drug trade under the supervision of the Pharmaceutical Society. Regrettably, the divisions within the Society's Council, exacerbated if not caused by the by-law dispute, made progress impossible. With great reluctance, Glyn-Jones agreed that the most satisfactory solution would be to have a friendly action brought against the Society in order to obtain an authoritative definition of the powers of the Society under its Charter.

As an experienced and successful barrister, Glyn-Jones must have been extremely reluctant to give judges the opportunity to determine what the Pharmaceutical Society could or could not do. He must have been fully aware that little good would come to the Society from the decision to invite the law courts to define the meaning of the Royal Charter. If

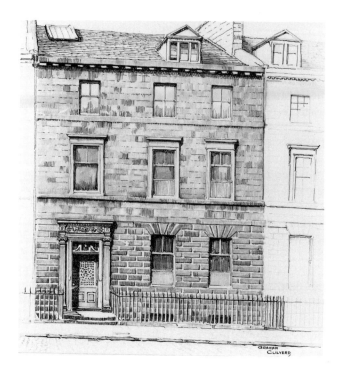

53   *Thirty-six, York Place, Edinburgh, the house of the Society's Scottish Branch.*

an outside body had challenged the right of the Society to perform certain acts, it might have been necessary to have the matter settled by law. But it was offering hostages to fortune to initiate a friendly action in this way. He may, of course, have made the mistake of thinking that the Pharmaceutical Society was bound to win. Both sides of the case were, after all, being prepared by the Society, and Jenkin's case was, to all except legal minds, incredibly feeble. The difficulty was that the Pharmaceutical Society was asking for too much. If the Society had won the case, any activity that it could conceivably have wished to undertake, would have been declared to be within its powers. Was it reasonable in that case for the Society to expect a favourable judgment?

The evidence suggests that Glyn-Jones did not leap before looking: he was pushed. There were Council members who wanted to stop him setting up the Joint Industrial Council. There were others who wanted to follow the Scots in setting up a separate organisation to further the commercial interests of proprietor pharmacists. Glyn-Jones was himself anxious to prevent this from happening. He saw the formation of the Scottish Pharmaceutical Federation not only as a threat to his vision of the Pharmaceutical Society as the all-inclusive organisation of pharmacists but, more immediately, as a danger to the continued existence of the Pharmaceutical Society. The Society was a voluntary organisation dependent on the subscriptions of those who joined primarily for the protection of their material interests. If new organisations were to be formed in Scotland and England to protect the trading and business activities of proprietor chemists, how could the Pharmaceutical Society survive? Could a Society which was held responsible for opening the register to unqualified dispensers and for imposing unwanted poisons regulations on chemists continue to attract pharmacists? What could be more frustrating for Glyn-Jones than to discover that just as he was preparing to merge the P.A.T.A. and the Chemists' Defence Association with the Pharmaceutical Society, the Scottish chemists were destroying the unity of the profession by setting up an independent and rival organisation?

The officers of the North British Branch of the Pharmaceutical Society were far from happy with the developments in Scotland. The Scottish Pharmaceutical Federation had its roots in the local "pharmaceutical associations" which flourished in many areas of Scotland, membership of which was not confined to members of the Pharmaceutical Society. The Federation was formed to "centralise and foster the general opinion of pharmacists" and "to do those things which it was said, owing to the limitations of the Charter, the Pharmaceutical Society could not do". The relationship between the Federation and the Society in Scotland was far from satisfactory. A Joint Committee of Reference had to be set up to "advise in any case of doubt or difficulty arising between the operations of the Executive of the North British Branch of the Pharmaceutical Society and the operations of the Scottish Pharmaceutical Federation". When J. Rutherford Hill, the secretary of the North British Branch, heard about the impending legal case in London, he wrote to George Mallinson, the assistant secretary of the Society, in terms which reveal his sympathy with Glyn-Jones' dilemma:

> Personally I regard this matter with very great regret. It is a sad and most melancholy state of affairs when members of any Society enter upon litigation of this kind which can only have originated in circumstances of hostility and ill-will. My experience has been that all such procedure leads to nothing but mischief, contention and injury to all parties and interests concerned.

The case of *Jenkin v. The Pharmaceutical Society* came before Mr. Justice Peterson in the Chancery Division of the High Court on Tuesday 19 October 1920.[5] Arthur Henry Jenkin had volunteered to act as plaintiff in the case and had been selected primarily because he was the only member of Council who was not connected with retail pharmacy. He was at the time the Head Dispenser of the City of London and East London Dispensary. In order to act as plaintiff he had to resign from the Council, but he was later re-elected and served as Treasurer of the Society from 1932 to his death in August 1934. He was secretary of the Guild of Public Pharmacists for the first ten years of its existence (1923–33). Although acting as plaintiff he did not allow the case to interfere with his annual holiday. Among the Society's records there is a picture postcard from France, dated 27 July 1920, addressed to Sir William Glyn-Jones. It reads:

> Do you mind sending me the result of the case to Hotel Chatelard, Montreux, Switzerland and I shall be there by the end of next week. Arthur H. Jenkin.

Sir William replied:

> I have just received an intimation that our case will not be reached this Session and that it will have to stand over until after the long vacation.

Jenkin sought an injunction to restrain the Council of the Pharmaceutical Society from undertaking certain activities. The Society had already applied part of its funds to promoting a Joint Industrial Council and proposed to spend further sums in its establishment and work. The Society also proposed to undertake various other activities, namely:

(1) to regulate the hours of business of members of the Society,

(2) to regulate the wages and conditions of employment as between masters and their employees who were members of the Society,

(3) to regulate the prices at which members shall sell their goods,

(4) to exercise the function of an employers' association,

(5) to insure and to effect insurance of members of the Society against errors, neglect and misconduct of employees, and against fire, burglary, damage to plate glass, and generally against insurable risks,

(6) to audit accounts, collect debts and take stock for its members,

(7) to provide and maintain an employment register and a register of unsatisfactory employees,

(8) to provide and supply information as to the commercial standing of persons and firms with whom members of the Society wish to transact business,

(9) to provide legal advice to members.

This list comprised all those activities already carried out by the P.A.T.A. and the Chemists' Defence Association and those intended to be performed by the new Scottish Pharmaceutical Federation. The list had been drawn up by Glyn-Jones to prepare the way for the fulfilment of his grand design to unite all pharmacists under the roof of the Pharmaceutical Society and thereby create a great voluntary professional organisation on the lines of the British Medical Association. He wanted the case to establish beyond doubt the Society's right to defend and promote the economic interests of its members. Yet it was not, in any way, his intention that the Society should devote itself exclusively to the task of safeguarding and improving the material rewards of the profession. On the contrary, he had equally ambitious plans to enhance the educational and scientific activities of the Society. He had, moreover, already done more to enlarge the Benevolent Fund than any previous member of the Society. But no one questioned the Society's right, under its Charter, to advance chemistry and pharmacy, to promote education, and to provide for a benevolent fund. The only object under scrutiny was "the protection of those who carry on the business of chemists and druggists".

Jenkin's case was presented by Sir Albion Richardson. The Pharmaceutical Society, he said, might be conveniently divided into two classes of members, whose interests were in conflict. The first class consisted of those chemists and druggists who were themselves proprietors of businesses; the second were those registered as qualified chemists and druggists who were employed by other people. The acts which the Society proposed to perform were things injurious to the employee class and solely for the benefit of the other class. A substantial part of the income of the Society consisted of subscriptions paid by its members, and the plaintiff sought to restrain the Society from applying this income to the benefit of one class only. The new powers which the Society sought, such as the formation of an Industrial Council, the insurance of members against fire, burglary, and other risks, the auditing of accounts, the keeping of an employment register, could only be for the benefit of the employer section of the Society's membership. The powers of the Society could not be used, as was now intended, for the protection of one class—the employers—against another class— the employed: the powers must be used for the protection of chemists and druggists as a whole.

The second line of argument was that the powers now sought had not been contemplated at the time the Charter was granted, and the majority of them, being in restraint of trade, would have been illegal in 1843. For seventy years the Society had made no attempt to do any of the things now proposed; it had never been suggested that the Society had the power to do them, nor, assuming that it had such power, that it was in the interests of the members to exercise it.

> Among the objects proposed was the formation of an Industrial Council . . . for the purpose of regulating wages, hours, and working conditions in the drug industry. That must mean a union with the powers of a trade union. There was no other way of regulating wages except by imposing penalties on people who accepted wages which were too low. That penalty might be expulsion from the society. With regard to the regulation of prices at which members should sell their goods, this pointed to a combination for controlling prices and providing that goods should not be sold under a certain price. That had not been contemplated by the Charter of Incorporation; it was quite a modern notion. It was a matter of common knowledge that in 1843 a combination to regulate prices would have been illegal. It was in restraint of trade, and did not become legal until after 1871.

"The real contest between plaintiff and defendants", concluded Sir Albion Richardson, "was as to whether the Pharmaceutical Society was entitled to convert itself into a trade union, with all the powers of a trade union, and all the purposes of a trade union".

The case for the Pharmaceutical Society had two distinct parts. In the first part an attempt was made to rebut the plaintiff's case. The second part queried the authority of the court to determine the question.

Alexander Macmorran, the Society's counsel, argued that the words in the Charter, "the protection of those who carry on the business of chemists and druggists", referred to a class of persons smaller than the total membership. There was, he said, no reason why a society democratically controlled by its members should not decide to take measures specifically to protect one section of the total membership.

> His submission was that there was a great distinction between the persons who carried on business as chemists and druggists and those who might be members of the Society; and the Society, governed as it was by the general meetings and by the Council, might very well, under its Charter, claim to have the right of protecting the interests of those who carried on the business of chemists and druggists, although that class was not the entire membership of the Society.

But very few of the activities the Society proposed to undertake would be restricted in their benefit to one section of the membership, and those that were so restricted, such as the regulation of prices, the effecting of insurance, and the auditing of accounts, "did not affect in any way the relation between employers and employees". Take, for example, the proposal to form a Joint Industrial Council, "within and under the control of the Society".

> If it is not within and under the control of the Society, it may be, and probably will be, undertaken by a body outside, and the Society, therefore, are in this position,

that they want to keep all the matters, so far as may be, which might be dealt with by an Industrial Council under their own control . . . That is really the inwardness of the suggestion with regard to the Industrial Council . . . The regulation of wages, hours, and working conditions does not operate only for the benefit of employers. The regulation of wages may be as much in the interests of those employed as in those of employers, and still more is that the case with regard to hours and working conditions. It is necessary to a very great extent in a trade like that of chemists and druggists that hours and working conditions should, as far as may be, be uniform—at least, uniform in particular districts. An Industrial Council might say to its members, "You shall not, except in cases of emergency and the like, keep open beyond a certain hour in the evening," or, "You may not employ your assistants for more than a certain number of hours a day." My Lord, it is for the protection of the business as a whole and the members of the business as a whole—or it may be so—that they should be prevented from undue competition with one another in the shape of wages, hours, and working conditions, the absence of which prevention might inflict serious injury upon persons employed as well upon the employers . . . Then the settlement of disputes between the different parties: surely it would be in the interests of all engaged in the business that the dispute, even if between employers and employees, should be settled as far as possible, and settled by an authoritative body . . . there was no suggestion that the Society's action in these directions was to be solely for the benefit of employers. With regard to the collection of statistics, clearly this was for the benefit of the whole of the trade; the improvement of health was rather for the benefit of persons employed than for employers, and the same observation might be made about the provision of special treatment, where necessary, for workers in the industry.

There was nothing in all this which could reasonably be said to be outside the functions of a Council who had undertaken to protect those who carried on the business of chemists and druggists, and all the Society sought to do was to establish such a committee under their own control and within the Society rather than allow the work to be done outside the Society and without their control, a control which had been exercised for the benefit of the public for a very great number of years. The same remark would apply to other powers it was sought to obtain.

The second part of the defendants' case concerned the validity of the plaintiff's action. It was argued that the doctrine of *ultra vires* cannot be applied to a corporation established by Royal Charter. If such a corporation exceeds its powers as set out in its charter, the remedy is not to apply to the Courts but to the Crown. Membership of the Society was perfectly voluntary. An ordinary member had the right to vote at general meetings and the right to vote in the election of members of Council who controlled the general government of the Society. If by any chance he found himself in a minority and felt aggrieved, his remedy was to leave the Society. In the present case, the plaintiff had actually been a member of the Council: but, instead of accepting the decisions of that body, he sought to come to the Court and restrain the rest of the Council from what they thought they were justified in doing in the conduct of the business of the whole Society. In so far as plaintiff sought to say that the proposed acts were *ultra vires* (beyond the powers), there was no such remedy open to him. If he had a remedy, it would be a remedy only resorted to in very serious cases; that was, to petition the Crown, under procedure similar to the old writ of *scire facias*, for the revocation of the Charter.

The other point ... was really a point of considerable substance—namely, assuming that in his Lordship's view some of the things were held to be *ultra vires*, whether or not there was any legal remedy ... The distinction between a statutory corporation and a chartered corporation was well known; a statutory corporation could do nothing except what it was expressly authorised to do, but a corporation by common law created by Charter could do everything that it was not forbidden to do ... Even if his Lordship had a doubt as to whether the purposes mentioned in the statement of claim were *ultra vires* in the ordinary sense in which the term was used, nevertheless, that did not entitle anybody, even a corporator, to come forward and say they were illegal because they were *ultra vires* and that he could take steps to prevent them being done ... There was no remedy in this or any court of law to restrain the acts complained of.

Mr. Justice Peterson gave his judgment on 27 October 1920.

The first question was whether a chartered society could be restrained from doing acts not prohibited but not expressly authorised by its Charter. Societies, whether incorporated or not, which owed their status to an Act of Parliament could not apply their funds to any purpose foreign to the purposes for which they had been established or embark on any undertaking in which they were not intended by Parliament to be concerned ... But corporations constituted by Royal Charter, and not dependent for constitution and status on an Act of Parliament, stood on a somewhat different footing. A corporation created by Charter at common law could do with its property all such things as an ordinary person could do, and even if the Charter expressly prohibited a particular act, the corporation could at common law do the act ... But if a corporation did anything which was prohibited or not authorised by the Charter, the Charter might be recalled by the Crown on proceedings under *scire facias*. Although there was this difference between a statutory company and a company incorporated by Charter, it did not follow that a member of a chartered company could not take proceedings to prevent the company doing acts outside the purpose of its Charter, which might lead to the destruction of the corporation by forfeiture of its Charter ... In my opinion the authorities justify me in holding that if the Society in the present case intends to do acts which are not authorised by its Charter, a member is entitled to ask for an injunction restraining the commission of acts outside the scope of the Charter, which may result in the forfeiture of the Charter and the destruction of the Society.

Mr. Justice Peterson then ruled that it was not within the powers or purposes of the Pharmaceutical Society to take part, or expend any of its funds, in the formation, establishment, maintenance or work of an Industrial Council. Moreover, the Society could neither undertake for its members, nor spend any part of its funds on, any of the following activities:
(1) the regulation of hours of business
(2) the regulation of wages and conditions of employment as between masters and their employees,
(3) the regulation of prices,
(4) the insurance of members.
By implication, the Society was prevented from acting as an employers' association.

There must be some legal justification for the judgment in the Jenkin case, but, from an historical point of view, it simply seems perverse. The manifest purpose of an Industrial Council was to regulate industrial relations fairly and justly. Its axiom was that neither employers nor employees should be disadvantaged. Its objectives were conciliation and social harmony. It would be difficult to conceive of an institution designed more explicitly to protect chemists and druggists as a whole. The Pharmaceutical Society, in terms of its Charter and by reason of its constitution, would seem to be the ideal organisation to establish and maintain an Industrial Council for the drug trade. By 1920 membership of the Pharmaceutical Society was available to all pharmacists on equal terms. When its Charter was granted in 1843, however, the Society was an association of proprietor chemists. One of its objectives, if not its primary objective, was to protect the trading interests of its members. From the time of its foundation onwards, it had consistently, but not exclusively, acted as the chemists and druggists' trade association. The Privy Council Office had no illusions about that. When Sir Almeric FitzRoy, the Clerk of the Privy Council, met Lord Rhondda, the President of the Local Government Board, in 1917, he "took occasion to impress upon him that his relations with the Pharmaceutical Society, and no less with the British Medical Association, must be governed by the fact that they were two of the closest trade unions to be found in the United Kingdom". Neither Sir Almeric FitzRoy nor his predecessor at the Privy Council for twenty years, Sir Charles Peel, had ever sought to challenge the Society's right to act in this way. They assumed its Charter gave it this function.[6]

There were many points in Mr. Justice Peterson's decision which might have formed the basis of an appeal. Several other chartered bodies, alarmed at the decision, pressed the Society to appeal against it, for it was a legal precedent applicable to all other chartered bodies. It established new law. Before the Jenkin case, chartered corporations assumed they could do as they pleased, that all their acts were valid. Mr. Justice Peterson's decision meant that, in future, any of their members would have the right to seek an injunction from the High Court to restrain the corporation from acting outside the terms of its charter or doing acts which infringed the general law. The Executive of the Society's North British Branch also pressed for an appeal. They pointed out that a decision of the Chancery Division of the High Court had no authority in Scottish law; it had only persuasive effect, unless an appeal were made to the House of Lords. The decision must also have been a bitter blow for Sir William Glyn-Jones. The decision meant that his immediate plans to establish a Joint Industrial Council for pharmacy had to be abandoned and that his long-term design to transform the Society into a great professional trade union like the B.M.A. would need to be reconsidered. Far from promoting the economic interests of proprietor chemists, the Pharmaceutical Society might now find itself competing for their allegiance and subscriptions with a new aggressive trade association, unshackled by professional statutory obligations.

Why did the Society not appeal? The answer must be that the majority of Council members had already got the decision they wanted. The proprietor chemists wanted to form their own independent trade union and follow the path taken by their Scottish confrères. They set about it with unseemly haste. A sub-committee of Council was immediately appointed to consider the Test case decision. Its terms of reference precluded the possibility of an appeal and assumed that a new national trade organisation would be established. The

368

sub-committee sat from 10.30 a.m. to 3.30 p.m. on Tuesday 9 November and drew up a report which was considered by a joint meeting of the Society's Council and the Local Associations Executive Committee on Wednesday 17 November. By the end of the year, only two months after the judge's decision, the Retail Pharmacists' Union had been formed.

Glyn-Jones did all he could to limit the damage that the Jenkin's decision might inflict on the Society. He worked hard to ensure that the Retail Pharmacists' Union remained in a close and co-operative relationship with the Pharmaceutical Society. He released the senior of the Society's two assistant secretaries, George A. Mallinson, to become secretary

---

The Jenkin Case 1920: The Pharmaceutical Society and the Retail Pharmacists' Union

---

After the decision in the Jenkin case, a sub-committee set up by the Council of the Pharmaceutical Society recommended the formation of a new organisation to handle the collective business interests of proprietor chemists and suggested that its "fundamental objects" should be distinguished from those of the Pharmaceutical Society in the following way:

Pharmaceutical Society

(a) Advancement of chemistry and pharmacy as science and art.

(b) Education of those who should practise chemistry and pharmacy.

(c) Benevolence.

(d) Anything that affects the qualification, functions or privileges which are, or should be, restricted to pharmacists.

(e) Administration, including examination and registration under the Pharmacy Acts.

(f) Protection other than as above of those carrying on business on their own account.

Trade Organisation

(a) The regulation of the relation
   (i) between employees and employers,
         or
   (ii) between employers and employers.

(b) The imposing of restrictive conditions on the conduct of trade or business.

(c) The provision of benefits to members.

(d) Matters generally affecting the trading interests of pharmacists carrying on business as such, distinguished from functions restricted by law to pharmacists.

---

of the R.P.U. And just as, in 1493, Pope Alexander VI divided the New World between Spain and Portugal, so, in 1920, Sir William Glyn-Jones drew a line of demarcation between the territory of the Pharmaceutical Society and that of the Retail Pharmacists' Union. The boundaries, created in 1920, still hold today, despite the occasional border dispute in the interval.

A few years after the Test case, Glyn-Jones recalled the events that followed the decision and concluded that all was for the best in a world where everything is a necessary evil. The Council of the Pharmaceutical Society, he pointed out, "could not have prevented the establishment of an independent, and perhaps rival, organisation" of master pharmacists on trade union lines.

> In fact, there was already in existence an organisation, the C.D.A., powerful by reason of its numbers and resources, which would not have stood aside and allowed the creation of a third national organisation of pharmacists. So far from adopting any dog-in-the-manger attitude, the Council took the initiative in the negotiations which led to the creation of the tripartite organisation of the P.A.T.A., C.D.A., and R.P.U. The respective activities of the old Society and the new body were mutually agreed upon on more or less well defined lines. Confusion of functions, overlapping activities, divided counsels, were avoided, and instead of rival organisations competing with each other for kudos, two powerful allies, each responsible for their sphere of work, are now working side by side, and between them are covering every need of the pharmacist, whatever may be his sphere, which can be met by national organisation. The division of labour based on the principle of specialisation has rendered possible a great advance both in the essential and fundamental chartered objects of the Society. Its statutory, legal, educational, and scientific work upon which all else in pharmaceutical organisation depends, has been advanced to a degree perhaps previously impossible, but the change has led to a wonderful increase in the protection and enhancement of the trading business interests which are being so well developed by the R.P.U. Never, taking the whole field of legitimate nationally organised effort, has pharmacy been so well served as it now is.

When the Retail Pharmacists' Union was first set up, it was housed in the offices of the Chemists' Defence Association and the P.A.T.A. in Temple Avenue, London, E.C.4. It was not only the same premises that the organisations shared. Since the R.P.U. would need to offer indemnity insurance and legal defence to proprietor chemists, it made sense, to avoid duplication and possible conflict of interest, to make use of the C.D.A., the existing and effective organisation in this field. To maintain continuity of administration for the C.D.A., some adjustment was necessary to the Central Executive Committee of the R.P.U. According to the original rules, the Committee was to consist of 21 (later reduced to 18) members elected on a territorial basis. It was agreed, however, to enlarge the Committee for the first three years, to include the original eight C.D.A. directors up to the expiry of their terms of office. As soon as a suitable building was found nearer Bloomsbury Square the R.P.U. and C.D.A. moved into 19 Tavistock Square, W.C.1. The P.A.T.A. settled in next door at Number 18. Ironically both buildings were later demolished to make way for the present headquarters of the British Medical Association.

The Retail Pharmacists' Union , later, in 1932, renamed the National Pharmaceutical Union, and, since 1977, the National Pharmaceutical Association, was, as its constitution and rules stated, "a union of retail employer chemists for the protection of trade interests". It covered much more than responsibility for wages, prices, hours of business and working conditions which had been denied to the Pharmaceutical Society by the Test case. It took over from the Society the representation of pharmacists in all matters coming under the National Health Insurance Act, including the Central Checking Bureau. The Executive Committee of the R.P.U. were permitted by the constitution to constitute themselves as a sub-committee to which the Company Chemists Association could nominate representatives for the purpose of dealing with wages and hours of labour and National Health Insurance matters, and it was through this provision that the Central N.H.S. (Chemist Contractors) Committee was formed in 1948. In 1976 this became the Pharmaceutical Services Negotiating Committee. Membership of the R.P.U. included membership of the P.A.T.A. and of the C.D.A. Among other benefits to members were a number of business services—trade mark registration, debt collection, help in stocktaking (previously a much neglected activity among pharmacists) and an enquiry service.

The early years of the R.P.U. were not free from storms and stress. George Mallinson had to fight opposition from without and within the R.P.U. He was an inspired choice as secretary. A few months after taking over he was called to the Bar after late night study. Within the Pharmaceutical Society he had gained a reputation for drive and organising ability in local association work which stood him in good stead in his new role. He built up a large membership in a very short time, by stumping the country, stirring up local initiative and organising conferences at heavy cost. For two years the R.P.U. showed a deficit, but Mallinson's effort was worth while. By 1925 the R.P.U. had 7,000 member shops and 115 branches and by 1930 the membership comprised nine-tenths of the chemists' shops in England and Wales.

Under Mallinson new services were continually being added. In 1922 the Chemists' Mutual Insurance Company was launched, providing cover at low premiums for the ordinary hazards of life such as fire, burglaries and flood, as the C.D.A. did for the special hazards of the chemist's business. Within five years the C.M.I. had prospered sufficiently to be able to offer policyholders a rebate on their premium renewal. In 1928 the chain of protection was completed by the creation of the Chemists' Sickness and Provident Society, offering sickness insurance and retirement provision. Mallinson was particularly energetic in looking after the business needs of the pharmacist. In October 1924 he launched a Business Training Course for chemists' assistants. For a fee of five guineas they received a five month correspondence course covering advertising, commercial law, retail selling, book-keeping, shop management and window dressing. In the same year, the chairman of the Business Services Section of the R.P.U. gave an address on salesmanship, which he described as the "weakest weapon in the pharmacist's armoury". What he said on that occasion neatly encapsulates the message of the R.P.U.

> If a customer walks into a chemist's shop and asks for some Epsom salts, he will probably be asked "Yes, Sir, about twopenny worth?" If he walks into a tobacconist's and asks for a packet of cigarettes he won't be asked, "Yes, Sir, twopenny Woodbines?" He will be shown an expensive variety about 2s. or 2s. 6d. The tobacconist is not out to help the customer to save money—that is not his job. But chemists do it over and over again. The salesmanship course deals with this subject as the ordinary trader sees it, and perusal by a pharmacist will be a wide education, and the adoption of the best principles will unquestionably react upon his pocket most beneficially.[7]

The formation of the Retail Pharmacists' Union left the Pharmaceutical Society free to concentrate on the furtherance of the professional as distinct from the commercial interests of pharmacists. The working agreement between the two organisations came into prominence again in 1951 when the Society was proposing to seek a Supplemental Charter.

371

The main change in the Charter was to replace the clause dealing with the protection of those carrying on the business of chemists and druggists by one which referred to maintaining the honour and safeguarding the interests of members in the exercise of their profession. The National Pharmaceutical Union had the idea that the change was being made to nullify the effect of the Jenkin decision and this was raised with the Society's Council. On 2 May 1951 F.W. Adams, then Secretary and Registrar of the Society, wrote to assure the N.P.U. that the Society would continue to adhere to the agreement of 1920 "in deciding what are the proper functions of the two bodies . . . whatever the terms of its Charter". The letters exchanged on the matter were published in the *Pharmaceutical Journal* in 1951. The Society's original Charter of 1843 was revoked, except insofar as it incorporated the Society, by a Supplemental Charter in 1953. The objects of the Society were slightly modified to reflect changes in its status and in the practice of pharmacy. The 1953 Charter now lays down the objects as (1) to advance chemistry and pharmacy, (2) to promote pharmaceutical education and the application of pharmaceutical knowledge, (3) to maintain the honour and safeguard and promote the interests of the members in the exercise of the profession of pharmacy, (4) to provide relief for distressed persons.

At the same time as the Society was acquiring its new Charter, Boots Cash Chemists were introducing new commercial practices into retail pharmacy. In 1952 they opened their first "super store" which incorporated the idea of self-service derived from the drug stores in the U.S.A. The Society immediately protested. Throughout its existence the Pharmaceutical Society has consistently maintained that

> drugs and medicines are not ordinary commercial articles for which the limit of the market may safely be the desire and capacity of the public to purchase them. It is not in the public interest that they should be subject to the ordinary conditions of trade and any and every method adopted to induce the public to purchase them.[8]

Encouraging customers to select their own medicines (including Part 1 poisons) from the shelves and take them to a cash desk was seen as a development which, at the very least, debased the image of pharmacy. A High Court action (*The Pharmaceutical Society v. Boots Cash Chemists (Southern) Ltd.*, 1953) was fought over the technical issue of whether the sale of medicines was being conducted under the supervision of a pharmacist. The Society lost the case and the Court of Appeal upheld the decision in favour of Boots.[9]

Two years later the Society's Council appointed a committee to examine the current state of the general practice of pharmacy with particular reference to the maintenance of professional standards. In 1961 the committee submitted its report of 75 paragraphs and 24 recommendations. The full report was published in the *Pharmaceutical Journal* in April 1963. Arising from the report and its recommendations, a motion was put to the Annual General Meeting in 1965 directing that new pharmacies must be situated in physically distinct premises and must confine their trading activity to the sale of pharmaceutical, professional and "traditional" chemists' goods, (i.e. toilet goods, cosmetics and photographic materials). Owing to the large attendance at the A.G.M. no vote could be taken and a special general meeting to consider the motion was arranged for 25 July 1965 in the Royal Albert Hall. R.C.M. Dickson, who was Retail Director of Boots at this time, sought an injunction to restrain the holding of the meeting. He also claimed that the motion was outside the scope of the Society's powers and, being in restraint of trade, had no legal force. His application

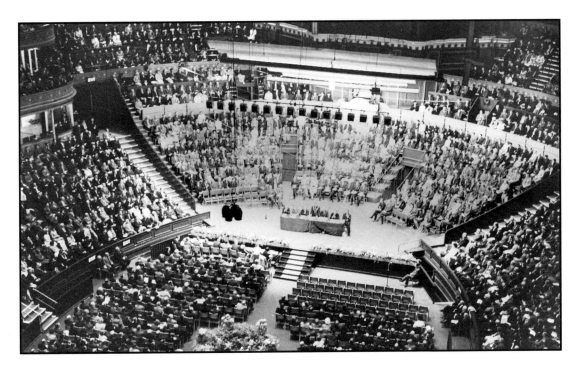

54 *Special General Meeting of the Pharmaceutical Society at the Albert Hall, 25 July 1965.*

for an injunction was refused by the High Court on an undertaking being given by the Society that no attempt would be made to give the motion effect until after the judgment in the action to determine whether the object of the motion was *ultra vires*. The meeting in the Albert Hall endorsed the Society's motion by 5020 votes to 1336.

The Society was unable during the hearing of the case *(The Pharmaceutical Society v. Dickson)* to satisfy the courts that the professional side of a pharmacy business was adversely affected by other activities. The High Court ruled that "it is not within the powers, purposes or objects of the Pharmaceutical Society . . . to enforce . . . the provisions of the motion . . . on the ground that the said provisions are in restraint of trade". The Court of Appeal upheld this decision and in 1968 the House of Lords affirmed it. The House of Lords held that the motion restricting the sale of certain goods in pharmacies was *ultra vires* as it was not related to the only relevant main object of the Society, namely, maintaining the honour and safeguarding and promoting the professional interests of members. Moreover, the proposed restrictions were in restraint of trade and had not been shown to be reasonable.

As in the Jenkin case, the Society's powers under its Charter had been challenged and the doctrine of *ultra vires* invoked. The case had no perceptible effect on the Society's functions: its control over the professional, as distinct from the trading, aspect of pharmacy was not in any way affected. The Society's Council had been made to recognise its limitations at heavy financial cost. Once again, other chartered bodies expressed concern and indignation at the ruling which affected them all. *The Pharmaceutical Society v. Dickson* was the first case where the courts have definitely stated that the doctrine of "restraint of trade" could apply to a profession. Lord Morris of Borth-y-Gest said:

> The fact that the society is incorporated by charter does not entitle it to impose on its members a restraint of trade that is unreasonable and unjustified.

* * *

No individual, other than Jacob Bell, has had a greater influence upon the development of the Pharmaceutical Society than Sir William Glyn-Jones. "Of all the leaders in the history of the organised pharmaceutical body politic in this country", wrote the editor of the *Pharmaceutical Journal*, "none has made so deep and lasting an impression on its structure and functions, alike on the business and professional side".[10] The seven years (1918-1926) of his secretaryship saw the establishment of compulsory courses of instruction for the examinations, the opening of schools of pharmacy under public authorities and the institution by the University of London of a degree in pharmacy. It was Glyn-Jones, in association with W.E. Dixon, who prepared the case that forced the General Medical Council in 1928 to appoint a Pharmacopoeia Commission (with Dr. C.H. Hampshire, formerly chief pharmacist at University College Hospital as full-time secretary) to take responsibility for the preparation of the new edition of the *British Pharmacopoeia*, with due recognition of the contribution of pharmacists. It was the vigour of Glyn-Jones that gave reality to Edmund White's advocacy of the establishment of the Society's Pharmacological Laboratories. In 1924 a Therapeutic Substances bill was being considered by parliament. That year Edmund White, the chairman of the British Pharmaceutical Conference, used his address to refer to "this newer materia medica" as "a sort of 'no man's land' between medicine and pharmacy" and asked:

> Is it not possible to foresee the Pharmaceutical Society recognised as the suitable public body to be put in charge of such work as is contemplated by the Therapeutic Substances Bill? At any rate, the Council should carefully explore the situation before the territory is staked out and the opportunity lost.

In the following year the bill was enacted. Glyn-Jones promptly took steps to set up a department for testing the substances mentioned in the schedules. The Society's pharmacological laboratories were formally opened on 16 June 1926 by the Minister of Health, Neville Chamberlain. The Therapeutic Substances Act (1925) and the Therapeutic Substances Regulations (1931) controlled the manufacture and importation of therapeutic substances such as vaccines, sera, toxins and insulin of which the manufacture for sale had to be conducted under licence from the Ministry of Health or other appropriate body.

Glyn-Jones was particularly pleased that a new edition of the *British Pharmaceutical Codex*, to keep pace with developments in therapeutics and with pharmaceutical practice, had been produced during his term as secretary. "Seven thousand copies were first printed and quickly sold, and over fifteen hundred of the next reprint of 5,000 have already been sold", he reported in 1924.

> The work has immensely increased the prestige of the Society amongst medical and scientific workers. Incidentally, it has produced a profit of between three and four thousand pounds, which the Council, instead of merging in its general funds, has set aside for purposes of research and systematic work in the preparation of future

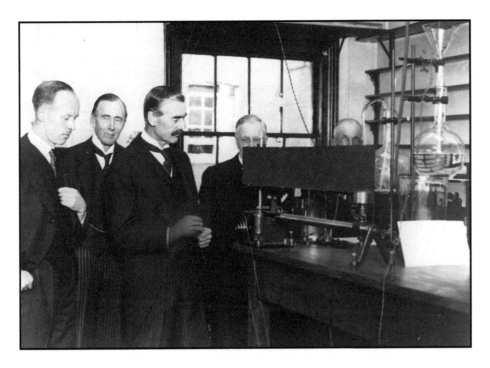

55 *The new pharmacological laboratories, 17 Bloomsbury Square, 16 June 1926, opened by the Rt. Hon. Neville Chamberlain, Minister of Health. With F.E. Bilson, President 1926 – 7, Dr J.H. Burn, Sir H. Rolleston and P.F. Rowsell.*

editions . . . the Council . . . has enlisted and co-opted leading pharmaceutical authorities on to its new Science Committee, to which it has delegated not only work, but large powers of initiation. The Society was never so well equipped for fulfilling one of its principal chartered objects, "The Advancement of Chemistry and Pharmacy," as it is today.

Glyn-Jones believed that it was the Society's duty to see that, as conditions changed, the position of pharmacists in new spheres of activity was secured. In 1924 he noted that pharmacy was being carried on more and more outside of chemists' shops— in school clinics, maternity centres, child-welfare centres, TB sanatoria, and VD clinics; and that private paying patients were receiving treatment increasingly in voluntary hospitals instead of at expensive private nursing homes. Pharmacists, he believed, must be ready to seize such opportunities. As medical practice became more reliant on pathological investigation, the pharmacist should become the laboratory diagnostician for the general practitioner. A growing number of pharmacists were being employed outside of retail business: it was the duty of the Pharmaceutical Society to look after the interests of all of them.

Sir William Glyn-Jones admired and envied the power and prestige of the British Medical Association. During his lifetime, the B.M.A. completely overshadowed all other professional associations in the field of medicine. By the end of the First World War, three-quarters of British medical practitioners were members. The success of the B.M.A. seemed to be directly related to its ingenious constitution, the unique feature of which was the pivotal role of its local organisation. The Pharmaceutical Society consisted of a council, in which the real power was vested, and a general meeting which was supposed to afford the members as a whole an opportunity of expressing their views. But the heavy commitment of time and energy demanded of council members meant that the councils were seldom truly representative and in touch with the members, and the general meeting was a cumbersome and untrustworthy method of ascertaining the trends of opinion. In Glyn-Jones' eyes, the B.M.A. had overcome these problems. Its local organisation consisted of divisions grouped in branches. The effective control of the Association lay with the Representative Body consisting chiefly of delegates elected by the divisions. The Representative Body, with between two and three hundred members, was the B.M.A.'s parliament. It was here that important issues facing the profession were raised: the attendance was always good, the debates keen.

When Glyn-Jones became secretary of the Pharmaceutical Society in 1918 he began the work of incorporating the best features of the B.M.A.'s constitution into the structure of the Pharmaceutical Society. The local associations of chemists and druggists had demonstrated their value during the parliamentary struggles of 1908 and 1911. The Local Associations Executive had helped the Society unstintedly during the Great War and had, until the creation of the Retail Pharmacists' Union , represented the chemists in the N.H.I. scheme. Their commitment and dynamism were waiting to be harnessed to the Society's chariot. By 1921 Glyn-Jones' strategy for achieving this was put into operation. An Organisation Committee was set up which submitted to Council a scheme for the formation of branches of the Society throughout the country. Early in 1922 the Council adopted the scheme and during that and the following year the existing local associations either converted themselves into Pharmaceutical Society branches or formed such branches by affiliation while retaining their own identity. By 1924 there were 114 branches and every member of the Society automatically became a member of one or other of these branches. "Every member is made conscious of his membership", wrote Glyn-Jones, "and pharmacists who are not members will feel more and more out of place. The Society will be recognised by all *more* as a living force and *less* as a paper organisation".

But Glyn-Jones' plan went much further than this. His idea was to graft onto the existing structure of the Pharmaceutical Society, an annual meeting of branch representatives and a peripatetic scientific jamboree in the style of the B.M.A.'s annual conference. He did not have to look beyond the already flourishing British Pharmaceutical Conference to find the solution to his problem. The British Pharmaceutical Conference was an independent organisation which had during its fifty-nine years consistently sponsored scientific research and had placed on record in its *Year-Book of Pharmacy* the principal results of original work that invariably attained a high standard. Its annual conferences celebrated the progress of scientific pharmacy in Britain.[11] Glyn-Jones simply decided to take it over. In January 1922 he sent a letter to its Executive informing them of the adoption by the Society's Council of the recommendations of the Organisation Committee.

> The Society shall organise at least once a year, a National Conference, not necessarily meeting in the same place each year, and the Conference shall consist of delegates officially appointed to represent Branches of the Society. The Conference shall deal with the Science and Practice of Pharmacy, and will be

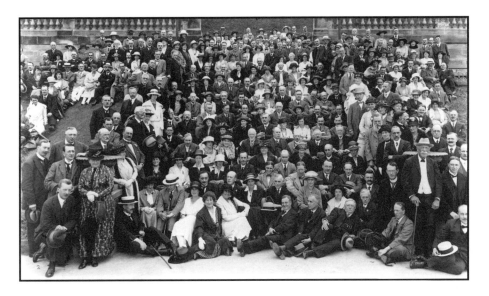

56 *Delegates at Scarborough, British Pharmaceutical Conference, 15 June 1921.*

concerned with the general advancement of the objects of the Pharmaceutical Society.

The letter went on to suggest that, since this development must "have a bearing on the work of the British Pharmceutical Conference", its Executive and the Council should get together to discuss it. Although the President of the Society and five other members of its Council were members of the Conference Executive, the letter from Glyn-Jones came as a bolt from the blue. Surprise soon turned to anger. At a meeting of representatives of both bodies on 1 February, the President of the Society, E.T. Neathercoat, outlined the Council's proposals: the crucial decisions had already been taken and were not subject to negotiation. As a result of the decision in the Jenkin case, he said, the Society was now free to devote more attention to the first of its chartered objects, the advancement of chemistry and pharmacy. Council had decided to form local branches of the Society and to hold a national conference which would deal with the domestic affairs of the Society as well as the subjects dealt with by the British Pharmaceutical Conference. There would, therefore, in future be two conferences, unless the members of the British Pharmaceutical Conference agreed to unite in forming one conference under the Society's auspices. If that were the case, the name "British Pharmaceutical Conference" would be retained. The Executive could then form an Expert Committee to which Council, while retaining the power of veto, would delegate the duty of running the Conference. Arrangements would be made for those who were not pharmacists to attend the Conference and assist in its work. The Society would take over responsibility for the production and publication of the *Year-Book of Pharmacy*, the terms of supply to members and others to be decided later. If these proposals were approved in principle, a small joint committee of Council and Executive would draw up a detailed scheme for presentation to the 1922 Conference in Nottingham. The Council "gratefully acknowledge the splendid work that has been done by members and non-members of the Society" in the Conference in the past, and were anxious to secure their active co-operation in the future.

A recent chairman of the Conference, H.G. Rolfe, has commented that if the Council had wished to arouse opposition to a merger, they could hardly have acted more effectively. The policy adopted by the Council—amalgamate or else, the decision has been taken—was, in his view, most unfortunate. One cannot, he adds, say the objective was undesirable, but the tactics employed were certainly unwise. This much cannot be denied. Nonetheless, Glyn-Jones' action achieved its objective swiftly and decisively. At the Nottingham meeting of the British Pharmaceutical Conference in the summer of 1922 the members voted by a large majority to accept the Pharmaceutical Society's main proposals and the merger went ahead.

Difficulties inevitably developed after such a "shot-gun wedding". One of the inducements for the amalgamation offered by Glyn-Jones was that the Society would send delegates from their branches to the Conference. However the arrangements for the meetings of branch representatives and for deciding the subjects to be discussed were handled directly by the Society and quite separately from other Conference matters. This produced an unfortunate dichotomy in the Conference and a declining attendance of delegates at the whole Conference, which was not remedied until 1956. The scientific status of the Conference continued to grow, however, and the holding of these annual meetings performed the invaluable function of presenting pharmacy as a scientific discipline to the general public. In 1928 the *Year-Book of Pharmacy* was incorporated in a quarterly journal—the *Quarterly Journal of Pharmacy and Allied Sciences*—the title being changed the following year to the *Quarterly Journal of Pharmacy and Pharmacology*. Facilities were thus provided for the publication of original scientific work other than that presented as papers at the annual Conference. Gradually the number of papers from other sources increased so that in 1949 the *Quarterly Journal* became the monthly *Journal of Pharmacy and Pharmacology*. At first the Conference papers were published over several monthly numbers but now they are published in one number as a supplement to the Journal. "The future of the Conference and its continuation as a useful body in the national life", declared its chairman, Dr. C.H. Hampshire, in 1933, "will rest principally upon its reputation as a means for the publication of scientific research in pharmacy, and for the discussion of technical problems". The reputation of the Conference and of its associated Journal has grown considerably since 1933.

In the spring of 1926 William Glyn-Jones threw away the security and routines of the secretaryship of the Pharmaceutical Society to take on the job of organising the Proprietary Articles Trade Association of Canada. At an age when most men would be well content to rest on their laurels, Glyn-Jones, with his usual dynamic intensity, threw himself into this new venture. This formidable undertaking, entered upon with characteristic buoyancy and hopefulness, was carried through with remarkable expedition and success. In just over a year, he had organised retail and wholesale druggists and drug manufacturers in Canada in a comprehensive organisation to maintain the retail prices of chemists' goods. The Canadian P.A.T.A. was to prove his last and least enduring success. On 9 September 1927 he died in Vancouver from cerebral haemorrhage. At the end of the year, the Commissioner

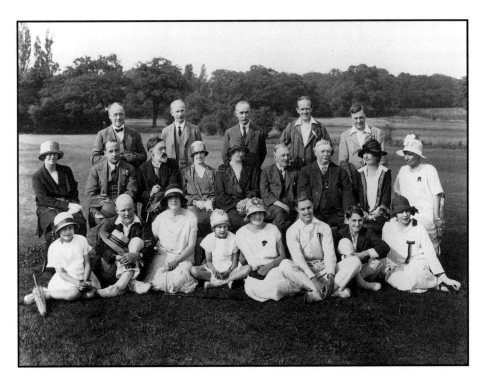

57   *Group including Sir William Glyn-Jones, participants, organisers and family members taking part in the annual event for the Maws Challenge Shield Competition, organised for pharmaceutical associations in London at the Maws Sports Ground, Monken Hadley Estate, New Barnet, 1925.*

under the Combines Investigation Act of 1910 declared the P.A.T.A. illegal, being a collusive arrangement to impose a system of resale price maintenance. Commenting on Glyn-Jones' work in creating the Canadian P.A.T.A., the editor of the *Pharmaceutical Journal* wrote:

> But this undertaking, an heroic one for a man who all his life through had been overwrought in mind and body, gave the finishing stroke to the busy brain that had seldom had a respite from strain and stress in all the years of Sir William's public life. And yet he died, as he would have wished, had there been any choice given to him, in full activity of mind, and with an undiminished zest for life and the labour which he loved.

* * *

In July 1926 Lord Balfour, Lord President of the Council, appointed a distinguished Departmental Committee "to consider and report whether any modifications are necessary or desirable in the Poisons and Pharmacy Acts".[12] On the request of the Committee, Sir William Glyn-Jones, at great inconvenience to himself, prepared a detailed memorandum on the Acts and their administration. His intimate experience of the working of the Acts invested his evidence with an especial value and authority, which were acknowledged by the

Committee at the time and which make his views worthy of careful study today.

The subject matter of the Poisons and Pharmacy Acts may be classified into (1) restrictions upon the sales of poisons and the practice of pharmacy and (2) the constitution and functions of the Pharmaceutical Society. Whether this law requires amendment or not, he wrote, "it most certainly needs codifying". Since its beginning in 1851 it has "been very much a matter of compromise between differing views and conflicting interests". The view that detailed regulations are necesary for the storage and sale of poisons has contrasted with the view that the safety of the public is best secured by having poisons dispensed and supplied only by suitably educated persons. It has not been easy to impose adequate restrictions on the sale of dangerous substances used in medicines without unduly hampering their use for non-medicinal purposes. In legislating it has always been difficult to reconcile the interests of medical men and pharmacists. The founders of the Pharmaceutical Society were primarily concerned to provide "an adequately trained body of persons qualified as efficient pharmacists", but the Poisons Acts were attempts to meet a demand for safeguards from the misuse of poisons.

The Departmental Committee, urged Glyn-Jones, should be exhaustive and comprehensive in its enquiry. It should consider the fundamental question, do we need pharmacists at all or can medical practitioners do the job?

> It should be decided whether there is, in connection with the science and art of medicine, need for a separate class of persons, constituting a profession allied with medicine, whose functions would be the manufacture and supply, including dispensing, of materia medica, by which I mean all the material used by the medical profession for purposes of diagnosis and treatment. If there is need of such a class of persons, what is to be their sphere of work, and should that work be confined to persons registered as having given evidence of their fitness and qualfication for it? Can the position of those to be engaged in that work be made sufficiently remunerative and attractive to justify the expenditure of the necessary time and money on the part of those who are to qualify for it? . . . On the other hand, can it be said that here, unlike other countries abroad, for the purposes of the practice of medicine there is not need for such a separate class or profession as pharmacists? Is the medical practitioner able and willing to undertake all the duties of the pharmacist, including pharmaceutical research, standardisation, both chemical and physiological, as well as the dispensing of the medicines which he and other physicians prescribe? If so, the course which the Pharmaceutical Society and the leaders in pharmacy are now following had better be abandoned.

Pharmacy and poison laws in this country will never be satisfactory, argued Glyn-Jones, until these main principles are settled.

> In my opinion . . . there is an amount of specialised work to be done which will justify the existence of a separate pharmaceutical profession, the members of which will need a fairly liberal general education, and will require a knowledge of , and training in, several sciences to the extent possessed by the present holders of University science degrees . . . To such persons exclusively should be entrusted the control of "chemists' shops" where alone, subject to exceptions to meet emergencies or the needs of sparsely populated areas, physicians' prescriptions should be dispensed and potent drugs and dangerous poisons sold by retail . . . What is needed is that the Legislature should decide what constitutes the business

of a "chemist and druggist" as distinct from other businesses and then prohibit its being undertaken by others than pharmacists.

The central authority for the purposes of the Poisons and Pharmacy Acts is at present the Pharmaceutical Society acting under the supervision, "or rather subject to the veto", of the Privy Council. The Society has administered the Acts well despite the complexities of the task created by their patchwork and makeshift character.

> For over eighty years, the Society has at considerable cost to itself, administered the Pharmacy Acts better ... than they could have been administered by any existing body or Government Department, seeing that there has been no such Department which has possessed the necessary technical knowledge and experience. In so doing the Society has rendered a material service to the State.

The basic dilemma of the Pharmaceutical Society is that it "has had to act as both the General Medical Council and the British Medical Association of Pharmacy". It has had to protect its members' professional and commercial interests and at the same time act as a registering, prosecuting, rule-making and disciplinary authority.

> In my opinion, the establishment of a Board of Pharmacy, with, generally speaking, somewhat similar powers and duties to those possessed by the G.M.C. and the Dental Board, is required. That Board, though not itself examining, would control the standard of training and examinations. It would make such regulations as are necessary for governing the storage and sale of poisons and the performance of the functions of the pharmacist. It would frame the Schedule of Poisons, and be the Prosecuting Authority for the enforcement of the provisions of the Pharmacy Acts and of the Regulations made thereunder. If such a body existed, it would be possible to make provision for needed disciplinary powers over those who are registered, and to give to that body the exercise of such powers. It is essential that such a Board should be mainly composed of pharmacists. The whole Board should be appointed by the Government. It might be well to arrange that some of the members should be the nominees of the Pharmaceutical Society, the General Medical Council, and the Universities. The bye-laws and regulations made by the Board would be subject to the approval of the Privy Council ... The expenses of the Board ... could be met out of registration fees, initial and annual.

The Board of Pharmacy would become the regulatory agency for the practice of pharmacy. Its authority would extend to all registered pharmacists whether or not they were members of the Pharmaceutical Society. Glyn-Jones was not in the least suggesting that pharmacists should be free from control, surveillance and discipline. On the contrary he was advocating a more effective regulatory system.

> It cannot, I think, be denied that a body consisting of members who have voluntarily joined it largely for the protection of their trade and professional interests, governed by a Council elected only by those members, is not suitable to act as an examining, registering, prosecuting and rule-making authority. There must always be at least a suspicion of partisanship.

Removing the Poisons Schedule from the control of the Council would end the accusations that the Society added substances to the list merely to enhance the chemists' monopoly of their sale. The establishment of a Board of Pharmacy would remove the main sources of friction between the Council and the members of the Society. The difficulties encountered in the past in trying to persuade the members to adopt the regulations for the storage and dispensing of poisons, and to agree to changes in the scope and character of the qualifying examination and to the imposition of curricula and periods of training would not recur. No longer would the Society have the odious task of disciplining and prosecuting its own members. The Society would be relieved of the incongruous obligation to devise and administer regulations, which have the force of law, not only for its own members but for all registered pharmacists. All these unpleasant and unpopular functions would be taken over by the Board of Pharmacy.

For Glyn-Jones the principal argument for the creation of a Board of Pharmacy was the effect it would have on the Pharmaceutical Society.

> If these changes were made, the Pharmaceutical Society would be free to protect and enhance the interests of its members, without the limitations at present imposed upon it as a body possessing statutory powers to be exercised primarily in the interest of the public as a whole.

The Pharmaceutical Society would be rejuvenated. The Council, untramelled by statutory obligations, could respond unashamedly to the members' demands. Dependent for its survival and prosperity upon its ability to recruit members, the Society would produce leaders who pursued policies attractive to the pharmaceutical constituency. The Pharmaceutical Society would be transformed into a great voluntary professional association. Once the Board of Pharmacy had been established, the Society would be left with all its major professional activities intact. It would still continue to conduct examinations but they would no longer be the only qualifying examinations.

> The Pharmaceutical Society would conduct examinations as also would any University where a curriculum and examination satisfactory to the Board of Pharmacy were provided.

The Society would remain an educational and scientific institution. The School of Pharmacy, the library and museum, the British Pharmaceutical Conference, the laboratories, the Society's publications (The *Pharmaceutical Journal*, the *British Pharmaceutical Codex*, The *Year-Book of Pharmacy*) and its involvement in the revision of the *British Pharmacopoeia* would not be adversely affected in any way. The Benevolent Fund would remain. The Society could pursue all of its chartered objectives. But it would also be able to take up again the commercial and trade union activities which had been removed after the decision in the Jenkin case.

> Such a change would make possible a fusion of the Society, the Retail Pharmacists' Union, and the Chemists' Defence Association, should the members of these respective bodies desire it.

The damage caused by the Jenkin case could be repaired. The whole of the resources of the Society could be brought into play to defend the professional and material interests of members wherever and however they practised pharmacy. The Pharmaceutical Society would become the pharmaceutical body militant here on earth. No pharmacist would be able to afford to be outside its ranks. The unity of the statutory register and the list of members of the Pharmaceutical Society would be achieved.

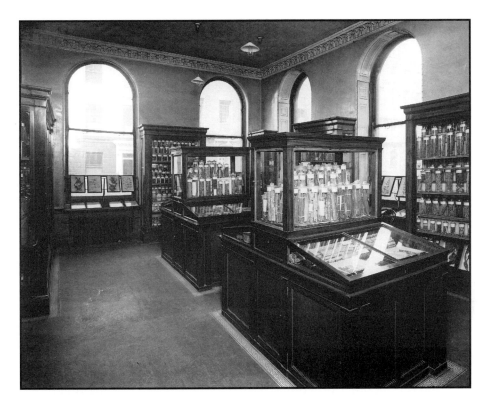

58 *Museum room no. 2, first floor, 17 Bloomsbury Square. Taken in 1931/2, displaying materia medica collections and mounted herbarium specimens.*

The agenda which Sir William Glyn-Jones had set for the Departmental Committee on the Poisons and Pharmacy Acts went way beyond the limits set by the Privy Council Office. The Committee owed its origin to poisons and not to pharmacy. At their first and second meetings the members of the Committee recorded their view that their terms of reference "did not permit the extension of their inquiry to matters unconnected with poisons, except in so far as those matters were implied in or were immediately subsidiary to questions connected with poisons". The principal consequence of this decision was the refusal of the Committee to consider the general question of dispensing medicine or to define what the proper function of the pharmacist should be. The Committee was anxious not to arouse the opposition of the medical profession. It studiously avoided recommending that the dispensing of medicines should be reserved to the pharmacist. In spite of lip-service to the ideal of protecting the public, there was no attempt to prevent a medicine containing poison being dispensed by the person who prescribed it. No provision was made to prevent the dispensing of poisons by unqualified persons in doctors' surgeries, nor to ensure the inspecting of doctors' surgeries and hospital dispensaries where poisons were stored and dispensed.

The Departmental Committee owed its existence to a desire by certain government departments to bring the scheduling of poisons under the control of Whitehall and at the same time to secure, for the benefit of leading chemical manufacturers, a wider distribution of agricultural, horticultural and industrial poisons. Following the concessions made to the chemical industry in 1908, the Committee's report marked a further significant retreat from the public health policies pursued by Sir John Simon in the nineteenth century. Although it was common knowledge that agricultural and horticultural preparations were the usual source of poison used in suicide and crime, the Committee, instead of suggesting increased restrictions on their sale, recommended extending the facilities for acquiring them.

The Departmental Committee was engaged for four years, from 1926 to 1930, in taking evidence and preparing its report. The Committee argued that the Pharmaceutical Society should be required to give up its statutory powers in the control of poisons. It was undesirable, especially with the increasing discovery of new poisons, that the Poisons Schedule should be open to amendment only on the proposal of the Society's Council. It was recommended that the Home Office should become the central authority for poisons and should appoint an Advisory Poisons Board. To secure the acquiescence of the Pharmaceutical Society in these changes, the Committee provided for reforms in the organisation of pharmacy which the Council considered highly desirable. This process of horse-trading eventually secured the passage of the Act.

The Committee's Report contained as an appendix the draft of a bill. Although it was very substantially recast during its progress through parliament, the general structure of the bill was reproduced in the Pharmacy and Poisons Act of 1933. Part I is headed "Pharmacy" and deals with membership of the Pharmaceutical Society, the appointment of Privy Council nominees to its Council, the registration of business premises, the removal of the necessity for a general meeting to approve by-laws, the setting up of a Statutory Disciplinary Committee, and certain other provisions related to the internal organisation of pharmacy. Part II, entitled "Poisons" introduces new regulations governing the sale of poisons, sets up a Poisons Board to act as an advisory committee to the Home Secretary for the preparation of a list of poisons and rules relating to their sale, and makes provision for the sale of certain poisons by persons other than "authorised sellers of poisons".

Soon after the publication of the Committee's report in the spring of 1930, the Council of the Pharmaceutical Society issued a statement welcoming some of the recommendations and rejecting others. The principal criticism of the bill was that it did not restrict the dispensing of physicians' prescriptions to pharmacists and that it did not sufficiently safeguard the position of chemists as the sole suppliers by retail of medicinal poisons. A committee of Council was set up to prepare amendments to the draft bill and in the following November the Council held a conference with representatives of the principal bodies connected with pharmacy. The bill and another draft bill were discussed at three meetings of Branch Representatives, two held in 1931 and one in 1932.

The Government's bill was introduced into the House of Lords and read a second time on 12 March 1931. It was in charge of Lord Ponsonby of Shulbrede, who claimed that the time had come when matters affecting poisons should be administered by a minister responsible to parliament. He emphasised that the aim of Part I of the bill was to raise the status of the Pharmaceutical Society, to extend its authority and to increase its powers of supervision. The rejection of the bill was moved by Lord Dawson of Penn, who had been chairman of the Consultative Council on Medical and Allied Services, on which Glyn-Jones had served, and which produced in 1920 ambitious plans for a comprehensive and unified

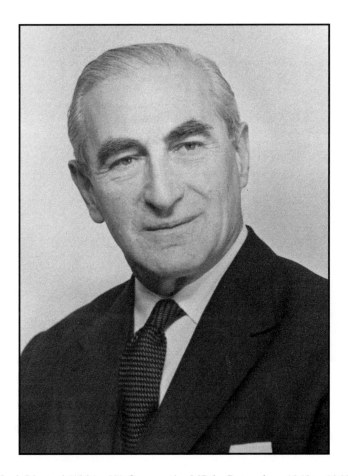

59   *Sir Hugh Linstead (1901–87) Conservative MP for Putney from 1942 to 1962 and secretary of the Pharmaceutical Society from 1926 to 1964. Following his retirement from the Society he became chairman of Macarthy plc from 1964 to 1980.*

health service. Lord Dawson, in an impressive speech, argued that the medical profession had not been consulted, that the Ministry of Health rather than the Home Office was the appropriate authority (drugs are a matter of medicine, not of crime and addiction), and that the dispensing of medicines should be undertaken by pharmacists or under the supervision of a doctor. The Pharmaceutical Society, he said, was " a body of expert pharmacists who are best fitted to decide whether a given substance should go into the schedule of poisons . . . On the whole, they do their work very well because they are a skilled body". Here is a body, he went on to say,

> which has been working for years most satisfactorily, under the control of the Privy Council, composed of expert pharmacists . . . people who spend their lives in association with the scientific aspects of drugs and the medicines that are mostly concerned with the use of poisons; and they are to be replaced by this extraordinary

385

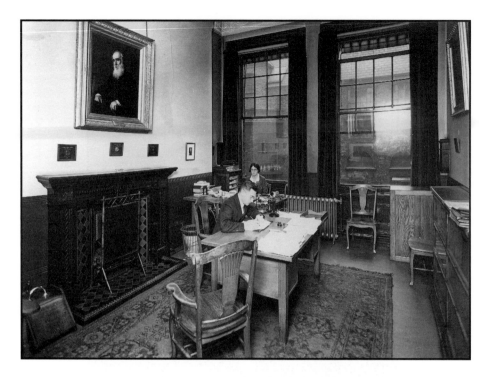

60 *Secretary's room, first floor, 16 Bloomsbury Square, 1928. With Hugh Linstead, the Secretary at that time, below a portrait of Elias Bremridge, former secretary, above the mantelshelf.*

body which aims at centralising all power inside the Home Office . . . I would point out the unwisdom of taking away from a profession, whose life is spent in dealing with these intimate problems, the authority which they have very well carried out in the past, and giving it to a small centralised authority, with an Advisory Committee, which has no real power and which can be completely over-ridden by a Secretary of State and by people with a very imperfect knowledge of the subject with which they are called upon to deal.

The Poisons Board, he added, is a sham: it "will be an out-and-out bureaucratic body". The Secretary of State has power to do almost anything. "It will be in the power of the Secretary of State to overrule them and to act entirely as he pleases . . . The real authority in regard to poisons will be transferred to permanent officials at the Home Office".

Several peers supported Lord Dawson, but on an assurance from Lord Ponsonby that the Government would consult representatives of the medical profession, his motion was withdrawn. The committee stage of the bill was taken on Thursday 26 March, when numerous amendments were considered. On a test division upon an amendment making the Poisons Board rather than the Secretary of State the final authority for deciding what should or should not be in the Poisons List, the Government won by 28 votes to 16. The Report stage was taken on 28 April, when certain additional amendments were inserted,

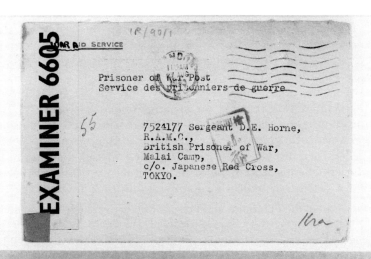

The Pharmaceutical Society of Great Britain

PATRON: HIS MAJESTY THE KING

TELEGRAMS: "BREMRIDGE, WESTCENT, LONDON."
TELEPHONE: HOLBORN 8967 (+LINES).

17, BLOOMSBURY SQUARE, LONDON. W.C.I.

SECRETARY & REGISTRAR: HUGH N. LINSTEAD, O.B.E., Ph.C.

26th. August 1943.

EL.

WAR AID SERVICE.

Dear Mr. Horne,

I was glad to learn from your wife that you are safe and well although a prisoner of war. I hope that you are as happy and comfortable as possible in the circumstances.

Under present conditions I am not able to write to you very frequently, but if I can be of any help to you or your family I shall be glad to do all that is possible.

Quite a number of members and former members of the Society are prisoners of war or internees in Japanese hands, and I believe that the following are in the same camp as yourself:- Corporal Alexander Cockburn and Sergeants Harry Hall and James Innes.

You may be interested to hear that for about three years we have been in constant touch with members and students of the Society who are prisoners of war and internees in Germany and Italy, and have been able to send them reference books and notes to aid them in keeping in touch with pharmaceutical matters. Recently also permission has been obtained to send the Pharmaceutical Journal each week. In several camps in Germany our members have formed little study groups, which apart from being a method of maintaining their efficiency in their work has served

61 *Letter from Hugh Linstead as Secretary of the Society, to Sergeant D. Horne RAMC whilst a British Prisoner of War. The letter was sent in August 1943, and received in December 1944.*

and the bill received its third reading on 30 April and was introduced into the House of Commons on the same day. It appeared in the orders for the day on several occasions in May and June but pressure of other business prevented its being reached and the Commons adjourned without the second reading being taken. During the summer "the economic blizzard", as the *Chemist and Druggist* called it, swept away the Labour Government and led to the return of its prime minister, Ramsay MacDonald, as the head of a National Coalition Government. The progress of the Pharmacy and Poisons bill came to an end.

Negotiations between the Pharmaceutical Society and the Home Office continued, however, and an agreement was reached on an amendment to clause 17 which would indicate to the Poisons Board how they were to differentiate between the poisons to be placed in Part I and the poisons to be placed in Part II of the Poisons List. Since persons other than "authorised sellers of poisons" were to be entitled to sell poisons in Part II, the economic welfare of every chemist was involved in this issue. On 5 March 1932 the Council of the Society passed a resolution indicating its revised attitude towards the bill:

> (a) That in the event of the Pharmacy and Poisons Bill (with the agreed amendment to clause 17) being introduced by the Government, the Council will withdraw its opposition and give such assistance to the passing of the bill as may be open to it;
> (b) that this policy be dependent upon there being no amendments made to the bill which affect pharmacists adversely, and upon the Government being prepared to oppose any such amendments should they be moved.

This decision was submitted to a Branch Representatives meeting held in London on 26 April 1932 and approved by a large majority. A resolution in similar terms was carried by a large majority at the Annual General Meeting of the Society on 18 May.

The bill was not reintroduced by the Government until 28 February 1933. It received its second reading in the Lords on 7 March when the Government was able to announce that the bill had been amended in consultation with the Pharmaceutical Society and was now practically an agreed measure. The Committee stage was taken on 8 March and the third reading on 23 March. The bill received its second reading in the Commons on 11 April and was considered by Standing Committee A on 9 and 11 May. The unanimity of the profession was dissolved by an unsuccessful attempt to introduce amendments designed to secure the representation of Scottish pharmacists on the Society's Council and on the Statutory Committee. On 15 June, however, the Government, with the agreement of the Society's Council, moved an amendment, which was accepted, providing that one member of the Statutory Committee should be a pharmacist resident in Scotland. The bill was read a third time and passed on that day. It received the Royal Assent on 28 June 1933.[13]

The main provisions of the Pharmacy and Poisons Act of 1933 were:

(1) Every person registered as a pharmacist became, by virtue of his registration, a member of the Pharmaceutical Society. The distinction between registration under the Pharmacy Acts and membership of the Pharmaceutical Society was ended. The Pharmaceutical Society became an obligatory association and the corporate representative of all who practise pharmacy in Great Britain.

(2) In addition to the fees payable on registration, members of the Society were required to pay an annual fee to retain their names on the register.

(3) The requirement that by-laws of the Society be confirmed and approved by a special general meeting of the Society was abolished.

(4) The Privy Council gained the right to appoint three additional members of the Society's Council who need not be pharmacists.

(5) A Register of Premises where poisons are sold was set up. The first Register was published by the Society in the spring of 1936.

(6) A disciplinary body (the Statutory Committee) was established with authority not only over pharmacists but also over companies carrying on business under the Pharmacy Acts. The Committee comprised a chairman and five members. The chairman, appointed by the Privy Council, must be a person having "practical legal experience". The chairman has, in fact, always been an eminent member of the legal profession. The five members are appointed by the Council of the Pharmaceutical Society: they need not all be pharmacists but one must be a pharmacist resident in Scotland. It has always been the practice to appoint pharmacists of wide experience. The six members of the first Statutory Committee were appointed in July 1934.

(7) The Statutory Committee was given the duty of inquiring into any case where a pharmacist or any "authorised seller of poisons" was alleged to have been guilty of misconduct or to have been convicted of a criminal offence. The Committee was given the power (a) to direct that the name of a pharmacist be removed from, or restored to, the register and (b) to disqualify an "authorised seller of poisons", e.g. a limited company, from acting in that capacity and to remove one or more of the premises of a corporate body from the Register of Premises.

(8) The Pharmaceutical Society was placed under a duty to enforce the 1933 Act and was authorised to appoint inspectors, who must be pharmacists, for the purpose. The inspectors had the task of inspecting the premises of those registered as "authorised sellers of poisons", the conditions under which poisons were stored and the registers kept for recording sales. Proceedings under the Act were to be taken in courts of summary jurisdiction and not, as under the 1868 and 1908 Acts, in the civil courts.

(9) The ultimate responsibility for the control of poisons was placed in the hands of the Home Secretary.

(10) A Poisons Board was established to advise the Home Secretary on what should be included in the Poisons List. Poisons in Part I of the list could be sold by retail only at pharmacies; poisons in Part II could be sold also by any shopkeeper subject to certain conditions. Poisons were further classified by means of schedules to the Poisons Rules made under the Act. Schedule Four comprised that group of poisons which could be supplied to the public only on the authority of a medical practitioner's prescription. The first Poisons Board was constituted on 1 November 1933. The Board prepared the Poisons List and draft Poisons Rules and presented them to the Home Secretary with its report in May 1935. The list as confirmed by him, with modifications, took effect on 1 January 1936 and the Poisons Rules came into operation on 1 May 1936.

The term "authorised seller of poisons" was used in the Act to describe persons permitted to sell poisons in Part I of the Poisons List: it included individual proprietor pharmacists as well as corporate bodies having a pharmacist registered as a superintendent. The term "pharmacy" came to be used to describe the registered premises of an authorised seller of poisons.

The immediate consequences of the 1933 Act was to increase the Pharmaceutical Society's income by over £11,000 a year and its membership from 13,800 to 20,900 (an

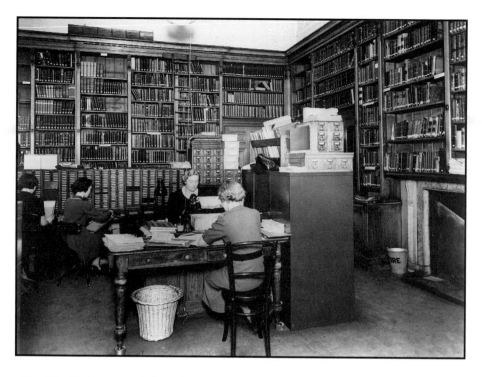

62   *The Registry, second floor, 16 Bloomsbury Square, 1931/2.*

increase of fifty per cent.) The new members paid an annual retention fee of £1-11s.-6d. (the amount of the former annual subscription) and in return enjoyed all the privileges of membership including the right to use the description "M.P.S". and to receive the *Pharmaceutical Journal* weekly. By no means all of the 7,000 new members were happy with this arrangement. Before the Act was passed, they enjoyed all the advantages of being registered without paying a penny. Now if they failed to pay their retention fee, they found themselves in the same position as an unqualified person. They ceased to be pharmacists and lost, *inter alia*, the right to sell Part I poisons and to dispense prescriptions under the National Health Insurance scheme. Moreover, both old and new members became subject after 1933 to the surveillance of the Society's inspectorate and of the new disciplinary committee. The 1933 Act implied a major change in the balance of power between the Society's Council and its members. The relatively ineffectual show of hands replaced the sound of departing feet as the sign of disaffection with Council policy.

What the Jenkin case had begun, the 1933 Act accomplished. The nail was driven into the coffin of Glyn-Jones' grand design for a British Medical Association of Pharmacy. Instead of the Pharmaceutical Society shedding its load of statutory duties, the 1933 Act added substantially to it. Professional regulation and control triumphed over protection and trade unionism. The amalgamation of the Pharmaceutical Society with the Retail Pharmacists' Union and the Chemists' Defence Association, so much desired by Glyn-Jones after 1920, was removed from the pharmaceutical agenda. The economic interests of pharmacists would continue to be served by a diversity of organisations. The needs of proprietor pharmacists were met by the National Pharmaceutical Union and those of hospital pharmacists by the Guild of Public Pharmacists. Other employed pharmacists became members of the Association of Pharmaceutical Employees or joined one of the three trade unions which accepted pharmacists, the Amalgamated Society of Pharmacists, Drug and Chemical Makers, the Shop Assistants Union, and the National Warehouse and General Workers Union.

* * *

When the Pharmaceutical Society was founded, any person in this country could sell and advertise practically any medicine he liked, could put into it whatever he pleased, could call it by any name he fancied and claim for it anything and everything he wished the public to believe. The public were likewise free to buy any drug or medicinal preparation they wished in any quantity without restriction from the chemist and without the necessity of a medical prescription. Even the doctor's prescription implied the minimum of medical control since it belonged to the patient and could be dispensed indefinitely. The Poisons and Pharmacy Acts mark the beginning of legislative restrictions on the sale and purchase of drugs and medicines. By present-day standards, the restrictions imposed by these Acts were minimal. Scheduled poisons could be sold only by registered chemists and the more dangerous poisons, listed in Part I of the schedule, could be sold only if the purchaser were

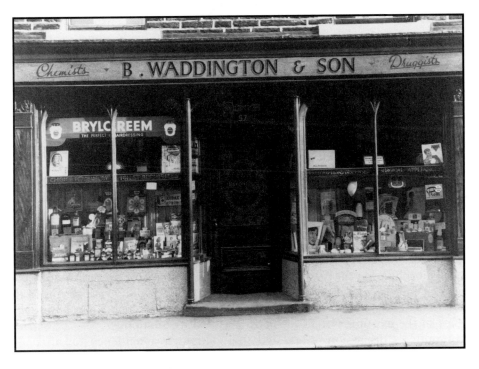

63   *B. Waddington & Son, 57 Market Street, Thornton, Yorkshire. Taken in 1951, this view depicts the traditional appearance of a typical provincial pharmacy.*

known to the seller or introduced by someone known to him and after an entry had been made in the poisons register. The attempts by Sir John Simon in 1868 and 1869 to prevent the sale of medicinal poisons except on the written order of a legally qualified medical practitioner were warded off by the Pharmaceutical Society's lobbying and the predilection of the House of Commons for free trade. A series of legal actions in the early 1890s extended the operation of the 1868 Pharmacy Act to proprietary medicines containing poisons. The list of poisons was recast in 1908. Cocaine, morphine, opium and derivatives containing more than one per cent of morphine were placed in the first, more restrictive, part of the Schedule and a revised British Pharmacopoeial formula for laudanum, the most widely used opium preparation, had the same effect. But not until 1916 were opium and cocaine regulated as narcotic drugs rather than as poisons.

A convergence of international and domestic factors account for this change of direction.[14] Instigated by the United States Government, a series of conferences which began at Shanghai in 1909 and continued at The Hague in 1911–12, 1913, and 1914 laid the foundations for the international control system that came to maturity in the 1920s. The International Opium Convention, signed at The Hague on 23 January 1912 committed the signatories to restricting the trade and consumption of drugs to "medical and legitimate uses" and to applying the necessary regulations to all preparations which contained more than 0.2 per cent. morphia or more than 0.1 per cent. of either heroin or cocaine. These specific commitments strongly influenced the shape of British drug regulation over the next decade. There was, however, no immediate enthusiasm for action. An interdepartmental committee met in May 1914 to frame the legislation which would ensure British compliance with the convention but the discussions were desultory with none of the Whitehall departments keen to take the initiative. Among the outside influences on the Committee were Dr. Alfred Cox of the B.M.A. and Uglow Woolcock, secretary of the Pharmaceutical Society. Dr. Cox was keen for British legislation to adhere strictly to the international guide lines.

> The advantage of restricting the sale of these substances in this way would be that the only legal way in which they could be obtained would be on the prescriptions of a body of men who by their education and training would on the whole, I think, respond to the responsibility.

Uglow Woolcock, supported by the Privy Council Office, advocated a less rigid approach and secured a compromise solution. Doctors got their "prescription-only" restriction for opiates and cocaine, as well as limitations on the currency of prescriptions and the total quantity of drugs to be dispensed. But these restrictions were to apply only to a range of preparations well above the limits set at The Hague. Only preparations containing over one per cent. of morphia, heroin or cocaine would require a doctor's prescription: it was left to the professional discretion of the pharmacist to decide if preparations under this limit were being bought for "legitimate and medical purposes". The control of retail sales would remain part of the existing system of pharmaceutical regulation.

The committee's discussions suggested that, although a tendency towards increasing regulation was discernible, the proposed legislation would not impose stringent controls on the every day sale and use of narcotics. The First World War changed this intention. Two separate issues were involved. By 1916 it had become apparent that Britain was the source of a considerable amount of smuggled drugs. Reports from government officials in India and Burma indicated that cocaine seized there came from Britain. Opium for smoking and morphine discovered in the Far East and the United States had been sent from Britain. With Britain under wartime emergency conditions, the smuggling of drugs on British ships was a considerable embarrassment for the Government. Meanwhile, on the home front, the influence of cocaine on the efficiency of the army was the problem. The question of the use of drugs by soldiers first emerged in February 1916 in two separate incidents. In the first, two respectable London stores, Harrods and Savory & Moore, were fined for selling morphine and cocaine without observing the Pharmacy Act regulations. The drugs had been sold in small packets in a handy case, advertised by Savory & Moore in the *Times* as a "useful present for friends at the front". William Glyn-Jones, who acted as prosecuting counsel in the Harrods case, pointed out that "it was an exceedingly dangerous thing for a drug like morphine to be in the hands of men on active service". In the same month, an ex-convict and a prostitute were convicted of selling cocaine to Canadian troops in Folkestone under Regulation 40 of the Defence of the Realm Act which made it an offence to supply intoxicants to members of the armed forces with intent to make them drunk or incapable. The officer in charge of the barracks hospital admitted that over forty Canadian soldiers were being treated there for the habit. The case attracted a great deal of publicity and increased the pressure on the Government to take action against narcotic drugs.

On 11 May 1916 the Army Council issued an order forbidding the sale or supply of cocaine, opium, codeine, heroin, Indian hemp, and morphine to any member of the forces unless ordered by a doctor on a written prescription, dated and signed by him and marked "not to be repeated". This order set a precedent for wider control and for the use of regulations rather than legislation to acheive it. The medical profession rejoiced. The *Lancet* was enthusiastic about "placing on the liberty of the subject a restriction of a nature that is novel to our poisons legislation". It welcomed "yet another instance of an innovation, long advocated in years of peace, being secured without controversy under the stimulus of a great war", and argued that "a measure now applied to one section of the community should be made applicable to all sections". "If we wait until the war is over", continued the *Lancet*, "we shall find ourselves confronted with all those pettifogging controversies and the clamouring of vested interests which always put a brake on progress". The march of progress was more inexorable than even the *Lancet* could have anticipated.

Although the Home Office admitted that the bearing of narcotics control "on the 'Defence of the Realm' is neither very direct nor important", the Army Council regulation was extended to the civilian population by an order-in-council on 28 July 1916. DORA 40B made it an offence for anyone except medical men, pharmacists and vets to be in possession of cocaine, to sell it, or to give it away. It could only be supplied on the written, non-repeatable prescription of a qualified medical practitioner. Similar provision, without the detailed prescription requirements, applied to raw and powdered opium. A proclamation prohibiting the import of all cocaine and opium except under Home Office licence was published at the same time. For the first time in the history of this country certain drugs became, under the DORA 40B regulation, available only with a doctor's prescription. It is not surprising that both the *British Medical Journal* and the *Lancet* welcomed the restriction enthusiastically. The *Pharmaceutical Journal* was considerably more restrained and the *Chemist and Druggist* wisely observed that "the Army Council order is a bad precedent for medicine and pharmacy".

Details which emerged from police surveillance after the regulations came into force failed to produce any evidence that DORA 40B was necessary. Although the police focussed their attention on enforcing the regulation, the number of prosecutions were minimal. In February 1917 a parliamentary committee demonstrated the inadequate basis on which DORA 40B had been founded.

> We are unanimously of opinion that there is no evidence of any kind to show that there is any serious, or, perhaps, even noticeable prevalence of the cocaine habit amongst the civilian or military population of Great Britain. There have been a certain number of cases amongst the overseas troops quartered in, or passing through, the United Kingdom, but there is hardly any trace of the practice having spread to British troops, and, apart from a small number of broken-down medical men, there is only very slight evidence of its existence amongst the general population.

The perceived needs of the war effort allowed the introduction, virtually without opposition, of quite unnecessary incursions into the freedom of the individual. Traditional safeguards were swept away by bureaucrats who believed that social problems could be solved by wrapping them up in a bundle of regulations, preferably of their own drafting.

With the end of the war and the expiration of the Defence of the Realm Act, the issue of narcotic drug control again came to the fore. Article 295 of the Treaty of Versailles committed its signatories to honour the agreements made in the pre-war Hague convention, and these became the basis of the Dangerous Drugs Act of 1920. Parliament showed little interest in the bill which passed without significant opposition. The Act came into force on 1 September 1920. The import of opium prepared for smoking was prohibited. The import, export and manufacture of raw opium, cocaine, heroin and morphia were prohibited except under licence. The manufacture, sale, possession and distribution of preparations containing more than 0.2 per cent. of morphia or more than 0.1 per cent. of either cocaine or heroin were strictly regulated. The sale of regulated drugs was restricted to pharmacists acting on a doctor's written prescription and to medical practitioners. The sale of narcotic drugs had to be recorded in books open to police inspection. Contravention of the Act was punishable by a fine of up to £200 or imprisonment for up to six months, or both.

The Pharmaceutical Society, although at first disappointed that it had not been consulted when the bill was first presented in May, gave the Act a cautious welcome after some of its suggestions had been incorporated. "Even at the cost of some circumspection of their liberties", commented the *Pharmaceutical Journal*, "we are confident that pharmacists as a class will loyally co-operate in making the new law effective". However, when the government drafted regulations spelling out specific details of the Act's enforcement, the Society's Council decided, in February 1921, to take all possible measures to obtain their withdrawal. The main objection to the draft regulations was that they made the sale of an important class of drugs dependent upon a doctor's prescription. The Council urged that this should be withdrawn and that the existing freedom of the chemist to sell drugs to known customers and to persons introduced by known customers upon the signing of the poisons book should remain. The Council pointed out that the Act subjected pharmacists to a plethora of regulations, which, if breached, even inadvertently, could lead to a criminal prosecution which might result in a large fine or even a prison sentence. Moreover, in spite of the apparent concern with public safety, doctors retained the right to both prescribe and dispense these dangerous drugs themselves. The Act required only that dispensing doctors, like chemists, keep a register of their sales.[15]

The Government was unsympathetic to these grievances and the Acts of 1923, 1925 and 1932 amended the Dangerous Drugs Act of 1920 in ways which hardly affected the pharmaceutical profession. The Pharmacy and Poisons Act of 1933, however, contained a Fourth Schedule which listed five poisons which could only be sold to the public in accordance with a prescription given by a doctor, a dentist, or a veterinary surgeon. The substances listed in the schedule were barbituric acid and its derivatives, amidopyrine, the dinitrophenol group, phenylcinchoninic acid and its derivatives, and the sulphonal group.

The Fourth Schedule owed its origin to Sir William Willcox, a member of the Departmental Committee on the Poisons and Pharmacy Acts, which deliberated from 1926 to 1930. Willcox, a leading authority on forensic medicine, was consulting physician to St. Mary's Hospital, London, and medical adviser, from 1919 to his death in 1941, to the Home Office. He spearheaded a campaign against the abuse of barbiturates and succeeded in convincing leading members of the medical profession that barbiturates should be treated as dangerous drugs. The difficulty, however, was that barbiturates could not be controlled under the Dangerous Drugs Acts without the authority of the League of Nations. It was to short-circuit this process that the Fourth Schedule was added to the Pharmacy and Poisons Act of 1933. The creation of Schedule Four and the enactment of the Dangerous Drugs Acts constituted a major increase in the medical profession's control of the supply of drugs to the general public. Since 1933 the chemotherapeutic revolution has led to further increases in that control. The introduction of an ever widening range of drugs of increased potency, efficacy and toxicity has heightened the risks to the individual of uncontrolled medication. The Poisons Board, responding to pressure for greater control of these new drugs, added them to Schedule Four, limiting their sale and supply to medical prescription. But as Schedule Four grew and grew, so did the view that poisons legislation was an inappropriate mechanism for the regulation of the new chemotherapy. Under the 1968 Medicines Act, a committee was appointed to examine all medicines and decide which should be available only on prescription. The Poisons Act of 1972 dealt with non-medicinal poisons.

The first Therapeutic Substances Act (1925) did not challenge the public's right of access to new medicines. It regulated by licence the manufacture, but not the sale, of a limited number of products the purity or potency of which could not be adequately controlled by chemical means. These products included vaccines, sera, toxins, antigens, insulin and certain other substances. At first it was not considered necessary to restrict the retail sale or supply of these substances, but when penicillin and other antibiotics became available for general use towards the end of the Second World War the question of regulating their manufacture and sale had to be tackled. The Penicillin Act of 1947 and the Therapeutic Substances (Prevention of Misuse) Act of 1953 recognised that antibiotics were substances "capable of causing danger to the health of the community if used without proper safeguards" and permitted their supply to the public only by medical practitioners or from pharmacies on the authority of a doctor's prescription. The Therapeutic Substances Act of 1956 replaced the earlier Acts and brought within a single statute the control of both the manufacture and the supply of therapeutic substances. It has now been replaced by the Medicines Act of 1968.

It was during the First World War that the effective regulation and restriction of

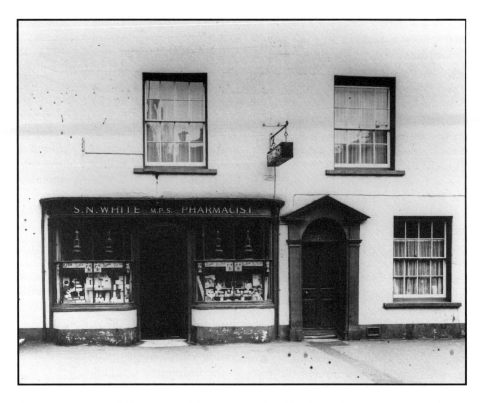

64 *The premises of S.N. White MPS, Pharmacist, Topsham, Devon. One of a series of images assembled by the Society's History Committee in the 1950s to record the rapidly disappearing traditional pharmacy.*

consumer purchases of drugs and medicines began in this country. The first significant abridgement of the public's right of self-medication was the promulgation of DORA 40B in 1916. The Venereal Diseases Act of 1917 was another wartime measure promoted to maintain the health and efficiency of the armed forces. The Act restricted the treatment of venereal disease to qualified medical practitioners and forbade anyone from making, by advertisement or other public notice, a claim to give advice on, prescribe for or treat such diseases. It made it unlawful for anyone other than a registered medical practitioner to recommend any medicine for the prevention, cure, or relief of venereal disease. One of the main aims of the Act was to prevent the sale of proprietary medicines and chemists' counter prescribing for venereal diseases.

The Food and Drugs Act of 1938 made it illegal for a person to provide with a drug sold by him a label which falsely described the drug or was in any way calculated to mislead as to the nature, substance or quality of the drug. It was also made unlawful to publish an advertisement having such characteristics. The effectiveness of these provisions was limited by the fact that the manufacturer of a proprietary medicine was not required to disclose its composition, provided he fixed the appropriate medicine stamp to each bottle or packet.

This state of affairs was changed by the Pharmacy and Medicines Act of 1941 which was the outcome of several years effort to institute some measure of legislative control over the advertising and sale of proprietary medicines. The Act abolished the medicine stamp duty as from 2 September 1941 and required the full disclosure on the label of the active ingredients in all proprietary medicines. It prohibited the advertisement, except to the medical profession, of any article in terms which were calculated to lead to its use in the treatment of certain diseases, namely, Bright's disease, cataract, diabetes, epilepsy or fits, glaucoma, locomotor ataxy, paralysis, or tuberculosis. The Act also restricted the channels of distribution of medicines. The retail sale of medicines was restricted to (1) registered medical practitioners and registered dentists (2) authorised sellers of poisons and (3) persons who had served a regular apprenticeship in pharmacy and who, at the time of the passing of the Act, were conducting on their own account a business comprising the retail sale of drugs. Such persons were permitted to sell medicines only at a shop (not from a stall) and the sales had to be under the personal control of the person concerned. The sale of vegetable drugs, natural and artificial mineral waters and proprietary medicines (except those sold under B.P. or B.P.C. titles) was not restricted to authorised persons.

After the Second World War rapid developments in pharmaceutical research led to the marketing of powerful new drugs which superseded most of the traditional medicines but gave rise to serious problems for which the existing legislation was never designed. The Poisons Board in 1959 expressed the view that further legislation was needed urgently to provide control over certain potent medicines which could cause serious damage to health if widely used in self-medication. In the same year the Interdepartmental Committee on Drug Addiction recommended that drugs having an effect on the central nervous system and liable to produce physical or psychological deterioration should be restricted to supply on prescription. After the devastating effects of thalidomide became known in 1962 there was widespread anxiety about the absence of safeguards to ensure that new drugs should not be put on the market before every possible step had been taken to bring the harmful side effects of new drugs to the notice of doctors. Proposals for new legislation were published in 1967 in a White Paper entitled *Forthcoming Legislation on the Safety, Quality and Description of Drugs and Medicines*. The Medicines Act of 1968 was based on the proposals in the White Paper and was designed to replace all earlier legislation relating to medicines.[16]

* * *

From its foundation the Pharmaceutical Society had an unbroken commitment to raising the standard of pharmaceutical education. Jacob Bell had an almost naive faith in the power of education to transform the trade of the chemist and druggist into the profession of the pharmaceutical chemist. The Society's School of Pharmacy was set up in 1842 to provide a complete course in the basic sciences and their application to pharmacy.[17] The School with its laboratories always had the first call on the financial resources of the Society. It was regarded as a beacon pointing the way forward to a more scientific and prestigious future. The School set standards of education and research which were far in advance of the needs and aspirations of the vast majority of chemists and druggists. By producing the men who became the leaders in scientific, academic and industrial pharmacy, the School inspired in each generation a vision of pharmacy that transcended the everyday reality of the chemist and druggist's world.

The 1868 Pharmacy Act made the Society's minor examination the portal through which all newcomers to the trade had to pass. The educational consequences of the Act are difficult

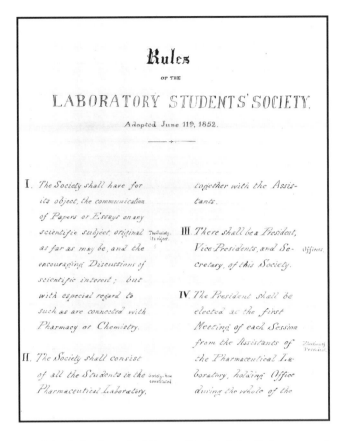

Rules

OF THE

LABORATORY STUDENTS' SOCIETY.

Adopted June 11th, 1852.

I. The Society shall have for its object, the communication of Papers or Essays on any scientific subject original as far as may be, and the encouraging Discussions of scientific interest; but with especial regard to such as are connected with Pharmacy or Chemistry.

II. The Society shall consist of all the Students in the Pharmaceutical Laboratory, together with the Assistants.

III. There shall be a President, Vice-Presidents, and Secretary, of this Society.

IV. The President shall be elected at the first Meeting of each Session from the Assistants of the Pharmaceutical Laboratory, holding Office during the whole of the

65 *First page of the Rules from the* Minute Book of the Laboratory Students Society, *founded in 1852.*

to evaluate. It provided a stimulus by creating a widespread demand, but the demand was for the rudimentary and mechanical knowledge required to pass the examination. The Minor examination had previously been the qualifying examination for assistants: after 1868 it became the test for admission to the register. The Major examination, previously the test for entry into business, became a higher qualification sought after only by the academically inclined.

Initially the passing of the 1868 Act, heralding as it did a compulsory examination for chemists and druggists, provided a needed stimulus to pharmaceutical education. The Society's School had few of its sixty benches unoccupied in the 1868–69 session while the following year 90 students entered for the chemical lectures, 93 for botany and as many as 96 for the laboratory course. There was a marked increase in the number of candidates for the examination. This increased demand brought the Council face to face with a difficulty which was not to be solved for half a century. The Council's report for the annual meeting in 1869 confidently observed that "the chemists and druggists of the present time will be succeeded by men better qualified to uphold pharmacy as a profession as well as practise it as a trade", but offered no solution to the problem of how professional pharmaceutical students were to receive their training. Apprenticeship was obviously the principal means but if proper emphasis was to be placed upon the sciences which are the foundation of pharmacy, apprenticeship alone would not suffice. Some academic training must accompany and supplement it. The fact that apprenticeship continued to be the principal method of initiation into the vocation of the chemist and druggist was a major impediment to pharmacy's claim to be a profession. Although apprenticeship was never formally abolished in the training of medical practitioners, it ceased to be a significant feature of medical education after 1858. Its survival as the basic form of training for the chemist and druggist associated him with the craftsman and the skilled manual worker.

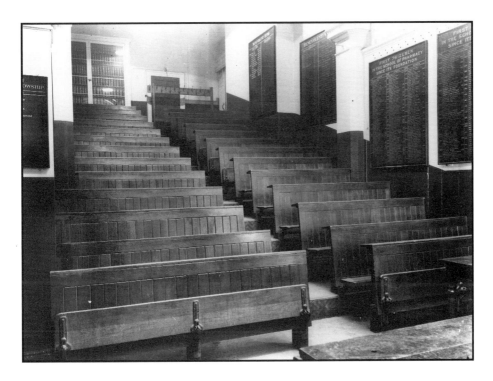

66 *Lecture Hall, School of Pharmacy, 17 Bloomsbury Square. The new benches with supports for students' notebooks were installed in 1928. The wall boards record legacies to the Benevolent Fund and Prizemen of the School of Pharmacy.*

Apprenticeship is essentially a conservative institution. It works well in a relatively static society in which social structures and practices are reproduced generation after generation: it maintains continuity and stability. But in a modern, industrial, dynamic society, where innovation and change are built into the fabric of social relationships, apprenticeship merely passes on to the new generation the obsolescent ideas and practices of an earlier age. Apprenticeship as a form of education was haphazard and unsystematic, so much depending upon the character and attainment of the master to whom the apprentice was attached. In pharmacy the quality of the apprentice's educational experience depended on the economic and social status of the establishment in which he served. Since medical practitioners did most of their own dispensing, it was only in a comparatively few shops that apprentices had opportunities for learning practical pharmacy and dispensing. The earlier the age at which apprenticeship was begun the more the preliminary scientific and general education of the initiate was neglected. Apprenticeship emphasised unduly the purely practical and empirical at the expense of the theoretical and scientific. Yet it is not difficult to understand why a Council dominated by and representing retail chemists should be reluctant to abandon apprenticeship: it was a source of cheap and well-motivated labour. Although it might be argued that apprenticeship sacrificed the future of the pharmaceutical profession to the commerical needs of the proprietor chemist, the absence of an alternative educational infrastructure meant there was little choice.

The School of Pharmacy in Bloomsbury Square provided the most modern course available in Great Britain, but its accommodation was limited, and the rest of the country had neither the means nor the will to follow the example of London. In the 1870s four-fifths of the students at "the Square" came from the provinces, and this fact suggests that the society might have been well advised to follow the example of the medical profession and concentrate its educational facilities in the metropolis, instead of trying to develop provincial

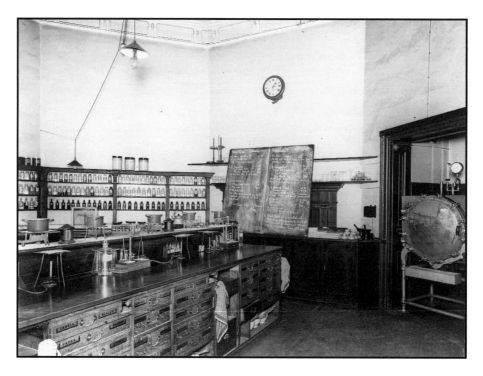

67   *The Dispensary, School of Pharmacy, 17 Bloomsbury Square, 1931/2.*

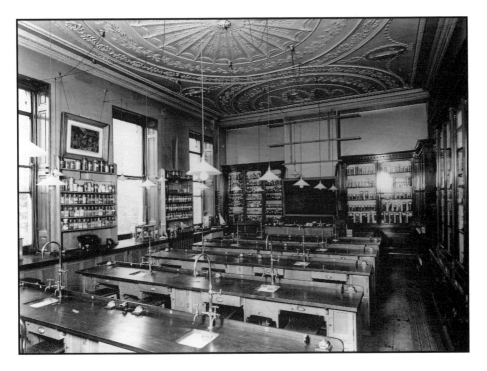

68 *Histological Laboratory, 17 Bloomsbury Square, 1931/2. The room was re-fitted in 1926, which included the installation of electric lights, water, sinks and gas at all the benches.*

schools. However that may be, the Council decided to encourage local associations of chemists to set up schools or at least to provide classes which apprentices could attend in their off-duty hours. In 1870 local associations were asked to report upon their needs and subsequently invited to apply for grants. In 1869 there were seventeen such associations in England and eleven of them had plans for some systematic teaching. A year later there were twenty-two associations of which fourteen had made provision for the instruction of apprentices, although only nine intended to hold classes in all three subjects of the Minor examination. In addition, there were four associations in Scotland, all of them with organised classes. Aberdeen was one of the first centres to receive a grant from the Society: £10 was donated to purchase apparatus for teaching chemistry, materia medica and botany. The grants were not regular subventions but offered for specific purposes such as the supply of books or the acquisition of apparatus and were usually of the value of £10 or £20. The last grant of which a record can be found is the payment in 1896 of £20 to the Liverpool Pharmaceutical Students' Society for the purchase of a materia medica cabinet and specimens, to be entrusted to Liverpool University College for use in the pharmaceutical classes held there.

There was little uniformity in the "schools" set up by the local associations.[18] In Bristol the pharmacy students studied in the science classes at the School of Mines; in Plymouth in the Science School; in Manchester at Owen's College; and in Glasgow in the Mechanics Institute. In Newcastle the Durham University College of Medicine made arrangements to run classes for pharmaceutical students. H.B. Proctor was appointed to a Chair (little more than a lectureship) in practical pharmacy and the University Reader in Chemistry gave the course in pharmaceutical chemistry. The medical school library was made available to the sixteen students of pharmacy who attended the first session in 1869–70. In Leicester, renowned in the nineteenth century for its radical nonconformity, the assistants and apprentices got together to form an educational co-operative in which the members prepared and read papers for each other's benefit. Later formal lectures were arranged and a library and materia medica cabinet were set up in permanent rooms.

The seventh annual meeting of the British Pharmaceutical Conference which met in Liverpool in 1870 discussed pharmaceutical education at the request of the Council of the Pharmaceutical Society. F. Baden Benger read a paper on "The Apprenticeship and Early Training of Pharmacists" in which the mixture of noble sentiments and practical unreality was typical of nineteenth-century discussion of the subject. He advocated that young men intending to become apprentices should receive, in various provincial centres, a sound elementary education in chemistry, botany and materia medica before apprenticeship. This would mean that the work of apprentices, which was usually irksome drudgery, would become interesting and instructive.

George F. Schacht did more than anyone to keep pharmaceutical education a subject for debate within the Society. His views veered from the severely practical to the wildly visionary. In 1871 he put forward a radical proposal which owed a great deal to the educational philosophy of "payment by results" adopted by the British government in 1862 as the basis for the distribution of grants to foster elementary and scientific education. Schacht suggested that the Society should give up its School of Pharmacy and distribute the money saved, some £2,000 a year, throughout the country in the form of premiums to teachers of successful candidates at the Society's examinations. In this way, the Society "would promote the scientific education of the whole body of which it is the professed head by a comprehensive scheme eminently practical and as eminently just". The scheme would bring "all schools, whether metropolitan or provincial, into one common arena, there to be estimated and supported solely according to the results they can accomplish". Not only "would that admitted difficulty, 'provincial education', disappear as a separate and distinct question, but local and individual enterprise throughout the whole country would receive an impetus that could not fail to result in a largely increased amount of good healthy work". In August 1881 Schacht was propounding another scheme, equally novel but rather more idealistic. He presented to the Society's Council a plan for remodelling the medical profession and making pharmacy an integral part of it. All students, whether of medicine or pharmacy, would have to obtain a degree in Arts and attain a certain proficiency in chemistry, botany and materia medica. After that, intending pharmacists would study practical pharmacy, dispensing and prescriptions in a registered pharmacy for three years and, after examination, would be awarded the degree of Bachelor of Pharmacy. Such graduates would have the right to represent pharmacy on the General Medical Council which would have the duty of prescribing curricula, appointing examining boards, and conferring titles on those who graduated. Eventually only graduates would have the right to dispense the prescriptions of medical men and sell poisons.

All professions harbour within their senior ranks members who like to indulge in fantasies about professional education. On the more mundane level, the great majority of students seek to obtain the necessary qualifications with the minimum expenditure of money, time and effort. It did not take long for the level of education to fall to the level of the examination. The Society's School of Pharmacy continued to demand high standards. Courses continued to be oriented towards the Major examination and the average period of attendance at the School was five months. This was, however, far in excess of the requirements for the Minor examination. By 1872 John Attfield, the professor of chemistry, was complaining that instead of attending the full course of lectures on chemistry, students wished only to learn facts regarding the "chemical bodies of the pharmacopoeia". Instead of the Minor examination testing the acquisition of a sound pharmaceutical education, education or rather "cramming" was being fitted to the examination requirements. In 1872 students were passing the qualifying examination after six weeks spent learning model answers to five hundred specimen questions. The corollary of "payment by results" was the emergence of privately owned schools with courses tailored to the bare essentials. One such establishment openly advertised that "the student's time will be principally employed in examination in which the questions are such as he may reasonably expect afterwards".

The most important educational development after 1868 was the collapse of the provincial schools and classes sponsored by the Society and the successful launch of proprietary schools. There were two such schools in 1870 and five by 1880. Four of them were established in London, a fact which suggests that the Society's concern to develop provincial education was literally misplaced. The first of the private schools was set up by J.C. Braithwaite, who had once been an instructor in the laboratories at Bloomsbury Square. In 1861 he had begun to give private instruction at his home in Kentish Town and within two years had moved to larger premises where he set up a laboratory to hold day and evening classes. In 1870 there was a sudden increase in the number of students, so he enlarged the laboratory by taking over adjoining buildings and laid out a plot of land as a botanic garden. At this point he felt justified in calling his school, "The North London School of Chemistry and Pharmacy". In the same year John Muter, M.A., a chemical analyst, opened "The South London School of Chemistry and Pharmacy" in Kennington Road.

Perhaps the most successful of all the private schools in the nineteenth century was Wills' Westminster College of Pharmacy. George Sampson Valentine Wills began his career as an educationalist by organising a correspondence course in pharmaceutical subjects, sending out manuscript notes to students and marking answers in return. In 1874 he fitted out two rooms in his house at Southwark as laboratories where he taught ten part-time students. Before long he was teaching full time in large premises in Lambeth Road. Students flocked to his door and soon another move became necessary, this time to Kennington Road, where two halls were fitted up as laboratories and lecture theatre. When even these premises became inadequate, Wills seized the opportunity to buy up the disused Trinity Baptist Chapel in Trinity Square. The galleries were converted into chemistry laboratories for 74 students and the nave into a lecture theatre. In 1899 it was estimated that 4,000 chemists and druggists owed their place on the register to the training they had received at Westminster College.

The encouragement given to private enterprise in pharmaceutical education was paralleled by the decision to privatise the Society's School. In 1873 the Council decided to

403

substantially reduce its control of and commitment to the School of Pharmacy and to hand over its administration to the professors. Previously admission to the lectures had been free and, with the exception of fees from students in the chemical laboratory, the entire cost had been borne by the Society. The professor of chemistry and pharmacy and the professor of botany and materia medica received a stipend of £300 a year. The professor of practical chemistry was paid £150 and a percentage of the laboratory fees. The Society subsidised the School at the rate of about £500 a year. In 1874 the School was put on a semi-autonomous and self-supporting basis. Each of the three professors was given an annual endowment of £100 and free use of the rooms but had to meet all other expenses. The professors had to supply all their own materials but pocketed all the fees.

The privatisation of the School of Pharmacy was an economy measure: the decision was taken simply to reduce expenditure. No one at the time sought to wrap the decision up in ideological clothing. It was left to later commentators to see the move as an attempt to provide incentives for better teaching. The new system, it was alleged, ensured that the fees of students attracted by alert and imaginative teaching went into the pockets of the professors whose personality and learning filled the lecture theatre. Since students would attend only the well-taught courses, the dull and incompetent lecturer would go to the wall. For the theory of consumer choice in education to work in practise, untrained minds must be capable of deferring immediate gratification for long term benefit. Such deferment may be an admirable end-product of an educational system: to assume its a priori existence is a form of educational infanticide.

The Society's School was an institution singularly unfit for privatisation, for it was not solely a teaching institution. Its professors were acknowledged to be eminent in their sciences; they were actively conducting and stimulating research; in their laboratories and under their supervision much of the practical work needed for the revision of the *British Pharmacopoeia* was undertaken. Yet the new system lasted for twenty-two years. It was abandoned in 1896 when it was revealed that certain members of the Staff had found it possible to combine teaching duties with a lucrative private analytical practice economically conducted in the Society's laboratories. A committee of the Council appointed in June 1895 reported, with a noticeable lack of enthusiasm, that the work of the research laboratory was "on the whole satisfactory". At the annual meeting in 1896 the members of the Society were briefly informed that the Council had "deemed it expedient to resume the direct control of its school of pharmacy".

Proprietary schools continued to flourish in the closing decades of the nineteenth century. In 1890 out of a total of seven such schools only two were outside London. The Manchester College of Chemistry and Pharmacy was owned by W. Spencer Turner, a pharmaceutical chemist. The Liverpool School of Pharmacy was closely linked to the local chemists' association whose council members acted as official visitors. By 1900 the number of private schools had increased to twenty-two; ten in London (including two for women students), three in Scotland, two in Birmingham, two in Manchester, and one each in Leeds, Liverpool, Newcastle, Sheffield and Southsea. Competition for students was keen. Advertisements described facilities in glowing terms and displayed lists of examination successes and "unsolicited" testimonials. Unlike the students in their advertisements, the schools did not all succeed. The South West London College in King's Road Chelsea and the Central School of Pharmacy in Marylebone Road were among the failures.

By 1900 the proprietary schools were not only in competition with each other but also with many public institutions. In 1899 courses in pharmacy were being offered in Mason's College, Birmingham, Owen's College, Manchester, Hartley College, Southampton, and in the University Colleges of Nottingham, Liverpool and Bristol. County councils in England and Wales were empowered by the Technical Instruction Act of 1889 to encourage technical and scientific education; and the 1890 Budget brought them the windfall of the "whisky money", the excise duty on spirits, to spend on it. By 1899 courses for pharmacy students were available in fifteen of the new technical schools. In 1881 the philanthropist, Quintin Hogg, one of the few people who felt that technical education should go beyond the elementary stage, founded Regent Street Polytechnic. Under the stimulus of the City and Guilds examinations, other polytechnics were soon established in London. In its first prospectus of 1895 the South West Polytechnic (later the Chelsea Polytechnic) declared its intention of offering, within the Chemistry Department, courses in subjects such as pharmacy, dyeing and brewing. Not long after, evening classes were organised in pharmaceutical chemistry, botany and materia medica. From this part-time course developed the Chelsea School of Pharmacy, now the Chelsea Department of Pharmacy, Kings College London, which is now one of the two remaining pharmacy schools in London.

Although by the end of the nineteenth century there were as many as forty-five institutions offering courses in pharmacy, the percentage of failures in the Minor examination increased during the last three decades. During the later 1870s half the candidates who presented themselves for the examination in London failed: by the beginning of the new century the failure rate had risen to seventy per cent. In their reports the Visitors appointed by the Privy Council to attend the examinations repeatedly stressed the need for compulsory courses of instruction to bring down the failure rate. "It is evident that many young men of defective education still unsuccessfully attempt to enter upon the business of pharmacy", wrote Dr. Thomas Stevenson in 1891.

For thirty years Professor John Attfield campaigned for the introduction of regulations requiring candidates for the qualifying examination to produce documentary evidence of having "diligently and deliberately" studied for an appropriate period at properly supervised and publicly recognised schools of pharmacy. Systematic training in approved institutions, he argued, should supersede mere cramming for examinations.[19] It is not surprising to find George Wills, the owner of the Westminster College, among Attfield's opponents. Such regulations, he argued, went against the principles of free trade and would not only give the Pharmaceutical Society a valuable but undesirable monopoly but also debar from the profession those who could not afford the inflated fees of a recognised school.

> In the name of reason, what can it matter to the examiners or to the public, where or how a candidate obtained his knowledge? Is he qualified, *that* is the all-important question.

Will's case was a strong one. It is certainly curious that neither Attfield nor any of his supporters considered the possibility of devising an examination system which would test the acquisition not of rote learning but of the competencies, aptitudes, and skills required of the qualified chemist.

The Council of the Pharmaceutical Society made every attempt to reform the educational and examination system: but, until 1908, their efforts were successively blocked by both chemists and druggists and, more significantly, by the Privy Council. A provision for dividing the qualifying examination into two parts, the practical and the scientific, and for establishing a curriculum with specified courses of study at recognised teaching institutions appeared for the first time in the Society's Pharmacy Act Amendment bill of 1881. In 1887 the Council introduced another bill into parliament to obtain powers to divide the examinations and impose compulsory courses of study. The bill passed the House of Lords and was read a second time in the Commons but was subsequently dropped. It was reintroduced without success in 1888 and 1889. In 1891 another bill was introduced with the same objectives but also making provision to admit all registered chemists to membership of the Society. The bill was not enacted. Further attempts to secure the educational powers were linked to attempts to regulate company trading. None was successful until the 1908 Act secured both objectives.

The return of demobilised servicemen at the end of the Great European War enabled the Pharmaceutical Society in 1919 to both divide the Minor examination and introduce the principle of compulsory courses of study. By 1920 the scheme of pharmaceutical education had reached the stage where the chemist and druggist qualifying examination was divided into two parts, a pure science section (chemistry, physics and botany) and an applied pharmaceutical section (materia medica, pharmacy, including posology and the translation and dispensing of prescriptions, and poisons law). The parts could be taken either together or separately. Attendance at approved courses of instruction was a necessary preliminary to entry for the examination. An apprenticeship of 4,000 hours was another essential and it might be served either wholly in retail pharmacy or half in retail and half in hospital pharmacy. The preliminary scientific syllabuses in chemistry, physics, and botany had been recast to bring them as nearly as possible in line with the first year syllabuses in those subjects in University science courses. In this way pharmacy students could be readily accommodated in existing ordinary science classes.

The first links of the Society's School of Pharmacy with the University of London came in 1901 when the three professors in post were given the status of recognised teachers of the University. Then in 1912 Henry George Greenish, professor of pharmaceutics, and A.W. Crossley, professor of chemistry, were appointed professors in the University. In 1922 Sir William Glyn-Jones made representations to the University with a view to instituting a degree in pharmacy. The proposal was accepted in principle by the Senate and a joint committee of the University and the Council was appointed to work out the details. By 1924 the final regulations had been drafted and submitted to the University for approval. These were originally for an internal degree but the possibility of instituting an external degree was immediately afterwards considered. A problem which arose early was that of the conditions under which graduates of the University could be admitted to the Pharmaceutical Register. A means of effecting this was neatly devised. The two pharmaceutical qualifications, pharmaceutical chemist and chemist and druggist, were set up by two separate statutes, the Acts of 1852 and 1868. It was possible, then, to alter the pharmaceutical chemist qualification so as to be obtainable after a three years academic course and an apprenticeship reduced from 4,000 to 2,000 hours and able to be taken either before or after the final University examination. By this means it was possible to recognise the intermediate B.Pharm. as the preliminary scientific examination and the B.Pharm. as the pharmaceutical chemist examination, except for forensic pharmacy, which the Society retained as an examination conducted by itself which had to be passed before the pharmaceutical chemist diploma was awarded. The London degree was the first to be recognised under this scheme and it was followed at intervals by the corresponding degrees of the Universities of Manchester, Glasgow and Wales. In 1924 the degree of bachelor of pharmacy was instituted in the University of London Faculty of Medicine and in the following year the School of Pharmacy was admitted, within that Faculty, as a school of the University.

At the same time as negotiations were proceeding with the University of London, a committee was set up by the Society's Council to draft by-laws and examination regulations which would raise the standard of the preliminary examination and secure more effective control by the Society over the two parts of the qualifying examination. This committee presented its report to the Council on Tuesday 2 December 1924. The president, F.P. Sargeant, explained to the Council that there were three principal changes involved. The standard of the preliminary examination would be raised. The preliminary scientific examination would be separated from the qualifying examination so that the two could no longer be taken at one sitting. Finally, the pharmaceutical chemist examination would be divorced from the chemist and druggist examination so that a student after obtaining his preliminary scientific examination would have the choice of proceeding by means of a one-year course to obtain the qualification of chemist and druggist or by means of a two-year course to obtain the qualification of pharmaceutical chemist.

These proposals were not well received by the members of the Society and in Scotland there was considerable hostility. Sir William Glyn-Jones arranged meetings in Birmingham, Leeds, Manchester and London where he and the president presented expositions of the changes and the reasons behind them. A memorandum was sent to each Branch explaining the changes. Opposition focussed on two points; first, the proposal to limit the period of apprenticeship for the pharmaceutical chemist qualification to 2,000 hours while that for the chemist and druggist qualification remained at 4,000 hours, and secondly, the proposal to permit candidates to proceed directly to the pharmaceutical chemist qualification without first qualifying as a chemist and druggist. Despite the opposition, the new regulations were passed in their original form by a special general meeting by 148 votes to 118. The Privy Council gave its approval and they came into force in August 1925. Written examinations were instituted in all subjects and practical examinations in all subjects except forensic pharmacy. Oral examinations were discontinued except in pharmacy in the chemist and druggist qualifying examination.

The difficulties experienced in amending the regulations in 1925 gave weight to the idea that regular revision should be undertaken at reasonably short intervals. It was with this in mind that in 1928 the Council appointed a committee consisting of E.S. Peck, Harry Berry and Dr. McCall to consolidate the regulations. Their report was issued in 1930. The principles set out in this report were based on the dangerous and erroneous notion that there was a widening gap developing between the requirements of the retail practice of pharmacy and those of hospital and industrial pharmacy. The report postulates that the chemist and druggist and the pharmaceutical chemist should be regarded as very different types of pharmacist. The chemist and druggist would become a retail pharmacist and his training should therefore be designed to produce a man highly proficient in dispensing, able to differentiate between good and bad samples of drugs and galenicals, be thoroughly grounded in the principles of sterilisation and have such acquaintance with biological therapeutic agents as would enable him to handle these substances intelligently. The pharmaceutical chemist, on the other hand, would normally find an outlet for his training in manufacturing laboratories and hospitals. In his training, therefore, special emphasis would need to be placed upon the manufacture of galenicals and the sterilisation of medicinal substances. He would also require a thorough knowledge of crude drugs and to be proficient in their examination and in pharmaceutical and chemical analytical work generally.

The main thrust of the Committee's report was that the education of the chemist and druggist should follow, from the outset, a different route from that of the pharmaceutical chemist. Fortunately, there were two major obstacles to the implementation of the report. First the opinion, strongly held in Scotland, that the normal road to the pharmaceutical chemist qualification should be by way of the chemist and druggist examination; second, the sheer impracticability of running two distinct first year courses in most schools of pharmacy. When the next set of examination changes was made in 1935 the philosophy of the 1928 Committee was rejected. The new regulations returned to the situation which had prevailed in the days of the old Major and Minor examinations. The obstacle, which had been created by the 1925 regulations, to a person who had taken the chemist and druggist course proceeding directly to the higher qualification was removed. Physiology was added to the subjects of the chemist and druggist qualifying examination, for which a course of one academic year was prescribed. The subjects of the London degree and the pharmaceutical chemist qualifying examination were altered to pharmaceutical chemistry, pharmacy, physiology, pharmacognosy and forensic pharmacy and the vocational character of the examination was thereby increased. This change of subjects facilitated the assimilation of the first year of the course for the higher qualifications to the course for the chemist and druggist qualifying examination. The 1935 regulations contained other significant changes. London University matriculation or its equivalent was adopted as the preliminary standard. Zoology was added to the preliminary scientific examination being combined with botany under the title of biology. The Council was given power to lay down conditions under which apprenticeship should be served.

In 1932 the Council reviewed the position of the various schools of pharmacy approved by them and particularly that of the privately owned schools. The view was taken that the private schools were by now an anachronism, an inheritance from the time when there was little pharmaceutical instruction available from public educational authorities. The schools owed their success largely to the personality and ability of their principal. Although they had served previous generations well, they were now finding it increasingly difficult to attain the progressively rising standards which revised syllabuses made it necessary for the Society to exact. In a declaration of policy the Council made clear its intention to deny recognition to new private schools and gradually to phase out existing ones. During the 1930s Manchester University absorbed the privately-owned schools in its neighbourhood [20] and, on the initiative of the Society, negotiations were set on foot which ultimately led to the schools in Bath and Leeds being taken over by the Merchant Venturers College and the University of Leeds. By 1938 only three proprietary schools survived, the London College, the South of England College and the Liverpool School of Pharmacy. The latter was the last to close, its work being taken over in 1949 by the city's technical college. The Society closed the South of England College by purchasing it at a generous price and the proprietor of the London College was persuaded to abandon educational management by being appointed the full-time secretary of the Society's Statutory Committee.

At the annual meeting of the Society in 1927 it was announced from the chair that "the whole question of the future of the Society's premises" was under consideration by the Council, and that £5,000 had been set aside as the nucleus of a building fund in preparation for the time when existing leases on Bloomsbury Square would expire. The annual report for 1930 showed that a block of houses in Brunswick Square, Bloomsbury had been purchased for demolition and the erection of the Society's new headquarters and school of pharmacy. Building work started in 1938 but had to be abandoned at the outbreak of war when the School was evacuated to Cardiff and the administration to Derbyshire. By 1945 it was clear that, because of escalating costs, the Brunswick Square project would need to be modified. An appeal for advice was made to the University of London which offered immediate assistance and later made the proposal to purchase the partially-completed building in Brunswick Square. The University and the Society agreed that the College of the Pharmaceutical Society (the title was acquired in 1932) should be reconstituted as an

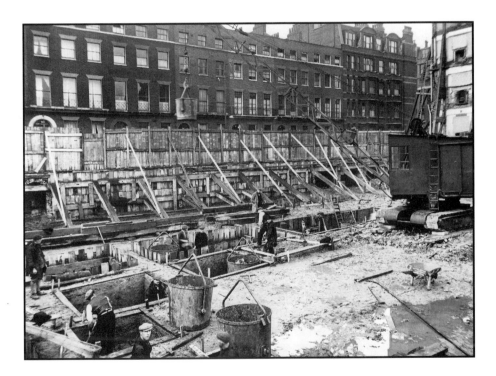

69 *Preparation of the site for the proposed new headquarters building of the Pharmaceutical Society, 25–35 Brunswick Square, January 1939. This eventually became the site of the School of Pharmacy of the University of London.*

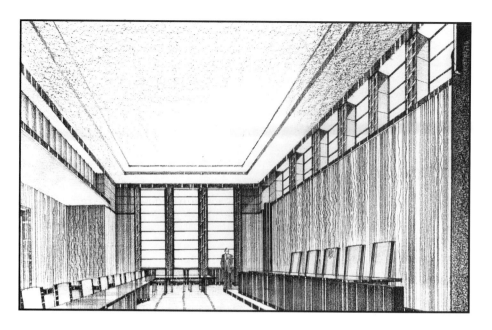

70 *Perspective sketch of the new Council Room, from the plans for the new Society headquarters, 1938.*

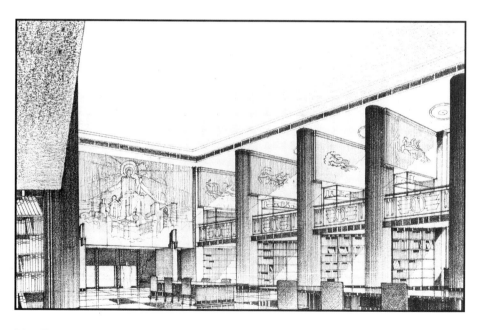

71 *Perspective sketch of the Library from the plans for the proposed new Society headquarters, 1938.*

independent body and this was accomplished in 1949 under the title of "The School of Pharmacy, University of London". A Royal Charter of Incorporation was granted in 1952. Whereas students had previously studied for diplomas of the Society or for a pass B. Pharm. degree, the honours degree in pharmacy, instituted in 1946, became the only course on offer from 1950. Building work recommenced in Brunswick Square in 1954. The pharmaceutics department moved to the new building in 1955 and other departments followed until the transfer was completed in 1960 when the building was officially opened.[21] The Society's headquarters remained at 17 Bloomsbury Square until September 1976 when they were transferred to a new building at No. 1, Lambeth High Street.

In the early days of the Second World War the Council of the Pharmaceutical Society issued a report which looked to the future of pharmaceutical education. Already by 1941 an all-graduate profession had become a realistic aspiration. In the immediate future the policy was to extend the course for the chemist and druggist qualification from one year to two to enable

> the holding of one examination which would be both the chemist and druggist qualifying examination and the pharmaceutical chemist qualifying examination. This would facilitate the establishment of one statutory register of persons eligible to practise pharmacy instead of two . . . Admission to the register would be either

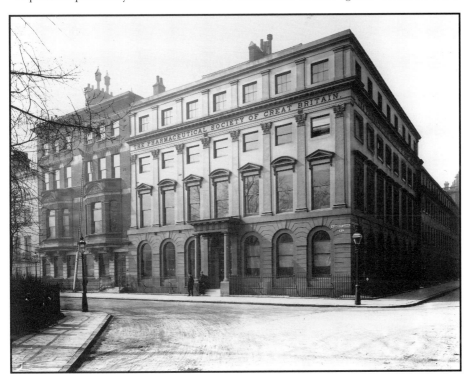

72 *The Society's headquarters in the 1890s. This shows the rebuilding carried out by the Society, including the additional storey and portico of number 17, and the construction of the adjacent building.*

411

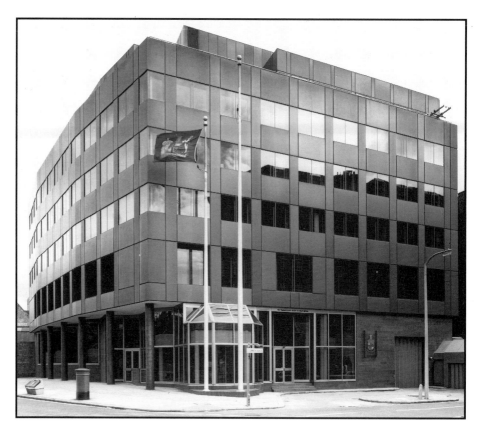

73   *Exterior of the Society's headquarters building, 1 Lambeth High Street, 1990.*

through the examination conducted by the Society or through a university degree
. . . but admission through a degree would be the rule rather than the exception.[22]

It was not until the early 1950s that the Council came to the conclusion that a three year period of academic study for all students of pharmacy, leading to the examination and award of the pharmaceutical chemist diploma as the only registrable qualification, apart from the degree, was justified and ought to be implemented. In 1953 a new Pharmacy Act became the starting point for a whole series of changes. The existing register of chemists and druggists was abolished and the names which had previously appeared on it were transferred to a new register of pharmaceutical chemists. The 1953 Act was intended merely as a transitional measure and remained in force only until a more comprehensive measure could be enacted. The profession of pharmacy is now regulated by the Pharmacy Act of 1954 which not only absorbed the 1953 Act but repealed the now outmoded Acts upon which the fabric of professional pharmacy had been constructed in the past, including the Pharmacy Acts of 1852, 1868 and 1908. A new register was compiled in which all pharmacists were included as pharmaceutical chemists. Alongside this change came an innovation in the designation of membership of the Society. Those whose names had previously been on the register of pharmaceutical chemists became fellows of the Society (F.P.S.) and those previously registered as chemists and druggists and all who would in the future come on to the register were designated members (M.P.S.). At the same time, the Council were empowered to designate as fellows members who have made outstanding contributions to pharmaceutical knowledge or who have attained distinction in the science, practice, profession or history of pharmacy.

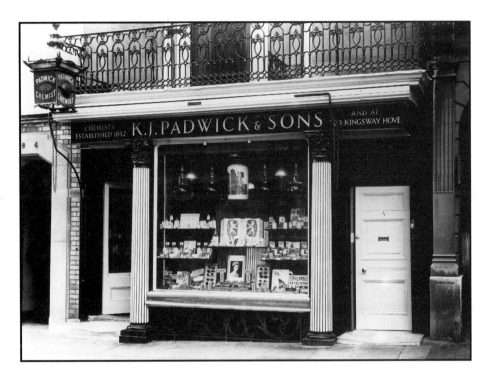

74   *K.J. Padwick & Sons, 5 Preston Street, Brighton, Sussex. This picture can be dated by the Queen Elizabeth II Coronation photograph and decorations in the shop window. A greater part of the original Regency shop front is preserved.*

Since 1 September 1967 all new pharmacy students have been required to read for a degree in pharmacy before being eligible for registration. In time, therefore, the profession will be composed entirely of graduates with similar training and qualifications. The current requirements for registration are a degree in pharmacy approved by the Pharmaceutical Society and a period of 12 months' supervised practical experience. Half of this experience must be in either hospital or community pharmacy, and the rest either there or in industry, in agricultural and veterinary pharmacy, or in a school of pharmacy. Degree courses in pharmacy leading to either a B. Pharm. or B.Sc. (Pharm.) degree are at present given in 16 schools of pharmacy in the United Kingdom. Of the ten universities one each is in

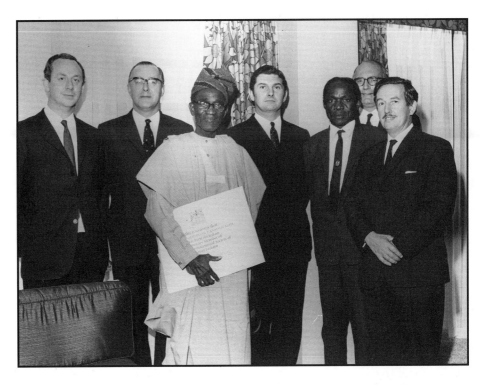

75 *Secretary and Registrar (1967–85) D.F. Lewis and W.M. Darling (member of Council 1962–) with Chief Azariah Ozusegun Ransome-Kuti of Nigeria, awarded an Honorary Membership of the Society, 8 October 1970.*

Scotland, Wales and Northern Ireland: the remaining seven are in England. Of the six non-university institutions there is one Scottish central institution and five English polytechnics. Two-thirds of all those graduating in pharmacy do so at universities.

NOTES AND REFERENCES TO CHAPTER SEVEN

1. The P.A.T.A. and Retail Price Maintenance 1896–1976

1. M.J. Winstanley, *The Shopkeeper's World 1830–1914* (1983) and J. Hood and B.S. Yamey, "The middle-class co-operative retailing societies in London, 1864–1900", *Oxford Economic Papers*, new series 9 (1957) 309–22.
2. *C. & D.* 50 (1897) 163
3. *C. & D.* 48 (1896) 643
4. Stanley Chapman, *Jesse Boot of Boots the Chemists* (1974)
5. *C. & D.* 43 (1893) 729, 775, 809, 841, 873, 875, 894–5, 903–4
6. *P.J.* 119 (1927) 283–7 *C. & D.* 107 (1927) 365–6
7. *P.J.* 113 (1924) 660
8. *C. & D.* 50 (1897) 803

9. *C. & D.* 48 (1896) 748
10. *C. & D.* 49 (1896) 287, 523
11. *C. & D.* 49 (1896) 297, 523–4, 666
12. *C. & D.* 49 (1896) 337
13. B.S. Yamey, "The origins of resale price maintenance: a study of three branches of retail trade", *Economic Journal* 62 (1952) 522–45
14. *C. & D.* 48 (1896) 630
15. *C. & D.* 49 (1896) 521
16. *C. & D.* 49 (1896) 523–4
17. *C. & D.* 48 (1896) 560
18. Henry W. Macrosty, *The Trust Movement in British Industry, A Study of Business Organisation* (1907) 244–54
19. *C. & D.* 49 (1896) 487
20. *C. & D.* 49 (1896) 124
21. *C. & D.* 52 (1898) 1016 : 50 (1897) 317
22. *C. & D.* 50 (1897) 118
23. *C. & D.* 51 (1897) 808
24. *C. & D.* 49 (1896) 487
25. *P.J.* 113 (1924) 660
26. *C. & D.* 48 (1896) 630
27. B.S. Yamey (ed.) *Resale Price Maintenance* (1966) Chapter 8.
28. 1920 (662) xxiii 483
29. Departmental Committee, Board of Trade. *Restraint of Trade* (1931)
30. *Report of the Committee on Resale Price Maintenance*, 1948–49 (7696) xx 383 paragraphs 160, 142, 84, 42, 81, 85.
31. 1950–51 (8274) xxvii 981 paragraph 43
32. *P.J.* 181 (1958) 285–90, 353–7, 445, 449–51
33. *Hansard* 691 (10 March 1964) 260
34. *P.J.* 204 (1970) 656–66

2. *National Health Insurance to National Health Service 1911–1948*

1. Bentley B. Gilbert, *The Evolution of National Insurance in Great Britain* (1966)
2. E.P. Hennock, *British Social Reform and German Precedents* (Oxford, 1986)
3. Pat Thane (ed.) *The Origins of British Social Policy* (1978)
4. David G. Green, *Working-Class Patients and the Medical Establishment* (1985)
5. *P.J.* 86 (1911) 706–7, 746
6. *P.J.* 86 (1911) 771: 87 (1911) 59–65
7. *Departmental Committee on the Supply of Medicines to Insured Persons*, 1913 (6853, 6854) xxxvi 777, 795
8. *P.J.* 87 (1911) 215
9. *P.J.* 86 (1911) 806: 88 (1912) 717
10. *P.J.* 88 (1912) 448–9
11. *P.J.* 87 (1911) 215
12. *P.J.* 86 (1911) 806
13. *P.J.* 88 (1912) 448
14. *P.J.* 87 (1911) 126
15. *P.J.* 87 (1911) 215
16. *P.J.* 87 (1911) 218
17. *P.J.* 87 (1911) 59–65

18. E. Halevy, *A History of the English People in the Nineteenth Century* (1961) volume 6
19. 1912–13 (6305) lxxviii 679
20. H. Eckstein, *The English Health Service* (1959) 127
21. J. Anderson Stewart, "Jubilee of the National Insurance Act", *P.J.* 189 (1962) 33–5
22. *The Drug Tariff under the National Insurance Acts,* 1914–16 (8062, 8063) xxix 657, 689
23. *Royal Commission on National Health Insurance* 1926 (2596) XIV 585–6
24. *Report of the Working Party on Differences in Dispensing Practice between England and Wales and Scotland* (1948) paragraphs 34,35
25. *The Times* 7 July 1958
26. Charles Webster, *The Health Services Since the War* (1988) I
27. Almont Lindsey, *Socialised Medicine in England and Wales* (Chapel Hill, 1962) Chapter 17
28. A.H.S. Hinchliffe, *Committee on the Cost of Prescribing,* Final Report 1959, 13–15, 84
29. H.A. Clegg and T. E. Chester, *Wage Policy and The Health Service* (Oxford, 1957) 59–60
30. *P.J.* 231 (1983) 338–40: *C. & D.* 220 (1983) 439–40 : J.W.B. Fish, *The Guild of Hospital Pharmacists, 1923–1983* (1983)
31. *P.J.* 115 (1925) 764–5 *C. & D.* 159 (1953) 619, 644, 670 : 160 (1953) 17,43
32. Brian Watkin, *Documents on Health and Social Services* (1975) 348–9

3. The Jenkin Case, 1933 Act, Dangerous Drugs and Education
1. Jose Harris, "Society and the state in twentieth-century Britain", in F.M.L. Thompson (ed.) *The Cambridge Social History of Britain 1750–1950* (Cambridge 1990) volume 3, chapter 2, 63–117
2. Sir William S. Glyn-Jones, *Ten Years of the Society's History 1913–1923* (1924)
3. *P.J.* 103 (1919) 9–10, 147–150
   C. & D. 91 (1919) 689, 873–6
4. *Committee on Relations between Employers and Employed,* 1917–18 (8606) xviii 415; 1918 (9002) x 659; 1918 (9153) vii 629
5. *P.J.* 105 (1920) 386–90, 405–6
6. Sir Almeric FitzRoy, *Memoirs* (1925) II 646–7
7. *P.J.* 113 (1924) 43
8. Pharmaceutical Society of Great Britain, *Report of the Committee of Enquiry,* Part II (1941) 8
9. J.R. Dale and G. E. Appelbe, *Pharmacy Law and Ethics* (4th edition, 1989) chapter 26, 336–350
10. *P.J.* 119 (1927) 283–7
11. H.G. Rolfe, "The British Pharmaceutical Conference, 1863-1963" *Journal of Pharmacy and Pharmacology* XV (1963) 10T-42T
12. *Departmental Committee on the Poisons and Pharmacy Acts,* 1929–30 (3512)xvi 979
13. Hugh N. Linstead, *Poisons Law* (1936)
14. Virginia Berridge, "War conditions and narcotics control: the passing of Defence of the Realm Regulation 40B", *Journal of Social Policy* 7 (1978) 285–304
15. *Committee on Draft Regulations under the Dangerous Drugs Act 1920* 1921 (1307) x 29
16. J.R. Dale and G. E. Appelbe, *Pharmacy Law and Ethics* (4th edition 1989) chapters 1–15
17. T.E. Wallis, *History of the School of Pharmacy* (1964)
18. M.P. Earles, "The Pharmacy Schools of the Nineteenth Century", in F.N.L. Poynter, *The Evolution of Pharmacy in Britain* (1965) 79–95
19. John Attfield, *A pamphlet on the relation to each other of Education and Examination, especially with regard to pharmacy in Great Britain* (second edition 1882)
20. Brian Robinson, *The History of Pharmaceutical Education in Manchester* (1986)
21. Frank Fish, "School of Pharmacy, Brunswick Square", *P.J.* 231 (1983) 120–2
22. Pharmaceutical Society of Great Britain, *Report of the Committee of Enquiry,* Part II (1941) 18

EPILOGUE

The Royal Pharmaceutical Society in 1991

When the Pharmaceutical Society received its charter in 1843, it was a voluntary association of proprietor chemists and druggists who had joined together to protect and enhance their economic and social status. From its foundation, the Society pursued a strategy of professionalisation designed to transform the drug trade into the profession of pharmacy. Central to this policy was the establishment of a system of education and qualification and the promotion of chemistry and pharmacy as practical sciences. A model school of pharmacy with a museum of materia medica and laboratories for practical chemistry was set up in conjunction with an examination system which provided qualifications for both principals (the Major examination) and assistants (the Minor). A programme of scientific meetings and the publication of a pharmaceutical journal completed the Society's prospectus.

The Pharmaceutical Society has not only survived 150 years of rapid and far reaching social change (in itself a considerable feat) but has also achieved to a remarkable extent the objectives sought by its founders. The Society has become the corporate representative of all who practise pharmacy in Great Britain. All registered pharmacists are members and take on the obligations and enjoy the privileges of such membership. Today all pharmacists undergo a thorough professional education and qualify by demonstrating their competence in rigorous and publicly accredited examinations. Dispensing medical prescriptions is now universally recognised, as Jacob Bell wished it might be, as the pharmacist's primary responsibility. Ninety-five per cent of the British population obtain their medicines from registered pharmacies. In 1984 the 11,000 pharmacies in Great Britain dispensed 380 million prescriptions.

Although the Pharmaceutical Society continues to pursue the same basic aims set for it in 1843 it is today a very different organisation. In 1843 the Society was an exclusive association of men: today, thirty-eight per cent of its members are women. Half the pharmacists under the age of thirty are women. In the year 1989–90 both the president and vice-president of the Society were women. In 1843 all but a handful of members were independent proprietor chemists and druggists: now fewer than one member in four is a proprietor pharmacist. Over two-thirds of pharmacies are owned by companies, partnerships and co-operative societies. One large multiple, Boots, has over a thousand branches. Even in community pharmacy, sixty per cent. of pharmacists are employees. The Pharmaceutical Society is no longer a voluntary organisation: since 1933 membership has been obligatory for all those on the Register. The number of members on 31 December 1988 was 36,779.

When the Pharmaceutical Society received its first charter, it was the only national organisation of pharmacists. At the end of the nineteenth century, William Glyn-Jones founded the Proprietary Articles Trade Association and the Chemists Defence Association. Since the Jenkin case in 1920 a number of organisations have emerged to protect the immediate economic interests of various groups of pharmacists. The National Pharmaceutical Association represents the owners of over 10,000 pharmacies throughout the United Kingdom: its membership of 7,400 proprietors includes the vast majority of independent community pharmacists. The Guild of Hospital Pharmacists, now a membership group of the recently formed trade union, Manufacturing, Science, Finance (M.S.F.), negotiates pay and conditions of service of some 4,000 pharmacists working in hospitals. The negotiation of terms of service with the Government on behalf of community pharmacy contractors under the N.H.S. is the function of the Pharmaceutical Services Negotiating Committee (P.S.N.C.), which is a separately constituted body. The Joint Boots Pharmacists Association and the Co-operative Pharmacy Technical Panel comprise pharmacists employed by the Boots Company and the Co-operative societies. The National Association of Women Pharmacists continues to promote their special interests.

Since the end of the Second World War the Pharmaceutical Society has lost both its School of Pharmacy and its examination system. For over a hundred years the Society was directly involved in both educating and examining those who sought to qualify as pharmacists. In 1949 the Society's School was transferred to the University of London and since 1970 the Society has ceased to hold its own examinations. Yet the Society remains deeply involved in the promotion of pharmaceutical education. The involvement begins in schools and colleges with the promotion of pharmacy as a career for young people. Most of the Society's branches have careers officers. The staff of the Society's Education Division work with the branches in providing advice and materials (booklets, posters, videos, and tape-slide presentations) to recruit students to schools of pharmacy. The Education Division organises an annual pharmacy careers convention for London and home counties schools and colleges. Although the media of presentation are modern, there is nothing new in the idea which lies behind such activity. The Pharmaceutical Society has always sought to raise the standard of entry into the profession. Jacob Bell spent much time considering how to improve the social and intellectual quality of pharmacy apprentices and for decades the Society tried to insist that apprentices should pass the preliminary examination before being indentured. Today the demand for places in schools of pharmacy exceeds the supply. Selection is on the basis of Advanced Level results (Highers in Scotland) in science subjects: only high calibre applicants are admitted. On average about two-thirds of the students are women and in some schools the proportion is as high as three-quarters.

Apprenticeship is a thing of the past. Before becoming a pharmacist now a student must obtain a degree at one of the sixteen schools of pharmacy in universities and polytechnics in the United Kingdom and undertake a year's preregistration experience in practice.

Present annual intakes of students into schools of pharmacy total approximately 1,350 (1990 data) up from a total intake of about 800 in 1967. The Pharmaceutical Society reviews and approves the pharmacy degree courses in Great Britain. Council members and senior representatives of the Society make quinquennial accreditation visits to all the British pharmacy schools. The Society's aim is to ensure that degree courses, supplemented by preregistration experience and further vocational training, produce competent pharmacists in whichever branch of the profession they choose to work. The Society requires that the courses should cover three areas of pharmaceutical science. These are pharmaceutics (which, including pharmaceutical microbiology, deals with the formulation, preparation, production and testing of medicines), pharmaceutical chemistry (which deals with the chemistry and analysis of drugs of synthetic and natural origin and drug-containing systems) and pharmacology (which deals with interaction between drugs and the living organism). In addition courses must include an element of pharmacy law, ethics and practice, so that students have a clear idea of the legal, ethical and social responsibilities involved in the professional practice of pharmacy in all its branches.

Before being registered as a pharmacist, a pharmacy graduate must spend a year, under supervision, gaining practical training and experience. The Pharmaceutical Society requires that the pharmacy premises where preregistration training is to take place satisfy minimum standards and be subject to inspection. Each student is placed under the supervision of a tutor approved by the Society. The Society's Education Division is responsible, on behalf of the Council, for the approval of premises, the placement of graduates and the appraisal scheme. It also organises seminars for tutors and study days for the students. It produces the preregistration experience manual which not only contains guidance and information for the student but is also used in the appraisal process. Major changes in the preregistration scheme are in the pipeline. Following recommendations in the Nuffield Report (1986) a registration examination and a competency based system of training are being developed.[1].

"Any profession, the members of which base their professional service on knowledge which is continually expanding and changing, must embrace the philosophy that continuing education is an integral part of professional practice". Fifteen years ago, the Council of the Pharmaceutical Society endorsed this statement from the report of its working party on postgraduate education and training. Continuing education is needed, as the Nuffield Report reiterated, to enable pharmacists to keep pace with changes in science and practice; to supplement the initial training of a pharmacist by dealing with matters not covered in the degree course or preregistration year; and to bring up to date the knowledge of pharmacists who may have qualified many years ago. In spite of the Department of Health's reluctance to help busy and isolated community pharmacists attend courses, the Society has devoted much time and effort to the introduction, administration and researching of continuing education programmes. The distance learning courses developed at the schools of pharmacy at Strathclyde and Leicester are good examples of imaginative initiatives which deserved greater financial and moral support.

In addition to its own activities in this field, the Pharmaceutical Society established in 1981 the College of Pharmacy Practice. The objectives of the College are to promote and maintain a high standard of practice, to advance education and training in all pharmaceutical disciplines and at all levels, to establish standards of vocational training, to advance knowledge of the application of pharmacy in total health care, and to conduct, promote and facilitate research into the practice of pharmacy and publish the results. It was decided that, for at least the first five years, the College should remain under the overall control of the Council of the Society and would receive financial and administrative support during that period. On 1 January 1986 the College became a separate and independent professional body.

It is vital for any profession to be involved in the production of new knowledge. The Nuffield Report drew attention to the fact that in Britain the system for funding research degrees puts pharmacy at a disadvantage: the interdisciplinary nature of pharmacy as an applied science weakens it against single subject "pure" disciplines in the contest for research funds. The system leads to a shortage of Ph.D. pharmacists both in industry and in the schools of pharmacy and limits the amount of basic pharmaceutical research being undertaken. Since the establishment of the Redwood research scholarship in 1887, the Pharmaceutical Society has been successful in attracting the endowment of an impressive number of research awards. Although the scholarships awarded by the Society cannot compensate for the low level of government funding, research in the pharmaceutical sciences has benefited from the financial and moral support of the Society.

When the School of Pharmacy was transferred to the University of London in 1949, the Society lost not only a teaching institution but also a centre of scientific work and research. Shortly after the loss of the School, however, two scientific departments were established at the Society's headquarters, one to prepare publications, the other to maintain the comprehensive museum of crude drugs and two herbaria. In addition, two laboratories were set up behind 17 Bloomsbury Square to undertake research related to the work of these departments. In 1958 the two departments with their laboratories were combined into the Department of Pharmaceutical Sciences, which was given additional functions including the organisation of scientific meetings and the preparation of exhibitions and recorded lectures. Soon the increased work undertaken in the laboratories required more space, so when practical examinations were discontinued in the Society's laboratories in Edinburgh, the pharmaceutics laboratory was moved there, leaving the analytical laboratory to take over the empty accommodation in London. Another part of the old examination laboratories was later turned into a second analytical laboratory to examine formal samples taken under the Scottish Drug Testing Scheme. In 1970 the original analytical research laboratory was transferred from London to Edinburgh.

In 1972 the Pharmaceutical Society entered into a contract with the Department of Health to undertake the examination and testing of samples arising from the work of the medicines inspectorate under the Medicines Act of 1968. This led to the establishment, at 36 York Place, Edinburgh, of the Medicines Testing Laboratory, designed to provide a broadly-based, independent, analytical service to the Medicines Division of the Department of Health. Its main function is to carry out both chemical and microbiological examination of samples submitted by the medicines inspectorate as part of the general surveillance programme of medicines sold or supplied in the United Kingdom. Investigational work and analysis of samples is also undertaken for government authorities in other countries, for international organisations including the World Health Organisation, and for the Society's Law Department in connection with its responsibility for law enforcement. The primary function of the Pharmaceutics Division of the Society's Edinburgh Laboratories is to provide authoritative guidance to the profession on pharmaceutics and applied aspects of the pharmaceutical sciences. Evaluated information is supplied to the Council, to the Medicines Testing Laboratory, to the Society's publications, and to government departments and other outside bodies . The Division has undertaken innovatory work on British standards related to pharmacy and provides a problem-solving and advisory service on technical and practical aspects of pharmacy. To support those activities the comprehensive information resources of the Society are selectively abstracted and maintained in a database.

The Pharmaceutical Society has an unbroken tradition, going back to Jacob Bell's day, of organising scientific meetings at its headquarters. Five-day postgraduate schools, formal symposia and workshops, and regular meetings of the Society's membership groups (Agricultural and Veterinary Pharmacists, Industrial Pharmacists, and Hospital Pharmacists) are organised by the Society's Scientific and Technical Services Division. The *Pharmaceutical Journal*, now the official weekly journal of the Society, was bequeathed to the Society by its owner Jacob Bell on his death-bed in 1859. It has been published without interruption since July 1841 and its contribution to the development of pharmacy as a profession cannot be separated from that of the Society itself. The Journal has always been the principal means of communication between the Council and the members: it has been the mainspring for the development of professional consciousness among pharmacists. "The Journal", declared Jacob Bell, "should never subside into a philosophical record of high science which apprentices and students could not understand". One of the Journal's great strengths is that it has always followed Jacob Bell's advice. All aspects of the practice of pharmacy—science, technology, business and politics—have been, and are, covered by the Journal in a style and in language geared to the diverse interests of all members of the Society. It has a weekly circulation of 40,000.

In contrast the *Journal of Pharmacy and Pharmacology* is a monthly research journal of international standing, circulating to individual research workers and to research and educational establishments, industrial laboratories, hospitals and government health departments in more than 90 countries. It is now in the top two percent of quoted journals and among the top five journals publishing pharmacy and pharmacology. Its content and presentation have changed radically since volume one. Its international reputation has strenghtened and each year it publishes work from more than 35 countries on all aspects of the sciences concerned with the discovery, detection, evaluation, mechanism of action, safety, development and formulation of drugs and medicines. The Journal still reports the scientific proceedings of the British Pharmaceutical Conference, but now as a supplement to the December issue.

The Pharmaceutical Society publishes a number of books which are widely used not only in Great Britain but in the Commonwealth and many other countries. From 1907 to 1973 ten editions of the *British Pharmaceutical Codex* were published. From 1934 the *B.P.C.* was a valuable source of standards for drugs and medicines and for substances not included in the *British Pharmacopoeia*. These standards were recognized by the 1968 Medicines Act and are recognized in Commonwealth and other countries. However, the recommendation of the Medicines Commission, that the *British Pharmacopoeia* should be the only compendium of standards for drugs and medicines for human and veterinary use, led to extensive changes in the new volume, published in 1979, and retitled *The Pharmaceutical Codex*. Very few of the analytical standards of the *British Pharmaceutical Codex* continue to have legal status, being replaced by those published in the *British Pharmacopoeia* of 1988. The role of the B.P.C. in setting standards has now effectively finished. The new edition of the *Pharmceutical Codex* which is being prepared by the Pharmaceutics Division in Edinburgh will present the concepts, practices and technology relevant to the application and development of pharmaceutics in the 1990s.

The *British National Formulary* is a joint publication of the British Medical Association and the Pharmaceutical Society. It is produced under the authority of a Joint Formulary Committee which has representatives of the medical and pharmaceutical professions and the Department of Health. It is under continuous revision and over 150,000 copies are sent every six months to doctors and pharmacists in the National Health Service. The *B.N.F.* has its origins in the health insurance formularies of the 1930s. During the Second World War these were united into a National War Formulary which provided formulas incorporating substitutes for scarce imported ingredients. The first *B.N.F.* proper was produced in 1949 following the inception of the N.H.S. In 1981 a new style *B.N.F.* was published to meet the need for a more comprehensive formulary incorporating a much wider range of preparations while still providing informed advice on their relative merits. The *B.N.F.* contains information on all the prescribable drugs and medicines available in the United Kingdom with notes on prescribing them, indications, cautions, contra-indications, doses, side-effects, and basic N.H.S. cost. The *British National Formulary* is an up-to-date pocket book intended for rapid reference by practising doctors and pharmacists designed to encourage prescribing which is both medically and cost effective.

The aim of *Martindale: The Extra Pharmacopoeia*, the twenty-ninth edition of which was published by the Pharmaceutical Society in February 1989, is, and always has been, to provide a concise and unbiased summary of the properties, actions, and uses of drugs and medicines for the practising medical practitioner and pharmacist. *Martindale* is now recognised as the world's most comprehensive source of drug information in a single volume and is used in many countries as an authoritative reference book. The contents of the current edition are divided into three parts. Part 1 (1,535 pages) contains monographs on nearly 4,000 substances arranged in 72 chapters which bring together drugs with similar actions or uses; thus, for example, antibiotics, sulphonamides, urinary antiseptics and the newer quinolones are all gathered together into a comprehensive chapter on antibacterial agents. Part 2 (95 pages) consists of a series of short monographs on supplementary drugs and other substances. These monographs include new drugs, drugs under investigation, drugs difficult to classify and obsolescent drugs. Part 3 (11 pages) provides the active-ingredient composition of some 670 proprietary medicines (excluding herbal medicines) sold over-the-counter in the United Kingdom. There are over two hundred pages of indexes. If *Martindale* did not exist, no one would think it possible to create it: its production is of that order of achievement. As a source of drug information it is as authoritative and comprehensive as the *Oxford English Dictionary* is for the English Language.

William Martindale, the originator and first editor of the *Extra Pharmacopoeia*, had been pharmacist and lecturer at University College Hospital before acquiring a pharmacy in New Cavendish Street, London. He became president of the Pharmaceutical Society in 1899. After the first edition in 1883, he published the *Extra Pharmacopoeia of unofficial drugs, chemicals and pharmaceutical preparations* in collaboration with Dr. W. Wynnn Westcott, who provided most of the medical information included. The book was so successful that it underwent ten editions in the nineteen years before Martindale's death in 1902. After that, his son William Harrison Martindale continued publication with the help of Westcott until 1925 and then alone until his own death in 1932. In that year the Pharmaceutical Society took the wise decision to acquire the copyright of the book, and has been responsible for each edition since. Electronic forms of *Martindale* have been available since the twenty-eighth edition and are supplemented by annual updates. The thirtieth edition is scheduled for 1994.

The Pharmaceutical Society has one of the leading libraries of pharmacy in the world with over 65,000 books, manuscripts and pamphlets comprising works on pharmacy, materia medica, pharmacology, chemistry, botany and allied subjects. It receives over 500 periodical publications, including 290 foreign pharmaceutical journals. Among its historical treasures is a collection of rare books which includes all the London Pharmacopoeias from 1618, many early foreign pharmacopoeias, and English and foreign herbals of which the earliest is the *Latin Herbarius* of 1485. The Library of Daniel Hanbury, a collection of some 550 volumes containing many rare illustrated botanical works, was presented to the Society by his brother Sir Thomas Hanbury in 1892. Although underfunded and understaffed, the Library provides an invaluable service to members and visiting scholars from many parts of the globe. Attached to the Library is the Technical Information Service which provides technical advice and information on all pharmaceutical problems. The Service is provided by expert information-pharmacists who deal, courteously and expeditiously, with over 16,000 inquiries each year from members employed in all branches of pharmacy and other bona fide enquirers.

Although the Society's collection of crude drugs and the herbaria were transferred in 1969 to the University of Bradford and subsequently to the Royal Botanic Gardens at Kew, the Society still has an impressive museum collection, which now covers a wide range of material relating to the development of pharmacy. The museum houses a fine collection of pharmaceutical ceramics, notably English tin-glaze drug jars and pill slabs, including the Howard collection and many 17th and 18th century dated examples. The ceramic collection also covers 18th and 19th century pharmaceutical Leedsware, creamware, stoneware, and earthenware, including a variety of feeders, leech jars and potlids. In 1953 E. Saville Peck bequeathed the greater part of his collection of English and Continental bell-metal mortars to the Society. The museum contains a substantial selection of dispensing apparatus and equipment used for storage, dispensing and display as well as microscopes, medicine chests, weights, scales and measures. These are complimented by a collection of manuscripts, paintings, prints, drawings, photographs and printed ephemera illustrating a wide range of subjects of pharmaceutical interest. The transformation of drug therapy and production is traced in the collection of materia medica and proprietary medicines dating from the 17th century to the present day. An illustrated catalogue of the Society's extensive collection of caricature prints and drawings was published in 1989, under the title *The Bruising Apothecary.* Similar catalogues of the Society's paintings, ceramics and photographs would prove useful publications.

In 1970 the responsibility for the organisation of the British Pharmaceutical Conference was transferred from the Conference Executive to the Council of the Pharmaceutical Society. The idea behind this move was to "modernise" the Conference by making it a more effective vehicle for public relations and to increase its political impact. Although the

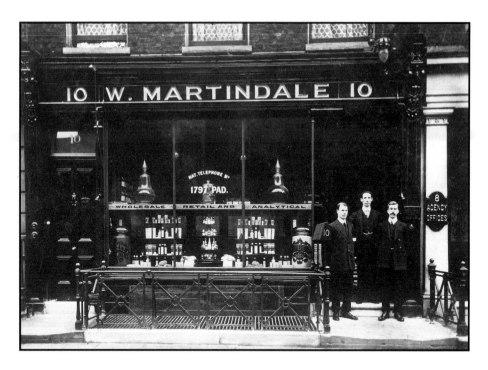

76   *The premises of W. Martindale, 10 Cavendish Street, London, in 1913.*

science content of the Conference was to remain the key feature of the meetings, attention was to be focussed in future upon Conference discussions of topical controversies to produce "press-worthy" items with a view to conveying conclusions to the public on an authoritative professional basis. The Conference was also intended now to provide opportunities for meetings between pharmacists in different types of practice, thereby emphasising and developing their common interests and disseminating the lessons of up-to-date practice across the boundaries of each specialty. The Conference would thus promote greater professional solidarity and development, while continuing to act as a forum for the discussion of advances in the pharmaceutical sciences. If they were alive today, Sir William Glyn-Jones would probably approve of the change but the founders of the British Pharmaceutical Conference might have very serious reservations.

The Constitution of the Pharmaceutical Society was revised on 1 January 1954 by the coming into operation of the 1953 Pharmacy Act and the granting of the Supplemental Charter. The objects of the Society are now (1) to advance chemistry and pharmacy (2) to promote pharmaceutical education and the application of pharmaceutical knowledge (3) to maintain the honour and safeguard and promote the interests of the members in the exercise of the profession of pharmacy and (4) to provide relief for distressed persons connected with the Society. It is the pursuit of these objects that gives the Society its character as a professional body. The Society is governed, as it has been since 1933, by a Council of twenty-four, twenty-one of whom are pharmacists elected by the members and three, who need not be pharmacists, appointed by the Privy Council. The Supplemental Charter gives formal recognition to the Scottish Department and to the Society's branches.

The North British Branch of the Society was founded in 1841 and was one of the first branches to be established. John Mackay, a close friend of Jacob Bell and the founder of John Mackay Ltd., manufacturing chemists, was its first secretary and held the post for forty years. From the outset the branch held regular scientific meetings and a library and museum were started in 1852. From 1851 the main activity of the branch was the organisation of the Society's examinations in Edinburgh which were conducted over a period of 118 years and attracted candidates from both Scotland and the North of England. In 1884 the branch obtained premises at 36 York Place and two years later the local committee became an Executive body conducting the affairs of the Society in Scotland. In July 1948 the North British Branch became the Scottish Department, which is now reponsible for the management of the Society's work in Scotland. The Welsh Executive of the Society was not formed until 1976. It replaced Rhanbarth Cymru, the Committee of the Society's Welsh region, and is now responsible for managing the Society's affairs in Wales.

The branch system is now the nucleus of the Society's organisation and affords an opportunity for every member to participate actively in the Society's work. The meeting of branch representatives following the annual meeting in May enables the views of the branches to be made known on important pharmaceutical issues. Since 1968 the branches have been organised into regions and since 1976 there have been 12 regions and 137 branches.

Since 1852 the Pharmaceutical Society has accumulated a number of statutory powers and duties. These place on the Society the obligation of administering and enforcing various aspects of the law in relation to pharmacy. Under the Pharmacy Act of 1954 the Society is responsible for maintaining the Register of Pharmacists. Under the Medicines Act of 1968 it maintains the Register of Pharmacy Premises. The same Act gives the Society the task of exercising disciplinary control over bodies corporate and others carrying on retail pharmacy businesses, whether or not they are professional pharmacists. The Medicines Act of 1968 is enforced by inspectors who are appointed by the Government but are members of the Society's staff. Their number fluctuates slightly: at present there are twenty-two.

The Statutory Committee of the Pharmaceutical Society is the disciplinary tribunal of pharmacy.[2] It consists of six persons, five appointed by the Council of the Society, and one, the chairman, who is always an eminent lawyer, appointed by the Privy Council. The Committee acts independently of the Society's Council even though the Society meets its costs. The Committee holds inquiries into cases reported to it, either directly or by the Society's Council, and decides the action to be taken. It has the power to remove from the Register the name of any pharmacist convicted of a criminal offence or guilty of misconduct. It may also disqualify a corporate body if an employee, an officer or member of the Board has been convicted or is guilty of misconduct. A body corporate which has been convicted of an offence under the relevant Acts (e.g. 1968 Medicines Act or 1971 Misuse of Drugs Act) may be disqualified from conducting retail pharmacy. In such cases, the Registrar would be directed by the Committee to remove from the Register all those premises at which the body corporate carries on the business of retail pharmacy. If a direction to disqualify is not given, there is power to give a direction for removal of one or more premises from the Register.

The Statutory Committee is essentially a judicial body although lacking in some respects the full powers of a court of law. It is concerned with acts or conduct which reflect upon the fitness of the person concerned from a professional pharmaceutical point of view, and is not a court for determining questions of private conduct. Thus it is concerned with a conviction for a criminal offence only insofar as the offence may have some bearing upon the person's fitness to act as a pharmacist, and similarly with misconduct only as it may affect the relationship of a pharmacist with his colleagues, or with his profession, or with the public. The Statutory Committee is not a general court of morals nor is it a substitute for the criminal courts.

The Council of the Pharmaceutical Society appoints each year an Ethics Committee, drawn entirely from Council members, which deals with matters relating to professional conduct. This Committee receives information and complaints and decides on the appropriate course of action, which can be to recommend to the Council reference to the Statutory Committee. Many of the complaints to the Statutory Committee alleging professional misconduct are made by the Council, and in considering such complaints the Statutory Committee takes into account the Society's Code of Ethics (formerly the Statement upon Matters of Professional Conduct). But it is not bound by it. The decision as to what conduct is misconduct justifying removal from the Register is one which only the Statutory Committee can make, and it is not bound by any code formulated by the Pharmaceutical Society. Nonetheless, in practice, the Committee uses the Society's Code of Ethics as a guide to standards of professional practice.

Cases of alleged professional misconduct arise in relation to several issues. Action has been taken by the Statutory Committee against advertising which implies invidious distinction between pharmacists or pharmacies, which is neither dignified nor discreet, and which is likely to bring the profession into disrepute. Pharmacists have appeared before the Committee for failing to exercise personal control of their pharmacy, for unsatisfactory general conduct in the pharmacy, and for maintaining their premises in a dirty and untidy condition. Pharmacists are required to exercise professional responsibility in the supply of drugs: the fact that the sale of certain medicines which are liable to abuse is not unlawful does not mean that the pharmacist is free to sell excessive quantities. Pharmacists who fail to take due care in dispensing and whose mistakes place the public at risk and bring the profession into disrepute may find themselves before the Statutory Committee.

Although most Statutory Committee cases deal directly with a pharmacist's professional and legal responsibilities and are related to his professional work, the Committee has jurisdiction, as far as pharmacists are concerned, in all cases of criminal conviction, whether they arise from offences under the Medicines Act or from offences of a general nature. Inquiries have been held relating to theft, motoring offences, forgery, receiving stolen goods, sexual offences, firearms offences as well as offences under the Misuse of Drugs Act and the Food and Drugs Act. It is not necessary for the offences to be connected with the pharmacist's professional work: the test applied by the Statutory Committee is whether the offence renders the person unfit to have his name on the Register. In 1982 Lord Justice May, in dismissing the appeal of Mr. Harari against a decision of the Statutory Committee, said:

> ... Mr. Harari stresses that the conduct, of which complaint was made, related in no way to his activity, experience or business as a pharmaceutical chemist. But ... it is not only conduct directly related to pharmacy and pharmacists of which the Statutory Committee is entitled and should properly take cognisance. When one is dealing with the activities of professional men and women it must be realised that there can be conduct on their part which although in no way directly referable to their profession, nevertheless, in the view of right minded members of that profession renders them unsuitable to continue to be members of the profession ...

Many of the Statutory Committee inquiries following criminal convictions, however, arise in connexion with pharmaceutical offences. Most common are those in which the sale or dispensing of medicinal products that are required by law to be supervised by a pharmacist take place in the pharmacist's absence. The Committee has always taken the view that supervision is a major responsibility of the pharmacist. In 1971 the chairman said:

> ... it is vitally important to ensure that the drugcounter and the dispensary are adequately covered by a qualified pharmacist at all times of the day with a real 100 per cent cover.

And in 1985 the Committee stated:

> ... we can point out that the sale of these medicines without any supervision by a pharmacist is a matter that is not only serious, but the cause of great possible and potential danger to the public.

For many pharmacists, particularly in community pharmacy, the most conspicuous aspects of the Pharmaceutical Society's work are the Inspectorate and the Statutory Committee. The Society makes its impact on them more as an instrument of surveillance and control than as an organisation for defending their interests and reputation. Some pharmacists complain that the Statutory Committee has a wider ambit and is more active than the disciplinary bodies of other professions. It is certainly the case that whereas a medical practitioner has to be found "guilty of serious professional misconduct" before losing his licence to practise, a pharmacist's name may be removed from the Register for any form of "misconduct". The General Medical Council has demonstrated, throughout its existence, extreme reluctance to expunge the names of the unworthy from the Medical Register. It seems to act more to protect the medical profession than the general public. The Statutory Committee of the Pharmaceutical Society, on the other hand, has not hesitated to exercise its powers to protect the public from pharmacists whose behaviour falls below the standards generally expected of members of a profession.

It is, perhaps, understandable that many pharmacists should feel aggrieved that their profession is subject to stricter professional regulation than others, especially when observers draw the false conclusion that misconduct is more frequent among pharmacists. On careful reflection, however, pharmacists should take pride in the work of the Inspectorate and the Statutory Committee. If professions are to retain their privileges at a time when free competition is widely touted like some patent medicine as the cure for all society's ills, they must be seen to exercise their powers of self-regulation in the public interest. The main public function of a professional association is to guarantee the competence and integrity of its members. This it does by imposing qualifying examinations and other conditions of

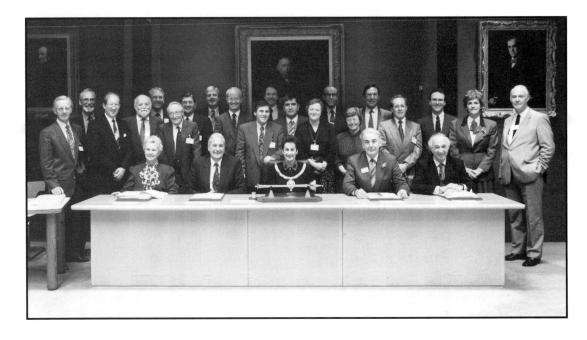

77   *The President and members of the Society's Council, 1990 – 91.*

membership on the one hand, and by the establishment and enforcement of professional codes of conduct on the other. It is the guarantee of integrity that is the main distinguishing mark of the professions. Non-professional occupations may have associations, training schemes and tests of competence; they do not have, because they do not need to have, codes of conduct. The Statutory Committee and the Ethics Committee of the Pharmaceutical Society represent the machinery through which the professional conscience of pharmacy finds expression. Their object is clear. It is to impose on the profession itself the obligation of maintaining the quality of the service and to prevent the common enterprise of pharmacy being frustrated by the moral turpitude or the unrestrained cupidity of a small minority. It is in every pharmacist's long-term interest to ensure that the public receives service of the highest possible standard from each member of the profession.

The Pharmaceutical Society is, however, more than an organisation for guaranteeing the competence and integrity of pharmacists. Pharmacists are today, as they have always been, a diverse collection of people, with widely differing aspirations, conditions of work, and positions within the medical division of labour. Membership of the Pharmaceutical Society is the fundamental bond that holds them together as members of a single profession. It is this membership which has created and which sustains the profession of pharmacy. Being members of the same profession engenders a unique type of human relationship which although less intense and pervasive than personal love or friendship is nonetheless the source of dedication and commitment. Membership of the Pharmaceutical Society provides pharmacists of all varieties with a common identity and a degree of protection which they would do well to cherish and defend.

REFERENCES TO THE EPILOGUE

1. *Pharmacy. The Report of a Committee of Inquiry appointed by the Nuffield Foundation* (1986)
2. J.R. Dale and G.E. Appelbe, *Pharmacy Law and Ethics* (4th.edition, 1989) Chapter 21

Presidents and Secretaries of the Pharmaceutical Society

PRESIDENTS

1841–43	Wm. Allen F.R.S	1909–11	John F. Harrington
1843–44	Charles Jas. Payne	1911–13	Charles B. Allen
1844–48	John Savory	1913–18	Edmund White
1848–49	Thos. N.R. Morson	1918–20	William L. Currie
1849–50	Peter Squire	1920–24	E.T. Neathercoat
1850–51	William Ince	1924–25	F. Pilkington Sargeant
1851–52	Thomas Herring	1925–26	Philip F. Rowsell
1852–53	Joseph Gifford	1926–27	Frederic E. Bilson
1853–55	Henry Deane	1927–29	Herbert Skinner
1855–56	Jn. T. Davenport	1929–30	L. Moreton Parry
1856–59	Jacob Bell	1930–32	A.R. Melhuish
1859–61	Thos. N.R. Morson	1932–33	F. Gladstone Hines
1861–63	Peter Squire	1933–35	John Keall
1863–69	G. Webb Sandford	1935–36	E. Saville Peak
1869–70	Henry S. Evans	1936–38	Thomas Marns
1870–71	G. Webb Sandford	1938–39	Thomas Guthrie
1871–73	Adolph F Haselden	1939–42	Walter Deacon
1873–76	Thos. Hyde Hills	1942–44	W.S. Howells
1876–79	John Williams	1944–45	F.G. Wells
1879–80	G. Webb Sandford	1945–46	J.C. Young
1880–82	Thomas Greenish	1946–47	G.R. Knox Mawer
1882–96	Michael Carteighe	1947–48	Mrs J.K. Irvine
1896–99	Walter Hills	1948–50	H. Clement Shaw
1899–1900	Wm. Martindale	1950–51	A.A. Meldrum
1900–03	G.T.W. Newsholme	1951–52	F.C. Wilson
1903–04	Sam. Ralph Atkins	1952–53	W.J. Tristram
1904–06	Richd. A. Robinson	1953–54	T. Heseltine
1906–09	J. Rymer Young	1954–55	E.A. Brocklehurst

1955–56	H. Steinman	1974–75	C.C.B. Stevens
1956–57	G. Shaw	1975–77	J.P. Bannerman
1957–59	D.W. Hudson	1977–78	Mrs E.J.M. Leigh
1959–60	G.H. Hughes	1978–79	John E. Balmford
1960–61	T. Reid	1979–81	D.N. Sharpe
1961–62	H.S. Grainer	1981–82	Professor A.H. Beckett
1962–63	Miss M.A. Burr	1982–83	W.H. Howarth
1963–65	C.W. Maplethorpe	1983–84	C.R. Hitchings
1965–67	J.C. Bloomfield	1984–85	Dr D.H. Maddock
1967–68	A. Aldington	1985–87	Dr T.G. Booth
1968–70	A. Howells	1987–89	B. Silverman
1970–72	W.M. Darling	1989–90	Mrs M. Rawlings
1972–73	J.P. Kerr	1990–	Mrs L.J. Stone
1973–74	D.E. Sparshott		

SECRETARIES

1841	R.W. Farmar | *Joint hon.* G.W. Smith / *secretaries*	1918–26	Sir William Glyn-Jones
		1926–64	Sir Hugh Linstead
1842–57	George Walter Smith	1949–67	F.W. Adams
1857–84	Elias Bremridge	1967–85	D.F. Lewis
1884–1913	Richard Bremridge	1985–	J. Ferguson
1913–18	W.J. Uglow Woolcock		

Index

Page numbers in *italic* refer to illustrations

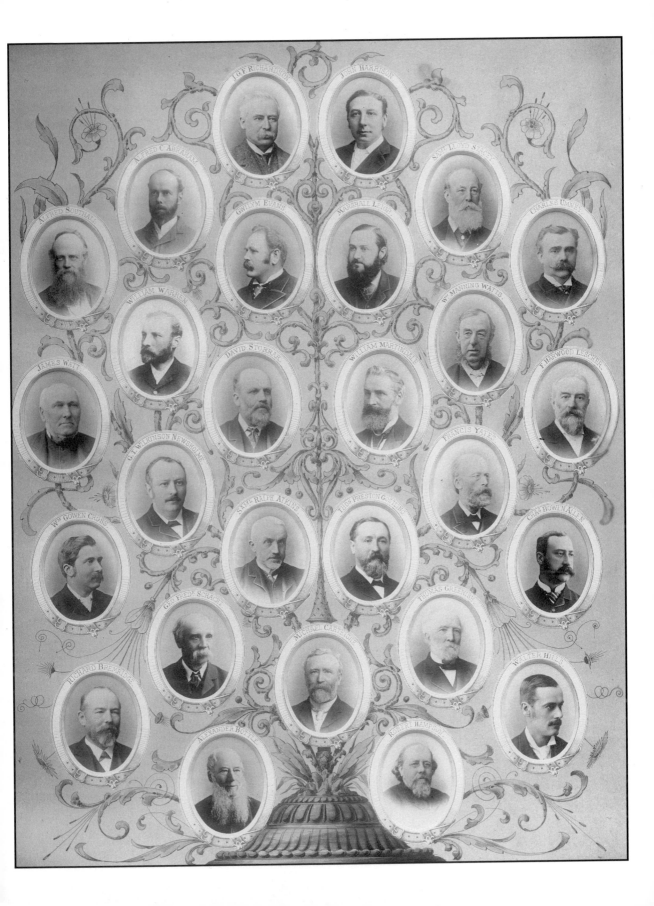